Instructional Course Lectures Spine

Edited by
Howard S. An, MD
The Morton International Professor of Orthopaedic Surgery
Director, Division of Spine Surgery and Spine Fellowship Program
Rush-Presbyterian-St. Luke's Medical Center
Chicago, Illinois

Published by the
American Academy
of Orthopaedic Surgeons
6300 North River Road
Rosemont, IL 60018

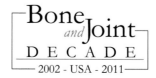

Editorial Board

Contributors

Nicholas U. Ahn, MD, Fellow in Spine Surgery, Department of Orthopedic Surgery, Rush-Presbyterian-St. Luke's Medical Center, Chicago, Illinois

Todd J. Albert, MD, Department of Orthopaedic Surgery, Rothman Institute, Thomas Jefferson University Medical College, Philadelphia, Pennsylvania

Gary M. Alegre, MD, Department of Orthopaedic Surgery, University of Louisville School of Medicine, Louisville, Kentucky

Howard S. An, MD, The Morton International Professor of Orthopaedic Surgery, Department of Orthopaedic Surgery, Rush-Presbyterian-St. Luke's Medical Center, Chicago, Illinois

Richard A. Balderson, MD, Chief, Scoliosis Service, Rothman Institute, Thomas Jefferson University, Philadelphia, Pennsylvania

Randal R. Betz, MD, Medical Director of Spinal Cord Injury Unit, Shriners Hospitals, Philadelphia Unit, Philadelphia, Pennsylvania

Oheneba Boachie-Adjei, MD, Director, Spine Deformity, The Hospital for Special Surgery, New York, New York

Robert K. Boyce, MD, Department of Orthopaedic Surgery, UCLA School of Medicine, Los Angeles, California

Keith H. Bridwell, MD, Asa C. and Dorothy W. Jones Professor, Chief, Pediatric and Adult Spinal Surgery, Department of Orthopedic Surgery, Washington University School of Medicine, St. Louis, Missouri

Daniel A. Capen, MD, Associate Clinical Professor,University of Southern California, Los Angeles, California Neuro-Trauma Service, Rancho Los Amigos Medical Center, Downey, California

Eugene J. Carragee, MD, Director, Orthopaedic Spine Center, Associate Professor, Functional Restoration, Spine Center, Stanford University School of Medicine, Stanford, California

In Sup Choi, MD, Department of Radiology, Lahey Clinic, Burlington, Massachusetts

Jerome M. Cotler, MD, The Everett J. and Marian Gordon Professor, Department of Orthopaedic Surgery, Jefferson Medical College of Thomas Jefferson University, Philadelphia, Pennsylvania

Rick B. Delamarter, MD, Medical Director, The Spine Institute, St. John's Hospital, Santa Monica, California

Thomas A. Einhorn, MD, Professor and Chairman, Department of Orthopaedic Surgery, Boston University Medical Center, Boston, Massachusetts

Frank E. Eismont, MD, Professor and Vice Chairman, Department of Orthopaedics & Rehabilitation, Co-director, Acute Spinal Cord Injury Unit, The University Miami School of Medicine, Miami, Florida

Jeffery S. Fischgrund, MD, Department of Orthopaedic Surgery, William Beaumont Hospital, Royal Oak, Michigan

Adam E. Flanders, MD, Associate Professor of Radiology, Department of Radiology/Neuroradiology, Thomas Jefferson University Hospital, Philadelphia, Pennsylvania

Steven R. Garfin, MD, Professor and Chairman, Department of Orthopaedics, University of California at San Diego, San Diego, California

Steven D. Glassman, MD, Assistant Professor of Orthopaedic Surgery, University of Louisville School of Medicine, Department of Orthopaedics, University of Louisville School of Medicine, Louisville, Kentucky

Robert N. Hensinger, MD, Professor of Surgery, Section of Orthopaedic Surgery, University of Michigan, Ann Harbor, Michigan

Harry N. Herkowitz, MD, Chairman, Department of Orthopaedic Surgery, William Beaumont Hospital, Royal Oak, Michigan

Richard J. Herzog, MD, FACR, Chief, Division of Teleradiology, Department of Radiology and Imaging, Hospital for Special Surgery, New York, New York

James D. Kang, MD, Assistant Professor of Orthopaedic Surgery, Department of Orthopaedic Surgery, University of Pittsburgh, Pittsburgh, Pennsylvania

Eubulus J. Kerr III, MD, Spine Fellow, University of Chicago Spine Center, Chicago, Illinois

David H. Kim, MD, Attending Surgeon, Boston Spine Group, Boston, Massachusetts

Mark A. Knaub, MD, Orthopaedic Surgery Resident, Department of Orthopaedic Surgery, University of Pittsburgh, Pittsburgh, Pennsylvania

John P. Kostuik, MD, Professor, Chief of Spine Surgery, Department of Orthopaedics, Johns Hopkins University, Baltimore, Maryland

Cyril F. Kruse, MD, Orthopedic Surgery Resident, Akron General Medical Center, Akron, Ohio

Lawrence G. Lenke, MD, The Jerome G. Gelden Professor of Orthopaedic Surgery, Department of Orthopaedic Surgery, Washington University School of Medicine, St. Louis, Missouri

Isadore H. Leiberman, BSc, MD, FRCSC, Orthopaedic and Spinal Surgery, The Cleveland Clinic Foundation, Cleveland, Ohio

John E. Lonstein, MD, Minnesota Spine Center, Minneapolis, Minnesota

John A. McCulloch, MD, FRCSC, Professor of Orthopedics, Northeastern Ohio Universities, College of Medicine, Rootstown, Ohio

Michael F. O'Brien, MD, Associate Clinical Professor, Orthopaedic Department, University of Colorado Health Sciences Center, Woodridge Orthopaedic and Spine Center P.C., Wheat Ridge, Colorado

James W. Ogilvie, MD, Interim Chair, Department of Orthopaedic Surgery, University of Minnesota, Minneapolis, Minnesota

Chetan K. Patel, MD, Spine Fellow, Department of Orthopaedic Surgery, William Beaumont Hospital, Royal Oak, Michigan

Artemis G. Pazianos, MD, Staff Endocrinologist, Department of Endocrinology, Lahey Clinic, Burlington, Massachusetts

Bernard A. Pfeifer, MD, Clinical Assistant Professor, Orthopaedic Surgery, Hospital of Orthopaedic Surgery, Boston University School of Medicine, Department of Orthopaedic Surgery, Lahey Clinic, Burlington, Massachusetts

Frank M. Phillips, MD, Associate Professor of Surgery, University of Chicago Spine Center, Chicago, Illinois

Raj Rao, MD, Director of Spine Surgery, Department of Orthopaedic Surgery, Medical College of Wisconsin, Milwaukee, Wisconsin

Wolfgang Rauschning, MD, PhD, Professor of Clinical Anatomy, Academic University Hospital, Uppsala, Sweden

Glenn R. Rechtine, MD, Professor, Department of Orthopaedics, University of Texas Southwestern Medical Center, Dallas, Texas

John Rhee, MD, Assistant Professor, Orthopaedic Surgery, Emory Spine Center, Emory University, Decatur, Georgia

K. Daniel Riew, MD, Assistant Professor, Department of Orthopaedic Surgery, Washington University School of Medicine, St. Louis, Missouri

Michael B. Shapiro, MD, Department of Orthopaedic Surgery, Johns Hopkins University, Baltimore, Maryland

Jeffery S. Silber, MD, Assistant Professor, Department of Orthopaedics, Long Island Jewish Medical Center, New Hyde Park, New York

Andrew Slucky, MD, Assistant Attending, Orthopaedic Surgery, The Hospital for Special Surgery, New York, New York

Patrick N. Smith, MD, Orthopaedic Resident, Department of Orthopaedic Surgery, University of Pittsburgh, Pittsburgh, Pennsylvania

Derek Snook, MD, Orthopaedic Surgery Resident, Akron General Medical Center, Akron, Ohio

Eeric Truumees, MD, Spine Surgeon, Department of Orthopaedic Surgery, William Beaumont Hospital, Royal Oak, Michigan

Alexander R. Vaccaro, MD, Associate Professor, Department of Orthopaedic Surgery, Thomas Jefferson University, Philadelphia, Pennsylvania

Jeffery C. Wang, MD, Chief, Spine Service, Assistant Professor of Orthopaedic Surgery, Department of Orthopaedic Surgery, Duke University, Durham, North Carolina

Bradley K. Weiner, MD, Assistant Professor of Orthopedics, Northeastern Ohio Universities, College of Medicine, Rootstown, Ohio

Robert B. Winter, MD, Minnesota Spine Center, Minneapolis and St. Paul, Minnesota

Preface

The Instructional Course Lecture (ICL) series published by the American Academy of Orthopaedic Surgeons (AAOS) has contained essential reading material for orthopaedic surgeons for decades. The articles in these volumes are written by leading authorities in the field, and the writing style and organization always have been of the highest quality. I was greatly honored when the Academy asked me to organize an ICL that focused on the spine. In this single volume text, the reader is presented with a review of current, state-of-the-art information about spine surgery.

It was not difficult to select articles for this volume, as most of the articles published for the past several years represent unsurpassed reviews in the literature. I have organized 34 articles into nine sections, including degenerative cervical disorders, herniated lumbar disk, lumbar spinal stenosis, pediatric spine, spondylolisthesis, adult spinal deformities, cervical spine trauma, thoracolumbar spine trauma, and osteoporotic spine. These topics cover virtually all aspects of spine surgery. I was very fortunate to recruit leading spine surgeons to review the articles in each section. Each reviewer did a spectacular job, describing the most important points of the article, adding supplementary or missing information, and commenting on the current treatment on the specific disorder. I am very grateful to these contributing reviewers; their comments and insights make this volume invaluable.

Dr. Frank Phillips, a well-known spine surgeon from Chicago, is currently an Associate Professor and the Director of Minimally Invasive Spine Surgery in the Department of Orthopaedic Surgery at Rush Medical College. I appreciate his succinct review of the articles on degenerative cervical disorders and current indications and techniques of anterior and posterior procedures for cervical spondylotic radiculopathy and myelopathy.

Dr. Ashok Biyani is an Assistant Professor at Medical College of Ohio and was a stellar spine fellow at Rush Medical College under my direction a few years ago. His comments on the herniated lumbar disk are excellent and germane to current surgical practice. I certainly agree with his comment on the necessity for strict patient selection criteria, the gold standard microdiscectomy, and the cautious approach to new and unproven techniques.

Dr. Lou Jenis is a spine surgeon in Boston who has written extensively on lumbar spinal stenosis. His review of the classic articles on the pathoanatomy of lumbar spinal stenosis, along with articles on conventional laminectomy and minimally invasive decompression techniques, reflects his expertise in this area.

Dr. John Lubicky, one of my colleagues at Rush Medical College, was recently honored with Ronald L. DeWald, MD, Professor of Spinal Deformity in the Department of Orthopaedic Surgery at Rush-Presbyterian-St. Luke's Medical Center. His review of the seminal articles on congenital spinal deformity and pediatric back pain is superb in that he discusses the essential points in the literature, as well as his preferences based on his extensive surgical experience in this area.

Dr. Christopher DeWald is another colleague at Rush Medical College who has extensive experience in all areas of spine, especially spondylolisthesis. He reviews articles on etiology, classification, clinical presentation, imaging studies, and treatment for both low- and high-grade spondylolisthesis. Even though this topic is controversial, Dr. DeWald's comments are mainstream with literature support.

Dr. Lawrence Lenke is the Jerome J. Gilden Professor of Orthopaedic Surgery at Washington University in St. Louis and Chief of Spinal Services at Shriners Hospital for Children. He is the most active surgeon and most prolific writer in the area of spinal deformity in the country; I feel fortunate to have his contribution. All of his comments are supported by the literature, most of which is his own work. The articles identify important issues of adult spinal deformity surgery, and Dr. Lenke's comments are both pertinent and insightful.

Dr. James Kang is a well-known spine surgeon from University of Pittsburgh and has contributed a great deal to the literature, especially in the areas of intervertebral disk degeneration and cervical spine surgery. Dr. Kang makes salient points on the acute management of cervical spine trauma. Although controversial, his comments on acute closed reduction based on neurologic status of the patient are sensible.

In my section, I reviewed a number of excellent articles on thoracolumbar spine trauma, including Dr. Cotler's introduction along with articles on imaging requirements, classification, and nonsurgical treatment. These articles will remain classics for many years. Surgical treatment of thoracolumbar spine trauma continues to evolve given the availability of anterior and posterior spinal implants that are both biomechanically sound and clinically effective. For thoracolumbar spine fractures, one method is not necessarily superior over another. Thus, the orthopaedic surgeon should have precise documentation of the patient's neurologic status and clearly understand the fracture mechanism and biomechanical stability of the fracture patterns. The combination of these factors determines the surgical approach and the type of spinal instrumentation used. Good fusion is paramount, as in all cases of spinal surgery that involve arthrodesis and instrumentation.

Finally, Dr. Timothy Yoon from Emory University, another superior fellow from Rush Medical College, did an outstanding job reviewing the contemporary articles on osteoporosis. As new technologies such as vertebroplasty and kyphoplasty are becoming available, the surgical indications are changing as well. However, as Dr. Yoon emphasizes, any new technology should be embraced only after well-designed clinical studies show its safety, efficacy, and specific indications. These advances in spine surgery definitely improve the quality of life in the elderly, and as more people live into their 80s and 90s, osteoporosis should take high priority for continued research.

Again, I am honored to work with these spine surgeons of great reputation, and it was a great pleasure to re-read these classic articles written by prominent authors. I am grateful to the reviewers and authors for providing the finest information in spine surgery today. I would also like to thank Lynne Shindoll, Managing Editor in the Academy's Publications Department. She coordinated article selection and edited all the reviews. I believe this volume should be part of the library of every surgeon, from residents to established surgeons, as invaluable reading material whether read from beginning to end or used primarily as a reference.

Howard S. An, MD
Editor

Contents

Section 9 Osteoporotic Spine

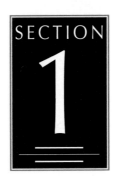

SECTION 1

Degenerative Cervical Disorders

Degenerative Cervical Disorders

The section on degenerative cervical disorders provides an overview of the diagnosis and management of cervical conditions encountered by orthopaedic spine surgeons. Dr. Raj Rao provides an excellent review of the often elusive sources of neck pain in patients presenting for spinal care, emphasizing the complex interactions of mechanical, biologic, and neurologic factors that might be responsible for the patient's clinical presentation. The degenerative cascade of the cervical spine is reviewed, and the clinical correlates of the various degenerative pathologies are discussed. Dr. Rao also reviews the literature regarding the natural history of symptoms in patients with cervical spine disease. Orthopaedic spine surgeons would be well advised to review the natural history of a particular condition so that appropriate and reasonable treatment options are recommended.

In an article on the evaluation of neck pain, radiculopathy, and myelopathy, Drs. Robert Boyce and Jeffery Wang emphasize the frequency that age-related degenerative findings are seen on imaging studies of the cervical spine. These findings, however, should not necessarily be assumed to cause the patient's symptoms. They also describe the relative benefits of various imaging modalities for the spine and the optimal imaging studies required in specific clinical situations. Correlating symptoms with concordant imaging findings remains crucial to predicting success with any type of surgical intervention. The advantages of combining CT myelography with MRI in situations in which surgical decision making may be complex are described. These studies are complementary, often providing more detailed anatomic visualization than would be provided by each of these studies individually. The authors also provide a reasonable nonsurgical approach to the management of neck pain. Although not discussed in this article, cervical diskography remains a controversial but potentially useful diagnostic test in the workup of patients with axial neck pain.

Dr. Patrick Smith and associates provide an excellent review of anterior cervical approaches for the treatment of cervical radiculopathy and myelopathy. Often described as the "workhorse," the anterior cervical approach has a long history of success in treating a variety of cervical conditions. The authors also supply a valuable discussion of some recent modifications to the standard anterior cervical decompression and arthrodesis procedure. The use of anterior cervical instrumentation is described, as is a well-balanced view of the advantages and potential disadvantages of the use of instrumentation. Although anterior instrumentation seems to increase radiographic fusion rates, the relative clinical advantage of instrumentation is unclear, and the cost effectiveness of instrumentation merits further study. The authors also list the relative merits of using substitutes for autograft for achieving anterior cervical fusion. Further study is required to more precisely define the indications for the use of both cervical instrumentation and allograft materials.

Drs. Chetan Patel and Jeffery Fischgrund focus on complications of anterior spinal surgery. Fortunately, most complications are extremely rare, but when they occur, they may have devastating consequences for the patient. The authors emphasize that many of these complications can be avoided by adhering to well-established surgical technique. They also describe a number of "tricks" that can be used during anterior cervical approaches to potentially reduce the likelihood of complications. Strategies for managing complications are outlined as well.

The article on posterior cervical spine procedures by Drs. Howard An and Nicholas Ahn is a timely review of these approaches. Results of posterior laminoforaminotomy are excellent in most patients who have primary radicular symptoms without prolonged and significant neck pain. For multiple-level (ie, more than three) cervical spondylotic myelopathy or radiculopathy requiring decompression and fusion, the anterior cervical approach has been commonly used for the last three to four decades. However, there has been a recent resurgence of interest in the posterior approach to cervical decompression and fusion. The posterior cervical spine also provides an advantageous biomechanical environment for placing instrumentation. For a posterior cervical neural decompression to be considered, sagittal alignment must be preserved. Despite the recently popularity of laminoplasty in the United States, the authors advised caution with this approach in patients with significant axial neck pain and when treating bilateral radicular symptoms. Multiple-level laminectomy and/or foraminotomy plus fusion with a lateral mass screw fixation system is preferred in these cases.

Combined anterior-posterior cervical surgery is also briefly discussed. This strategy has become more popular recently, combining the advantages of anterior direct neural decompression with the use of the lateral masses to obtain improved cervical fixation. The most obvious scenario for this approach is postlaminectomy kyphosis in which multiple-level corpectomy and strut grafting may be required. Posterior lateral mass screw systems provide secure segmental fixation to prevent graft dislodgement anteriorly. Anterior plating in these long strut grafting cases is associated with an unacceptable rate of graft and instrument failures. Although a combined approach may be a useful strategy, in most cases a well-designed and executed surgical plan using either an anterior or a posterior approach will achieve the goals of surgery and avoid the added morbidity associated with combined approaches.

Dr. K. Daniel Riew and associates describe the use of microsurgery for degenerative conditions of the cervical spine. The late Dr. John McCulloch, a coauthor of this article, was a pioneer in the use of the operating microscope for treating spinal conditions. The article explains Dr. McCulloch's philosophy and the microsurgical approach that he taught and championed for many years. The goals of microsurgery in the spine are to achieve adequate spinal decompression and stabilization, when necessary, in a safe and predictable fashion while minimizing soft-tissue dissection. Proponents of the use of the operating microscope cite their ability to perform surgery with more precision and a lower risk of neurologic injury as a consequence of the improved visualization and illumination afforded by the operating microscope. Although this argument seems plausible, the clinical benefits associated with the use of the operating microscope have yet to be scientifically substantiated. Currently there is much interest in minimally invasive approaches to the treatment of spine conditions, and the operating microscope is a useful adjunct to many of these treatments. The more limited dissection typically associated with the use of the operating microscope may reduce morbidity and has provided much of the impetus to developing less invasive approaches to surgically treat spine problems.

Frank M. Phillips, MD
Associate Professor, Department of Orthopaedic Surgery
Rush Medical College
Rush-Presbyterian-St. Luke's Medical Center
Chicago, Illinois

Neck Pain, Cervical Radiculopathy, and Cervical Myelopathy: Pathophysiology, Natural History, and Clinical Evaluation

Raj Rao, MD

Abstract

Degenerative cervical disk disease is a ubiquitous condition that is, for the most part, asymptomatic. When symptoms do arise as a result of these degenerative changes, they can be easily grouped into axial pain, radiculopathy and myelopathy. While the pathophysiology of radiculopathy and myelopathy is better understood, the source of neck pain remains somewhat controversial. A discussion of the mechanisms of neck and suboccipital pain, and the chemical and mechanical factors responsible for neurologic symptoms is warranted. Examination of the patient with these symptoms will reveal variations in the clinical presentation. A thorough understanding of the natural history of these conditions will allow appropriate treatment to be carried out. The natural history of these conditions suggests that for the most part patients with axial symptoms are best treated without surgery, while some patients with radiculopathy will continue to be disabled by their pain, and may be candidates for surgery. Myelopathic patients are unlikely to show significant improvement, and in most cases will show stepwise deterioration. Surgical decompression and stabilization should be considered in these patients.

Cervical spondylosis is a common and occasionally disabling condition, occurring as a natural consequence of aging in the vast majority of the adult population. A clinical approach to symptomatic cervical spondylosis can be simplified by dividing the findings at presentation into the categories of axial neck pain, radiculopathy, myelopathy, or some combination of these three. While the pathogenesis of radiculopathy and myelopathy in cervical spondylosis is better understood, the source of neck pain remains controversial. The aim of this chapter is to review the pathophysiology and natural history of each of these conditions and to describe the pertinent clinical features of cervical disk pathology.

Pathophysiology
Neck Pain

In a substantial number of patients, axial neck pain is a result of muscular or ligamentous factors related to posture, poor ergonomics, stress, and/or chronic muscle fatigue. Neck muscle pain can develop secondarily as a result of postural adaptations to a primary source of pain in the shoulder, the craniovertebral junction, or the temporomandibular joint. The phys-

iology of this pain process in the involved muscles is unclear. Patients with chronic myofascial pain have been shown to have a lower level of high-energy phosphates in the involved muscle tissue.[1] It is unclear whether this causes the pain or is a result of the pain. Unencapsulated free nerve endings in muscle serve as chemonociceptive and mechanonociceptive units. Chemonociceptive nerve endings may respond to metabolites that accumulate during anaerobic metabolism in fatigued muscle, or they may respond to nonneurogenic pain mediators released by injury or ischemia, such as bradykinin, histamine, serotonin, and potassium ions. Mechanonociceptive nerve endings respond to stretch or pressure. Sensitization of these nerve endings may be a primary source of muscle pain.

Attributing axial neck pain to degenerative changes in the cervical disks or facet joints is a source of controversy, primarily because of the ubiquitous nature of such changes in the spine. Nevertheless, it does appear that cervical disks and facet joints can be pain generators. Nerve fibers and nerve endings found in the peripheral portions of the disk[2,3] offer a possible mechanism by which degenerated cervical disks can produce pain directly.

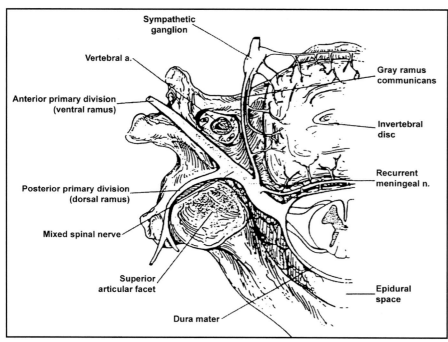

Fig. 1 Cross-sectional view showing the cervical nerve root, dorsal and ventral primary rami, recurrent meningeal or sinuvertebral nerve, and sympathetic plexus. Note the proximity of the disk space, vertebral artery, and facet joints. (Reproduced with permission from: Cramer GD, Darby SA (eds): *Basic and Clinical Anatomy of the Spine, Spinal Cord and ANS.* St. Louis, MO, Mosby Year-Book, 1995, p 141.)

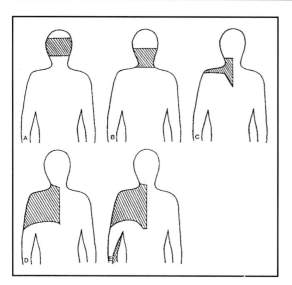

Fig. 2 Axial pain patterns provoked during diskography at each cervical level. A = level between second and third cervical vertebrae, B = level between third and fourth cervical vertebrae, C = level between fourth and fifth cervical vertebrae, D = level between fifth and sixth cervical vertebrae, and E = level between sixth and seventh cervical vertebrae. (Reproduced with permission from Grubb SA, Kelly CK, Bogduk N: Cervical discography: Clinical implications from 12 years of experience. *Spine* 2000;25:1382-1389.)

The disk is innervated by the sinuvertebral nerve, formed by branches from the ventral nerve root and the sympathetic plexus[3] (Fig. 1). Once formed, the nerve turns back into the intervertebral foramen along the posterior aspect of the disk, supplying portions of the anulus, the posterior longitudinal ligament, the periosteum of the vertebral body and pedicle, and the adjacent epidural veins. A recent review of the findings of cervical diskography performed over a 12-year period suggested that reliable patterns of pain are produced by stimulation of each cervical disk[4] (Fig. 2). The authors reported a high percentage of patients in whom multiple disks were concurrently responsible for axial neck pain.

The facet joint is also recognized as a source of axial neck pain. Provocative injections into the facet joints in asymptomatic volunteers produced a reproducible pattern of axial neck pain and pain in the shoulder girdle[5] (Fig. 3). This pattern of facet joint-induced pain can be accurately treated by anesthetic injections into the facet joint,[6] or by blocking the dorsal primary rami,[7] further suggesting that the facet joints do indeed play a role in the development of axial neck pain.

Patients with degenerative arthritis in the upper cervical joints can present with severe suboccipital pain that radiates down into the neck or to the back of the ear. Injection of the atlanto-occipital and atlantoaxial joints results in a reproducible pain pattern in this region.[8] Wächli and associates[9] reported unilateral headaches and atypical facial pain as a result of degenerative changes at the second and third cervical level. In some patients, suboccipital headaches are presumed to be a result of irritation of the greater occipital nerve, which originates from the posterior rami at the second, third, and fourth cervical levels. Another potential source of suboccipital pain is the sinuvertebral nerves from the first, second, and third cervical levels, which ascend cephalad to innervate the atlantoaxial ligaments, the tectorial membrane, and the dura mater of the upper cervical cord and posterior cranial fossa.[3]

Cervical Radiculopathy and Myelopathy

Neurologic symptoms in cervical spondylosis are the result of a cascade of degenerative changes that most likely begin at the cervical disk. Age-related changes in the chemical composition of the nucleus pulposus and anulus fibrosus result in a progressive loss of their viscoelastic properties. The disk loses height and bulges posteriorly into the canal. With this loss of height, the vertebral bodies drift toward one another. Posteriorly, there is infolding of the ligamentum flavum and facet joint capsule, causing a decrease in canal and foraminal dimensions. Osteophytes form around the disk margins and at the uncovertebral and facet joints. The posteriorly protruded disk material, osteophytes, or thickened soft tissue within the canal or foramen results in extrinsic pressure on the nerve root or spinal cord.

Mechanical distortion of the nerve root may lead to motor weakness or sensory deficits. The exact pathogenesis of radicular pain is unclear, but it is generally thought that, in addition to the compression, an inflammatory response of some kind is necessary for pain to develop. Within the compressed nerve root intrinsic blood vessels show increased permeability, which secondarily results in edema of the nerve root. Chronic edema and fibrosis within the nerve root can alter the response threshold and increase the sensitivity of the nerve root to pain.[10] Neurogenic chemical mediators of pain released from the cell bodies of the sensory neurons and nonneurogenic mediators released from disk tissue may play a role in initiating and perpetuating this inflammatory response[11] (Table 1). The dorsal root ganglion has been implicated in the pathogenesis of radicular pain. Prolonged discharges originate from the cell bodies of the dorsal root ganglion as a result of brief pressure. In addition to the chemicals produced by the cell bodies of the dorsal root ganglion, the membrane surrounding the dorsal root ganglion is more permeable than that around the nerve root, allowing a more florid local inflammatory response.

Certain positions of the arm may decrease stress within the nerve root and relieve radicular pain. Davidson and associates[12] described the shoulder abduction sign—for example, relief of severe radicular pain when the patient rests the hand

on the top of the head. Davidson and associates theorized that, in addition to decreasing tension within the nerve root, this position may lift the sensory root or dorsal root ganglion directly cephalad or lateral to the source of compression, and decompression of epidural veins may contribute to pain relief. Cervical spondylotic myelopathy is the manifestation of long tract signs resulting from a decrease in the space available for the cervical spinal cord. In addition to the spondylotic processes that contribute to the extrinsic pressure (Fig. 4), certain factors are thought to be important in the development of myelopathy; these include the anterior-posterior diameter of the spinal canal, dynamic cord compression, dynamic changes in the intrinsic morphology of the spinal cord, and the vascular supply of the spinal cord.

A congenital decrease in the anterior-posterior diameter of the spinal canal can play a role in the development of cervical myelopathy. The anterior-posterior diameter of the subaxial spine in normal adults measures 17 to 18 mm, and the diameter of the spinal cord is approximately 10 mm in this region. Individuals with an anterior-posterior diameter of the spinal canal of less than 13 mm are considered to have congenital cervical stenosis. There is a strong association between flattening of the cord within the narrowed spinal canal and the development of cervical myelopathy. Penning and associates[13] believed that symptoms of cord compression occurred when the transverse area of the cord was less than 60 mm². Houser and associates[14] thought that the shape and degree of flattening of the spinal cord could be an indicator of neurologic deficit; 98% of their patients with severe stenosis and a banana-shaped spinal cord had clinical evidence of myelopathy. Ono and associates[15] described an anterior-posterior cord compression ratio that was calculated by dividing the anterior-posterior diameter of the cord by the transverse diameter of

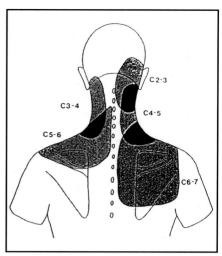

Fig. 3 Composite map of axial pain patterns produced by injections into the facet joints at the second through seventh cervical levels. (Reproduced with permission from Dwyer A, Aprill C, Bogduk N: Cervical zygapophyseal joint pain patterns: I. A study in normal volunteers. *Spine* 1990;15:453-457.)

Table 1	
Chemical Mediators of Spinal Pain[7]	
Neurogenic	**Non-Neurogenic**
Substance P	Bradykinin
Somatostatin	Serotonin
Cholecystokinin-like substance	Histamine
Vasoactive intestinal peptide	Acetylcholine
Calcitonin gene-related peptide	Prostaglandin E$_1$
Gastrin-releasing peptide	Prostaglandin E$_2$
Dynorphin	Leukotrienes
Enkephalin	DiHETE
Gelanin	
Neurotensin	
Angiotensin II	

the cord (Fig. 5). Patients with substantial flattening of the cord, suggested by an anterior-posterior ratio of less than 0.40, tended to have worse neurologic function. Ogino and associates[16] thought that an increase in this ratio to 0.40 or greater, or an increase in the transverse area to more than 40 mm² was a strong predictor

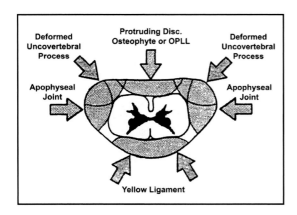

Fig. 4 Degenerative changes that contribute to compression of the spinal cord in cervical myelopathy. OPLL = ossification of the posterior longitudinal ligament. (Reproduced with permission from Bernhardt M, Hynes RA, Blume HW, White AA: Current concepts review: Cervical spondylotic myelopathy. *J Bone Joint Surg Am* 1993;75:119-128.)

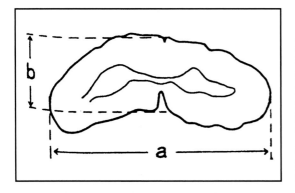

Fig. 5 Determination of the anterior-posterior compression ratio (AP) in patients with myelopathy. AP = b/a × 100. (Reproduced with permission from Ono K, Ota H, Tada K, Yamamoto T: Cervical myelopathy secondary to multiple spondylotic protrusion: A clinico-pathologic study. *Spine* 1977;2:109-125.)

of recovery following surgery.

Dynamic factors in the cervical spinal column affect the degree of cord compression. Hyperextension narrows the spinal canal by shingling the laminae and buckling the ligamentum flavum. Translation or angulation between vertebral bodies in flexion or extension can result in narrowing of the space available for the cord. Patients who do not have cord compression statically may compress the cord dynamically, leading to the development of myelopathic symptoms.[17] Retrolisthesis of a vertebral body can result in pinching of the spinal cord between the inferior-posterior margin of a vertebral body and the superior edge of the lamina caudad to it (Fig. 6). This compression may be aggravated in extension, and it may be relieved in flexion as the retrolisthesis tends to reduce. Forward slippage of a vertebral body may cause compression of the spinal cord between the supe-

rior-posterior margin of the vertebral body below and the lamina above. This is aggravated by flexion of the spinal column. Hypermobility cephalad to a degenerated and stiffened segment is commonly seen at the third and fourth cervical levels in elderly individuals, and it may result in myelopathy.[18]

Morphologic changes also occur within the spinal cord itself with flexion and extension. Breig and associates[19] showed that the spinal cord stretches with flexion of the cervical spine and shortens and thickens with extension. Thickening of the cord in extension makes it more susceptible to pressure from the infolded ligamentum flavum or lamina. In flexion, the stretched cord may be prone to higher intrinsic pressure if it is abutting against a disk or a vertebral body anteriorly.

In 1924, Barre[20] was apparently the first to propose that vascular factors play a

role in the development of cervical myelopathy. Acute or subacute development of myelopathy in the absence of a mechanical compression of the spinal cord is thought to be pathognomonic in these patients.[21] There is some experimental evidence to support a role for vascular factors in the pathogenesis of myelopathy. Cervical cord ischemia superimposed on compression of the cord resulted in dramatic neurologic findings in two separate experiments involving canines.[22,23] The effects of compression and ischemia were thought to be additive and responsible for the clinical manifestation of myelopathy. In a separate study, obstruction of the peripheral arterial plexus in dogs caused structural changes within the spinal cord.[24] The classic study by Breig and associates[19] showed that blood flow through the anterior spinal artery and anterior radicular arteries may be reduced when those vessels are tented over a disk or a vertebral body, but flow through the tortuous posterior spinal arteries is not substantially affected in this position. Vessels that are thought to be most prone to reduced flow are the transverse intramedullary arterioles arising from the anterior sulcal arteries. These vessels perfuse the gray matter and adjacent lateral columns.[25]

Severe compression results in degenerative changes in the spinal cord. The central gray matter and the lateral columns show the most changes, with cystic cavitation, gliosis, and demyelination most prominent caudad to the site of compression. The posterior columns and posterolateral tracts show wallerian degeneration cephalad to the site of compression. These irreversible changes may explain why some patients do not recover following decompressive surgery.

Natural History

There are few population-based studies on the prevalence of neck pain. A recent study of a Saskatchewan adult population showed that neck pain is more prevalent than commonly perceived: 66% of adults experienced neck pain during their lifetime, with 54% having experienced it during the past 6 months and 5% highly disabled by it.[26] Another population study demonstrated a 9% point prevalence of neck and shoulder pain.[27] The prevalence of neck pain appears to be higher in better educated individuals with a history of injury, headaches, or low back pain.[28]

DePalma and associates[29] found that most patients with axial symptoms from cervical spondylosis do reasonably well. They reported that, following 3 months of nonsurgical care, 21% of patients had complete relief of symptoms, 49% had partial relief, and 22% had no relief. Rothman and Rashbaum[30] found that 23% of a similar group of patients remained partially or totally disabled at the end of 5 years. In the same study, they found no substantial difference between that group of nonsurgically treated patients and another group of patients with "predominantly" axial neck pain who had undergone surgery. They recommended nonsurgical management for axial symptoms.

In 1963, Lees and Turner[31] reported on the natural history and prognosis of cervical spondylosis. Fifty-one patients in their "nonmyelopathic group" had pain in the neck, shoulders, arms, or hands. Patients were treated with a collar, exercises, traction, manipulation, and rest. Of 10 patients who were followed for 10 to 19 years, 3 had no symptoms after the first few months of treatment, 3 continued to have mild symptoms, and 4 had more troublesome symptoms. Of 41 patients who were followed for 2 to 10 years, 19 had no symptoms, 12 had intermittent symptoms, and 10 had moderate disability. Myelopathic symptoms did not develop in any of the patients during the course of the 19-year follow-up period. It appears that, while approximately 45% of patients with nonmyelopathic symptoms have good resolution of those symptoms shortly after onset, the remaining 55%

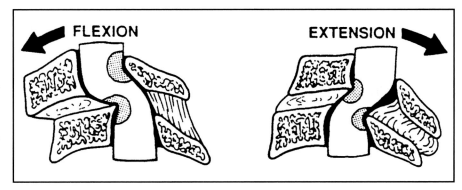

Fig. 6 Dynamic compression of the spinal cord with flexion and extension of the spinal column. (Reproduced with permission from Bernhardt M, Hynes RA, Blume HW, White AA: Current concepts review: Cervical spondylotic myelopathy. *J Bone Joint Surg Am* 1993;75:119-128.)

continue to have minor or moderate long-term morbidity. Nonsurgical treatment appeared to alleviate symptoms without influencing the eventual outcome.

Gore and associates[32] carried out a clinical and radiographic study of 205 patients who had presented with axial neck pain or radicular symptoms in the upper extremities. One hundred sixty-one of these patients were treated with rest, traction, a collar, medications, or combinations of these modalities. At the time of follow-up at 10 to 25 years, 43% had complete resolution of pain, 25% had mild residual pain, and 32% had moderate or severe residual pain. Patients with radicular symptoms or findings had a less favorable prognosis. Treatment did not appear to influence the eventual outcome. The pain could not be correlated to the degenerative changes seen on radiographs. Gore and associates concluded that many patients with this condition have long-term symptoms that may be moderately disabling.

The true natural history of cervical myelopathy may be difficult to determine because in the vast majority of cases the symptoms are attributed to age or other neurologic conditions. Thus, knowledge of the natural history of this condition has been derived from a select population in whom the disease was already diag-

nosed and possibly was well established. In 1952, Spillane and Lloyd[33] reported that the course of cervical myelopathy in their patients appeared to be one of progressive disability. In a 1956 report on 120 patients with cervical spondylotic myelopathy, Clarke and Robinson[34] stated their belief that, once the disorder was recognized, neurologic function never returned to normal. Of their patients, 75% had episodic progression, 20% showed slow steady progression, and 5% had a rapid onset of symptoms followed by a lengthy period of stability. Sensory and bladder changes tended to be transient, but motor changes tended to persist and to progress over time. A soft collar helped to decrease nerve root symptoms and improve gait for 50% of their patients.

Lees and Turner[31] reported on a group of 44 patients who had had symptoms of myelopathy for 3 to 40 years. They thought that long periods of nonprogressive disability were the rule and progressive deterioration was the exception. Neither the age at the onset of symptoms nor treatment with a collar or surgery appeared to influence the eventual prognosis. Nurick[35] reported similar findings: he observed that the disability was established early in the course of the disease and was followed by static periods lasting many years. The prognosis was better for patients who presented with mild disease, and disability tended to progress in patients older than 60 years of age. Symon and Lavender[36] reviewed the results reported by Lees and Turner and found that, when disability was used as a criterion, only 18% of patients showed improvement. In their own series, they reported steady, progressive deterioration in 67% of patients with cervical spondylotic myelopathy. Phillips[37] also thought that the prognosis was poor; only one third of his patients obtained improvement from treatment with a soft collar, and patients who had had symptoms for more than 2 years showed no improvement. A recent multicenter, nonrandomized study by the Cervical Spine Research Society suggested a similarly poor outcome of nonsurgical management of cervical myelopathy.[38] In that study of 43 patients, 20 underwent surgery and 23 received medical treatment. The surgically treated patients had decreased neurologic symptoms and overall pain and improved functional status, but the nonsurgically treated patients had a decrease in their ability to perform activities of daily living with worsening of neurologic symptoms.

Clinical Evaluation
Axial Neck Pain
Neck pain is an extremely common but nonspecific presenting symptom. The pain or soreness is usually in the paramedian neck muscles posteriorly, with radiation toward the occiput or into the shoulder and periscapular regions. The patient reports stiffness in one or more directions, and headaches are common.[39] The neck pain may be accompanied by radiating "referred" pain in the shoulder or arm that does not follow a dermatomal distribution. Referred pain can be associated with a sensation of warmth or tingling and with autonomic phenomena such as piloerection and sweating. Localized areas of tenderness in the muscle may be present. Deep palpation of

some of these areas, known as trigger points, results in reproducible patterns of referred pain.

In the absence of radicular symptoms or findings, determining the source of neck pain can be a diagnostic challenge. Identifying a position of maximal discomfort may provide a clue to the underlying pathology. Anterior neck pain along the sternocleidomastoid muscle belly that is aggravated by rotation to the contralateral side is most often a result of muscular strain. Pain in the posterior neck muscles that is worsened by flexion of the head suggests a myofascial etiology. Pain in the posterior aspect of the neck that is aggravated by extension, especially with rotation of the head to one side, suggests the possibility of a discogenic component. Patients who present with severe pain in the suboccipital region often have pathological changes in the upper cervical spine. The pain in these patients may radiate to the back of the ear or the caudad part of the neck. Rotation of the neck is often markedly restricted.

Pain in the neck and shoulder girdle can develop as a result of adaptations stemming from an initial source of pain. The initial source of pain may resolve, but postural adaptations and compensatory overuse of normal tissues in the neck and shoulder girdle can result in new pain patterns. It is important to obtain an accurate history regarding how the pain initially presented and how it might have changed with time.

Pathologic changes in the shoulder can present with localized pain or pain referred to the neck. The pain may radiate down the anterior or lateral aspect of the arm. Careful examination of the shoulder will help to differentiate this cause from pathologic changes in the neck. Pain in the neck and shoulder girdle can also be referred from the heart, lungs, viscera, and temporomandibular joint. A detailed and accurate history and physical examination will help to rule out the possibility that pain in the neck is

being referred from another region. Morning stiffness, polyarticular involvement, rigidity, or cutaneous manifestations suggest an inflammatory arthritic component. Fever, weight loss, or nonmechanical neck pain may point to an infectious or neoplastic process.

Cervical Radiculopathy
Cervical radiculopathy refers to symptoms in a specific dermatomal distribution in the upper extremity. Patients describe sharp pain and tingling or burning sensations in the involved area. There may be sensory or motor loss corresponding to the involved nerve root, and reflex activity may be diminished.

Patients typically have severe neck and arm pain that prevents them from getting into a comfortable position. They may hold the arm over the head, typically resting the wrist or forearm on top of the head (the shoulder abduction sign[12]) and sometimes tilting the head to the contralateral side. The symptoms are usually aggravated by extension or lateral rotation of the head to the side of the pain (the Spurling maneuver). Aggravation of the symptoms by neck extension often helps to differentiate a radicular etiology from muscular neck pain or a pathological condition of the shoulder with secondary muscle pain in the neck. It is also important to remember that multiple sources of pain in the neck and upper extremity are common and that the nerve structures may be compressed at more than one site.[40,41] Patients with metabolic disorders, such as diabetes, who have neuropathy may be more susceptible to radiculopathy and compressive neuropathy. Adaptations to the initial radiculopathy may result in secondary pathologic changes in the shoulder, carpal tunnel syndrome, or ulnar nerve irritation, which may persist long after the initial radiculopathy has resolved. Henderson and associates[42] reviewed the clinical presentations of cervical radiculopathy in 736 patients: 99.4% had arm pain, 85.2% had sensory deficits, 79.7% had neck pain, 71.2% had reflex deficits, 68% had motor deficits, 52.5% had scapular pain, 17.8% had anterior chest pain, 9.7% had headaches, 5.9% had anterior chest and arm pain, and 1.3% had left-sided chest and arm pain (cervical angina). Neurologic deficits corresponded with the offending disk level in approximately 80% of patients.

Radiculopathy of the third cervical nerve root results from pathologic changes in the disk between the second and third cervical levels and is unusual. The posterior ramus of the third cervical nerve innervates the suboccipital region, and involvement of that nerve causes pain in this region, often extending to the back of the ear. An isolated motor deficit from radiculopathy of the third cervical nerve root cannot be detected clinically.

Radiculopathy of the fourth cervical nerve root may be an unexplained cause of neck and shoulder pain. Numbness extending from the caudad aspect of the neck to the superior aspect of the shoulder may be present. Diaphragmatic involvement may result from involvement of the third, fourth, and fifth cervical nerve roots.[43,44] Motor deficits in the diaphragm manifest as paradoxical respiration, and they may be confirmed by fluoroscopic evaluation of the abdomen.

Radiculopathy of the fifth cervical nerve root can present with numbness in an "epaulet" distribution, beginning at the superior aspect of the shoulder and extending laterally to the midpart of the arm. The deltoid muscle is innervated primarily by the fifth cervical nerve, and involvement of that nerve can result in profound weakness of this muscle. The absence of pain with a range of motion of the shoulder and the absence of impingement signs at the shoulder help to differentiate radiculopathy of the fifth cervical nerve root from a pathologic shoulder condition. The biceps reflex is innervated by the fifth and sixth cervical nerves and may be affected.

Radiculopathy of the sixth cervical nerve root presents with pain radiating from the neck to the lateral aspect of the biceps, to the lateral aspect of the forearm, to the dorsal aspect of the web space between the thumb and index finger, and into the tips of those digits. Numbness occurs in the same distribution. Motor deficits are best elicited in the wrist extensors, but they also may be elicited by elbow flexion and forearm supination. The brachioradialis and biceps reflexes may be lost or diminished. The sensory symptoms may mimic carpal tunnel syndrome, which typically involves the radial three and a half digits and causes weakness in the thenar musculature.

The seventh cervical nerve root is the most frequently involved by cervical radiculopathy. The patient has pain radiating along the back of the shoulder, often extending into the scapular region, down along the triceps, and then along the dorsum of the forearm and into the dorsum of the long finger. The patient usually pronates the forearm while trying to describe the location of the symptoms, and this is a useful observation when the physician is trying to differentiate the hand symptoms from those of sixth cervical radiculopathy and carpal tunnel syndrome. Motor weakness is best appreciated in the triceps, wrist flexors, and finger extensors. The triceps reflex may be lost or diminished. Entrapment of the posterior interosseous nerve may be mistaken for the motor component of seventh cervical radiculopathy and presents with weakness in the extensor digitorum communis, extensor pollicis longus, and extensor carpi ulnaris. Sensory changes are absent, however, and the triceps and wrist flexors show normal strength.

Radiculopathy of the eighth cervical nerve root usually presents with symptoms extending down the medial aspect of the arm and forearm and into the medial border of the hand and the ulnar two digits. Numbness usually involves the dorsal and volar aspects of the ulnar two digits

and hand and may extend up the medial aspect of the forearm. The patient reports difficulty with using the hands for routine daily activities. It is important to differentiate eighth cervical radiculopathy from ulnar nerve weakness. The function of the flexor digitorum profundus in the index and long fingers and of the flexor pollicis longus in the thumb can be affected by eighth cervical radiculopathy, but they are not affected by ulnar nerve entrapment. With the exception of the adductor pollicis, the short thenar muscles are spared with ulnar nerve involvement but involved with eighth cervical or first thoracic radiculopathy. Entrapment of the anterior interosseous nerve may masquerade as eighth cervical or first thoracic radiculopathy, but it does not cause the sensory changes or have thenar muscle involvement. Patients occasionally present with symptoms that simulate radiculopathy but result from nonspondylotic pathologic changes (Table 2). Schwannomas usually arise from the intradural portion of the sensory root and may cause severe pain in a dermatomal distribution. Meningiomas can similarly cause radicular or myelopathic symptoms, depending on their size and precise location. Benign or malignant vertebral body tumors usually present with nonmechanical neck pain that progresses to severe radiculopathy, and even myelopathy, as the amount of bone destruction increases. A Pancoast's tumor of the apical lung can involve the caudad cervical nerve roots and, additionally, involve the sympathetic chain. Idiopathic brachial plexus neuritis is thought to be viral in nature and presents with severe arm pain that resolves and leaves behind polyradicular motor deficits. Polyradicular involvement may also be seen with epidural abscesses. Reflex sympathetic dystrophy occasionally occurs following trauma to the upper extremity, and it presents as diffuse burning pain or paresthesias accompanied by discoloration, edema, or other autonomic phenomena.

Table 2
Differential Diagnosis of Radiculopathy

Peripheral entrapment syndromes

Rotator cuff/shoulder pathology

Brachial plexitis

Herpes zoster

Thoracic outlet syndrome

Sympathetic mediated pain syndrome

Intraspinal or extraspinal tumor

Epidural abscess

Cardiac ischemia

Table 3
Nurick[35] Classification of Disability From Cervical Myelopathy

Grade I	No difficulty in walking
Grade II	Mild gait involvement not interfering with employment
Grade III	Gait abnormality preventing employment
Grade IV	Able to walk only with assistance
Grade V	Chairbound or bedridden

Cervical Spondylotic Myelopathy

Cervical spondylotic myelopathy is the most common cause of acquired spastic paraparesis in adults. The patient may present with subtle findings that have been present for years or with quadriparesis that developed over the course of a few hours. Perhaps the most unique feature of the condition is its subtle and varied presentation, and the fact that its diagnosis requires a high index of suspicion.

The clinical picture varies, depending on the anatomic portion of the cord that is primarily involved. Crandall and Batzdorf[45] described five broad categories of cervical spondylotic myelopathy: (1) transverse lesion syndrome, in which the corticospinal, spinothalamic, and posterior cord tracts were involved with almost equal severity and which was associated with the longest duration of symptoms, suggesting that this category may be an end stage of the disease; (2) motor system syndrome, in which corticospinal tracts and anterior horn cells were involved, resulting in spasticity; (3) central cord syndrome, in which motor and sensory deficits affected the upper extremities more severely than the lower extremities; (4) Brown-Séquard syndrome, which consisted of ipsilateral motor deficits with contralateral sensory deficits and which appeared to be the least advanced form of the disease, and (5) brachialgia and cord syndrome, which

consisted of radicular pain in the upper extremity along with motor and/ or sensory long-tract signs.

Ferguson and Caplan[21] divided cervical spondylotic myelopathy into four syndromes: (1) medial syndrome, consisting primarily of long tract symptoms; (2) lateral syndrome, consisting primarily of radicular symptoms; combined medial and lateral syndrome, which is the most common clinical presentation; and (4) vascular syndrome, which presents with a rapidly progressive myelopathy and is thought to represent vascular insufficiency of the cervical spinal cord.

The findings in cervical spondylotic myelopathy vary from patient to patient. Patients typically present with the insidious onset of clumsiness in the hands and lower limbs. They may report worsening handwriting in the past few months or weeks, difficulty with grasping and holding, or diffuse numbness in the hands. They frequently have had increasing difficulty with balance that they attribute to age or arthritic hips, and relatives may volunteer that their gait has become increasingly awkward. Nurick[35] developed a system for grading the disability in cervical spondylotic myelopathy on the basis of gait abnormality (Table 3). On physical examination, the findings that establish the diagnosis are brisk reflexes, clonus, or pathologic reflexes confirming an upper motor neuron lesion. Myelopathy resulting from a region of the cord cephalad to the third cervical level may result in a hyperactive scapulohumeral

reflex,[46] for example, tapping of the spine of the scapula or acromion results in scapular elevation and/or abduction of the humerus. This is thought to be a stretch reflex of the trapezius muscle. Superficial reflexes such as the abdominal or cremasteric reflex are often diminished or absent in the presence of upper motor neuron lesions. The pathologic reflexes that are typically elicited are the inverted radial reflex, the Hoffmann reflex, and the extensor plantar reflex. Muscle weakness and wasting in the lower extremities with superimposed loss of proprioception result in an unsteady, broad-based gait.

Sensory findings in cervical spondylotic myelopathy vary. Pain, temperature, proprioception, and vibratory and dermatomal sensations may all be diminished, depending on the exact area of the cord or the nerve root that is compromised. Sphincter disturbances are not usually presenting symptoms. Patients may complain of urinary urgency, hesitation, and frequency and rarely of urinary incontinence or retention. Fecal incontinence is unusual. In a study of 62 patients with cervical spondylotic myelopathy by Crandall and Batzdorf,[45] neck pain was present in fewer than half of the patients and associated radicular pain was present in 38%. The Lhermitte's sign with shocklike sensations in the torso and limbs resulting from quick flexion or extension of the neck was present in 27% of the patients, and sphincter disturbances were present in 44%.

Hand dysfunction in cervical spondylosis has, in the past, been attributed primarily to radicular pathology. Several recent reports have shown findings specific to the "myelopathy hand."[47,48] Diffuse numbness in the hands is extremely common and is often misdiagnosed as peripheral neuropathy or carpal tunnel syndrome. Clumsiness of the hands results in an inability to carry out fine motor tasks. Marked wasting of the intrinsic hand muscles is usually present.[49]

Ono and associates[47] described two specific signs of myelopathy hand: (1) the finger-escape sign (when the patient is asked to fully extend the digits with the palm facing down, the ulnar digits tend to drift into abduction and flexion) and (2) the grip-and-release test (weakness and spasticity of the hand result in a decreased ability to rapidly open and close the fist). Many neurologic conditions can mimic cervical spondylotic myelopathy (Table 4). Multiple sclerosis, a demyelinating disorder of the central nervous system, causes both motor and sensory symptoms, but it typically has remissions and exacerbations, involvement of the cranial nerves, and characteristic plaques that can be seen on MRI of the brain and spinal cord. Amyotrophic lateral sclerosis results in upper and lower motor-neuron symptoms, with no alteration in sensation. Subacute combined degeneration seen with vitamin B_{12} deficiency results in corticospinal tract and posterior tract symptoms, with greater sensory involvement in the lower extremities. Patients with metabolic or idiopathic peripheral neuropathy have sensory symptoms that mimic those of myelopathy.

Atypical Presentations of Cervical Spondylosis

Cervical angina, a symptom constellation mimicking ischemic heart disease but produced by cervical radiculopathy, is a well-known entity. Women with pain of cervical radicular origin may present with chronic breast pain.[50] Facial pain or paresthesias may be secondary to involvement of the spinal nucleus of the trigeminal nerve and may result from pressure on the cephalad and middle parts of the cervical spinal cord. Marked spurring along the anterior aspects of the vertebral bodies as a result of proliferative degenerative changes may manifest as dysphagia, dyspnea, or dysphonia as a result of pressure on the esophagus, larynx, or trachea. Similar hypertrophic spurs resulting

from the uncovertebral joints and facet joints can occlude the vertebral artery in its foramen and result in thrombosis of the vertebral artery. If the thrombosis spreads to the posterior inferior cerebellar artery, it may lead to palsy of the ipsilateral V, IX, X, and XI cranial nerves, Horner's syndrome, cerebellar ataxia, and possibly death—a constellation known as Wallenberg's syndrome. Sympathetic chain involvement can result in atypical symptoms such as dizziness, blurring of vision, tinnitus, retroocular pain, facial pain, or jaw pain.[51] Cervical spondylotic myelopathy has also been reported to present with hemiparesis.[52]

Radiculopathy occasionally presents in association with myelopathy. It is important not to let overriding radicular deficits obscure an underlying myelopathy. Patients with cervical myelopathy occasionally may have concomitant peripheral neuropathy or lumbar stenosis,[53] which might mask the lower extremity hyperreflexia typically expected from the myelopathy.

Summary

Degenerative cervical disk disease is a common condition that is, for the most part, asymptomatic. When symptoms do develop, they can be easily grouped into axial neck pain, radiculopathy, and myelopathy. An understanding of the pathophysiology of these conditions makes it possible to determine clinically whether the symptoms are likely a result of cervical spinal pathology and, in many cases, to further localize a specific level within the neck. The natural history of these conditions suggests that patients with axial symptoms usually are best treated nonsurgically, although some patients with radiculopathy continue to be disabled by pain and may be candidates for surgical treatment. Patients with myelopathy are unlikely to have substantial improvement and, in most cases, show stepwise deterioration. Surgical decompression and stabilization should

Table 4
Differential Diagnoses of Cervical Spondylotic Myelopathy
Peripheral polyneuropathy
Motor neuron disease
Multiple sclerosis
Cerebrovascular disease
Syringomyelia

be considered for these patients.

References

1. Bengtsson A, Henriksson KG, Larsson J: Reduced high-energy phosphate levels in the painful muscles of patients with primary fibromyalgia. *Arthritis Rheumat* 1986;29:817-821.

2. Ferlic DC: The nerve supply of the cervical intervertebral discs in man. *Bull Johns Hopkins Hosp* 1963;113:347-351.

3. Bogduk N, Windsor M, Inglis A: The innervation of the cervical intervertebral discs. *Spine* 1988;13:2-8.

4. Grubb SA, Kelly CK. Cervical discography: clinical implications from 12 years of experience. *Spine* 2000;25:1382-1389.

5. Dwyer A, Aprill C, Bogduk N. Cervical zygapophyseal joint pain patterns: I. A study in normal volunteers. *Spine* 1990;15:453-457.

6. Aprill C, Dwyer A, Bogduk N: Cervical zygapophyseal joint pain patterns: II. A clinical evaluation. *Spine* 1990;15:458-461.

7. Bogduk N, Marsland A: The cervical zygapophysial joints as a source of neck pain. *Spine* 1988;13:610-617.

8. Dreyfuss P, Michaelsen M, Fletcher D: Atlantooccipital and lateral atlanto-axial joint pain patterns. *Spine* 1994;19:1125-1131.

9. Wächli B, Dvorak J, Grob D: Cervical spine disorders and headaches. Read at the Annual Meeting of the Cervical Spine Research Society, New York, 1993.

10. Cooper RG, Freemont AJ, Hoyland JA, et al: Herniated intervertebral disc-associated periradicular fibrosis and vascular abnormalities occur without inflammatory cell infiltration. *Spine* 1995;20:591-598.

11. Chabot MC, Montgomery DM: The pathophysiology of axial and radicular neck pain. *Semin Spine Surg* 1995;7:2-8.

12. Davidson RI, Dunn EJ, Metzmaker JN: The shoulder abduction test in the diagnosis of radicular pain in cervical extradural compressive monoradiculopathies. *Spine*. 1981;6:441-6.

13. Penning L, Wilmink JT, van Woerden HH, Knol E: CT myelographic findings in degenerative disorders of the cervical spine: clinical significance. *AJR Am J Roentgenol* 1986;146:793-801.

14. Houser OW, Onofrio BM, Miller GM, Folger WN, Smith PL: Cervical spondylotic stenosis and myelopathy: evaluation with computed tomographic myelography. *Mayo Clin Proc* 1994;69:557-63.

15. Ono K, Ota H, Tada K, Yamamoto T: Cervical myelopathy secondary to multiple spondylotic protrusions: A clinicopathologic study. *Spine* 1977;2:109-125.

16. Ogino H, Tada K, Okada K, et al: Canal diameter, anteroposterior compression ratio, and spondylotic myelopathy of the cervical spine. *Spine* 1983;8:1-15.

17. Bernhardt M, Hynes RA, Blume HW, White AA III: Current concepts review: Cervical spondylotic myelopathy. *J Bone Joint Surg Am* 1993;75:119-128.

18. Mihara H, Ohnari K, Hachiya M, Kondo S, Yamada K: Cervical myelopathy caused by C3-C4 spondylosis in elderly patients: a radiographic analysis of pathogenesis. *Spine* 2000;25:796-800.

19. Breig A, Turnbull I, Hassler O: Effects of mechanical stresses on the spinal cord in cervical spondylosis. *J Neurosurg* 1966;25:45-56.

20. Barre JA: Troubles pyramidaux et arthrite vertebrale chronique. *Medecine Paris* 1924;5:358-360.

21. Ferguson RJ, Caplan LR: Cervical spondylotic myelopathy. *Neurol Clin* 1985;3:373-382.

22. Gooding MR, Wilson CB, Hoff JT: Experimental cervical myelopathy: Effect of ischemia and compression of the canine cervical spinal cord. *J Neurosurg* 1975;43:9-17.

23. Hukuda S, Wilson CB. Experimental cervical myelopathy: effects of compression and ischemia on the canine cervical cord. *J Neurosurg* 1972;37:631-52.

24. Shimomura Y, Hukuda S, Mizuno S: Experimental study of ischemic damage to the cervical spinal cord. *J Neurosurg* 1968;28:565-581.

25. Doppman JL: The mechanism of ischemia in anteroposterior compression of the spinal cord. *Invest Radiol* 1975;10:543-551.

26. Cote P, Cassidy JD, Carroll L: The Saskatchewan health and back pain survey: The prevalence of neck pain and related disability in Saskatchewan adults. *Spine* 1998;23:1689-1698.

27. Lawrence JS: Disc degeneration: Its frequency and relationship to symptoms. *Ann Rheum Dis* 1969;28:121-137.

28. Cote P, Cassidy JD, Carroll L: The factors associated with neck pain and its related disability in the Saskatchewan population. *Spine* 2000;25:1109-1117.

29. DePalma AF, Rothman RH, Lewinnek GE, Canale ST: Anterior interbody fusion for severe cervical disc degeneration. *Surg Gynecol Obstet* 1972;134:755-758.

30. Rothman RH, Rashbaum RF: Pathogenesis of signs and symptoms of cervical disc degeneration. *Instr Course Lect* 1978;27:203-215.

31. Lees F, Turner JWA: Natural history and prognosis of cervical spondylosis. *Br Med J* 1963;2:1607-1610.

32. Gore DR, Sepic SB, Gardner GM, Murray MP: Neck pain: a long-term follow-up of 205 patients. *Spine* 1987;12:1-5.

33. Spillane JD, Lloyd GHT: The diagnosis of lesions of the spinal cord in association with 'osteoarthritic' disease of the cervical spine. *Brain* 1952;75:177-186.

34. Clarke E, Robinson PK: Cervical myelopathy: A complication of cervical spondylosis. *Brain* 1956;79:483-510.

35. Nurick S: The pathogenesis of the spinal cord disorder associated with cervical spondylosis. *Brain* 1972;95:87-100.

36. Symon L, Lavender P: The surgical treatment of cervical spondylotic myelopathy. *Neurology* 1967;17:117-127.

37. Phillips DG: Surgical treatment of myelopathy with cervical spondylosis. *J Neurol Neurosurg Psychiat* 1973;36:879-884.

38. Sampath P, Bendebba M, Davis JD, Ducker TB: Outcome of patients treated for cervical myelopathy: A prospective, multicenter study with independent clinical review. *Spine* 2000;25:670-676.

39. Travell JG, Simons DG: *Myofascial Pain and Dysfunction: The Trigger Point Manual.* Baltimore, MD, Williams and Wilkins, 1983, pp 59-63.

40. Upton AR, McComas AJ: The double crush in nerve entrapment syndromes. *Lancet* 1973;2:359-362.

41. Massey EW, Riley TL, Pleet AB: Coexistent carpal tunnel syndrome and cervical radiculopathy (double crush syndrome). *South Med J* 1981;74:957-959.

42. Henderson CM, Hennessy RG, Shuey HM Jr, Shackelford EG: Posterior-lateral foraminotomy as an exclusive operative technique for cervical radiculopathy: a review of 846 consecutively operated cases. *Neruosurgery* 1983; 13:504-512.

43. Cloward RB: Diaphragm paralysis from cervical disc lesions. *Br J Neurosurg* 1988;2:395-399.

44. Buszek MC, Szymke TE, Honet JC, et al: Hemidiaphragmatic paralysis: an unusual complication of cervical spondylosis. *Arch Phys Med Rehabil* 1983;64:601-603.

45. Crandall PH, Batzdorf U: Cervical spondylotic myelopathy. *J Neurosurg* 1966;25:57-66.

46. Shimizu T, Shimada H, Shirakura K: Scapulohumeral reflex (Shimizu):Its clinical significance and testing maneuver. *Spine* 1993;18:2182-2190.

47. Ono K, Ebara S, Fiji T, Yonenobu K, Fujiwara K, Yamashita K: Myelopathy hand: New clinical signs of cervical cord damage. *J Bone Joint Surg Br* 1987;69:215-219.

48. Good DC, Couch JR, Wacaser L: "Numb clumsy hands" and high cervical spondylosis. *Surg Neurol* 1984;22:285-291.

49. Ebara S, Yonenobu K, Fujiwara K, Yamashita K, Ono K: Myelopathy hand characterized by muscle wasting: A different type of myelopathy hand in patients with cervical spondylosis. *Spine* 1988;13:785-791.

50. LaBan MM, Meerschaert JR, Taylor RS: Breast pain: a symptom of cervical radiculopathy. *Arch Phys Med Rehabil* 1979;60:315-317.

51. Clark CR: Cervical spondylotic myelopathy: history and physical findings. *Spine.* 1988;13:847-849.

52. Wallack EM, Ng KW, Lockhart WS: Hemiparesis in cervical spondylosis. *JAMA* 1976;236:2524-2525.

53. Edwards WC, LaRocca SH: The developmental segmental sagittal diameter in combined cervical and lumbar spondylosis. *Spine* 1985;10:42-49.

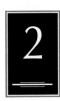

Evaluation of Neck Pain, Radiculopathy, and Myelopathy: Imaging, Conservative Treatment, and Surgical Indications

Robert H. Boyce, MD
Jeffrey C. Wang, MD

Abstract
Neck pain is a common complaint that typically represents a spectrum of disorders affecting the cervical spine. The clinical history and examination of patients with neck pain dictate the proper timing and selection of diagnostic studies such as plain radiography, MRI, and myelography with CT. Most neck pain is self-limiting and will resolve with appropriate conservative care. Nonsurgical treatment is the most appropriate first step in almost all cases of cervical radiculopathy. In contrast, the conservative care of cervical spondylotic myelopathy with measures such as physical therapy, spinal manipulation, medications, collars, and traction is limited.

Neck pain is a common complaint that reportedly affects as many as 70% of individuals at some point in their lifetime.[1] It can represent a spectrum of disorders affecting the cervical spine ranging from acute to chronic, and benign to pathologic. The cervical spine is a complex region, involving bone, disk, ligaments, neural elements, facet joints, and the paraspinal musculature. In an aging population, neck pain is commonly a result of arthritis, degenerative disk disease, instability, facet degeneration, or muscle pain.

Several factors determine the evaluation and management of patients with neck pain and a smaller subset of patients with the symptoms and signs of radiculopathy and myelopathy. As in other areas of the practice of spinal surgery, the implementation of specific tests and the application of specific therapies, including surgery, is driven by a detailed history and physical examination. This chapter provides the most current recommendations for the imaging, conservative care, and surgical indications for patients with neck pain, radiculopathy, and myelopathy.

Diagnostic Imaging
The timing and selection of diagnostic studies is dependent on the patient's clinical history and examination. Important considerations include the age of the patient, the onset and duration of symptoms, and the presence of any underlying disorders such as rheumatoid arthritis or ankylosing spondylitis.

Plain Radiographs
Two issues influence the appropriate timing of diagnostic studies: (1) the favorable natural history of neck pain and the fact that most neck pain will resolve with conservative measures; and (2) the possibility that many symptomatic and asymptomatic patients can have false positive imaging studies that may be unrelated to the current symptomatology. In a study of 200 asymptomatic patients, 95% of men and 70% of women had at least one degenerative change on plain films by age 60 to 65 years.[2] Friedenberg and Miller[3] reported that 25% of men and women have degenerative changes of the cervical spine by the fifth decade of life increasing to 75% by the seventh decade. More significant changes were seen in a matched group of asymptomatic patients, but there were no other significant differences between the two groups. Fenlin[4] reported degenerative changes in 70% of patients older than age 70 years. The C5-C6 level is most commonly affected by degenerative changes.[5]

In a population of 205 patients with neck pain who were assessed at 10-year follow-up, two thirds of the patients had a favorable long-term result, while one third continued to experience moderate to severe pain.[6] The presence or severity of pain was not correlated with any radiographic findings, and only the initial severity of symptoms correlated with residual pain at 10-year follow-up. In the

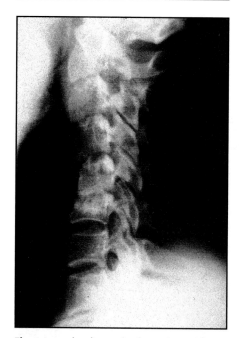

Fig. 1 Lateral radiograph of a patient with degenerative disk disease and neck pain. Narrowing of the disk space at C5-C6 and loss of normal lordosis of the cervical spine are seen. Posterior osteophytes at C5-C6, which decrease the sagittal dimension of the spinal canal, are also seen.

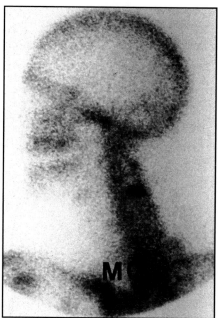

Fig. 2 Technetium bone scan of a patient with neck pain and normal plain radiographs. Increased uptake in the region of C4 reveals an osteoid osteoma involving the posterior elements.

absence of urgent findings (trauma, suspicion of neoplasm, infection, worsening neurologic deficit), a minimum 4-week period of conservative treatment is recommended prior to plain film radiographic evaluation. Other authors suggest a 6- to 8-week trial of conservative therapy.[7,8] The typical routine cervical spine series includes AP, lateral, and oblique views. These radiographs can demonstrate congenital stenosis, spondylotic segments, intraforaminal narrowing, degenerative subluxation, congenital malformations, and autofused spine segments.[9] Flexion and extension views can be added to evaluate the dynamic properties of the cervical spine, although in the setting of traumatic injuries, their utility and high false negative rate has come into question.[10] In the past certain authors have suggested that radiographs are indicated in only selected circumstances such as malignancy, infection, trauma or inflammatory arthritides; however, plain radiography is inexpensive, readily available, and noninvasive.[11,12] Other authors have considered it to be an extension of the physical examination and use plain radiography routinely. Plain radiography is extremely valuable and should be considered the first radiographic study performed during the evaluation of patients with cervical disorders.

Osteochondrosis in the nucleus pulposus region, spondylosis affecting the anulus fibrosus, disk space height loss, vacuum phenomenon, reactive sclerosis in the end plates, and Schmorl's nodes are degenerative changes that can be readily seen on plain radiographs.[5]

In patients with cervical disorders, symptom complexes are a result of instability, malalignment, intervertebral disk degeneration, and/or herniation or spinal stenosis.[13] In cervical spondylosis the most commonly affected level is C5-C6

followed by C6-C7[3] (Fig. 1). The least commonly affected level is C2-C3. "Normal" cervical lordosis has been reported to vary from $21° \pm 13°$ depending on patient age and degenerative changes.[2] A comparison of vertebral body width and canal size can be made to obtain the Pavlov's ratio, which is useful in determining spinal stenosis and the potential for clinically significant neurologic compression. A normal ratio is 1.0, and a ratio of less than 0.85 indicates stenosis. A ratio of less than 0.80 predisposes the patient to spinal cord or nerve root injury even with minor trauma.[14] Although this ratio is clinically useful, the absolute diameter of the cervical canal can also provide some valuable information and may be a more sensitive indicator of clinically significant cord compression. The normal adult cervical canal diameter is greater than 17 mm and is measured on the lateral radiograph from the posterior cortex of the vertebral body to the spinous process/lamina junction. Significant cord impingement begins when this measured space is less than 13 mm and the patient is considered to have congenital or acquired spinal stenosis.

Plain radiography may be useful in detecting the above factors; however, in order to visualize soft-tissue structures, and neural elements in particular, advanced imaging studies are required.

Radionuclide Imaging and MRI
Radionuclide imaging is a sensitive and nonspecific examination to assess for changes in bone metabolism or blood flow. It may detect degenerative joint disease, healing fracture, osteomyelitis, or neoplasm (Fig. 2). Radionuclide imaging is a useful screening tool to assess for generalized but typically not specific pathologic entities. Follow-up studies are often needed to pinpoint the exact diagnosis.

MRI is useful because of its ability to assess soft-tissue structures, neural elements, and sagittal alignment, as well as the space available for the neural elements, spinal cord and nerve root morphology, and signal changes within the disks, vertebral bodies, and the posterior soft-tissue elements[8] (Fig. 3).

MRI is indicated in the patient with progressive neurologic deficit, disabling weakness, or long tract signs.[7] It is also indicated in the patient with cervical radiculopathy who fails to improve after a 6-week trial of conservative therapy, and is also helpful for further evaluation in the presence of vertebral destruction or instability detected on plain films.[7] The principal limitations of MRI are the difficulty in distinguishing hard and soft disk herniation[15] and failure to detect foraminal disease because of osseous impingement. Because the distinction between the disk material and osteophytes at the vertebral end plates is often difficult to distinguish with MRI studies, additional imaging studies may be helpful to fully define the structures associated with neurologic impingement.

MRI using T1, T2, and three-dimensional sequences is at least as effective as CT scans with myelography in detecting compressive pathology.[16,17] Gadolinium enhanced images provide no additional benefit in the setting of spondylotic radiculopathy, although the use of gadolinium is quite helpful when differentiating scar tissue in patients with prior spinal surgery. The addition of gadolinium is also indicated when a neoplasm or spinal infection is suspected. MRI is the imaging study of choice in detecting or evaluating a spinal infection or spinal tumor.

In a study of 63 asymptomatic volunteers, 19% had an abnormality on MRI. Fourteen percent of subjects were younger than age 40 years and 28% were older than 40 years. A variety of pathology was identified: herniated nucleus pulposus, foraminal stenosis, and disk degeneration.[18] It cannot be emphasized enough that diagnostic tests must be closely matched with clinical signs and symptoms to minimize the significance of false

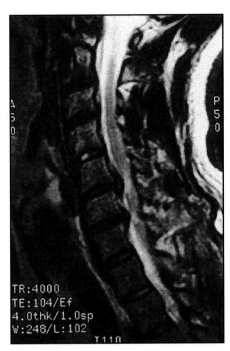

Fig. 3 Sagittal T2-weighted MRI of a patient with radiculopathy. Two large disk herniations are present at C5-C6 and C6-C7. Note the decreased signal in these diseased disks compared with adjacent levels and the cord signal at both levels.

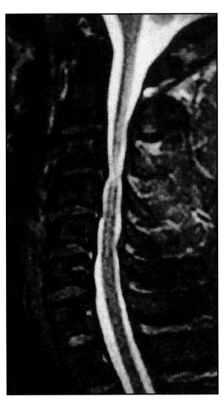

Fig. 4 Sagittal T2-weighted MRI of a patient with myelopathy. Increased cord signal at C3-C4 and degenerative disk space loss are findings consistent with cervical spondylotic stenosis.

positive studies. When MRI findings are incompatible with the clinical findings (the false negative rate for MRI is 5%), then imaging studies such as a CT scan with myelography may be indicated.[7,13,16]

MRI is superior to myelography and CT for evaluating intramedullary changes produced by spinal cord compression such as syringomyelia and myelomalacia,[13] along with intramedullary neoplasm, demyelinating disease, and various forms of myelitis. In a study of 100 patients with cervical spondylotic myelopathy (CSM), those with signal changes in the cord were more likely to have severe impairment of ambulation and sensory and motor disturbance[19] (Fig. 4). Another MRI study of 115 Japanese patients with CSM showed significant correlation between severity of myelopathy, the anterior posterior diameter of the spinal column, and the degree of compression of

the spinal cord. Forty-seven patients underwent both preoperative and postoperative MRI. Twenty-four of these patients (51%) had evidence of cord atrophy that predicted a poor clinical result.[20]

CT Myelography
Myelography paired with CT scanning provides excellent detail and differentiation of lesions of bone versus soft tissue (disk or ligament).[13] CT myelography is the study of choice in the presence of severe degenerative changes and in the presence of significant end plate osteophytes (Fig. 5). Disadvantages are the invasive nature of administering intrathecal contrast and the exposure to radiation.

In a prospective evaluation of 28 patients undergoing cervical surgery at 39 levels, Modic and associates[21] found MRI

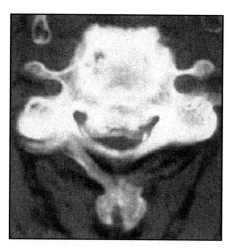

Fig. 5 A postmyelogram CT section through the cervical spine of a patient with myelopathy is shown. Large anterior and posterior osteophytes dramatically reduce the canal diameter. Bony detail and contour of the canal are seen.

to be as sensitive as CT myelography at detecting disease level, but less specific in terms of distinguishing bony from soft-tissue impingement. In this study MRI was at least as effective as plain myelography at detecting disease.

CT myelography can be considered a complementary study to a MRI scan. In a study by Shafaie and associates,[22] only a moderate degree of concordance was found between MRI and CT myelography in the evaluation of cervical myelopathy and radiculopathy in a group of 20 patients.[22] The authors concluded that the two methods are complementary rather than interchangeable or exclusive and can be used together in patient evaluations.

Electrodiagnostic modalities such as needle electromyography, somatosensory evoked potentials, and cervical root stimulation in the evaluation of neck pain, radiculopathy, and myelopathy are generally used when clinical examination and imaging fail to provide a clear diagnosis or perhaps conflicting diagnoses. This is often the case in patients with polyradiculopathy or peripheral nerve compression syndromes.

In a study of intraoperative somatosensory evoked potentials, a focal conduction block was accurately localized in 42 of 44 patients age 65 years or older with multilevel compression by MRI. Ninety-five percent of these conduction blocks occurred at C3-C4 or C4-C5 and these findings were useful in directing surgical intervention to the appropriate level.[23] Although these studies can be operator-dependent and can vary with technique, they can provide valuable information in the evaluation of cervical disorders and may help to differentiate primary cervical disorders from peripheral nerve entrapments syndromes or pain emanating from the intrinsic shoulder pathology.

Conservative Treatment

Most neck pain is self-limiting and will resolve with appropriate conservative care. Gore and associates[6] reported results of minimum 10-year follow-up on 205 patients with neck pain without any surgical intervention. Forty-three percent were free of pain, 79% had a decrease in pain, and 32% had moderate to severe residual pain.[6] The presence or severity of disease was unrelated to degenerative changes, the diameter of the spinal canal, degree of lordosis, or to any changes in measurements of these parameters over time. The initial treatment of acute neck pain is primarily directed at control of symptoms by means of anti-inflammatory medications and physical therapy.

Medications may provide relief of symptoms as in the use of low dose, short course narcotic analgesics; however, medications may be more effectively used to address the underlying pathophysiology.[24] Both corticosteroids and nonsteroidal anti-inflammatory drugs are effective at decreasing inflammation and resultant pain associated with acutely painful degenerative disk disease, radiculopathy, myelopathy, and rheumatoid arthritis.[24] Despite the common use of these medications, careful attention must be paid to their administration and possible side effects. In addition, patients treated routinely on long-term medications should be watched very closely for the possible deleterious effects on other organ systems.

Other potentially useful but less commonly applied medications include tricyclic antidepressants and muscle relaxants. In a randomized, double-blind crossover study of amitriptyline in the treatment of chronic low back pain, Pheasant and associates[25] showed a 46% decrease in the use of analgesics, an improvement in effect, but no improvement in activity level.

Muscle spasms are, at least in part, a protective mechanism potentiated by osseous or neural irritation. Muscle relaxants such as carisoprodol, metaxalone, and methocarbamol act on the central nervous system by decreasing transmission through spinal and supraspinal polysynaptic pathways with a resultant decrease in fasciculations and muscle stretch reflexes.[26] Benzodiazepines such as diazepam have a more selective action on the reticular neuronal mechanism that controls muscle tone. Cyclobenzaprine is another commonly used muscle relaxant with an as-yet undefined mechanism of action but with pharmacologic properties similar to the tricyclic antidepressants. It has been shown to be more effective than placebo at relieving muscle spasm in patients with neck and back pain.[27] The usefulness of these agents is limited by side effects such as central nervous system depression and the potential for addiction. The use of these types of medications only should be considered for short-term relief of the pain phase, with a rapid transition to the rehabilitation phase after the first week of symptoms. No role has been found for the long-term use of muscle relaxants in the treatment of most types of cervical disorders.

Physical therapy in the acute phase

uses passive modalities such as ice or heat, electrical stimulation, and manual techniques. After acute symptoms subside, dynamic and isometric strengthening exercises, neck and shoulder stretching, and aerobic conditioning (walking, cycling, and aquatic exercise) are instituted.[28] In a randomized prospective trial of 119 patients with chronic neck pain, intensive training, physical therapy, and cervical manipulation all produced meaningful improvement in pain, disability, medication use, and objective measures; however, there was no significant difference between the three treatments.[29]

Despite several randomized trials reported in the literature, the efficacy of spinal manipulation for neck and back pain over other treatments has not been shown.[30] In a randomized, parallel group clinical trial of 191 patients with chronic mechanical neck pain, rehabilitative neck exercises were superior to spinal manipulation alone. Patients treated with a combination of manipulative therapy and exercises showed greater gains in strength, motion, and endurance. Patient-rated outcomes after 11 weeks of treatment were no different between the three groups.[31]

Treatment of Cervical Radiculopathy
Nonsurgical Treatment
Nonsurgical treatment is the most appropriate first step in almost all cases of cervical radiculopathy.[7] In a longitudinal cohort study of the nonsurgical treatment of cervical disk herniation causing radiculopathy, Saal and associates[32] described 24 of 26 patients who were treated with traction, specific physical therapy exercises, oral anti-inflammatory medications, and patient education and experienced no neurologic loss. In another study, 57 patients with cervical radiculopathy were followed for up to 19 years. Forty-five percent had only one pain episode with no recurrence, 30% reported mild symptoms, and 25% complained of persistent or worsening symptoms.[33]

The use of a soft collar for a short period within 2 weeks of the onset of symptoms can reduce the acute inflammatory response and associated pain. Immobilization can also aid in the treatment of severe muscle spasms and soft-tissue strains, and it may help lessen the need for pain medications in the acute phase. Prolonged immobilization is to be avoided because of the deconditioning that may occur. Gradual weaning from the collar followed by physical therapy yields optimal results.

The efficacy of traction in the treatment of cervical radiculopathy is unclear; however, short-term relief of radicular symptoms is observed in patients using 8- to 10-lb home traction for 15- to 20-min periods.[34] The optimum recommended angle is 24° of flexion.[35] Traction should not be applied until acute muscle spasms have subsided, and thorough patient education in the proper use and techniques is essential.

Epidural steroids are most beneficial in patients with painful radiculopathy. In a well-designed study of selective nerve root injections for 55 patients with lumbar radiculopathy, Riew and associates[36] reported 29 patients who improved significantly enough to avoid surgical intervention. There was a significant difference in this study in favor of a combined bupivacaine and betamethasone injection over bupivacaine alone. A similar conclusion might be drawn for cervical radiculopathy, although to date no such study has been reported. The anatomy is different in the cervical region, than in the lumbar area, and only a highly trained individual should administer these injections in the region of the spinal cord.

Surgical Treatment
Surgical indications for cervical radiculopathy include progressive neurologic deficit, disabling motor deficit at presentation, persistent or recurrent radicular symptoms despite at least 6 weeks of conservative treatment, or segmental insta-

bility combined with radicular symptoms.[37] Before surgery is considered, imaging studies should clearly demonstrate pathologic findings that correlate with the distribution of the radicular symptoms.

In a prospective randomized study comparing surgery, physical therapy, or a cervical collar for long-standing (at least 3 months' duration) cervical radicular pain in 81 patients, Persson and associates[38] showed equal effectiveness between the three groups at 12-month follow-up; however, the surgical group reported less pain at early follow-up. Patients with radiculopathy should be carefully examined for any long tract signs, which may indicate spinal cord compression in addition to the nerve root compression.

Treatment of Cervical Spondylotic Myelopathy
Nonsurgical Treatment
The conservative care of CSM is limited. Observation of myelopathy caused by soft disk herniation is acceptable, with close attention paid to progression of signs or symptoms. Immobilization of the neck with an orthosis and rest may reduce neural irritation and may provide some relief of myelopathic symptoms; however, some authors caution against the use of cervical traction or epidural steroids in the treatment of this disease.[9,34] Ultimately CSM is a surgical condition and all reasonable efforts should be undertaken to decompress the spinal cord before significant functioning is lost. The natural history of this disorder, which can have a painless, insidious onset, is deterioration of neurologic function, paralysis, and possible death. Although this condition may plateau for some time, once deficits develop, irreversible nerve damage can lead to permanent impairment. The key to the treatment of cervical myelopathy is early diagnosis, careful observation, and early intervention before significant deterioration arises.

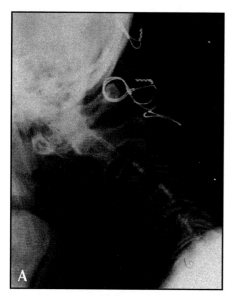 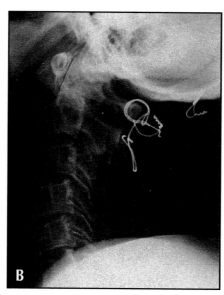

Fig. 6 Lateral flexion-extension radiographs of a patient with rheumatoid arthritis who underwent a prior attempt at posterior fusion. **A,** Flexion view shows a 5 mm atlanto-dens interval that decreases to normal limits on extension view **(B)**. Note the change in the relationship of the posterior elements of C1 on C2.

Surgical Treatment

Current surgical techniques for the cervical spine have elements of three basic goals: (1) decompression of neural elements, (2) stabilization of unstable segments, and (3) the ablation of painful articulations via fusion, which entails removal of bone or soft-tissue elements from the neurologic structures either with or without fusion. Particularly important indications for surgery include progression of signs or symptoms, presence of myelopathy for 6 months or longer, and a canal/vertebral body diameter ratio approaching 0.4.[39] Indications for surgery include difficulty walking, loss of balance, bowel or bladder incontinence, and severe spinal cord compression.[9] Signal changes within the substance of the spinal cord along with any signs of cervical myelopathy should prompt the surgeon to recommend early intervention before permanent deficits arise.

As in the low back, the decision to operate for neck pain in the absence of neural element compression is less defined than for radiculopathy or myelo-pathy. Cervical spondylosis presents a surgical challenge because it typically involves multiple levels. Only in cases of intractable axial neck pain where clinical findings can be well correlated with radiologic studies should surgical fusion be considered. Degenerative disease of the atlantoaxial facet often manifests itself more as suboccipital pain, and possibly headaches. If conservative measures fail, atlantoaxial fusion is the recommended treatment.[40]

Another indication includes atlanto-axial instability (AAI) as commonly seen in rheumatoid arthritis. AAI may be manifested by intractable pain or neurologic dysfunction and can develop from traumatic injuries, or in patients with inflammatory arthritis. The cervical spine is one of the most commonly affected areas in patients with rheumatoid arthritis and evaluation requires a high index of suspicion (Fig. 6). One third of patients with AAI and one half of those with vertical migration will develop long tract signs within 5 years of presentation, and if left untreated, the natural history of this dis-order is sudden death.[41,42] Although these patients sometimes have a relatively higher complication rate, occiput-cervical fusion to stabilize the area and arrest the cranial settling is beneficial. This treatment can be combined with posterior decompression and possibly an anterior resection of the odontoid.

In the subaxial spine, segmental instability can lead to intractable neck pain, and patients with significant subluxation may benefit from cervical fusion to stabilize the area. The presence of neck pain in the setting of degenerative disk disease alone may also be treated with cervical fusion if the pain can be truly defined and attributed to distinct levels of the spine that correlate with the imaging studies. Also, fusions are commonly performed in the lumbar spine for significant disk degeneration, but this practice is not yet widely applied to the cervical region.

Summary

Neck pain is commonly reported by patients and is associated with several disorders involving the cervical spine. A careful patient history and examination will dictate the appropriate selection of advanced diagnostic studies and nonsurgical and surgical treatment options. Most neck pain will resolve with appropriate nonsurgical care. Nonsurgical treatment is the first step for almost all patients with cervical radiculopathy; however, the results of nonsurgical treatment for patients with cervical spondylotic myelopathy are limited.

References

1. Cote P, Cassidy JD, Carroll L: The Saskatchewan Health and Back Pain Survey: The prevalence of neck pain and related disability in Saskatchewan adults. *Spine* 1998;23:1689-1698.

2. Gore DR, Sepic SB, Gardner GM: Roentgenographic findings of the cervical spine in asymptomatic people. *Spine* 1986;11:521-524.

3. Friedenberg ZB, Miller WT: Degenerative disc disease of the cervical spine: A comparative study of asymptomatic and symptomatic patients. *J Bone Joint Surg Am* 1963;45:1171-1178.

4. Fenlin JM Jr: Pathology of degenerative disease of the cervical spine. *Orthop Clin North Am* 1971;2:371-387.

5. Resnick D, Niwayama G (eds): *Diagnosis of Bone and Joint Disorders,* ed 2. Philadelphia, PA, WB Saunders, 1988.

6. Gore DR, Sepic SB, Gardner GM, Murray MP: Neck pain: A long-term follow-up of 205 patients. *Spine* 1987;12:1-5.

7. Levine MJ, Albert TJ, Smith MD: Cervical radiculopathy: Diagnosis and nonoperative management. *J Am Acad Orthop Surg* 1996;4:305-316.

8. Levine MJ, Boden SD: Diagnostic imaging of the spine, in An HS (ed): *Principles and Techniques of Spine Surgery.* Baltimore, MD, Williams & Wilkins, 1998, pp 103-127.

9. Bohlman HH: Cervical spondylosis and myelopathy. *Instr Course Lect* 1995;44:81-97.

10. Wang JC, Hatch JD, Sandhu HS, Delamarter RB: Cervical flexion and extension radiographs in acutely injured patients. *Clin Orthop* 1999;365:111-116.

11. Heller CA, Stanley P, Lewis-Jones B, Heller RF: Value of x-ray examinations of the cervical spine. *Br Med J (Clin Res Ed)* 1983;287:1276-1278.

12. Johnson MJ, Lucas GL: Value of cervical spine radiographs as a screening tool. *Clin Orthop* 1997;340:102-108.

13. Modic MT, Ross JS, Masaryk TJ: Imaging of degenerative disease of the cervical spine. *Clin Orthop* 1989;239:109-120.

14. Pavlov H, Torg JS, Robie B, Jahre C: Cervical spinal stenosis: Determination with vertebral body ratio method. *Radiology* 1987;164:771-775.

15. Sengupta DK, Kirollos R, Findlay GF, Smith ET, Pearson JC, Pigott T: The value of MR imaging in differentiating between hard and soft cervical disc disease: A comparison with intraoperative findings. *Eur Spine J* 1999;8:199-204.

16. Bartlett RJ, Hill CR, Gardiner E: A comparison of T2 and gadolinium enhanced MRI with CT myelography in cervical radiculopathy. *Br J Radiol* 1998;71:11-19.

17. Yousem DM, Atlas SW, Goldberg HI, Grossman RI: Degenerative narrowing of the cervical spine neural foramina: Evaluation with high-resolution 3DFT gradient-echo MR imaging. *AJNR Am J Neuroradiol* 1991;12:229-236.

18. Boden SD, McCowin PR, Davis DO, Dina TS, Mark AS, Wiesel S: Abnormal magnetic-resonance scans of the cervical spine in asymptomatic subjects: A prospective investigation. *J Bone Joint Surg Am* 1990;72:1178-1184.

19. Puzzilli F, Mastronardi L, Ruggeri A, Lunardi P: Intramedullary increased MR signal intensity and its relation to clinical features in cervical myelopathy. *J Neurosurg Sci* 1999;43:135-139.

20. Nagata K, Kiyonaga K, Ohashi T, Sagara M, Miyazaki S, Inoue A: Clinical value of magnetic resonance imaging for cervical myelopathy. *Spine* 1990;15:1088-1096.

21. Modic MT, Masaryk TJ, Mulopulos GP, Bundschuh C, Han JS, Bohlman H: Cervical radiculopathy: Prospective evaluation with surface coil MR imaging, CT with metrizamide, and metrizamide myelography. *Radiology* 1986;161:753-759.

22. Shafaie FF, Wippold FJ II, Gado M, Pilgram TK, Riew KD: Comparison of computed tomography myelography and magnetic resonance imaging in the evaluation of cervical spondylotic myelopathy and radiculopathy. *Spine* 1999;24:1781-1785.

23. Tani T, Yamamoto H, Kimura J: Cervical spondylotic myelopathy in elderly people: A high incidence of conduction block at C3-4 or C4-5. *J Neurol Neurosurg Psychiatry* 1999;66:456-464.

24. Dillin W, Uppal GS: Analysis of medications used in the treatment of cervical disk degeneration. *Orthop Clin North Am* 1992;23:421-433.

25. Pheasant H, Bursk A, Goldfarb J, Azen SP, Weiss JN, Borelli L: Amitriptyline and chronic low-back pain: A randomized double-blind crossover study. *Spine* 1983;8:552-557.

26. Baldessarini RJ: Drugs and the treatment of psychiatric disorders, in Goodman LS, Gilman A, Gilman AG (eds): *Goodman and Gilman's: The Pharmacological Basis of Therapeutics,* ed 7. New York, NY, MacMillan, 1985, pp 387-445.

27. Bercel NA: Cyclobenzaprine in the treatment of skeletal muscle spasm in osteoarthritis of the cervical and lumbar spine. *Curr Ther Res* 1977;22:462-468.

28. Garfin SR: Cervical degenerative disorders: Etiology, presentation, and imaging studies. *Instr Course Lect* 2000;49:335-338.

29. Jordan A, Bendix T, Nielsen H, Hansen FR, Host D, Winkel A: Intensive training, physiotherapy, or manipulation for patients with chronic neck pain: A prospective, single-blinded, randomized clinical trial. *Spine* 1998;23:311-319.

30. Koes BW, Assendelft WJ, van der Heijden GJ, Bouter LM, Knipschild PG: Spinal manipulation and mobilisation for back and neck pain: A blinded review. *BMJ* 1991;303:1298-1303.

31. Bronfort G, Evans R, Nelson B, Aker PD, Goldsmith CH, Vernon H: A randomized clinical trial of exercise and spinal manipulation for patients with chronic neck pain. *Spine* 2001;26:788-799.

32. Saal JS, Saal JA, Yurth EF: Nonoperative management of herniated cervical intervertebral disc with radiculopathy. *Spine* 1996;21:1877-1883.

33. Lees F, Turner JWA: Natural history and prognosis of cervical spondylosis. *Br Med J* 1963;2:1607-1610.

34. Murphy MJ, Leiponis JV: Nonoperative treatment of cervical spine pain, in The Cervical Spine Research Society Editorial Committee (eds): *The Cervical Spine,* ed 2. Philadelphia, PA, JB Lippincott, 1989, pp 670-677.

35. Colachis SC Jr, Strohm BR: A study of tractive forces and angle of pull on vertebral interspaces in the cervical spine. *Arch Phys Med Rehabil* 1965;46:820-830.

36. Riew KD, Yin Y, Gilula L, et al: The effect of nerve-root injections on the need for operative treatment of lumbar radicular pain: A prospective, randomized, controlled, double-blind study. *J Bone Joint Surg Am* 2000;82:1589-1593.

37. Albert TJ, Murrell SE: Surgical management of cervical radiculopathy. *J Am Acad Orthop Surg* 1999;7:368-376.

38. Persson LC, Carlsson CA, Carlsson JY: Long-lasting cervical radicular pain managed with surgery, physiotherapy, or a cervical collar: A prospective, randomized study. *Spine* 1997;22:751-758.

39. Law MD Jr, Bernhardt M, White AA III: Evaluation and management of cervical spondylotic myelopathy. *Instr Course Lect* 1995;44:99-110.

40. Grob D: Surgery in the degenerative cervical spine. *Spine* 1998;23:2674-2683.

41. Mathews JA: Atlanto-axial subluxation in rheumatoid arthritis. *Ann Rheum Dis* 1969;28:260-266.

42. Lipson SJ: Rheumatoid arthritis in the cervical spine. *Clin Orthop* 198;239:121-127.

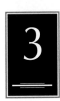

Anterior Cervical Approaches for Cervical Radiculopathy and Myelopathy

Patrick N. Smith, MD

Mark A. Knaub, MD

James D. Kang, MD

Abstract

Compression of the spinal cord and nerve roots caused by spondylotic changes or disk herniations is the most common etiology for cervical myelopathy, radiculopathy, or myeloradiculopathy. Surgical intervention in treating these conditions has been very successful. Anterior approaches to the cervical spine are being used for the treatment of cervical radiculopathy and myelopathy. The technical aspects of anterior diskectomy and corpectomy, methods of fusion, and the use of instrumentation are important treatment considerations.

Compression of the spinal cord and nerve roots from spondylotic changes or disk herniations is the most common cause of cervical myelopathy, radiculopathy, or myeloradiculopathy.[1,2] The majority of these pathologic changes occur in the lower cervical spine because of the greater mobility and smaller neural foramen in this region. In addition, the larger size of the lower cervical nerve roots makes them more vulnerable to compression from osteophytes or intervertebral disk material.

The natural history of myelopathy and radiculopathy has been extensively reported in the literature over the past 40 years. Clark and Robinson[3] reported that spontaneous regression of cervical myelopathy was highly uncommon. In a 1963 study, Lees and Turner[4] showed that 57%

of patients with radiculopathy experienced little or no regression of their symptoms within the first 3 months. In the early 1960s, Robinson and Smith[5] described the anterior surgical approach for treatment of spondylotic deformities and disk disease of the lower cervical spine. Over the years, modifications have been made to Robinson's original procedure for anterior decompression. With these changes, anterior decompression in the form of diskectomy or corpectomy has been shown repeatedly to provide good or excellent results in the treatment of radiculopathy or myelopathy.[6-11] For example, Emery and associates[12] reported long-term follow-up results from 118 patients undergoing anterior decompression for myelopathy. Thirty-eight of the 82 patients with a gait abnormality preop-

eratively achieved normal gait after surgery, with only one patient experiencing continued deterioration.

The Anteromedial Approach

The anteromedial approach to the cervical spine is the workhorse approach for cervical diskectomy and corpectomy procedures, allowing excellent exposure of the lower cervical spine from C3 to C7. With the patient supine on the operating table, a roll is placed under the scapula to facilitate positioning of the cervical spine in a neutral or slightly extended position. In those patients with severe stenosis or myelopathy, hyperextension should be avoided to prevent infolding of the ligamentum flavum and further narrowing of the spinal canal. For anterior cervical corpectomy and fusion (ACCF), Gardner-Wells tongs are used to assist in positioning the head and neck in the desired position as well as to immobilize the spine during the procedure. The shoulders are taped down to allow for adequate visualization for the marker x-ray to confirm the level(s) to be operated. Skin landmarks will assist the surgeon in making the appropriate skin incision. The C1-C2 interspace is located at the angle of the

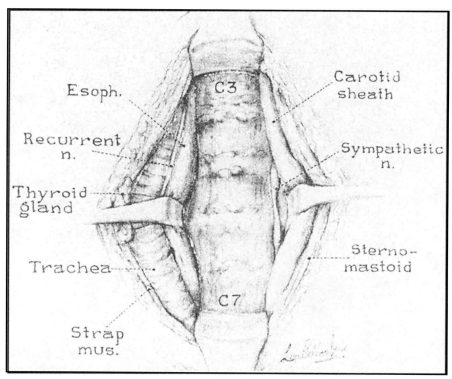

Esoph.
C3
Carotid sheath
Recurrent n.
Sympathetic n.
Thyroid gland
Trachea
Sterno-mastoid
C7
Strap mus.

Fig. 1 Exposure of the anterior surface of the vertebral bodies and disk spaces via a left-sided anteromedial approach. The esophagus and trachea are retracted medially and the carotid sheath laterally. (Reproduced with permission from Zdeblick TA, Bohlman HH: Cervical kyphosis and myelopathy. *J Bone Joint Surg Am* 1989;71:170-182.)

mandible whereas the hyoid bone is located at the level of C3 vertebral body. The C4-C5 interspace can be localized using the superior border of the thyroid cartilage. The cricoid cartilage and the carotid tubercle are located at the C6 vertebral body. The carotid tubercle arises from the anterior portion of the transverse process of C6 and can be palpated in the interval between the sternocleidomastoid muscle and the medial musculovisceral column.

A transverse incision in line with the skin creases of the neck will provide adequate exposure for most single- and two-level procedures. The transverse incision allows for better cosmesis, although it may limit exposure for multilevel procedures. An oblique incision may be used for procedures involving more than two levels. The decision to approach the cervical spine from the right or left side is usually based on the surgeon's preference and training. The advantage of approaching the cervical spine from the left is the consistent course of the left recurrent laryngeal nerve in the carotid sheath between the trachea and esophagus, rendering it less vulnerable to injury. Other surgeons, however, advocate a right-sided approach to facilitate operating with the right hand and to avoid the potential risk of injury to the thoracic duct in lower cervical procedures.

After making the appropriate skin incision, the first layer encountered will be the paired platysma muscle, which runs from the lower border of the mandible to the superficial fascia over the chest. It extends from just short of midline to the medial border of the sternocleidomastoid. The platysma is transected perpendicular to the orientation of the muscle fibers to expose the deep cervical fascia. The platysma is undermined on its superior and inferior surfaces to facilitate exposure in the cephalocaudal directions. The superficial layer of the deep cervical fascia is sharply dissected off of the medial border of the sternocleidomastoid to expose the middle layer of the deep cervical fascia. The remaining deep cervical fascia is bluntly dissected using the natural plane between the sternocleidomastoid and the trachea and esophagus. The carotid pulse should be palpated just deep to the sternocleidomastoid to assure its protection. The final two layers encountered are the pretracheal and prevertebral fascias that are bluntly dissected using a Kittner dissector, exposing the anterior aspects of the vertebral bodies and intervertebral disks (Fig. 1). At this point, an 18-gauge needle is placed into the intervertebral disk and a lateral radiograph is taken to identify the level of exposure. A discussion of the remainder of the approach follows in subsequent sections.

Dissection during the approach places several vital structures at risk if dissection strays from the appropriate anatomic planes. The carotid artery and jugular veins lie within the carotid sheath in the middle layers of deep cervical fascia. These structures must be identified by palpation of the carotid pulse and retracted laterally. The thyroid gland, located beneath the superficial layer of the deep cervical fascia, is vulnerable to injury with inadvertent medial dissection. Within the medial musculovisceral column are the trachea and esophagus. The exact location of these structures must be known at all times to avoid injury by retractors or electrocautery. The hypoglossal nerve runs in the most cephalad aspect of the approach and must be protected. The superior thyroid artery and vein and the external laryngeal nerve are also in the superior portion of the approach and should be identified and protected. The cervical sympathetic chain and stellate ganglion are at risk for injury with lateral dissection of the longus colli

The pseudarthrosis rate decreased to 4.4%. Although graft settling increased, this was not clinically significant and clinical outcomes between the two techniques were equivalent. Although clinical outcomes were equivalent in these two studies, pseudarthrosis is a known factor in poor outcomes and the incidence of this condition is an important consideration in patient treatment.

The alternative to anterior decompression for the treatment of cervical myelopathy and radiculopathy is posterior decompression either by laminectomy or laminoplasty. Phillips[17] compared the clinical outcomes of ACDF and posterior laminectomy in the treatment of cervical spondylotic myelopathy. Of those patients with symptoms for less than 1 year, 86% of the anterior diskectomy group showed improvement based on Nurick grade, compared to 67% improvement in the posterior group. Crandall and Batzdorf[18] compared ACDF with posterior laminectomy in the treatment of myelopathy. Although the early results were similar, long-term follow-up showed a tendency for continued improvement with ACDF and eventual deterioration with laminectomy. Herkowitz[19] compared the results of three different procedures: ACDF, laminectomy, and laminoplasty. All patients had at least three-level disease. Good or excellent results were found in 92% of the ACDF group, 86% of the laminoplasty group, and 66% of the laminoplasty group.

Autograft Versus Allograft

Anterior cervical arthrodesis after diskectomy diminishes neurologic irritation by limiting motion, restoring a more normal cervical alignment, and preventing collapse into kyphosis.[14] Pseudarthrosis rates for single-level ACDF range from 3% to 4%, and rise to approximately 27% following multilevel fusions. Although nonunions do not preclude a favorable outcome, pseudarthrosis has been correlated with less than optimal results. White

and associates[20] reported a 53% good or excellent outcome in 17 patients with pseudarthrosis compared with a 75% good or excellent rating in those with solid fusions. Similarly, Bohlman and associates[15] found that of the 122 patients who underwent ACDF, those who developed a nonunion had significantly worse arm and neck pain. Several factors contribute to pseudarthrosis, including surgical technique and number of levels fused. The use of allograft and its impact on union rates continues to be a topic of debate. The advantages of allograft include shorter surgical time and no graft-site morbidity. The advantages of autograft include better vascularization and ossification based on animal models and no immunologic reaction. Several authors have reported comparable results with the use of allograft in anterior cervical spine surgery.[21-23] Young and Rosenwasser[24] reported a 92% fusion rate with the use of fibular allograft for ACDF. The allograft group had shorter hospital stays and less postoperative pain. Shapiro[25] reported on 88 consecutive patients who underwent ACDF using allograft with a mean follow-up of 22 months. There were no pseudarthroses and no settling of the graft. Moreover, patients receiving allograft returned to work 5 weeks sooner than patients receiving autograft when compared to a previously reported series of 100 patients by the same author. Donor site morbidities such as seroma, hematoma, infection, and meralgia paresthetica have been reported to be as high as 20%.[26] Other studies have shown that pain at the donor site can last for up to 1 year in a third of patients.[27] Conversely, several studies have demonstrated superior results with autograft. Bishop and associates[28] supported the use of autograft when they compared iliac crest autograft and allograft in 132 patients undergoing interbody fusions. They found higher nonunion rates and higher subsidence rates with allograft in both single level and multilevel fusions. An and associ-

ates[29] compared iliac crest autograft with freeze-dried allograft. They found a 46% nonunion rate in the allograft group versus a 26% nonunion rate in the autograft group. Again, subsidence was higher in the allograft population.

Other biomechanical spacers acting as bone graft substitute have been used to stabilize the intervertebral disk space. These devices include threaded titanium cages, porous hydroxyapatite ceramics, and carbon fiber implants. Although early reports have been encouraging, long-term prospective studies are needed before conclusions can be made regarding these devices.

Instrumentation

The use of anterior plating with ACDF remains controversial as well. The theoretical benefits of anterior plating is its ability to stabilize and immobilize the intended segment, prevent graft migration, and facilitate fusion (Fig. 3). Biomechanical studies have shown that plating significantly adds stability to the construct, which may be important in increasing the likelihood of a solid fusion.[30] The higher fusion rates associated with plate fixation make it an attractive option. Despite potential complications, instrumentation for single level and multilevel ACDF has been widely accepted by many surgeons. Wang and associates[27] reported on 80 patients undergoing single level ACDF followed for 6 years. Plating was performed in 44 patients, resulting in a 4.5% pseudarthrosis rate compared with an 8.3% pseudarthrosis rate in the 36 patients without plating. There was a significant difference in graft collapse and patient outcome based on Odoms criteria between the two groups. In another study, Wang and associates[31] reported on two-level fusions with and without plating. Those patients without plates had a 25% pseudarthrosis rate compared to 0% in those treated with instrumentation. No complications directly related to instrumentation were reported. Historically, however, earlier cervical plates were associated with screw backout and potential catastrophic injury to the esophagus. Technical advancements in implant design, including screw locking mechanisms, have decreased the potential for this dreaded complication.

Anterior Cervical Corpectomy and Fusion

ACCF is considered by many to be the treatment of choice in patients with myelopathy and/or multilevel disk disease. It allows for a more thorough decompression of the spinal cord, and in some respects, may be safer than decompressing the cord through a single or multiple disk spaces. Attempting to decompress the spinal cord in a myelopathic patient through a narrow degenerated disk space may be dangerous, in that overdistraction of the disk space for visualization prior to removal of the spondylotic osteophytes may lead to neurologic deterioration. In patients with involvement of three or four disk levels, there may be additional theoretical advantages of ACCF versus a multiple level ACDF (Fig. 4). Emery and associates[32] demonstrated a direct correlation between pseudarthrosis rates and the number of fused segments. Of the 16 patients undergoing three-level ACDF, only 9 showed complete fusion of all segments. Of the seven patients with nonunions, two had severe neck pain and required revision. Swank and associates[33] compared the pseudarthrosis rates between two-level ACDF and one-level corpectomy and between three-level ACDF and two-level corpectomy. There was a significant increase in pseudarthrosis rates with ACDF surgeries as compared to the corpectomies. A possible explanation for this increasing pseudarthrosis rate may be a result of altered biomechanics with multiple diskectomies as demonstrated by Yoo and associates.[34]

The approach for corpectomy surgery is similar to that for diskectomy.

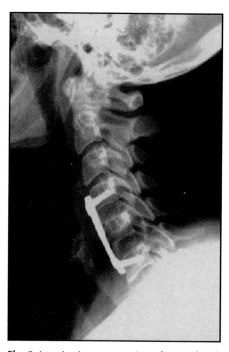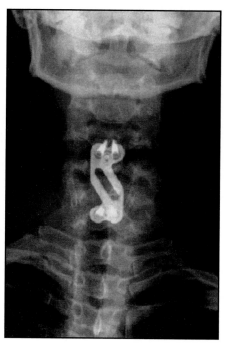

Fig. 3 Anterior instrumentation of a two-level ACDF using an anterior plate with a locking mechanism to prevent screw backout.

Although a transverse incision can be used, an oblique incision should be considered in cervical corpectomies to assure the needed exposure of two or three consecutive vertebral bodies. Patients should be placed in cervical traction for immobilization with Gardner-Wells tongs using 5 to 10 lb of weight. This will help maintain the head and neck alignment and facilitate graft insertion. Once the cervical spine is exposed, lateral dissection of the longus colli muscles is performed using electrocautery. Three millimeters of lateral dissection of the longus colli muscles is the maximum dissection needed to provide adequate visualization and still avoid vertebral artery injury. Caspar self-retaining retractors are then inserted in both the mediolateral and cephalocaudal directions. Using the operating microscope or loupe mignification, all intervening disks are removed in a similar manner as just described. The uncovertebral joints serve as important anatomic landmarks during a corpectomy. Symmetrical resection of the body requires staying within the boundary of the uncovertebral joints to avoid injury to the nearby vertebral artery. Using a high-speed burr, the vertebral bodies are removed to the depth of the posterior cortex. The remaining bone can be removed using fine-angled curets and micro-Kerrison rongeurs. The posterior longitudinal ligament should be visualized in the depth of the trough. The width of the trough should generally be three fifths of the vertebral body width. This usually measures 15 to 18 mm in width. Excessive lateral dissection beyond the uncovertebral joint may result in vertebral artery injury and should be avoided. Preoperative MRI scans should be reviewed carefully to evaluate for anatomic anomalies of the vertebral arteries. Details of the complications of cervical spine surgery will be discussed in chapter 38. At this point, posterior and posterolateral spondylotic osteophytes should be removed with micro-Kerrison rongeurs and fine-angled curets to provide adequate decompres-

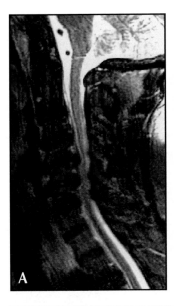 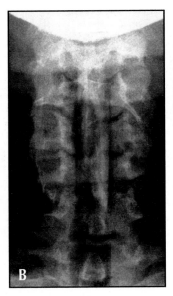 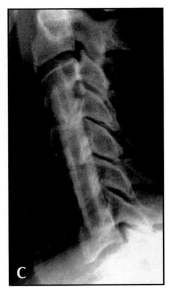

Fig. 4 A, Preoperative MRI showing multiple level stenosis with cord impingement. **B** and **C,** Postoperative AP and lateral radiographs showing a healed fibular autograft spanning the involved levels.

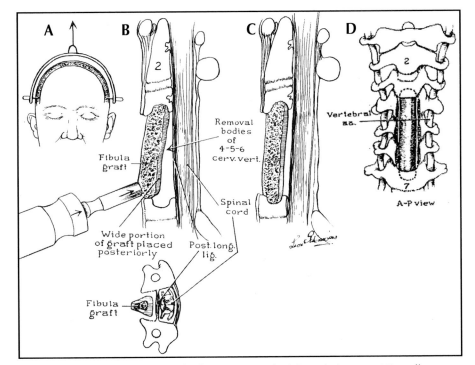

Fig. 5 After the decompression, skeletal traction is applied through the tongs (**A**) to allow placement of the fibula graft. Seating holes are fashioned into the superior and inferior end plates of the intact vertebral bodies with a high-speed burr (**B**). The ends of the graft are rounded and the graft is tamped into place (**C**). Release of the traction locks the graft into place (**D**). (Reproduced with permission from Zdeblick TA, Bohlman HH: Cervical kyphosis and myelopathy. *J Bone Joint Surg Am* 1989;71:170-182.)

caudal vertebral body (Fig. 5). These troughs will allow the strut graft to lock into place, reducing the likelihood of displacement or dislocation of the graft. The choice of graft is based on surgeon preference and number of levels involved. A tricortical iliac crest autograft or allograft can be used for one- or two-level corpectomies. If more than two levels are involved, a fibular strut autograft or allograft is recommended. The fibula is prepared by making convex surfaces at the ends of the graft matching the concave troughs made in the end plates. Additional traction is applied and the graft is inserted (Fig. 5). Traction is then removed, locking the graft in place. Instrumentation, if desired, is applied at this time. The patient is immobilized in a rigid cervical collar after surgery.

The success of anterior corpectomy is well documented in the literature. In 1987, Bernard and Whitecloud[9] reported their series of 21 ACCFs for cervical spondylotic myelopathy and myeloradiculopathy. Based on Nurick's classification, 16 of the 21 patients improved one function grade with the greatest improvement seen in patients treated within 1 year. In 1999, Fessler and associates[35] reported on 93 patients with a primary diagnosis of cervical spondylotic

sion of the spinal cord. Resection of the PLL provides a more radical decompression of the spinal cord, but whether it improves clinical outcomes is uncertain.

In preparation for bone graft insertion, two concave troughs are created in the inferior aspect of the cephalad vertebral body and the superior aspect of the

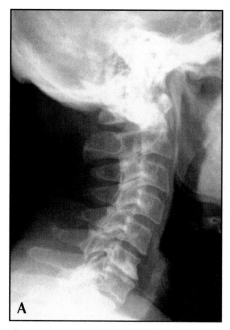 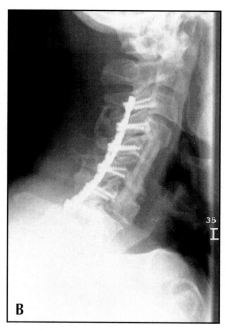 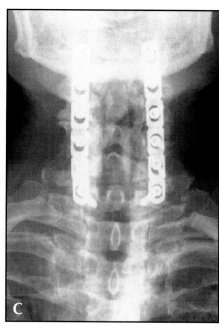

Fig. 6 Preoperative lateral radiograph (**A**) showing loss of the normal cervical lordosis in the lower cervical spine. Because of the risk of kyphosis after an isolated anterior procedure, this ACCF was supplemented with an instrumented posterior lateral mass fusion (**B** and **C**).

myelopathy. After ACCF, 86% of the patients showed improvement of at least one Nurick score grade, with deterioration occurring in only one patient. This result is significantly better than the outcomes reported by Nurick[36] for posterior surgical treatment for myelopathy, which showed only 33% improvement and 18% deterioration. Although some reports have noted regression of favorable results with longer follow-up, none have reported immediate worsening of symptoms following surgery as seen with posterior procedures.

Ossification of the Posterior Longitudinal Ligament

Ossification of the posterior longitudinal ligament (OPLL) has been described as a cause of cervical myelopathy and radiculopathy.[37,38] It can be identified on lateral radiographs as an abnormal radiodensity along the posterior margins of the vertebral bodies. There is an increased incidence of OPLL in the Asian population. Neither the etiology nor the pathogenesis is entirely understood. Hypertrophy of

the PLL is believed to be involved in the initial stages, followed by endochondral ossification of the ligament. Almost all patients with OPLL have at least some subjective complaints, such as hand numbness or neck pain.[39] Diagnosis can be made by plain radiographs, although CT scan will better differentiate OPLL and posterior osteophytes of the vertebral body. Regarding the natural history of OPLL, Matsunaga and associates[40] noted no clinical improvements in 207 patients with OPLL with nonsurgical treatment. In addition, there was deterioration in 13% of the patients. Conservative treatment, therefore, has a limited role in the treatment of symptomatic OPLL. Anterior corpectomy with removal of the ossified ligament followed by fusion is an option for treatment, although posterior procedures such as laminoplasty have become popular. Matsuoka and associates[41] reported on 107 patients with OPLL treated with anterior decompression and fusion. Seventy-one percent of the patients had improved Japanese Orthopaedic Association scores at 6.5 year follow-up.

Allograft Versus Autograft

Unlike single-level diskectomy, there is less information for comparison of autograft to allograft in corpectomy surgery. Macdonald and associates[42] reported on their series of 36 corpectomies with fibular allograft. By 24 months, they reported a 96% osseous union at both ends of the allograft. Subsidence occurred in two patients. Anterior plating was performed in 15 patients and halo immobilization applied in all but one patient. Eleraky and associates[43] reported on 185 corpectomies, including 141 cases with autogenous iliac crest graft and 44 cases using allograft. There was a 98.8% fusion rate with no significant difference between the two groups. Anterior plating was performed in all but six patients. Despite these results, autogenous bone graft is the preferred material for many surgeons. In Bernard and Whitecloud's[9] series of 21 ACCFs, all patients received fibular autograft, resulting in a 100% fusion rate. The number of levels decompressed in that series was three levels in 13 cases, four levels in four cases, and two levels in the remaining

muscles. Injury to these structures may result in Horner's syndrome.

Anterior Cervical Diskectomy and Fusion

For the majority of anterior cervical diskectomies, the anteromedial approach provides adequate exposure. If multiple levels are involved, a more oblique incision may be used to provide better exposure in the cephalocaudal direction. After the soft-tissue dissection, a spinal needle is placed into the exposed disk and a lateral radiograph confirms the correct disk space. After confirmation of the disk level, the longus colli muscles are undermined using electrocautery. A self-retaining retractor is placed underneath the longus colli muscles and opened to retract the muscles laterally. At this point, the entire disk space should be adequately visualized. Depending on the preference of the surgeon, an operating microscope or loupe magnification should be used to more safely decompress the neural elements. A scalpel is used to incise the anterior anulus fibrosus to allow removal of the disk contents with a pituitary rongeur. Downward pressure on the posterior longitudinal ligament should be avoided during removal of the disk material. Overhanging osteophytes on the anterior edge of the superior vertebral body should be removed to facilitate visualization of the entire disk space. To facilitate better exposure of the posterior regions of the disk near the spinal cord, the disk space should be distracted using the Caspar vertebral body screw distraction system (Aesculap Inc, San Francisco, CA). A 3-0 curet is used to remove any remaining disk fragments and to expose the bony end plates. A high-speed burr (3 to 4 mm) is used to shave the bony end plates of both the superior and inferior vertebral bodies until there is punctate bleeding. This procedure serves to prepare the vertebral end plates for the bone graft.

The uncovertebral joints will define the lateral margins of dissection within the disk space. If the patient's radiculopathy is caused by a soft disk herniation, the disk fragment may be found by exploring close to the posterior longitudinal ligament (PLL). Most disk herniations are contained within the margins of the PLL, but not infrequently, herniations may be transligamentous, with fragments of disk within the epidural space. In these cases, a rent in the PLL can be seen and the PLL must be taken down to retrieve the fragment. Resecting the PLL facilitates a thorough exploration of the epidural space. In cases where the herniation is contained by the PLL, it need not be resected. If the patient's radiculopathy is caused by uncovertebral spondylotic osteophytes, it is recommended that these osteophytes be removed for immediate relief of the patient's symptoms. These are removed by burring into the uncovertebral joints and carefully resecting the osteophytes using small, micro-Kerrison rongeurs and microcurets. Dissection laterally, past the uncovertebral joints, is dangerous because of the position of the vertebral arteries and should be avoided.

After adequate preparation of the disk space, either tricortical iliac crest autograft or banked allograft is placed into the disk space. Prior to placement of the bone graft into the disk space, all soft tissue should be removed from it and the graft cut to the appropriate size. Insertion of the graft is aided by increasing the distraction through the Caspar retractors. The graft is then tamped into place and recessed 1 to 2 mm from the anterior cortex of the vertebral bodies (Fig. 2). Care must be taken to remove all anterior osteophytes at the operated levels, which allows for accurate assessment of the depth of the graft and assures that an anterior cervical plate will sit flat across the disk space. Several graft configurations have been described, including the Robinson-Smith horseshoe graft, the Cloward dowel graft, the keystone graft

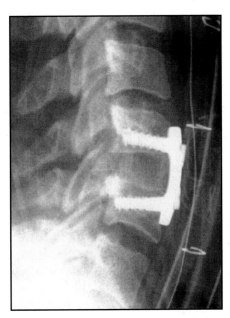

Fig. 2 An immediate postoperative lateral radiograph showing the placement of the autograft iliac crest graft recessed posterior to the anterior cortex of the vertebral bodies.

of Simmons, and the iliac strut graft of Bailey and Badgley. The Robinson-Smith graft is a tricortical graft that provides good structural support and excellent cancellous bone to facilitate fusion. The dimensions of the graft should measure a minimum of 7 mm in height or 2 mm greater than the original disk height as reported by An and associates.[13] If instrumentation is preferred, an anterior cervical plate is placed at this time.

In Robinson's original description involving 56 patients undergoing anterior cervical diskectomy and fusion (ACDF), removal of anterior osteophytes and complete removal of the osseous end plates were not performed. No instrumentation was used. Pseudarthrosis developed in 13% of the patients.[14] Bohlman and associates[15] reported on 122 patients using a technique similar to that described by Robinson, resulting in similar rates of pseudarthrosis. Emery and associates[16] reported on a modification of the Robinson technique in which the end plates were burred to expose subchondral bone.

four cases. In Emery and associates'[44] long-term follow-up of anterior decompression for cervical myelopathy, only one of the 36 ACCFs with fibular autograft went on to nonunion. Moreover, the authors found that an unsatisfactory outcome with respect to pain had a significant association with pseudarthrosis.

Instrumentation

Graft dislodgment has been reported as the most common complication after cervical corpectomy, occurring in 10% to 29% of cases. In an attempt to address these complications, anterior plating has been used to stabilize the graft.[45] Although anterior plating is believed to decrease the risk of graft dislodgment and lower the pseudarthrosis rate, its use is controversial. Recently, DiAngelo and associates[46] compared the biomechanical properties of cervical strut grafts with and without anterior plating. In this cadaveric study, anterior plating resulted in increased stiffness and decreased local cervical motion. It also resulted in reversal of graft loading with excessive loading of the construct in extension. The authors concluded that excessive loading in extension may result in pistoning and eventual failure of the construct. Epstein[47] compared the reoperation rate due to graft extrusion and pseudarthrosis in one-level ACCF with and without plating. Of the 48 non-instrumented cases, 3 resulted in immediate graft extrusion requiring replacement of the graft. Two more resulted in pseudarthrosis at 6 months requiring posterior wiring and fusion. In comparison, 1 of the 35 instrumented ACCFs had graft extrusion and 3 developed pseudarthrosis requiring posterior wiring and fusion. The author concluded that anterior plating did not significantly reduce the rates of graft extrusion or pseudarthrosis rate. Some studies have shown an increased pseudarthrosis rate with anterior plating, where it is believed that plating distracts the constructs, preventing settling of the graft into the end

plates.[48] Riew and associates[49] reported their series of 14 patients who had ACCF with buttress plating. One patient had complete extrusion of the graft on post-operative day three resulting in death, and three had pseudarthrosis; two requiring revision surgery. Vanichkachorn and associates[50] reported on 11 patients treated with fibula or iliac strut graft with buttress plating. No incidence of plate or graft migration or dislodgement occurred. All patients, however, in this series underwent posterior segmental fixation. Supplemental posterior fusion, particularly in those patients with kyphotic deformities, will decrease the pseudarthrosis rates and prevent graft or hardware migration (Fig. 6).

Summary

Anterior cervical spinal procedures yield good to excellent results in the majority of patients with cervical radiculopathy, myelopathy, and myeloradiculopathy. The anterior approach allows for direct decompression of the neural elements by removal of the offending pathologic disk material or osteophyte, whereas posterior procedures indirectly decompress the impaired neural structures. Concerns with the possible connection between allografts and nonunions have led to the use of autograft iliac crest bone grafts for all ACDF and some one-level corpectomies. Fibular strut autografts are used for all ACCF procedures except in the setting of trauma, in which an allograft fibular strut may be used. Anterior plates with screw-locking mechanisms are used in all one- and two-level ACDF procedures. Three- and four-level cervical disk disease is usually treated with a multilevel corpectomy and fibular strut fusion in an attempt to avoid the high rate of pseudarthrosis at one or more of the attempted fusion sites. All ACCF procedures are performed without plate fixation. Shaping the graft to key into the prepared end plates provides stability of the construct. With both ACDF and

ACCF procedures, the patients are placed into a semirigid cervical orthosis.

References

1. Montgomery DM, Brower RS: Cervical spondylotic myelopathy: Clinical syndrome and natural history. *Orthop Clin North Am* 1992;23:487-493.

2. Heller JG: The syndromes of degenerative cervical disease. *Orthop Clin North Am* 1992;23:381-394.

3. Clarke E, Robinson PK: Cervical myelopathy: A complication of cervical spondylosis. *Brain* 1956;79:483-510.

4. Lees F, Turner JWA: Natural history and prognosis of cervical spondylosis. *Br Med J* 1963;2:1607-1610.

5. Robinson RA, Smith GW: Abstract: Anterolateral cervical disc removal and interbody fusion for cervical disc syndrome. *Bull Johns Hopkins Hosp* 1955;96:223-224.

6. Cloward RB: The anterior approach for removal of ruptured cervical disks. *J Neurosurg* 1958;15:602-617.

7. Klein GR, Vaccaro AR, Albert TJ: Health outcome assessment before and after anterior cervical discectomy and fusion for radiculopathy: A prospective analysis. *Spine* 2000;25:801-803.

8. Bohlman HH: Cervical spondylosis with moderate to severe myelopathy: A report of seventeen cases treated by Robinson anterior cervical discectomy and fusion. *Spine* 1977;2:151-162.

9 Bernard TN Jr, Whitecloud TS III: Cervical spondylotic myelopathy and myeloradiculopathy: Anterior decompression and stabilization with autogenous fibula strut graft. *Clin Orthop* 1987;221:149-160.

10. Okada K, Shirasaki N, Hayashi H, Oka S, Hosoya T: Treatment of cervical spondylotic myelopathy by enlargement of the spinal canal anteriorly, followed by arthrodesis. *J Bone Joint Surg Am* 1991;73:352-364.

11. Saunders RL, Bernini PM, Shirreffs TG Jr, Reeves AG: Central corpectomy for cervical spondylotic myelopathy: A consecutive series with long-term follow-up evaluation. *J Neurosurg* 1991;74:163-170.

12. Emery SE, Bohlman HH, Bolesta MJ, Jones PK: Anterior cervical decompression and arthrodesis for the treatment of cervical spondylotic myelopathy: Two to seventeen-year follow-up. *J Bone Joint Surg Am* 1998;80:941-951.

13. An HS, Evanich CJ , Nowicki BH, Haughton VM: Ideal thickness of Smith-Robinson graft for anterior cervical fusion: A cadaveric study with computed tomographic correlation. *Spine* 1993;18:2043-2047.

14. Robinson RA, Walker AE, Ferlic DC, Wiecking DK: The results of anterior interbody fusion of the cervical spine. *J Bone Joint Surg Am* 1962;44:1569-1587.

15. Bohlman HH, Emery SE, Goodfellow DB, Jones PK: Robinson anterior cervical discectomy and arthrodesis for cervical radiculopathy: Long-term follow-up of one hundred and twenty-two patients. *J Bone Joint Surg Am* 1993;75:1298-1307.

16. Emery SE, Bolesta MJ, Banks MA, Jones PK: Robinson anterior cervical fusion: Comparison of the standard and modified techniques. *Spine* 1994;19:660-663.

17. Phillips DG: Surgical treatment of myelopathy with cervical spondylosis. *J Neurol Neurosurg Psychiatry* 1973;36:879-884.

18. Crandall PH, Batzdorf U: Cervical spondylotic myelopathy. *J Neurosurg* 1966;25:57-66.

19. Herkowitz HH: A comparison of anterior cervical fusion, cervical laminectomy, and cervical laminoplasty for the surgical management of multiple level spondylotic radiculopathy. *Spine* 1988;13:774-780.

20. White AA III, Southwick WO, Deponte RJ, Gainor JW, Hardy R: Relief of pain by anterior cervical spine fusion for spondylosis: A report of sixty-five patients. *J Bone Joint Surg Am* 1968;55:525-534.

21. Brown MD, Malinin TI, Davis PB: A roentgenographic evaluation of frozen allografts versus autografts in anterior cervical fusions. *Clin Orthop* 1976;119:231-236.

22. Cloward RB: Gas-sterilized cadaver bone grafts for spinal fusion operations: A simplified bone bank. *Spine* 1980;5:4-10.

23. Hanley E, Harvell J, Shapiro D, Kraus D: Use of allograft bone in cervical spine surgery. *Semin Spine Surg* 1989;1:262-270.

24. Young WF, Rosenwasser RH: An early comparative analysis of the use of fibular allograft versus autologous iliac crest graft for interbody fusion after anterior cervical discectomy. *Spine* 1993;18:1123-1124.

25. Shapiro S: Banked fibula and the locking anterior cervical plate in anterior cervical fusions following cervical discectomy. *J Neurosurg* 1996;84:161-165.

26. Whitecloud TS III: Complications of anterior cervical fusion. *Instr Course Lect* 1978;27:223-227.

27. Wang JC, McDonough PW, Endow K, Kanim LE, Delamarter RB: The effect of cervical plating on single-level anterior cervical discectomy and fusion. *J Spinal Disord* 1999;12:467-471.

28. Bishop RC, Moore KA, Hadley MN: Anterior cervical interbody fusion using autogeneic and allogeneic bone graft substrate: A prospective comparative analysis. *J Neurosurg* 1996;85:206-210.

29. An HS, Simpson JM, Glover JM, Stephany J: Comparison between allograft plus demineralized bone matrix versus autograft in anterior cervical fusion: A prospective multicenter study. *Spine* 1995;20:2211-2216.

30. Griffith SL, Zogbi SW, Guyer RD, Shelokov AP, Contiliano JH, Geiger JM: Biomechanical comparison of anterior instrumentation for the cervical spine. *J Spinal Disord* 1995;8:429-438.

31. Wang JC, McDonough PW, Kanim LE, Endow KK, Delamarter RB: Increased fusion rates with cervical plating for three-level anterior cervical discectomy and fusion. *Spine* 2001;26:643-647.

32. Emery SE, Fisher JR, Bohlman HH: Three-level anterior cervical discectomy and fusion: Radiographic and clinical results. *Spine* 1997;22:2622-2625.

33. Swank ML, Lowery GL, Bhat AL, McDonough RF: Anterior cervical allograft arthrodesis and instrumentation: Multilevel interbody grafting or strut graft reconstruction. *Eur Spine J* 1997;6:138-143.

34. Yoo JU, Zou D, Bayley JC, Yuan J, Edwards TE: Alterations in the loading characteristics of the tricortical cervical graft in the anterior cervical fusion. *Orthop Trans* 1992;16:792.

35. Fessler RG, Steck JC, Giovanini MA: Anterior cervical corpectomy for cervical spondylotic myelopathy. *Neurosurgery* 1998;43:257-267.

36. Nurick S: The natural history and the results of surgical treatment of the spinal cord disorder associated with cervical spondylosis. *Brain* 1972;95:101-108.

37. Bakay L, Cares HL, Smith RJ: Ossification in the region of the posterior longitudinal ligament as a cause of cervical myelopathy. *J Neurol Neurosurg Psychiatry* 1970;33:263-268.

38. Gui L, Merlini L, Savini R, Davidovits P: Cervical myelopathy due to ossification of the posterior longitudinal ligament. *Ital J Orthop Traumatol* 1983;9:269-280.

39. Nakanishi T, Mannen T, Toyokura Y: Asymptomatic ossification of the posterior longitudinal ligament of the cervical spine: Incidence and roentgenographic findings. *J Neurol Sci* 1973;19:375-381.

40. Matsunaga S, Sakou T, Taketomi E, Yamaguchi M, Okano T: The natural course of myelopathy caused by ossification of the posterior longitudinal ligament in the cervical spine. *Clin Orthop* 1994;305:168-177.

41. Matsuoka T, Yamaura I, Kurosa Y, Nakai O, Shindo S, Shinomiya K: Long-term results of the anterior floating method for cervical myelopathy caused by ossification of the posterior longitudinal ligament. *Spine* 2001;26:241-248.

42. Macdonald RL, Fehlings MG, Tator CH, et al: Multilevel anterior cervical corpectomy and fibular allograft fusion for cervical myelopathy. *J Neurosurg* 1997;86:990-997.

43. Eleraky MA, Llanos C, Sonntag VK: Cervical corpectomy: Report of 185 cases and review of the literature. *J Neurosurg* 1999;90(suppl 1):35-41.

44. Emery SE, Bohlman HH, Bolesta MJ, Jones PK: Anterior cervical decompression and arthrodesis for the treatment of cervical spondylotic myelopathy: Two to seventeen-year follow-up. *J Bone Joint Surg Am* 1998;80:941-951.

45. Ebraheim NA, DeTroye RJ, Rupp RE, Taha J, Brown J, Jackson WT: Osteosynthesis of the cervical spine with an anterior plate. *Orthopedics* 1995;18:141-147.

46. DiAngelo DJ, Foley KT, Vossel KA, Rampersaud YR, Jansen TH: Anterior cervical plating reverses load transfer through multilevel strut-grafts. *Spine* 2000;25:783-795.

47. Epstein NE: Reoperation rates for acute graft extrusion and pseudarthrosis after one-level anterior corpectomy and fusion with and without plate instrumentation: Etiology and corrective management. *Surg Neurol* 2001;56:73-81.

48. Curtin SL, Heller JG: Abstract: Multilevel anterior cervical reconstructions: Pseudoarthrosis and complication rates. *63rd Annual Meeting Proceedings.* Rosemont, IL, American Academy of Orthopaedic Surgeons, 1996, p 118.

49. Riew KD, Sethi NS, Devney J, Goette K, Choi K: Complications of buttress plate stabilization of cervical corpectomy. *Spine* 1999;24:2404-2410.

50. Vanichkachorn JS, Vaccaro AR, Silveri CP, Albert TJ: Anterior junctional plating in the cervical spine. *Spine* 1998;23:2462-2467.

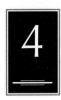

Complications of Anterior Cervical Spine Surgery

Chetan K. Patel, MD
Jeffrey S. Fischgrund, MD

Abstract
The anterior approach to the cervical spine is often used to treat many afflictions of the cervical spine. Although many complications can occur, the incidence of these complications is relatively low, especially when the physician has a thorough knowledge of spine anatomy and uses meticulous surgical technique.

The anterior approach to the cervical spine is one of the most common surgical approaches used in spine surgery. A relatively high rate of good results and a relatively low rate of complications can be expected from anterior cervical surgery. The complications can be considered chronologically as those occurring in the intraoperative, early postoperative, and late postoperative periods.

Intraoperative Complications
Neurologic Injury
An injury to the spinal cord or nerve roots is one of the most feared complications of any spine surgery. In a survey of 5,356 cases by the Cervical Spine Research Society, the incidence of neurologic complications was 1.04%, with a lower incidence of neurologic injury in anterior compared with posterior approaches.[1] The majority of the neurologic injuries anteriorly involved a nerve root, as opposed to the cord injuries noted with a posterior approach. The rate of spinal cord injury has been reported at a rate of 0.2% to 0.4%.[2-4] In more than 30,000 anterior cervical interbody fusions performed by over 700 neurosurgeons, 100 cases of significant myelopathy or myeloradiculopathy were noted. Seventy-five percent of these deficits were noted immediately postoperatively, while the others were noted in the early postoperative period.[2] Intraoperative mechanical compression with a Kerrison rongeur or other instruments, drill impaction, graft retropulsion, and vascular ischemia are some of the identifiable causes of cord and nerve injury. If a spinal cord injury is noted postoperatively, an immediate CT myelogram or MRI scan should be obtained. If a correctable radiographic finding is noted, urgent reexploration is recommended. Exploration may be considered to look for an epidural hematoma. In the absence of radiographic findings, re-exploration is unlikely to improve the neurologic status of the patient.[2] Steroids, according to the National Acute Spinal Cord Injury III spinal cord injury protocol, should be considered for cord injuries.[5] This protocol consists of a methylprednisolone bolus of 30 mg/kg followed by an infusion of 5.4 mg/kg for 23 hours if diagnosis of the injury is made within 3 hours and for 48 hours if the injury is identified within 8 hours. Intraoperative monitoring can be useful in reducing neurologic injury. Somatosensory-evoked potentials and motor-evoked potentials can help monitor the cord function, while spontaneous electromyography can be used to monitor individual nerve function. Injury to the recurrent laryngeal nerve (RLN) is the most common nerve injury after anterior cervical approach.[2] Whether a left-sided approach to the anterior cervical spine results in a decreased incidence of RLN palsy is a topic of debate that will be discussed further with the early postoperative complications.

Sympathetic Chain Injury
The cervical sympathetic chain is located on the anterolateral surface of the longus

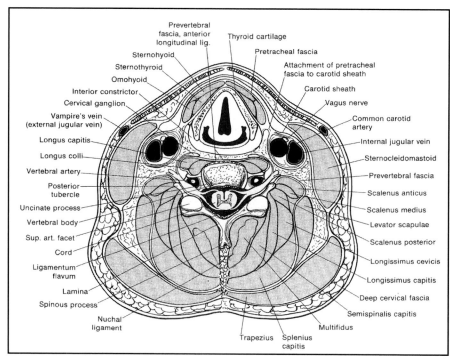

Fig. 1 Cross section of the neck at the level of C5 showing relevant anatomy. (Reproduced with permission from Hoppenfeld S, deBoer P (ed): *Surgical Exposures in Orthopaedics: The Anatomic Approach*. Philadelphia, PA, JB Lippincott, 1994, p 259.)

colli muscles, putting it at risk during retraction of the deepest layer of dissection (Fig. 1). Improper placement of retractors or vigorous retraction of longus colli muscles can lead to a Horner's syndrome from injury to the sympathetic chain. Classic postoperative symptoms from this injury are ptosis, meiosis, and anhydrosis.

Vascular Injury

Injury to the carotid or vertebral artery is rare. Trauma to the carotid artery can be minimized by the use of blunt retractors and constant vigilance while using sharp instruments. Intraoperative bradycardia may result from a vasovagal response caused by vigorous retraction of the carotid sheath. The vertebral artery is injured most often during corpectomy when the decompression extends lateral to the uncovertebral joints. Because the artery travels through the bony foramen, control of bleeding can be difficult.

Thrombin-soaked Gelfoam, along with manual pressure, can be used as a tamponade. If needed, direct exposure and control of the artery proximal and distal to the injury should be pursued.[6] A cerebrovascular accident can result from ligating the vertebral artery. Anatomic variations of the vertebral artery can be appreciated on the preoperative CT and may help avoid injuries and assist in exposure for the repair.[7] Careful identification of the midline and the uncovertebral joints can help prevent the surgeon from drifting too laterally during decompression and hardware placement. Plates that are not positioned straight can lead to placement of lateral screws that increase the risk of injury to the vertebral artery.

Esophageal Perforation

Although a direct injury to the esophagus is rare, it is important that the injury is recognized intraoperatively because this injury can be life threatening. An inci-

dence of 0.2% to 0.9% has been reported with one third of the injuries occurring intraoperatively in the largest study.[8-10] Intraoperative injuries were caused by sharp retractors and motorized instruments. A rough anterior spine construct from bone, cement, or prominent hardware was implicated as the cause of esophageal perforation recognized in the late postoperative period. Dysphagia, wound discharge, fever, leukocytosis, or complaint of neck fullness should raise suspicion for this injury. Plain radiographs, esophogram possibly augmented with a CT scan, endoscopic visualization, and direct exploration can assist in the diagnosis. Consequences of this injury include dysphagia, malnutrition, wound dehiscence, osteomyelitis, mediastinitis, sepsis, and death. Irrigation and débridement, direct repair of the defect, wound drainage, parenteral nutrition, and triple intravenous antibiotics are the essential elements of treatment. Few cases of late perforation have been treated successfully without surgical intervention; however, this is not the mainstay of treatment.[8]

Dural Tear

When a cerebrospinal fluid leak is noted, the site of the dural tear should be identified, and a direct repair of the dura should be performed when possible. Otherwise, fibrin glue and a subarachnoid drain may be used to close the tear. Ossification of the posterior longitudinal ligament can extend into and through the dura, a finding that can often be seen on preoperative CT scan.[11,12] When the dura is absent, a repair is difficult but can be facilitated by fascia lata and other dural substitutes.

Other Considerations

Injury to the superior thyroid artery, inferior thyroid artery, superior laryngeal nerve, and the thoracic duct in the left lower cervical approaches can occur; therefore, a thorough knowledge of the anatomy is required for prevention and management. Finally, wrong-level surgery is a complication that can easily be avoided. There is no substitute for a good quality marker radiograph to correctly identify the surgical level. Ensuring neutral rotation of the head at the time of the radiograph and the use of multiple markers can be helpful in achieving this goal.

Early Postoperative Complications

Recurrent Laryngeal Nerve Injury

Along with sore throat and difficulty swallowing, RLN injury is one of the most common complications to occur after anterior cervical surgery.[2] Damage to the RLN can produce hoarseness and vocal fold paralysis. The rate of injury has been reported in the range of 1% to 11%.[13-23] The anatomy of the RLN is different on the left and right side of the body. The right nerve recurs around the subclavian artery, while the left loops around the aorta. The right RLN is therefore shorter and has a more oblique course than its left counterpart, and this has been implicated as an important factor in its injury.[24] The inferior thyroid artery on the right enters the lower pole of the thyroid where the RLN enters the tracheoesophageal groove and can serve as a useful landmark in identification and protection of the RLN.[25] Retractor placement during a right-sided approach is more likely to stretch the shorter oblique nerve, which can decrease the perineural blood flow and cause injury.[26] This concept has led to strong surgeon preferences in terms of the laterality of the approach. However, in the few studies that have noted the laterality of the approach, the data do not support any statistical correlation between the side of the approach and the risk of RLN injury.[13,18,20,21] In most cases of RLN injury, spontaneous recovery can be expected as early as 6 weeks but may take as long as 6 months. If the symptoms do not resolve, an otolaryngologic consultation should be obtained to consider laryngoscopy and possible injection of the vocal folds. With a revision anterior cervical spine surgery, a higher rate of RLN injury has been reported.[13,27] Subclinical vocal fold paralysis can occur with the first operation that may be difficult to recognize with history alone. A preoperative inquiry should assess for any vocal problems, and consideration should be given to a preoperative laryngoscopic examination. This workup is vital if the repeat anterior approach will be performed contralateral to the original approach because fatal bilateral vocal fold paralysis can occur in this scenario.[28] It is important to remember that surgeries performed for reasons other than spinal pathology can also cause an RLN injury. Patients with previous thyroidectomy, carotid endarterectomy, thoracic aortic aneurysm repair, patent ductus arteriosus ligation, or a history of prolonged intubation can have RLN dysfunction.[29] Endotracheal (ET) tube cuff pressure is another important factor in RLN and pharyngeal injury. The duration of intubation, the size of the ET tube, the area of ET tube contact with the trachea, and the increased cuff pressure with retraction have all been shown to correlate with postoperative hoarseness and throat pain.[30-33] Thus, adjusting the ET tube cuff pressure with retraction, less vigorous retraction, decreased time of retraction, and minimizing surgical time would all be expected to decrease postoperative hoarseness and sore throat.

Dysphagia

Dysphagia can occur as a result of edema from retraction, hematoma, injury to the pharyngeal plexus, or rarely from an injury to the hypoglossal nerve during approach to the upper cervical spine.[34-37] Most cases are transient but can take up to 8 months to resolve.[38] Dysphagia persisting more than 1 to 2 months may require an otolaryngologic consultation in addition to a barium swallow and possible laryngoscopy.[39]

Respiratory Distress

Acute respiratory distress in the early postoperative period can be caused by a hematoma. Meticulous hemostasis and use of a drain postoperatively may help reduce the risk of this dire complication. Once discovered, the hematoma must be released urgently to avoid respiratory arrest.[25] Other causes of respiratory distress in the acute postoperative period such as edema, laryngospasm, vocal fold paralysis, congestive heart failure, pulmonary edema, and allergic reaction should not be overlooked. Long surgical time, preexisting pulmonary disease, and history of smoking are the main risk factors for reintubation in the postoperative period.[40] Patients with long intubation and retraction times thus should be considered for mechanical ventilation for 1 to 3 days postoperatively to allow edema to subside and to avoid urgent reintubation.[40]

Infection

As with any other surgical procedures, the risk of infection is higher for patients with diabetes mellitus, immunosuppression, chronic malnutrition, and obesity. The incidence of infection after anterior cervical spine surgery is relatively low and is lower than that associated with posterior cervical spine procedures. Prophylactic antibiotics given perioperatively for 24 hours can help reduce the risk of infection. Superficial infections such as cellulitis can be treated with a 10- to 14-day course of oral antibiotics, but these infections are difficult to distinguish from deep infections. Thus, close monitoring and a high index of suspicion must be used while treating cellulitis. Once a deep infection is diagnosed, irrigation and débridement should be followed by a course of parenteral antibiotics. Hardware should be left in place until solid fusion has occurred.[41] A successful fusion can be achieved even in the face of a deep infection. In cases of osteomyelitis, a fusion rate as high as 96% has been obtained with autogenous bone graft.[42]

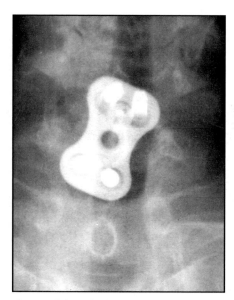

Fig. 2 Malaligned plate after anterior cervical diskectomy and fusion.

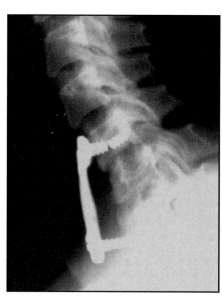

Fig. 3 Example of pseudarthrosis and hardware failure after a two-level anterior cervical diskectomy and fusion with local kyphosis.

Hardware Failure

In the early postoperative period, the incidence of hardware failure increases as the number of levels fused increases. Proper techniques for placement of graft and hardware can help decrease this complication.[43] Disk spaces must be avoided during placement of screws into bone. Careful attention should be paid to avoiding lateral placement of hardware that may injure the vertebral arteries (Fig. 2). Asymptomatic hardware loosening can be monitored closely without surgical intervention.

Late Postoperative Complications
Pseudarthrosis

As in other areas of spine and fracture healing, bone healing and clinical results are retarded with smoking.[44] Improper surgical technique can lead to early graft extrusion and failure with a higher rate of pseudarthrosis, especially in multilevel procedures[43] (Fig. 3). Looking beyond the early failures, the rate of nonunion increases with the number of levels that are fused.[21,45-48] Without instrumentation, nonunion rates are higher for allograft as compared with autograft for multilevel diskectomies and fusions.[48] Fusion rate for a single-level and multilevel diskectomies appears to be higher with the addition of a plate, although data from randomized prospective placebo-controlled trials are lacking.[49-51] It should be kept in mind, however, that a patient may be asymptomatic despite pseudarthrosis and may not require intervention.[45] When repair of pseudarthrosis is being considered for axial symptoms, considerable controversy exits with regard to the anterior versus posterior approach. Several studies have reported good results with a posterior fusion.[52-54] When radicular symptoms are present, posterior decompression accompanying posterior spinal fusion can provide good relief of radicular symptoms in addition to treating the axial symptoms.[53] Revision anterior surgery can be considered for patients with pseudarthrosis with or without radicular symptoms, myelopathy, or kyphosis. Although some studies have reported inferior results with the anterior approach, others have reported good success in treating both the radicular and axial symptoms.[52,54-56] No prospective randomized studies of note are available to help resolve this controversy.

Summary

The anterior approach to the cervical spine is the most frequently used approach for treatment of pathology of the cervical spine. The potential complications of this approach include neurologic and vascular injury, esophageal perforation, dysphagia, dysphonia, respiratory distress, infection, pseudarthrosis, and hardware failure. Fortunately, the incidence of the more serious complications is low, while the procedures result in a high rate of success. Meticulous preoperative planning and the use of the proper intraoperative techniques are the keys to minimizing complications.

References

1. Graham JJ: Complications of cervical spine surgery: A five-year report on a survey of the membership of the Cervical Spine Research Society by the Morbidity and Mortality Committee. *Spine* 1989;14:1046-1050.

2. Flynn TB: Neurologic complications of anterior cervical interbody fusion. *Spine* 1982;7:536-539.

3. Lunsford LD, Bissonette DJ, Zorub DS: Anterior surgery for cervical disc disease: Part 2. Treatment of cervical spondylotic myelopathy in 32 cases. *J Neurosurg* 1980;53:12-19.

4. Sugar O: Spinal cord malfunction after anterior cervical discectomy. *Surg Neurol* 1981;15:4-8.

5. Bracken MB, Shepard MJ, Holford TR, et al: Administration of methylprednisolone for 24 or 48 hours or tirilazad mesylate for 48 hours in the treatment of acute spinal cord injury: Results of the Third National Acute Spinal Cord Injury Randomized Controlled Trial: National Acute Spinal Cord Injury Study. *JAMA* 1997;277:1597-1604.

6. Smith MD, Emery SE, Dudley A, Murray KJ, Leventhal M: Vertebral artery injury during anterior decompression of the cervical spine: A retrospective review of ten patients. *J Bone Joint Surg Br* 1993;75:410-415.

7. Heary RF, Albert TJ, Ludwig SC, et al: Surgical anatomy of the vertebral arteries. *Spine* 1996;21:2074-2080.

8. Newhouse KE, Lindsey RW, Clark CR, Lieponis J, Murphy MJ: Esophageal perforation following anterior cervical spine surgery. *Spine* 1989;14:1051-1053.

9. Capen DA, Garland DE, Waters RL: Surgical stabilization of the cervical spine: A comparative analysis of posterior spine fusions. *Clin Orthop* 1985;196:229-237.

10. Tew JM Jr, Mayfield FH: Complications of surgery of the anterior cervical spine. *Clin Neurosurg* 1976;23:424-434.

11. Epstein NE: Identification of ossification of the posterior longitudinal ligament extending through the dura on preoperative computed tomographic examinations of the cervical spine. *Spine* 2001;26:182-186.

12. Hida K, Iwasaki Y, Koyanagi I, Abe H: Bone window computed tomography for detection of dural defect associated with cervical ossified posterior longitudinal ligament. *Neurol Med Chir (Tokyo)* 1997;37:173-175.

13. Beutler WJ, Sweeney CA, Connolly PJ: Recurrent laryngeal nerve injury with anterior cervical spine surgery risk with laterality of surgical approach. *Spine* 2001;26:1337-1342.

14. Bulger RF, Rejowski JE, Beatty RA: Vocal cord paralysis associated with anterior cervical fusion: Considerations for prevention and treatment. *J Neurosurg* 1985;62:657-661.

15. Cloward RB: New method of diagnosis and treatment of cervical disc disease. *Clin Neurosurg* 1962;8:93-132.

16. Dohn DF: Anterior interbody fusion for treatment of cervical-disk conditions. *JAMA* 1966;197:897-900.

17. Grisoli F, Graziani N, Fabrizi AP, Peragut JC, Vincentelli F, Diaz-Vasquez P: Anterior discectomy without fusion for treatment of cervical lateral soft disc extrusion: A follow-up of 120 cases. *Neurosurgery* 1989;24:853-859.

18. Heeneman H: Vocal cord paralysis following approaches to the anterior cervical spine. *Laryngoscope* 1973;83:17-21.

19. Lunsford LD, Bissonette DJ, Jannetta PJ, Sheptak PE, Zorub DS: Anterior surgery for cervical disc disease: Part I. Treatment of lateral cervical disc herniation in 253 cases. *J Neurosurg* 1980;53:1-11.

20. Morpeth JF, Williams MF: Vocal fold paralysis after anterior cervical diskectomy and fusion. *Laryngoscope* 2000;110:43-46.

21. Robinson RA, Walker AE, Ferlic DC, Wiecking DK: The results of anterior interbody fusion of the cervical spine. *J Bone Joint Surg Am* 1962;44:1569-1587.

22. Watters WC III, Levinthal R: Anterior cervical discectomy with and without fusion: Results, complications, and long-term follow-up. *Spine* 1994;19:2343-2347.

23. Yamamoto I, Ikeda A, Shibuya N, Tsugane R, Sato O: Clinical long-term results of anterior discectomy without anterior interbody fusion for cervical disc disease. *Spine* 1991;16:272-279.

24. Netterville JL, Koriwchak MJ, Winkle M, Courey MS, Ossoff RH: Vocal fold paralysis following the anterior approach to the cervical spine. *Ann Otol Rhinol Laryngol* 1996;105:85-91.

25. Guyer RD, Delamarter RB, Fulp T, Small SD: Complications of cervical spine surgery, in Herkowitz HN, Eismont FJ, Garfin SR, Bell GR, Balderston RA, Wiesel SW (eds): *Rothman-Simeone, The Spine*, ed 4. Philadelphia, PA, W B Saunders, 1999, pp 541-552.

26. Weisberg NK, Spengler DM, Netterville JL: Stretch-induced nerve injury as a cause of paralysis secondary to the anterior cervical approach. *Otolaryngol Head Neck Surg* 1997;116:317-326.

27. Coric D, Branch CL Jr, Jenkins JD: Revision of anterior cervical pseudoarthrosis with anterior allograft fusion and plating. *J Neurosurg* 1997;86:969-974.

28. Winslow CP, Meyers AD: Otolaryngologic complications of anterior approach to the cervical spine. *Am J Otolaryngol* 1999;20:16-27.

29. Manski TJ, Wood MD, Dunsker SB: Bilateral vocal cord paralysis following anterior cervical discectomy and fusion: Case report. *J Neurosurg* 1998;89:839-843.

30. Jellish WS, Jensen RL, Anderson DE, Shea JF: Intraoperative electromyographic assessment of recurrent laryngeal nerve stress and pharyngeal injury during anterior cervical spine surgery with Caspar instrumentation. *J Neurosurg* 1999;91(suppl 2):170-174.

31. Loeser EA, Machin R, Colley J, Orr DL II, Bennett GM, Stanley TH: Postoperative sore throat: Importance of endotracheal tube conformity versus cuff design. *Anesthesiology* 1978;49:430-432.

32. Sperry RJ, Johnson JO, Apfelbaum RI: Endotracheal tube cuff pressure increases significantly during anterior cervical fusion with the Caspar instrumentation system. *Anesth Analg* 1993;76:1318-1321.

33. Stout DM, Bishop MJ, Dwersteg JF, Cullen BF: Correlation of endotracheal tube size with sore throat and hoarseness following general anesthesia. *Anesthesiology* 1987;67:419-421.

34. Saunders RL, Bernini PM, Shirreffs TG, Reeves AG: Central corpectomy for cervical spondylotic myelopathy: A consecutive series with long-term follow-up evaluation. *J Neurosurg* 1991;74:163-170.

35. Sengupta DK, Grevitt MP, Mehdian SM: Hypoglossal nerve injury as a complication of anterior surgery to the upper cervical spine. *Eur Spine J* 1999;8:78-80.

36. Watkins RG: Cervical, thoracic, and lumbar complications: Anterior approach, in Garfin SR (ed): *Complications of Spine Surgery*. Baltimore, MD, Williams & Wilkins, 1989, pp 211-247.

37. Welsh LW, Welsh JJ, Chinnici JC: Dysphagia due to cervical spine surgery. *Ann Otol Rhinol Laryngol* 1987;96:112-115.

38. Clements DH, O'Leary PF: Anterior cervical discectomy and fusion. *Spine* 1990;15:1023-1025.

39. Winslow CP, Meyers AD: Otolaryngologic complications of the anterior approach to the cervical spine. *Am J Otolaryngol* 1999; 20:16-27.

40. Emery SE, Smith MD, Bohlman HH: Upper-airway obstruction after multilevel cervical corpectomy for myelopathy. *J Bone Joint Surg Am* 1991;73:544-551.

41. Gepstein R, Eismont FJ: Postoperative spine infections, in Garfin SR (ed): *Complications of Spine Surgery*. Baltimore, MD, Williams & Wilkins, 1989, pp 302-322.

42. McGuire RA, Eismont FJ: The fate of autogenous bone graft in surgically treated pyogenic vertebral osteomyelitis. *J Spinal Disord* 1994;7:206-215.

43. Vaccaro AR, Falatyn SP, Scuderi GJ, et al: Early failure of long segment anterior cervical plate fixation. *J Spinal Disord* 1998;11:410-415.

44. Hilibrand AS, Fye MA, Emery SE, Palumbo MA, Bohlman HH: Impact of smoking on the outcome of anterior cervical arthrodesis with interbody or strut-grafting. *J Bone Joint Surg Am* 2001;83:668-673.

45. Bohlman HH, Emery SE, Goodfellow DB, Jones PK: Robinson anterior cervical discectomy and arthrodesis for cervical radiculopathy: Long-term follow-up of one hundred and twenty-two patients. *J Bone Joint Surg Am* 1993;75:1298-1307.

46. Emery SE, Fisher JR, Bohlman HH: Three-level anterior cervical discectomy and fusion: Radiographic and clinical results. *Spine* 1999;22:2622-2624.

47. Emery SE, Bohlman HH, Bolesta MJ, Jones PK: Anterior cervical decompression and arthrodesis for the treatment of cervical spondylotic myelopathy: Two to seventeen-year follow-up. *J Bone Joint Surg Am* 1998;80:941-951.

48. Zdeblick TA, Ducker TB: The use of freeze-dried allograft bone for anterior cervical fusions. *Spine* 1991;16:726-729.

49. Geer CP, Papadopoulos SM: The argument for single-level anterior cervical discectomy and fusion with anterior plate fixation. *Clin Neurosurg* 1999;45:25-29.

50. Bose B: Anterior cervical instrumentation enhances fusion rates in multilevel reconstruction in smokers. *J Spinal Disord* 2001;14:3-9.

51. Wang JC, McDonough PW, Kanim LE, Endow KK, Delamarter RB: Increased fusion rates with cervical plating for three-level anterior cervical discectomy and fusion. *Spine* 2001;26:643-646.

52. Brodsky AE, Khalil MA, Sassard WR, Newman BP: Repair of symptomatic pseudoarthrosis of anterior cervical fusion: Posterior versus anterior repair. *Spine* 1992;17:1137-1143.

53. Farey ID, McAfee P, Davis RF, Long DM: Pseudoarthrosis of the cervical spine after anterior arthrodesis: Treatment by posterior nerve-root decompression, stabilization, and arthrodesis. *J Bone Joint Surg Am* 1990;72:1171-1177.

54. Lowery GL, Swank ML, McDonough RF: Surgical revision for failed anterior fusions: Articular pillar plating or anterior revision? *Spine* 1995;20:2436-2441.

55. Phillips FM, Carlson G, Emery SE, Bohlman HH: Anterior cervical pseudoarthrosis: Natural history and treatment. *Spine* 1997;22:1585-1589.

56. Zdeblick TA, Hughes SS, Riew KD, Bohlman HH: Failed anterior cervical discectomy and arthrodesis: Analysis and treatment of thirty-five patients. *J Bone Joint Surg Am* 1997;79:523-532.

Posterior Decompressive Procedures for the Cervical Spine

Howard S. An, MD
Nicholas U. Ahn, MD

Abstract

Cervical degenerative disease encompasses a complex array of pathologies. Before considering surgical intervention, the surgeon should have a complete understanding of the indications for surgery and should have conducted a thorough physical examination and evaluation of radiologic studies. In general, unless myelopathy is present, surgery should be the treatment of last resort, used only after conservative measures have failed.

The indications for posterior cervical decompression include both radiculopathy and myelopathy. However, these conditions alone are not sufficient to indicate that a posterior procedure is appropriate. Other factors, such as bilaterality of symptoms, presence or absence of cervical lordosis, number of levels involved, and presence of axial neck pain, should also be considered when deciding whether an anterior procedure or posterior decompression is more appropriate.

The posterior approaches to the lower cervical spine (C3 through C7) are generally reserved for degenerative disorders for which decompression of the thecal sac or nerve roots is warranted. The neurologic compromise can reflect diverse pathologies, including osteophytes at the facet or the uncovertebral joint, a herniated nucleus pulposus, and/or canal stenosis. Different approaches have been developed to address these different types of pathology. In addition, the posterior approach to the cervical spine is used for instrumentation and fusion in cases of instability, which may be traumatic, pathologic, or, in rare cases, degenerative.

Posterior decompression may be indicated for the patient with cervical radiculopathy or myelopathy. The indica-tions for surgical intervention in cervical radiculopathy include: (1) an unaccept-able or progressive neurologic deficit and (2) failure of a 3-month trial of conserva-tive therapy to relieve radicular arm pain with or without a neurologic deficit. The indications for surgical intervention in cervical myelopathy include (1) progres-sive myelopathy or neurologic deficit; (2) moderate to severe myelopathy that is stable and which has not improved over a 6-week to 3-month period; and (3) myelopathic symptoms that interfere with activities of daily living. With both myelopathy and radiculopathy, it is criti-cal that the surgeon correlate the patient's clinical symptoms with neuroradiogra-phic findings when choosing a surgical procedure. In addition, the patient must understand the goal of surgery, whether it be the prevention of further neurologic deterioration or the relief of pain, so that the surgeon is assured that the patient regards the planned surgical intervention as warranted.

The patient who presents with neck pain, cervical radiculopathy, or mild cer-vical myelopathy should first be evaluat-ed with a thorough physical examination, including a neurologic examination of the upper and lower limbs. Motor and sensory function as well as reflexes must be tested and documented. Plain radio-graphs may be obtained at the time of ini-tial presentation. Unless a dramatic abnormality is found, such as tumor, fracture, or dislocation, more advanced imaging studies such as CT or MRI are generally reserved until the patient has been symptomatic for at least 6 weeks.[1,2]

Severe spinal instability, which may damage the cord, or an unacceptable or progressive neurologic deficit, such as in cases of moderate to severe cervical myelopathy, are generally treated more aggressively. In these cases, surgical inter-vention should not be delayed because the neurologic deficit is less likely to resolve.[2,3]

This chapter addresses the surgical approaches to the cervical spine, but it must be emphasized that, except for few cases in which significant neurologic com-

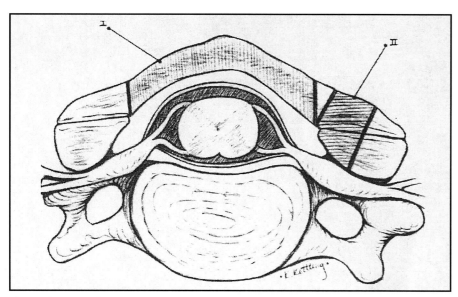

Fig. 1 Schematic of posterior cervical foraminotomy and laminectomy. Bone that is excised in a laminectomy is denoted by the numeral I. Bone that is excised in a foraminotomy is denoted by the numeral II. (Reproduced with permission from An HS, Riley LR III (eds): *An Atlas of Surgery of the Spine*. London, England, Martin Dunitz, and Philadelphia, PA, Lippincott-Raven, 1998, pp 13-54.)

promise is present, surgery should be considered the treatment of last resort. The vast majority of patients seen in clinical practice should be treated nonsurgically.

Posterior Approach to the Lower Cervical Spine

In the posterior approach to the cervical spine, correct positioning of the patient before an incision is made is critical. The head must be stabilized in the prone position. This can be accomplished easily with the Mayfield skull tongs, which have the added benefit of leaving the face free of external sources of pressure. Incorrect positioning of the patient may result in pressure ulcers, difficult exposure, and increased risk of neurologic injury. The internervous plane that lies in the midline of the posterior aspect of the neck is used; the approach involves dissecting between the layers of paraspinal muscles that are innervated by the right and left posterior rami of the cervical nerves. Once the deep fascia separating this muscular interval is split, the liga-

mentum nuchae is identified and incised in the midline. Subperiosteal dissection is carried down on both sides of the spinous processes to both laminae. In the cervical spine, the laminae of adjacent vertebrae do not overlap one another as much as they do in the thoracic spine. This leaves gaps between the laminae of adjacent levels, and great care must therefore be taken not to accidentally penetrate the interlaminar space and damage or puncture the dura or cord. The exposure is performed out to the lateral masses. If fusion is not being performed, care must be taken not to damage the facet joint capsules to prevent deterioration of the intervertebral motion segment. If fusion is anticipated, then the surgeon may dissect out and remove the facet capsules because no motion will be expected at the iatrogenically destroyed facet joints.

Posterior Foraminotomy

Posterior foraminotomy, also known as posterolateral or keyhole foraminotomy, is a simple procedure that is indicated in

cases of radiculopathy from nerve root compression from a herniated disk or osteophyte. Thus, the ideal candidate is the patient with radicular arm pain with little or no axial neck pain and no loss of cervical lordosis. Foraminotomy should also be strongly considered in cases of multilevel unilateral radiculopathy, especially if three or more levels are involved, because multilevel anterior procedures have higher failure rates. Other strong indications for foraminotomy, because anterior exposure in these instances is very difficult, are previous anterior surgery; a short, wide neck; and stenosis at the C7-T1 level.

Patients with significant axial neck pain in addition to radiculopathy have a less predictable response to isolated posterior foraminotomy; in these patients, an anterior diskectomy and fusion combined with anterior foraminotomy is the procedure of choice. If three or more levels are involved, then posterior foraminotomies with posterior fusion should be considered, as multilevel anterior procedures have a higher failure rate. Patients with loss of cervical lordosis are also poor candidates for posterior foraminotomy, as the posterior decompression may lead to increased instability and kyphotic deformity. In these patients, too, an anterior procedure or a posterior procedure with fusion should be considered.

As mentioned previously, radiographic and clinical findings must always be correlated before surgery is planned. If the correct indications are met, posterior foraminotomy has a high chance of success.

Surgical Technique

Because of the potential to damage neural structures during foraminotomy, careful preparation is necessary (Fig. 1). Visual magnification with either a 3.5× loupe or an operating microscope and lighting, with or without the use of a headlight, are critical for adequate visualization. These factors should be worked out well before the start of surgery.

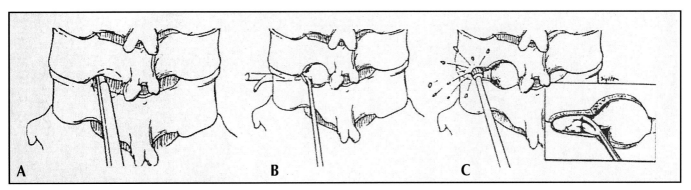

Fig. 2 Posterior cervical foraminotomy. **A,** A Kerrison rongeur is used to perform a laminotomy. **B,** A burr is used to perform medial facetectomy or foraminotomy, and a nerve hook is passed through the foramen to check for adequacy of decompression. **C,** A foraminotomy should be extended laterally until the nerve root is decompressed. (Reproduced with permission from An HS, Riley LR III (eds): *An Atlas of Surgery of the Spine.* London, England, Martin Dunitz, and Philadelphia, PA, Lippincott-Raven, 1998, pp 13-54.)

The steps involved in a posterior foraminotomy are shown in Figure 2. A Kerrison rongeur is initially used to remove a portion of the superior and inferior laminae. The foramen is entered by thinning the medial edge of the facets with a power burr. To avoid damaging the exiting nerve root at the level of the foramen, great care must be taken using the burr. Holding the instrument with both hands and resting the wrists or forearms on the patient will provide proprioceptive feedback to the surgeon and prevent inadvertent and potentially dangerous motions. The lamina and thinned facet are then gently lifted off the nerve root and dura using a small angled curet. The Kerrison rongeur should not be used to remove the facet because sliding this thicker instrument under the lamina may result in injury to the nerve root and cord. With the bone removed, the dura and nerve root are exposed, and bipolar cautery may be necessary to stop bleeding from the extensive venous plexus within the cervical canal. Maintaining meticulous hemostasis is of utmost importance because bleeding can lead to epidural hematoma formation and root or cord damage from poor visualization.

The nerve root is assessed after removal of the overlying facet to ensure that it is mobile and has been completely decompressed. The path of the root is visualized all the way out the foramen. A Woodson dental instrument or ball-tipped probe is passed through the foramen to ensure that adequate space is available in the foramen to allow the nerve root to freely pass through.

Removal of the disk is not routinely necessary to adequately decompress the nerve root. However, if diskectomy is deemed necessary, the nerve root is gently retracted in a cephalad direction with a Penfield periosteal elevator or nerve root retractor to allow the disk tissue to be removed. Great care must be taken not to retract the root too far because this may cause neurologic injury.

Results

Although earlier reports demonstrated inferior results with posterior foraminotomy as opposed to anterior cervical diskectomy and fusion (ACDF) for isolated cervical radiculopathy, more recent studies have shown otherwise. The inferior results may have been a result of incomplete understanding of adequate decompression when this procedure was still relatively new.[4]

It is currently accepted that excellent results can be expected following foraminotomy provided that the procedure is done for appropriate indications,

as outlined earlier. In a review of 60 patients without evidence of instability, Silveri and associates[5] reported that 98% of patients at mean 6-year follow-up had good to excellent results, with relief of preoperative pain symptoms in all patients. Likewise, in a large series of 846 consecutive cases of foraminotomy for cervical radiculopathy, Henderson and associates[6] demonstrated relief of arm pain in 96% of patients and relief of preoperative motor weakness in 98% of patients. These studies demonstrate that this simpler surgical technique may consistently yield good results without the need for the more dangerous and extensive anterior dissection and bone graft harvest necessary in ACDF.

Laminectomy

The primary indication for cervical laminectomy is in patients with spinal canal stenosis who have multilevel (three or more involved levels) spondylotic myelopathy with or without radiculopathy. If fewer than three levels are involved, anterior corpectomy and strut fusion is recommended. Patients must have preserved cervical lordosis if laminectomy alone is to be performed, or postlaminectomy kyphosis may result. Laminectomy can also be performed in patients with a flexible loss of lordosis, but the procedure

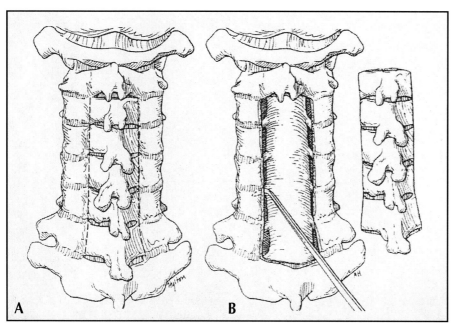

Fig. 3 Cervical laminectomy. **A,** The junction between lamina and lateral mass is burred down to perform a laminectomy. **B,** Following a laminectomy, the foramen is checked to ensure that there is space for the nerve roots. (Reproduced with permission from An HS, Riley LR III (eds): *An Atlas of Surgery of the Spine.* London, England, Martin Dunitz, and Philadelphia, PA, Lippincott-Raven, 1998, pp 13-54.)

must then be combined with lateral mass fusion to prevent postlaminectomy kyphotic deformity. Laminectomy increases the space available for the cord by excision of the impinging ligamentum flavum and bony structures. The cervical lordosis should be maintained, as this will also aid in indirectly decompressing the cord by allowing the cord to translate posteriorly. Thus, if there is any evidence of instability, laminectomy should be combined with lateral mass fusion to prevent kyphotic deformity.

Laminectomy and fusion should also be considered in cases of myelopathy with multilevel stenosis and significant neck pain. Anterior procedures should be avoided in these cases because of higher failure rates with anterior cervical fusions involving three or more levels.

Surgical Technique

Figure 3 shows the steps followed in performing a cervical laminectomy. After appropriate initial exposure, the cortices at the junction of the laminae and the lateral masses are thinned bilaterally with a power burr. A small Kerrison rongeur is then used to complete the cut, and a small angled curet is used to elevate the laminae. Somatosensory-evoked potentials should be monitored in most cases to ensure that no damage is done to the nerve roots. The adherent underlying venous plexus is cauterized to prevent formation of an epidural hematoma. If radicular symptoms are present, foraminotomies can be added to the procedure.

If fusion is necessary, the facet capsules are dissected and destroyed with the Bovey electrocautery device and then decorticated with power burr, curet, or small rongeur. The most stable means of internal fixation is accomplished by using lateral mass screws and plates (Fig. 4). Although different techniques have been used, the safest technique for screw placement from C3 through C6 has been described by An and Xu.[7] These authors described starting 1 mm medial to the center of the lateral mass and angulating the screw 15° cephalad and 25° to 30° lateral. Placement of screws in this direction allows for maximum clearance of the nerve root and facet joints.

Results

With laminectomy for spondylotic myelopathy, reported success rates have ranged from 68% to 85%. Herkowitz[8] compared ACDF with laminectomy for the treatment of multilevel spondylotic radiculopathy and found 66% good to excellent results with laminectomy versus 92% with ACDF. However, significant rates of postlaminectomy kyphosis (25%) and anterior subluxation (40%) compromised the results. These complications were most likely caused by a loss of adequate posterior structural support.

Guigui and associates,[9] in a retrospective review of 58 patients, demonstrated that destabilization following cervical laminectomy occurred only in patients with hypermobility on preoperative dynamic radiographs; preoperative listhesis witout hypermobility was not a risk factor. They therefore stressed the importance of preoperative flexion/extension radiographs in determining whether fusion is necessary when performing cervical laminectomy.

Zdeblick and associates[10] demonstrated in a biomechanical study of 12 human cadaver cervical spines that instability is more likely to develop following complete unilateral facetectomy or following bilateral partial facetectomy in which less than 50% of total facet remains. In addition, particularly high rates of postlaminectomy kyphosis and subluxation[11] have been reported in pediatric patients. Thus, in these cases the surgeon should strongly consider fusion at the time of decompression because this may improve overall outcome.

Laminaplasty

Laminaplasty is indicated in the treatment of multilevel (three or more levels) spondylotic myelopathy, myeloradiculopathy, or multilevel radiculopathy in patients with minimal axial neck pain. If fewer than three levels are involved, anterior corpectomy and strut fusion is recommended. An alternative procedure in patients with myelopathic disease at three or more levels would be laminectomy and foraminotomy with posterior lateral mass fusion to prevent destabilization. Laminaplasty achieves similar results while obviating the need for cervical fusion, thereby preventing loss of motion and risk of future development of transition syndrome.

While multilevel bilateral radiculopathy can also be treated with laminaplasty, many surgeons prefer anterior diskectomy and fusion in this situation. Another option would be to perform laminectomy, foraminotomy, and lateral mass fusion to prevent destabilization. Laminaplasty achieves decompression in these situations while again preserving motion.

Laminaplasty involves decompression of the central canal while preserving the posterior bony elements (Fig. 5). This is opposed to laminectomy, in which the posterior elements are removed and discarded. In laminaplasty, the lamina are detached at the lamina-facet junction on one side and hinged on the contralateral side to widen and decompress the canal. The rationale behind the development of laminaplasty was to prevent postlaminectomy kyphosis and instability that can result from laminectomy. Thus, laminaplasty is preferred in younger patients and in those with preoperative instability.

Laminaplasty should be avoided in the patient with significant neck pain in addition to multilevel stenosis. In these cases, laminectomy and foraminotomy combined with lateral mass fusion is the procedure of choice. As is true with all posterior cervical procedures, laminaplasty should not be performed if a preoperative kyphotic deformity is present. In these cases, an anterior procedure

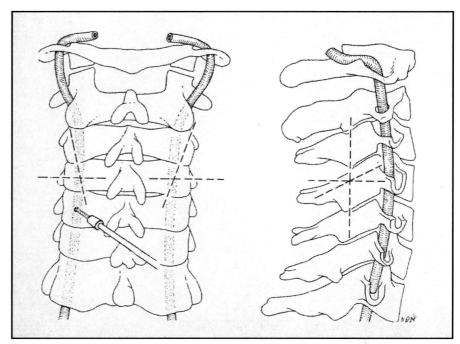

Fig. 4 Placement of lateral mass screws as described by An and Xu.[7] Starting 1 mm medial to the center of the lateral mass, the screw is angulated 15° cephalad and 25° to 30° lateral. Placement of screws in this direction allows for maximum clearance of the nerve root and facet joints. (Reproduced with permission from An HS, Riley LR III (eds): *An Atlas of Surgery of the Spine*. London, England, Martin Dunitz, and Philadelphia, PA, Lippincott-Raven, 1998, pp 13-54.)

is required to prevent angular instability and progression of kyphosis.

Surgical Technique
Several methods of laminaplasty have been described. They vary by the location of the hinge and the means of maintaining an open position; however, the fundamental concept of decompression with preservation of posterior elements is common to all the methods.

The "open door" laminaplasty is a simple and effective means of performing this procedure and is the method we prefer. The surgeon must first use clinical information to decide which side will be hinged and which side will be opened. The symptomatic side is generally chosen as the open side. Next, using a high-speed burr, the cortex is thinned at the junction of the lamina and lateral mass bilaterally to the inner cortex. The hinged side is thinned without completing the

cut such that the inner cortex is intact. The osteotomy is completed on the opening side. The lamina is then gently and gradually opened on the opening side by lifting the lamina on the opening side and closing the hinge on the opposite side. The thinned inner cortex of the hinged side is plastically deformed and the posterior elements are held open using a variety of different methods. We prefer to use bone graft at the open side to hold the posterior elements in position. The bone graft should be carefully shaped such that grooves are created and securely fit between the edge of the opened lamina and the edge of the lateral mass. Typically, three bone grafts are placed at C3, C5, and C7.

Results
Laminaplasty has been widely studied by Japanese researchers as a means of treating ossification of the posterior longitudinal

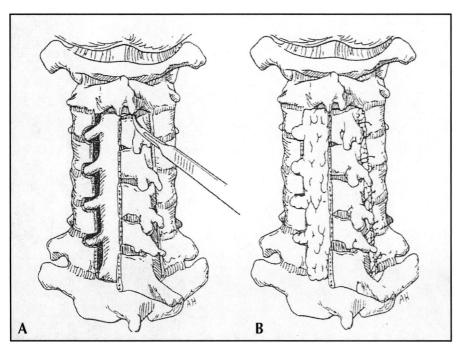

Fig. 5 Cervical laminaplasty. **A,** If necessary, a foraminotomy is performed on the opening side, before a laminaplasty. The interspinous ligament is divided at C2-3 and C7-T1, prior to lifting the lamina for laminaplasty. **B,** The opened lamina may be maintained by inserting bone grafts on the opening side or suturing the spinous processes to the facet capsules on the hinged side as shown. (Reproduced with permission from An HS, Riley LR III (eds): *An Atlas of Surgery of the Spine*, London, England, Martin Dunitz, and Philadelphia, PA, Lippincott-Raven, 1998, pp 13-54.)

ligament (OPLL) and multilevel cervical stenosis without destabilizing the cervical spine.[12-15] The results of this procedure have been relatively good. While there is still a risk of developing instability, it is significantly reduced in laminaplasty as compared with laminectomy. In a comparison between laminaplasty and laminectomy for the treatment of myelopathy or myeloradiculopathy, Herkowitz[16,17] reported 86% good to excellent results for laminaplasty as compared with 66% for laminectomy; the difference is attributed to the increased incidence of instability with laminectomy. The favorable results of laminaplasty have, for the most part, held up after long-term follow-up. Seichi and associates[14] demonstrated that up to 84% of patients undergoing cervical laminaplasty for multilevel spondylotic myelopathy maintained good results in a 10-year follow-up study.

Patients undergoing laminaplasty for multilevel stenosis secondary to OPLL also did reasonably well, with 78% maintaining improvement on long-term follow-up.

Uematsu and associates[18] demonstrated that in patients with bilateral disease, bilateral foraminotomy after laminaplasty may not be necessary, as the radicular pain on the hinged side seems to abate without foraminotomy. Although the mechanisms for this are not proven, improved vascular supply to the nerve root after decortication and thinning of the hinged side may be involved.

Combined Anterior and Posterior Approach

The combined approach in treating degenerative cervical spine disease is used less often than either the anterior or posterior approach. However, in some situations both anterior and posterior surgery is warranted, as either a single-day or a staged procedure. One such situation is when infection is present on one side, which may lead the surgeon to débride the infected side and use instrumentation for the other side. Other indications include situations where fixation was inadequate. This can occur when the bone quality is excessively poor due to tumor, infection, osteoporosis, or fracture or when technical problems arise during surgery on one side and adequate stabilization cannot be achieved.

Combined surgery may also be indicated in cases of severe spinal cord compression, if inadequate decompression has been obtained with the posterior approach because of compressive pathology anterior to the cord (large osteophytes, diffuse idiopathic skeletal hyperostosis, or OPLL). In addition, if kyphotic deformity of the cervical spine occurs after posterior laminectomy, the surgeon should perform anterior decompression and fusion, followed by posterior fusion and stabilization.

In summary, the indications for combined anterior and posterior cervical spine surgery are limited. However, the surgeon must be prepared to perform this more extensive procedure if necessary.

Complications

While generally less dangerous than the anterior Smith-Robinson approach to the cervical spine, posterior approaches are associated with complications as well. Hematoma formation may occur, which in severe cases may cause cord compromise requiring emergent decompression. The risk of hematoma can be diminished with careful dissection within the ligamentum nuchae and laterally subperiosteally on the laminae.[19]

As mentioned above, cervical spinal instability with development of postlaminectomy kyphosis may occur. This is more common after laminectomy but also occurs to a lesser extent after laminaplasty. Reattachment of the paraspinal muscles, especially to the C2 spinous process, may prevent loss of cervical lordosis following posterior decompression.[7]

Neurologic injuries are rare during the posterior approach, although they are more common than with anterior surgery. The risk of neurologic injury can be minimized by avoiding the placement of instruments into the spinal canal. Performing the decompression by using the burr to thin the outer cortices followed by using the curet to gently lift off the offending bone may also help to diminish the risk of neurologic injury. As mentioned previously, the surgeon should avoid using a Kerrison rongeur for posterior decompression, as this may result in neural impingement and compromise. In addition, the surgeon performing laminaplasty must make sure that the opened laminae remain secure. Praharaj and associates[20] describe cases in which either the open door "closed shut" or there was underriding of the lamina on the hinged side. Finally, C5 nerve root paresis may occur following laminectomy or laminaplasty because of tethering of the nerve root after posterior migration of the spinal cord. For this reason, the C5 foramen should be patent at the conclusion of the laminectomy or laminaplasty procedure.

Summary

Cervical degenerative disk disease presents a complex diagnostic and therapeutic challenge. The clinician must determine the relative contributions of neck pain, radicular pain, and myelopathy in the patient's presentation. Diagnostic studies such as conventional radiographs, CT scans, or MRI scans must be performed and interpreted within the context of the clinical presentation. Once the diagnosis is established, an individualized treatment plan should be formulated. Nonsurgical treatment may be successful in many situations, but when it is refractory or recurrent, surgical treatment should be considered. In general, patients with cervical spondylotic myelopathy should be treated aggressively to prevent potentially permanent loss of neurologic function.

Surgical options include posterior decompressive procedures. The surgical treatment is individualized based on the patient's symptoms, the location of the pathology, the levels of involvement, the sagittal alignment, and the surgeon's preference. Relative contraindications to posterior procedures include loss of sagittal lordosis, presence of severe axial neck pain, and bilateral radicular symptoms. However, for isolated radiculopathy or single-level or multilevel myelopathy with maintainance of cervical lordosis, a high rate of success can be expected with the posterior techniques of cervical foraminotomy, laminectomy, and laminaplasty.

References

1. Emery SE: Cervical disc disease and cervical spondylosis, in An HS (ed): *Principles and Techniques of Spine Surgery* ed 1. Philadelphia, PA, Williams & Wilkins, 1998, pp 401-412.

2. Grob D: Surgery in the degenerative cervical spine. *Spine* 1998;23:2674-2683.

3. Truumees E, Herkowitz HN: Cervical spondylotic myelopathy and radiculopathy. *Instr Course Lect* 2000;49:339-360.

4. Herkowitz HN, Kurz LT, Overholt DP: Surgical management of cervical soft disc herniation: A comparison between the anterior and posterior approach. *Spine* 1990;15:1026-1030.

5. Silveri CP, Simpson JM, Simeone FA, Balderston RA: Cervical disk disease and the keyhole foraminotomy: Proven efficacy at extended long-term follow up. *Orthopedics* 1997;20:687-692.

6. Henderson CM, Hennessy RG, Shuey HM Jr, Shackelford EG: Posterior-lateral foraminotomy as an exclusive operative technique for cervical radiculopathy: A review of 846 consecutively operated cases. *Neurosurgery* 1983;13:504-512.

7. An HS, Xu R: Posterior cervical spine procedures, in An HS, Riley LR III (eds): *An Atlas of Surgery of the Spine*. London, UK, Martin Dunitz, 1998, pp 13-54.

8. Herkowitz HN: A comparison of anterior cervical fusion, cervical laminectomy, and cervical laminaplasty for the surgical management of multiple level spondylotic radiculopathy. *Spine* 1988;13:774-780.

9. Guigui P, Benoist M, Deburge A: Spinal deformity and instability after multilevel cervical laminectomy for spondylotic myelopathy. *Spine* 1998;15:440-447.

10. Zdeblick TA, Zou D, Warden KE, McCabe R, Kunz D, Vanderby R: Cervical stability after foraminotomy: A biomechanical in vitro analysis. *J Bone Joint Surg Am* 1992;74:22-27.

11. Mikawa Y, Shikata J, Yamamuro T: Spinal deformity and instability after multilevel cervical laminectomy. *Spine* 1987;12:6-11.

12. Hirabayashi K, Toyama Y, Chiba K: Expansive laminaplasty for myelopathy in ossification of the longitudinal ligament. *Clin Orthop* 1999;359:35-48.

13. Matsunaga S, Sakou T, Nakanisi K: Analysis of the cervical spine alignment following laminaplasty and laminectomy. *Spinal Cord* 1999;37: 20-24.

14. Seichi A, Takeshita K, Ohishi I, et al: Long-term results of double-door laminaplasty for cervical stenotic myelopathy. *Spine* 2001;26:479-487.

15. Tomita K, Nomura S, Umeda S, Baba H: Cervical laminaplasty to enlarge the spinal canal in multilevel ossification of the posterior longitudinal ligament with myelopathy. *Arch Orthop Trauma Surg* 1988;107:148-153.

16. Herkowitz HN: Cervical laminaplasty: Its role in the treatment of cervical radiculopathy. *J Spinal Disord* 1988;1:179-188.

17. Herkowitz HN: The surgical management of cervical spondylotic radiculopathy and myelopathy. *Clin Orthop* 1989;239:94-108.

18. Uematsu Y, Tokuhashi Y, Matsuzaki H: Radiculopathy after laminaplasty of the cervical spine. *Spine* 1998;23:2057-2062.

19. Wellman BJ, Follett KA, Traynelis VC: Complications of posterior articular mass plate fixation of the subaxial cervical spine in 43 consecutive patients. *Spine* 1998;23:193-200.

20. Praharaj SS, Vasudev MK, Kolluri VR: Laminaplasty: An evaluation of 24 cases. *Neurol India* 2000;48:249-254.

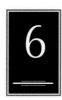

Microsurgery for Degenerative Conditions of the Cervical Spine

K. Daniel Riew, MD
John A. McCulloch, MD, FRCSC
Rick B. Delamarter, MD
Howard S. An, MD
Nicholas U. Ahn, MD

Abstract

Although the operating microscope has been used for spine surgery for more than 20 years, its use is still not widely accepted by orthopaedic spine surgeons. Nevertheless, surgeons who have used the operating microscope are well aware of its many advantages in performing spine surgery. Most notably, the superior visualization it provides allows for faster, safer, and more extensive decompressions. The reluctance of many surgeons to use the operating microscope often has to do with trepidation regarding new technology. The use of the operating microscope when performing anterior and posterior cervical spine surgery makes these procedures easier to carry out and decreases the risk of complications during decompression of the spinal cord.

Two events have had a permanent impact on the surgical treatment of degenerative spine conditions. The first was the adaptation of the microscope as an operating tool, first used in this manner by European otolaryngologists in the 1920s.[1] A commercial surgical microscope was introduced in 1953, and by 1978 it had been used in lumbar disk surgery.[2-4] The second event to impact surgical treatment of degenerative spine conditions was the advent of CT myelography and MRI, which provided the means to precisely localize pathologic conditions. The combination of the operating microscope with CT myelography and MRI has made surgery faster, safer, and technically easier and minimally invasive surgery requiring limited resection is now possible.

In this chapter, the advantages of using the operating microscope, the microanatomy of the cervical spine, and anterior and posterior cervical procedures done under the operating microscope will be discussed.

The Operating Microscope in Cervical Spine Surgery

Because of the increased emphasis on surgical precision (less invasive surgery) and the decreasing use of hospital resources (based on the rise in outpatient cervical and lumbar procedures), the advantages of the operating microscope far outweigh any minor disadvantages associated with the initial learning curve. These advantages are no direct hand-eye coordination (because the operating microscope is positioned between the surgeon's eyes and most of the shaft of the operating instrument), limited field of vision (facilitating excellent visualization of pathology), and enhanced line of vision (making positioning of the operating microscope and surgical instrument easier.)

In addition, the use of the operating microscope over loupe magnification is advantageous for several reasons. Magnification on the operating microscope can be easily decreased or increased. Three-dimensional vision can be maintained, the light source is perfectly coaxial to the line of vision, and observation of the surgical procedure is possible for operating room personnel.

The operating microscope is especially helpful when repairing dural tears in the cervical spine. With loupe magnification, only one person can stare into a small hole. During the repair of a dural tear, it is very difficult to provide mean-

One or more of the authors or the departments with which they are affiliated have received something of value from a commercial or other party related directly or indirectly to the subject of this chapter.

ingful assistance if what is going on in the depths of the wound cannot be visualized. The operating microscope enables the assistant to become a true co-surgeon.

Draping and Positioning of the Operating Microscope

A sterile plastic drape is used to cover the operating microscope during surgery. This drape has a plastic lens cover that fits over the microscope lens. The viewing ports are also covered. Once the operating microscope is brought into the proper position, the covering of the eyepieces is torn off at its serration. The eyepieces can be adjusted to accommodate the surgeon's interpupillary distance and to accommodate the particular surgeon's refraction if he or she does not have 20/20 vision. It is possible to have as many as four viewing ports on modern operating microscopes. Alternatively, there can be three viewing ports and a camera attached to the fourth port.

Once the operating microscope is brought into the field, the surgeon guides the head of the microscope to the surgical site. The base of the operating microscope is brought in only as close as necessary to place the head of the operating microscope in the proper position. In older microscopes, the base frequently had to be covered with a sterile drape so that it did not contaminate the surgical field. In the newer microscopes, however, a longer boom arm permits the microscope to be kept at a safe distance.

A surgeon may need to perform approximately 5 to 10 microsurgery cases to become comfortable with microsurgical techniques. Although the use of the operating microscope may prolong the procedure by several minutes at first, with experience, it is likely to decrease overall surgical times.

Instruments Used During Microsurgery of the Cervical Spine

Most of the tools used for microsurgery are used for loupe magnification surgery.

There are a few instruments that are absolutely essential for performing both posterior and anterior cervical decompressions. Foremost among these is a high-speed burr. It is absolutely essential that the burr have a high rotational speed, usually greater than 70,000 rpm, to be able to safely remove bone around neural and vascular structures. The use of burrs operated with a foot pedal is recommended. The burrs should be held with the dominant hand while suction is held with the opposite hand. The assistant can provide irrigation to prevent thermal injuries to the neural structures or bone.

When performing anterior procedures in patients with an intact posterior longitudinal ligament (PLL), a high-speed carbide burr under good visualization will safely remove all of the bony material without violating the PLL. A diamond burr, which usually increases the duration of surgery, is not necessary. In addition, the diamond burr has a greater potential for causing thermal injury. With microscopic visualization and constant palpation with the suction tip to determine if all of the bony material has been removed, it becomes readily apparent when all of the bone has been removed and the PLL has been located.

A set of microcurets is also very helpful in performing microsurgical procedures. These curets have a curved tip and are thin enough to squeeze into small spaces such as the neuroforamen. They come in sizes ranging from 1 to 5 mm. The most commonly used sizes are between 1 and 3 mm.

A 1-mm Kerrison rongeur is also very helpful for performing both anterior and posterior foraminotomies. These can only be used after thinning the osteophytes down to less than 1 or 2 mm. A Penfield-4 dissector can be used to palpate the lateral margin of the uncinate process when performing anterior operations. A small nerve hook can also be used to palpate the neuroforamen for

both anterior and posterior procedures; it can also be used to palpate the lateral margin of the pedicle, which ensures that an adequate foraminotomy has been performed. (Fig. 1, A).

Along with small nerve hooks, microneedle holders, fine-tipped bayonet forceps, angled pick-ups, and a knot pusher can be helpful when repairing dural tears (Fig. 1, B).

Anterior Cervical Procedures

The operating microscope enhances lighting and visualization in anterior cervical procedures, which helps the surgeon avoid complications during decompression of the spinal cord and nerve roots. It probably is an overstatement to say that use of a microscope is mandatory for these procedures. Many if not all of these cases can be accomplished with fiberoptic head light and loupe magnification. Depending on the surgeon's preference, the microscope may be used at the time of skin incision, at the time of diskectomy, or during dissection of the PLL, dura, and nerve roots. If fusion is necessary following diskectomy or corpectomy, it is generally performed without the operating microscope because a broader view of the anatomy is necessary for placement of the graft and instrumentation.

Surgical Approach

Exposure The Smith-Robinson anteromedial approach is most commonly used for the exposure of the middle and lower cervical spine, but other surgical approaches may be useful in special circumstances.[5,6] Understanding of the anatomical landmarks and adequate exposure are essential in the uncomplicated execution of the microsurgical procedure.

The patient is positioned supine with Gardner-Wells traction to the head. A reverse Trendelenburg position is recommended to allow venous drainage and reduce bleeding during surgery. The cervical spine is extended and slightly rotated toward the opposite side. If a plate is

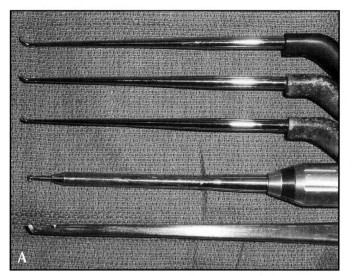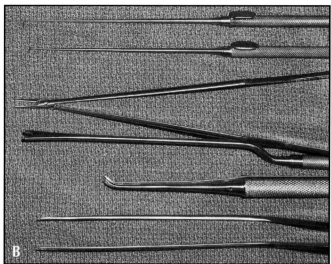

Fig. 1 A, Instruments used for microsurgery (from top to bottom) include 3-mm, 2-mm, and 1-mm microcurets; 2-mm carbide-tip burr; and a 1-mm Kerrison punch. **B,** Instruments for dural repair include (from top to bottom) right-angle bolted probe, micro nerve hook, Castro-Viejo needle driver, knot pusher, curved microforceps, and fine-tipped micro bayonet forceps.

used, the neck must be returned to a neutral position before placing the plate to prevent a permanent rotation of the segment. A rolled towel may be placed between the scapulae to enhance cervical lordosis. In order to minimize injury to the recurrent laryngeal nerve, the lower cervical spine is approached from the left, as the path of this nerve is more predictable and consistent on the left.

The anatomic landmarks include the hyoid bone overlying C3, the thyroid cartilage overlying the C4-C5 intervertebral disk, and the cricoid ring and carotid tubercle at C6. Great care must be taken to make sure that landmarks are palpated and that the incision is made in the appropriate location. A horizontal incision can be used for multiple levels provided it is long enough.

A transverse incision in line with the skin crease is made from the midline beyond the anterior aspect of the sternocleidomastoid muscle. The skin and subcutaneous tissue are undermined slightly, and division of the platysma muscle is completed. The platysma muscle may be divided either horizontally or vertically. Retraction of the divided muscle exposes the sternocleidomastoid muscle laterally and strap muscles medially. The deep cervical fascia is divided between the sternocleidomastoid muscle and strap muscles, and blunt finger dissection is done through the pretracheal fascia while palpating and retracting the carotid sheath laterally. The omohyoid muscle may be divided if necessary. Further blunt dissection toward the midline leads to the prevertebral fascia and longus colli muscles.

The superior thyroid artery is encountered above C4 and the inferior thyroid artery is seen below C6. These vessels should be identified and ligated as necessary. The prevertebral fascia is divided longitudinally to expose the disk and vertebral body. The longus colli muscles are mobilized laterally with a Cobb elevator or curet. The self-retaining retractors are repositioned under the longus colli muscles. The use of a self-retaining retractor with sharp edges should be avoided to prevent potential perforation of the esophagus medially. Once the prevertebral fascia is split, the cervical spine can be seen. Disk margins are prominent and make up the "hills," and the vertebral bodies are concave and make up the "val-leys." A bent 18-gauge needle is placed in the disk space and a lateral radiograph is taken to confirm the correct level.

The anterior approaches of the cervical spine involve dissections of related vital structures around the neck. The carotid sheath is an investment of the internal and common carotid arteries, the internal jugular vein, and the vagus nerve. It is adherent to the thyroid sheath and the fascia under the sternocleidomastoid. The carotid artery in the sheath can be palpated for pulsation and retracted laterally with the sternocleidomastoid. The carotid sheath should not be entered but rather retracted as a single unit when performing the Smith-Robinson approach.

During the left-sided approach to the lower cervical spine, the thoracic duct may also be encountered. The thoracic duct lies posterior to the carotid sheath and terminates at the junction of the left internal jugular and subclavian veins. The thoracic duct lies anterior to the subclavian artery, vertebral artery, thyrocervical trunk, and the prevertebral fascia, which separates the duct from the phrenic nerve and anterior scalene muscle.

The larynx performs important func-

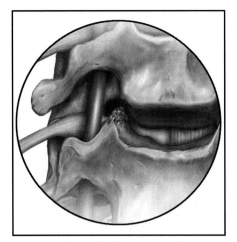

Fig. 2 Anatomy of the foramen, uncovertebral joint, and lateral disk space. Note that the uncovertebral joint serves as a landmark for lateral margins of exposure and for identification of foramen for decompression. The vertebral artery lies just lateral to the uncovertebral joints and must be avoided by using the curet to remove cartilage and osteophytes in a circular fashion away from lateral to medial.

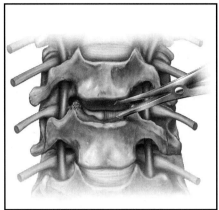

Fig. 3 Disk space after excision of cervical disk. Note that the PLL can be identified by the vertical striations (right side). Deep to the PLL lies the dural sac (left side). The PLL does not need to be excised unless it is perforated by offending disk material.

tions in respiration and vocalization. The cricothyroid muscle is innervated by the external laryngeal branch of the superior laryngeal nerve of the vagus nerve, and the other intrinsic muscles of the larynx are innervated by the recurrent laryngeal nerve. The superior laryngeal nerve is a branch of the inferior ganglion of the vagus nerve and travels along side the superior thyroid artery. The inferior laryngeal nerve is a recurrent branch of the vagus nerve that innervates all laryngeal muscles except the cricothyroid.

The anatomy of the recurrent laryngeal nerve is important to understand because the nerve's path may be encountered during the anterior cervical approach, and failure to protect the nerve may result in permanent hoarseness. On the left side, the recurrent laryngeal nerve loops under the arch of the aorta and is protected in the left tracheoesophageal groove. On the right side, the recurrent nerve travels around the subclavian artery, passing dorsomedial to the side of the trachea and esophagus. It is vulnerable as it passes from the subclavian artery to the right tracheoesophageal groove. Because this nerve is more susceptible to injury if the cervical spine is approached from the right, the left-sided approach is favored by most surgeons.

The recurrent laryngeal nerve should always be located when working from C6 downward on the right side. The best landmark for the surgeon to use is the inferior thyroid artery. The nerve usually enters the tracheoesophageal groove where the inferior thyroid artery enters the lower pole of the thyroid. It is also more common for the right inferior laryngeal nerve to be nonrecurrent where it travels directly from the vagus nerve and carotid sheath to the larynx.

Anterior Cervical Diskectomy and Corpectomy

The proper techniques of diskectomy and corpectomy cannot be overemphasized because outcome and complications are often associated with intraoperative factors. Proper lighting and magnification of the surgical field are essential during diskectomy, and for this reason, use of the operating microscope is recommended.

When performing an anterior cervical diskectomy, the cervical spine is first approached using the previously described exposures. Once the cervical spine is exposed, the operating microscope is brought into the field. The anterior anulus fibrosus is incised sharply and removed with a rongeur. The nucleus pulposus is removed using curets and a rongeur. The lateral margins of the anulus fibrosus are often inadequately dissected by the inexperienced surgeon. It is important to mobilize the longus colli muscles laterally in order to thoroughly remove the disk tissues laterally. If monopolar electrocautery is used to do so, great care must be taken not to damage the sympathetic chain; if damaged, it may cause a Horner's syndrome.

Great caution should be taken to avoid injury to the vertebral artery when removing disk or bone laterally. A small curet is used to dissect the disk tissues in a circular manner away from the lateral margin to safeguard the vertebral artery. The uncovertebral joints should also be identified on both sides as landmarks of lateral margins of exposure and for later decompression of the foramen (Fig. 2). Complete removal of cartilage material about the uncovertebral joints should be performed again using a small, curved curet, dissecting in a circular fashion away from the vertebral artery. If an anterior osteophyte is causing impingement on the nerve root, it is excised at this time.

All of the disk material is removed down to the PLL. The PLL has characteristic vertical striations that are clearly visualized under the operating microscope (Fig. 3). If the PLL is perforated by the offending disk material, further decompression should be done to expose the dura. The dura has a shiny surface and a slightly blue color. Use of the operating microscope and microsurgical instruments is especially important during dissection around the PLL and the dura. The PLL is usually entered in the midvertical

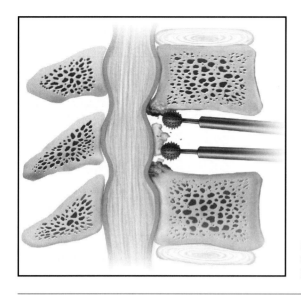

Fig. 4 Use of power burr to thin the posterior margin of vertebral body.

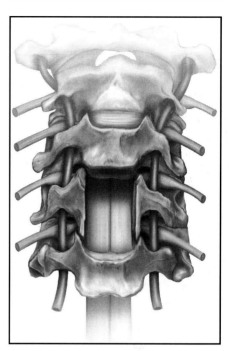

Fig. 5 View of excised vertebral body after corpectomy. Note that corpectomy has been successfully completed with all bone excised down to the PLL. The surgeon must make sure that the osteophytes at the posterior edges of the intervertebral disk are carefully and completely removed because these are often causes of severe cord compression.

line, and a microscopic probe is used to separate the PLL from the dura. The PLL is carefully removed using microscopic Kerrison rongeurs or a fine curet.

Frequently, osteophytes limit the exposure of the PLL and dura. The osteophytes tend to be more prominent at the inferior end plate of the vertebra or superior aspect of the disk space. A power burr should be used to thin the end plate and osteophytes, and a small, curved curet may be used to remove the bone from the spinal canal. Laterally, uncovertebral joints may be thinned using a power burr, and the foramen may be decompressed under direct vision using curets and Kerrison rongeurs. Again, the surgeon should always be aware of the location of the vertebral artery and nerve root during decompression of the intervertebral foramen.

For cervical spondylotic myelopathic cases, burst fractures, or tumors, corpectomy is most commonly performed. Following thorough diskectomy above and below the vertebra, corpectomy is initiated with a rongeur. The posterior margin of the vertebral body is thinned with a power burr (Fig. 4). The posterior shell is then removed with an angled curet using lifting motions aimed away from the dura. The osteophytes at the

posterior edges of the intervertebral disk are the frequent cause of spinal cord compression. Careful removal of these osteophytes must be done by extending the corpectomy cephalad or caudad. Again, the power burr is helpful to thin the bone and osteophytes before using the curet to pull the remainder of the osteophyte away from the dura. When the corpectomy is completed, the only visible structure lying anteriorly should be the PLL (Fig. 5). The vertebral arteries are most vulnerable during corpectomy, and the surgeon must always be aware of their location. The location of the vertebral arteries and any possible anomalies should be accurately determined preoperatively. The lateral extent of corpectomy generally should be in line with the medial aspect of the uncovertebral joint.

Anterior Cervical Fusion Techniques
When performing the Smith-Robinson technique of interbody fusion, the graft height should be about 2 mm greater than the degenerated disk space or at least 6 mm in total height to obtain adequate compressive strength and to enlarge the neural foramina.[7] Overdistraction of the intervertebral space may result in graft collapse and pseudarthrosis. The distraction of the disk space may be achieved by

skull traction, laminar spreader, or vertebral screws. Traction using Gardner-Wells tongs is temporarily increased to between 30 and 40 lb to distract the degenerative level while the graft is placed. Either a laminar spreader or a vertebral screw distractor is also placed for further distraction. The end plates in the disk space should be burred to create flat surfaces on both sides. Additionally, a 3- to 4-mm hole may be created in the middle of the end plate to promote vascularization of the graft. After measuring the depth and width of the disk space, the tricortical graft is obtained from the anterior iliac crest region; allograft bone may be a good alternative. The graft is gently placed 2 mm under the anterior cortical margin of the vertebral body (Fig. 6, *A*). The tricortical graft may be reversed so that the cortical margin is placed posteri-

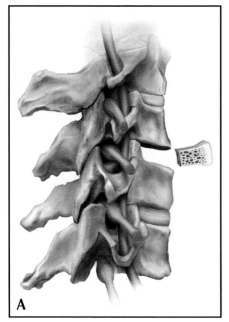

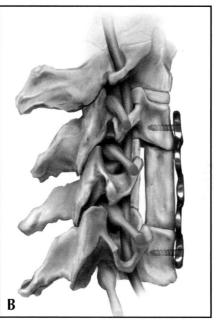

Fig. 6 A, Placement of bone graft into disk space for anterior cervical diskectomy and fusion using Smith-Robinson technique. **B,** Placement of strut graft after corpectomy. The source of the strut graft may be from the iliac crest or fibula in cases of multilevel reconstruction. The strut graft must be countersunk to prevent graft dislodgement, and anterior plating is often used to supplement the construct to prevent this potentially devastating complication.

Fig. 7 CT scan of a 54-year-old man showing unilateral spondylotic right foraminal narrowing (arrow). The patient had right arm pain, numbness, and tingling; microforaminotomy as an outpatient procedure was successful in relieving symptoms. A patient with this CT scan and presenting with these symptoms is the ideal candidate for posterior microforaminotomy.

orly. The traction is then reduced to 5 lb, and the laminar spreader is removed. The graft should be stable with compression forces from the end plates. Additional cancellous chips may be inserted into defects in the disk space.

Following corpectomy, strut grafting is performed (Fig. 6, *B*). The source of the strut graft is usually the iliac crest, but the fibula may be used for cases involving multiple-level reconstruction. The strut graft must be countersunk in order to prevent graft dislodgement. The bone graft may be placed between the inferior end plate of the superior vertebra and the superior end plate of the inferior vertebra, particularly if anterior plating is planned. A longer strut graft that is slotted between the superior end plate of the superior vertebra and the inferior end plate of the inferior vertebra provides greater stability.[8,9] The slots are created in the vertebral bodies using the power burr and curets. A correctly sized tricortical

bone graft is obtained from the iliac crest. The anterior wall of the inferior vertebra is notched to create a window defect. The graft is inserted into the slot in the superior vertebra first, and the graft is placed into the window in the inferior vertebra. While interspace distraction is being applied, the graft is then rotated and tapped into the slot in the inferior vertebra. The distraction is discontinued, and the graft should be stable with compression forces from the superior end plate of the superior vertebra and the inferior end plate of the inferior vertebra. A similar technique may be used to insert a longer fibular strut graft.

Posterior Cervical Microscopic Laminotomy/Foraminotomy and Laminaplasty

The operating microscope provides greatly improved magnification and illumination of the surgical site during laminoforaminotomy and laminaplasty. As a

result, these procedures are easier to perform and there is a greater degree of safety.

Cervical radiculopathy, in general, can be isolated to single nerve-root compression. If this compression is isolated to the foramen by either disk herniation or spondylotic changes, a simple posterior microforaminotomy can be the procedure of choice, giving complete relief of the radiculopathy without requiring a fusion (Fig. 7). In a neutral or lordotic cervical spine with cervical myelopathy or myeloradiculopathy requiring multilevel decompression, a microscopic cervical laminaplasty can be the procedure of choice, giving excellent relief of the spinal cord compression and allowing foraminotomies, if necessary, also without requiring a fusion.

"Cervical spondylotic myeloradiculopathy" is a term that tends to encompass all neural compressive disorders related to cervical spondylosis. This term may have a confusing clinical picture because of the differing clinical manifestations of myelopathy versus radiculopathy and the combination of the two in many clinical situations. Understanding the need for spinal cord decompression versus nerve-root decompression is critical in determining the rationale for posterior versus anterior approaches to the cervical spine. Both anterior and posterior cervical approaches play a role in the management of cervical spondylosis.

Posterior surgical approaches to the neural foraminal and spinal canal have been established as safe and efficacious.[5,7,10-15] Although details regarding the rationale for the posterior versus anterior approach in cervical spondylosis are beyond the scope of this chapter, it is important to point out two factors that determine which patients are most likely to benefit from a posterior approach. The first is the presence of kyphosis. Patients with cervical kyphosis have a higher likelihood of surgical failure when a posterior decompressive procedure is used.[5,7,8,12,16] Although a simple microforaminotomy may be acceptable in a kyphotic cervical spine, a laminectomy or laminaplasty is contraindicated in a kyphotic cervical spine. The second is stability of the cervical spine. The literature clearly shows the destabilizing effects of certain posterior cervical decompressive procedures, particularly wide laminectomies with resection of part or all of the facet joints.[7,8,17] Indeed, if more than half of the facet joints are resected in bilateral lateral foraminotomies or laminectomies, fusion of the involved cervical segments should be considered.[17]

The most common scenario for using the posterior cervical microforaminotomy is that of unilateral radiculopathy, either from spondylotic foraminal narrowing or lateral disk protrusion. Although radiculopathy is most frequently from unilateral one-level disease, bilateral one-, two-, or three-level foraminotomies can be easily accomplished using the operating microscope.

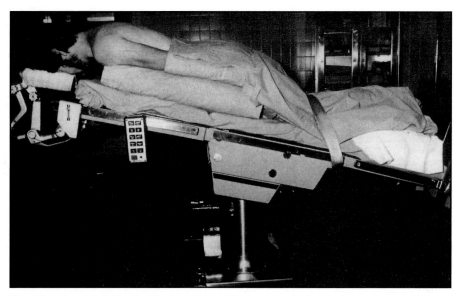

Fig. 8 The prone position used for posterior cervical surgery. Note that the neck is neutral to slight flexion.

Surgical Technique

Laminotomy/Foraminotomy The patient is placed in the prone position using a Mayfield three-point head holder with the neck kept in fairly neutral position, although slight flexion can be used (extreme flexion and extreme extension are to be avoided). The patient's shoulders are then taped to the operating table, and the patient is placed in approximately 15° to 20° of reverse Trendelenburg position (Fig. 8). The area is shaved, sterilized, and draped, and a radiograph or fluoroscopic evaluation is obtained to determine the level or levels to be addressed. For a single-level foraminotomy, a 2- to 3-cm incision can be made in midline over the appropriate surgical level. Unilateral subperiosteal elevation of the spinous process, lamina, and medial facet joint is done. A repeat radiograph or fluoroscopic evaluation will confirm the appropriate level.

The operating microscope is brought in and used for the remainder of the procedure. The caudal aspect of the upper lamina and rostral aspect of the lower lamina are cleaned of soft tissue as is 2 to 4 mm of the medial aspect of the inferior facet. A high-speed burr is used to remove 2 to 3 mm of the medial aspect of the inferior facet and to thin the caudal aspect of the upper lamina (Fig. 9). Using a 4-0 (or 2-mm) microcuret, the ligamentum flavum is freed from the undersurface of the upper and lower lamina as well as from the medial aspect of the superior facet. A 2-mm Kerrison punch is then used to underbite the upper and lower lamina and to remove approximately 2 mm of the medial aspect of the superior facet. The surgeon can then palpate the upper and lower pedicles (allowing precise anatomic location of the foramen) (Fig. 10). Depending on the amount of surgical decompression needed to decompress the exiting nerve root, underbiting the foramen can be done with a 1- or 2-mm Kerrison rongeur or even by thinning the roof of the foramen with the high-speed burr and flicking the bone off the exiting nerve root with a 4-0 microcuret. Minimal bleeding can be controlled with thrombin-soaked Gelfoam and a small cottonoid or by using a hemostatic sealant, such as Proceed (Fusion Medical, Fremont, CA). Although the bipolar cautery can be considered, minimal cau-

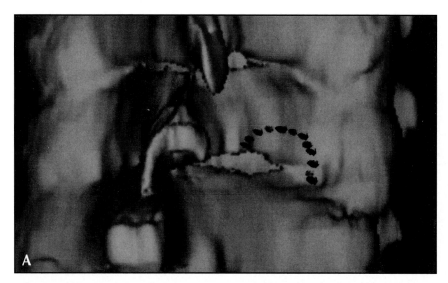

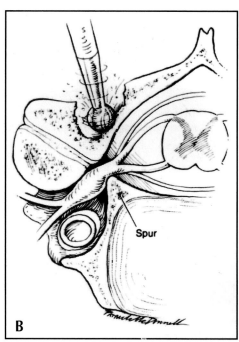

Fig. 9 A, Three-dimensional CT scan of the posterior cervical bony anatomy. Note the black marks outlining the bone to be removed. **B,** Drawing of the posterior cervical bony anatomy showing removal of 2 to 3 mm of the medial aspect of the inferior facet and thinning the caudal upper lamina with a high-speed burr.

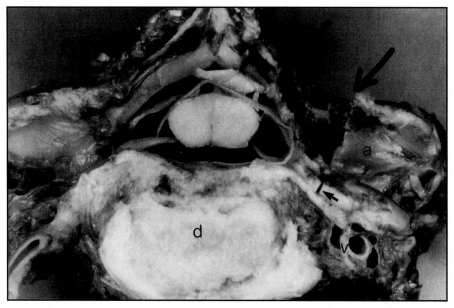

Fig. 10 Cadaver section showing proper bony resection (large arrow) for a posterior microforaminotomy. (d = disk; a = remaining facet and lateral mass; v = vertebral body; small arrow = nerve root.)

If a lateral disk herniation requires removal, it is performed following the completion of the foraminotomy. Disk herniation removal is begun by finding the lower pedicle and teasing the nerve root upward off the pedicle and disk. This generally exposes either the disk herniation or the bony spur requiring decompression (Fig. 11). Occasionally, the disk herniation is beneath the PLL, and the ligament can be incised with a No. 11 blade. Extreme caution is necessary to protect the nerve root and dural sac, requiring the ligament/anulus incision with the No. 11 blade to be down and lateral away from the cord and nerve root. Once the PLL is open, the 4-0 microcuret or micro nerve hook can be used to free the herniated fragments, and a small micropituitary rongeur is used to remove the fragments. If a bony spur is on the floor of the foramen requiring decompression, this can be removed again with the microcurets or a 2-mm high-speed burr (Fig. 12). Care should be taken not to retract the spinal cord or place instruments into the spinal canal underneath the spinal cord. Disk hernia-

terization around the nerve root should be used. A drain is generally not used for a single-level microforaminotomy.

This procedure can be done on an outpatient basis, but many patients are kept for a 23-hour stay. A soft cervical collar is used for comfort only for 7 to 10 days until the incision is healed. Most patients are able to return to desk work within 4 to 7 days, although physical therapy and sports activities are not permitted for 2 to 3 weeks.

tions in the canal should be removed from the anterior approach.

Laminaplasty Cervical laminaplasty was developed by the Japanese as a treatment alternative to laminectomy because of the fear of developing postlaminectomy kyphosis. The advantages of laminaplasty over laminectomy include retention of the lamina with a decreased potential for surgically induced instability and decreased perineural scarring. Several variations of laminaplasty have been described over the past 3 decades.[18-20]

The patient is placed in the prone position in a Mayfield three-point head holder with care taken to keep the neck in a neutral position. The posterior elements are exposed from a midline approach, taking care not to damage the facet joint capsules or interspinous ligaments (Fig. 13, *A*). The entire area of stenosis is exposed, including one level above and below the affected area, generally C3 to C7. Extending the dissection lateral to the facet joints may denervate the local musculature and should be avoided. Only the medial 50% of the facet is exposed. The soft tissue surrounding the lateral half of the joint is later needed to suture the lamina open with No. 1 nonabsorbable suture. Alternatively, small bone suture anchors can be imbedded in the lateral mass and attached to the suture. At this point, the operating microscope is brought into the field, and the rest of the procedure is performed under its magnification. Decompressive foraminotomies may be performed as needed for radiculopathy. The laminaplasty grooves are then prepared.

We prefer to perform the laminaplasty grooves with a high-speed burr. Excellent visualization afforded by the operating microscope allows for precise removal of the exact amount of bone necessary to perform this procedure. A trough extending the length of the stenosis is made through both laminar cortices at the junction of the lamina and facet joint (Fig.13, *B*). A bicortical trough is created

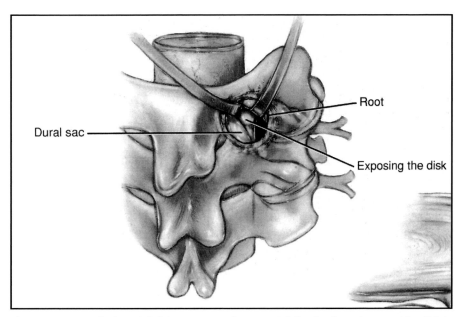

Fig. 11 Exposure of a lateral disk herniation (or bone spur) following foraminotomy. The disk is exposed by finding the lower pedicle and teasing the nerve root upward.

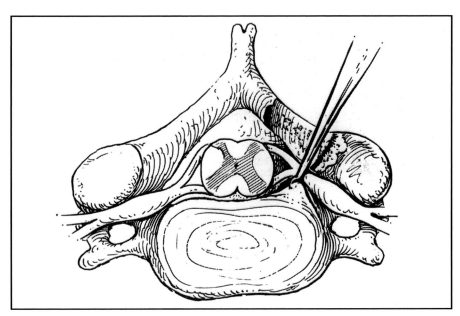

Fig. 12 Cervical cross-section illustrating removal of a lateral foraminal bone spur with a small curet. Disk or spur removal is performed only after proper foraminotomy has been accomplished.

on the open-door side of the lamina facet junction and a 2-mm Kerrison rongeur, and/or forward-angled curets, can be used to remove any continued bony connections or to free the ligamentum flavum and any dural adhesions. Bleeding is controlled with bone wax, bipolar cautery, and thrombin-soaked collagen foam and/or Proceed hemostatic sealant.

A unicortical trough created on the opposite side acts as an opening hinge upon canal expansion (Fig. 13, *C*). The

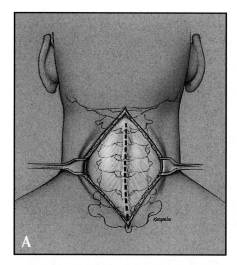

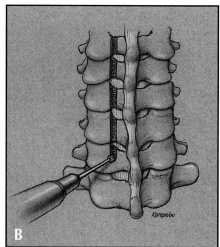

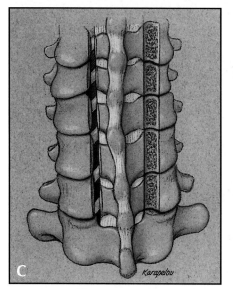

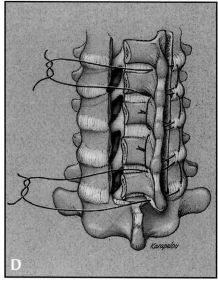

Fig. 13 Laminaplasty technique. **A,** Laminaplasty midline exposure of the posterior cervical spine. The entire area of stenosis is exposed, including one level above and below the affected area. **B,** A bicortical trough is created on the open-door side at the junction of the lamina and facet joint. A high-speed burr is used to create the trough. **C,** A unicortical trough is created on the opposite (hinge) side. The hinge-side trough is created 2 mm wider and 1 to 2 mm more lateral than the open-door trough. **D,** Nonabsorbable sutures are placed through the lateral facet capsule and tied around the spinous process to maintain the laminaplasty opening at approximately 40° to 45°.

to approximately 40° to 45° by creating a greenstick fracture at the unicortical trough. This procedure should be performed slowly and carefully to avoid complete fractures of the cortical hinge. If the lamina completely fractures on the hinge side, the lamina may displace into the spinal canal, producing nerve root compression and radiculopathy.

The stay sutures are then passed around or through the spinous processes and tied to the facet capsule to keep the laminaplasty opened at approximately 40° to 45° (Fig. 14). The dural sac can be freed from any adhesions or ligamentum flavum with a small forward-angled curet. All bleeding should be meticulously controlled throughout the procedure. A careful multilevel closure is performed by closing the deep cervical muscular fascia with 0-Vicryl interrupted sutures, the subcutaneous level with 2-0 sutures, and the skin with subcutaneous sutures or skin staples.

The postoperative course following laminaplasty is somewhat controversial. Some surgeons immobilize patients in a semirigid collar (such as the Aspen or Philadelphia) for approximately 8 weeks, then allow a light physical therapy course. Other surgeons prefer to begin range-of-motion therapy as early as 2 to 3 weeks after surgery. Early range of motion may increase ultimate motion but tends to also increase postoperative pain. On the other hand, immobilizing patients with a semirigid collar for 8 weeks decreases postoperative pain but may also decrease range of motion.

Finally, one of the attractive aspects of the laminaplasty procedure is the ease of converting it into a laminectomy. By simply turning the hinge side into a complete trough and removing the lamina en bloc, a safe, easy laminectomy can be achieved.

Summary

The procedures outlined were all initially described as nonmicroscope-visualized procedures. Many surgeons continue to

trough is started slightly (1 to 2 mm) more lateral than the opening groove on the opposite side and needs to be wide enough to allow space for the opening hinge maneuver such that the dorsal lamina cortices do not abut with the facet complex until adequate opening of the spinal canal has been attained. Before opening the laminaplasty, the ligamen-

tum flavum and interspinous ligaments should be released above and below the end lamina, and stay sutures (No. 1 nonabsorbable) should be placed through the facet capsule and muscle at each level on the hinged side (Fig. 13, *D*). Placement of these sutures is more difficult after the laminaplasty has been opened. The laminaplasty is then gently and slowly opened

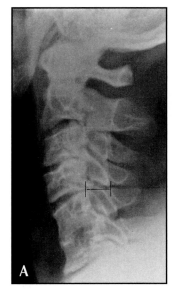
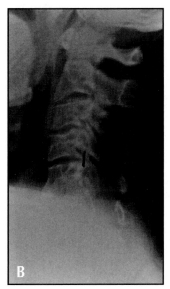
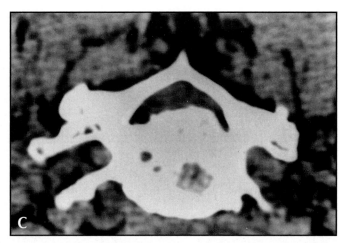
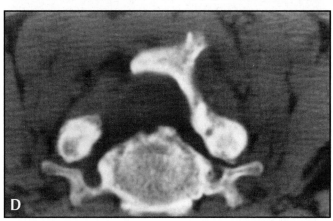

Fig. 14 Radiographs of the cervical spine of a 58-year-old man with a 2-year history of progressive loss of hand function and stumbling gait. **A,** Lateral radiograph reveals congenital spinal stenosis (C4-5 level measures 10 mm). **B,** Following C3-C7 laminaplasty, lateral postoperative radiographs reveal the open spinal canal (C4-5 level measures 20 mm). **C,** Preoperative CT scan showing marked spinal stenosis. The congenital spinal stenosis in conjunction with the posterior vertebral body osteophytes narrowed the spinal canal to 6 to 7 mm at the C4-5 level. **D,** CT scan at C5 level 1 year following C3-C7 laminaplasty. Note the wide-open canal, the well-healed laminaplasty hinge, and the approximate 40° laminaplasty opening.

perform these procedures without the benefit of any magnification or with only loupe magnification. It is the opinion of the authors that the use of the operating microscope vastly improves the visualization of the neural structures, which can result in more rapid decompressions and improved safety. The ability to see with great clarity the difference between the PLL and the dura, or between the ligamentum flavum and the nerve root, makes it less likely that the neural structures will inadvertently be lacerated or burred through. Although the use of the operating microscope requires some practice before proficiency is achieved, we believe that the learning curve is relatively short and that most surgeons accustomed to performing cervical spine surgery can master the required techniques within a short period of time.

References

1. Lang WH, Muchel F (eds): *Zeiss Microscopes for Microsurgery*. Berlin, Germany, Springer-Verlag, 1981.

2. Yasargil MG: Microsurgical operation of herniated lumbar disc. *Adv Neurosurg* 1977;4:81-82.

3. Caspar W: A new surgical procedure for lumbar disc herniation causing less tissue damage through a microsurgical approach. *Adv Neurosurg* 1977;4:74-80.

4. Williams RW: Microlumbar discectomy: A conservative surgical approach to the virgin herniated lumbar disc. *Spine* 1978;3:175-182.

5. Herkowitz HN: A comparison of anterior cervical fusion, cervical laminectomy, and cervical laminoplasty for the surgical management of multiple level spondylotic radiculopathy. *Spine* 1988;13:774-780.

6. Nakano N, Nakano T, Nakano K: Comparison of results of laminectomy and open-door laminoplasty for cervical spondylotic myeloradiculopathy and ossification of the posterior longitudinal ligament. *Spine* 1988;13:792-794.

7. Batzdorf U, Batzdorff A: Analysis of cervical spine curvature in patients with cervical spondylosis. *Neurosurgery* 1988;22:827-836.

8. Bohlman HH: Acute fractures and dislocations of the cervical spine: An analysis of three hundred hospitalized patients and review of the literature. *J Bone Joint Surg Am* 1979;61:1119-1142.

9. Verbiest H: Anterolateral operations for fractures and dislocations in the middle and lower parts of the cervical spine: Report of a series of forty-seven cases. *J Bone Joint Surg Am* 1969;51:1489-1530.

10. Benzel EC, Lancon J, Kesterson L, Hadden T: Cervical laminectomy and dentate ligament section for cervical spondylotic myelopathy. *J Spinal Disord* 1991;4:286-295.

11. Carol MP, Ducker TB: Cervical spondylitic myelopathies: Surgical treatment. *J Spinal Disord* 1988;1:59-65.

12. Ducker TB: Cervical radiculopathies and myelopathies: Posterior approaches, in Frymoyer JW (ed): *The Adult Spine: Principles and Practice*. New York, NY, Raven Press, 1991, vol 2, pp 1187-1206.

13. Henderson CM, Hennessy RG, Shuey HM Jr, Shackelford EG: Posterior-lateral foraminotomy as an exclusive operative technique for cervical radiculopathy: A review of 846 consecutively operated cases. *Neurosurgery* 1983;13:504-512.

14. Krupp W, Schattke H, Muke R: Clinical results of the foraminotomy as described by Frykholm for the treatment of lateral cervical disc herniation. *Acta Neurochir (Wien)* 1990;107:22-29.

15. Williams RW: Microcervical foraminotomy: A surgical alternative for intractable radicular pain. *Spine* 1983;8:708-716.

16. Callahan RA, Johnson RM, Margolis RN, Keggi KJ, Albright JA, Sourthwick WO: Cervical facet fusion for control of instability following laminectomy. *J Bone Joint Surg Am* 1977;59: 991-1002.

17. Zdeblick TA, Zou D, Warden KE, McCabe R, Kunz D, Vanderby R: Cervical stability after foraminotomy: A biomechanical in vitro analysis. *J Bone Joint Surg Am* 1992;74:22-27.

18. Hirabayashi K, Satomi K: Operative procedure and results of expansive open-door laminoplasty. *Spine* 1988;13:870-876.

19. Hirabayashi K, Miyakawa J, Satomi K, Maruyama T, Wakano K: Operative results and postoperative progression of ossification among patients with ossification of cervical posterior longitudinal ligament. *Spine* 1981;6:354-364.

20. Yoshida M, Otani K, Shibasaki K, Ueda S: Expansive laminoplasty with reattachment of spinous process and extensor musculature for cervical myelopathy. *Spine* 1992;17:491-497.

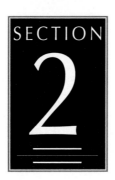

Herniated Lumbar Disk

Herniated Lumbar Disk

Lumbar disk herniation is an extremely common cause of low back pain, and symptoms of sciatica are frequent on presentation. Most patients respond well to nonsurgical treatment; over time, pain and radicular symptoms usually resolve. However, some patients require surgical treatment. The lifetime prevalence of lumbar disk surgery in the United States is believed to approach 3%. In this section, Drs. Carragee, Delamarter, and McCulloch and associates review the indications for surgical treatment of lumbar disk herniation and the surgical techniques of microdiskectomy.

Dr. Eugene Carragee reviews the indications for lumbar microdiskectomy. Absolute indications for surgical treatment include cauda equina syndrome and significant progressive neurologic deficit. Microdiskectomy, however, is more commonly performed for intractable radicular pain despite nonsurgical treatment for 6 weeks, especially in patients who need to return to work earlier and to avoid permanent disability. Before surgery is attempted, physical examination should reveal a positive tension sign or straight leg raising test, and imaging studies such as MRI should reveal nerve root compression that corresponds to the patient's radicular symptoms.

The main advantage of microdiskectomy over conventional diskectomy is significantly reduced morbidity and earlier return to work. The mean time to return to work can be reduced to 1.2 weeks, and approximately 25% of patients are able to return to work within 3 days. Despite the high success rate associated with conventional diskectomy, with immediate improvement in radicular pain postoperatively, as many as 20% to 40% of patients may continue to experience significant discomfort. The type of disk herniation and the status of the anulus after diskectomy may also have a predictive value in the clinical outcome and in the rates of recurrent or persistent sciatica and revision surgery. Patients with extruded disks and anular fissure have the best outcome, while those with extruded disks and anular defect have the greatest risk of frank reherniation requiring revision surgery. Treatment of anular prolapse without a discreet disk fragment is generally unsatisfactory; therefore, surgery should be avoided in this group of patients. Patients with certain psychosocial factors also frequently have an adverse outcome and are considered poor surgical candidates.

Dr. Rick Delamarter describes the microsurgical technique of lumbar diskectomy. The identification of the correct anatomic level and visualization and protection of the traversing nerve root are key factors in minimizing the risk of a poor clinical outcome. A great deal of attention is given to ways in which to minimize formation of postoperative scar tissue. A ligamentum flavum sparing approach is recommended in which the ligamentum flavum is detached from the medial border of the superior facet and upper and lower laminae. The nerve root is retracted medially along with the epidural fat and the ligamentum flavum, providing excellent exposure of the herniated disk. This approach decreases the risk of dural tear, nerve root injury, and epidural fibrosis. Loose disk fragments should be removed, and damage to the end plate should be avoided. Meticulous hemostasis at the end of the procedure is important to minimize the risk of epidural hematoma and formation of scar tissue.

Dr. John McCulloch's tragic demise has left a huge void in the field of spinal microsurgery. Dr. McCulloch was the undisputed leader and a visionary who probably contributed the most to the advancement of our knowledge and understanding of the microscopic anatomy of the lumbar spine. His article on microsurgery in the intertransverse interval is yet another outstanding review of microscopic anatomy. Attending to anatomic landmarks is key to avoiding complications and ensuring successful surgical outcome. The intertransverse interval provides access to the foraminal and extraforaminal disk herniation at all lumbar levels except L5-S1; at this level the herniated disk is best approached from within the canal. An extracanalicular anastomosis frequently exists between lumbar nerve roots in the intertransverse space; the most important is the anastomotic branch between the L4 and L5 nerve roots called the furcal nerve. Familiarity with the anatomy in the intertransverse interval is also helpful in transpedicular instrumentation.

Dr. McCulloch was very passionate about the use of

operative microscope, and in the final chapter of this section, he reviews the advantages of the operative microscope over conventional loupe magnification. Traditionally, neurosurgeons have preferred the operative microscope for spinal decompression, while many orthopaedic spine surgeons have tended to rely on loupe magnification. Today, most microdiskectomy is done on an outpatient basis, and successful outcomes are in the 90% to 95% range on carefully selected patients. Emerging new technologies, such as endoscopic diskectomy, are more likely to become popular with orthopaedic spine surgeons who have developed arthroscopic skills. However, all principles of microscopic spinal surgery will continue to be relevant. Moreover, microdiskectomy remains the gold standard, and the newer technologies such as microscopic endoscopic diskectomy should be compared to microdiskectomy to establish their safety and efficacy. Other emerging technologies such as nucleoplasty and laser diskectomy are aimed at patients with a contained herniated disk with radicular symptoms, but these procedures should not be widely adopted until clear indications, benefits, and complications are better defined with prospective randomized studies.

Ashok Biyani, MD
Assistant Professor
Department of Orthopedic Surgery
Medical College of Ohio
Toledo, Ohio

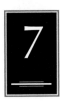

Indications for Lumbar Microdiskectomy

Eugene Carragee, MD

Introduction

Sciatica is a very common symptom; one author[1] suggests that 35% to 50% of adults develop sciatica. In young and middle-aged patients, sciatica usually is associated with lumbar disk irritation of lumbar roots. Most patients who develop sciatica recover spontaneously with time; many recover without medical attention. When treatment is indicated, diskectomy using a minimally invasive approach may be considered.

Microdiskectomy

The absolute indication for disk excision is serious neurologic injury due to a root or cauda equina compression; however, only a small number of disk excisions are done for this reason. More commonly, diskectomy is considered because of acute intractable pain; mild paresis; persistent, less severe pain; or the possibility of permanent disability. In patients without severe neurologic loss or symptoms, sciatica has been shown to resolve with time with either expectant care or aggressive rehabilitation. However, studies by Weber[2] and Saal and Saal[3] indicated a mean work loss of 4 months or longer in nonsurgical patients. Many patients request surgical intervention because it is perceived that surgery will more quickly relieve pain and allow an early return to usual activities.

Microsurgical techniques can achieve these goals in most patients. A smaller incision, improved lighting, and magnification optics have allowed less traumatic decompression of the root. In patients without coexisting stenosis, facetectomy is not needed.[4,5] The use of a limited diskectomy technique, as described by Spengler and associates,[6] shortens the surgical time and decreases the intraoperative risk of visceral injury and postoperative pain. Biomechanical studies indicate that a minimal laminotomy alone does not destabilize the vertebral segment and that activities may be rapidly resumed.[7]

In that sense, the short-term outcomes of microsurgery have redefined the indications for diskectomy. In the past, when the postoperative course required several months of convalescence, the benefits of surgery compared with the morbidity of traditional laminectomy needed to be carefully weighed. With microsurgical techniques used by experienced surgeons, intraoperative morbidity has been minimized. Activity restrictions recommended after microdiskectomy have varied but are uniformly shorter than those after conventional laminectomy. As a benchmark, it is worth reviewing the often-cited 1983 study by Weber,[2] which compared randomized surgical and nonsurgical treatment in a selected cohort of patients with lumbar disk herniation. Patients with severe sciatica and serious motor loss were excluded from this study. All patients had been treated conservatively, mainly with bed rest for at least 3 weeks. The average sick leave after surgery in this "subacute" group was reported to be approximately 12 weeks. These surgeries were mainly done in the 1970s and included decompressions that were prob-ably more destabilizing than the usual microsurgical techniques used today.

In contrast, developers of microdiskectomy techniques[5,8,9] have recommended earlier, aggressive mobilization and shorter postoperative convalescence. My group at Stanford University Medical Center recommends that patients return to full occupational, domestic, and recreational activities as soon as they feel able to after microdiskectomy. Patients also are told to expect some back and leg pain postoperatively but that this is "normal" and that the presence of some discomfort should not be cause to curtail or limit their activities. As a result of this practice, the sick leave time after surgery has been markedly reduced. The mean duration of sick leave in 152 consecutive working patients after microdiskectomy was found to be 1.2 weeks.[4,10] Approximately 25% of patients returned to work within 3 days.

Diagnosis and Imaging

Advanced MRI has revolutionized the treatment of sciatica. Although a typical large, paramedial extruded fragment can be satisfactorily seen with CT or myelography, MRI has largely supplanted these methods because of its superior resolution and ease of imaging. More importantly, smaller herniations and foraminal herniations or far lateral herniations are much more clearly defined with MRI.

A CT scan may still be recommended for some patients because of their size or intolerance of confined spaces.

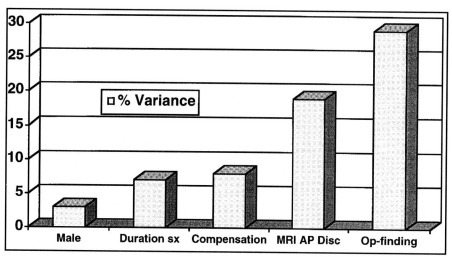

Fig. 1 Percent contribution to clinical outcomes of preoperative variables in a microdiskectomy model of 247 consecutive patients. Duration sx = duration of symptoms; Compensation = involvement in workers' compensation claims; MRI AP Disc = anteroposterior disk size; Op-finding = surgical finding.

More commonly, these obstacles can be overcome with open MRI scans and mild conscious sedation. Sometimes spinal deformities are more difficult to evaluate with MRI because of the difficulty of maintaining an oriented plane of reference. CT myelography with imaging cuts along the disk axis may allow a less complex view of the disk pathology in three dimensions. Similarly, sciatica in the presence of hypertrophic spondylosis may be difficult to interpret with MRI because of the relatively poor resolution around dense cortical bone. Again, CT alone or with myelography may provide a better view of bony impingement in this circumstance.

Diskography is most commonly used to discern the cause of axial pain in the spine. Less commonly, diskography has been used to delineate a disk rupture and the extruded fragment,[11] particularly in the postoperative spine, where scarring may obscure detail.

Diskography also may be used as a provocative test in some patients with atypical sciatica and back pain. The intention of this procedure is to reproduce the patient's pain with disk injection when other methods have failed to discern a clear root compression. In some patients, annular tears can be seen that may reproduce back and leg pain as the dye tracks to the outer anulus fibrosus. Care must be taken, however, in evaluating provocative pain results in diskography. Recent work has shown that subjects with no low back pain or sciatica may have significant pain produced by disk injection.[12-14] Furthermore, disk-injection pain intensity seems to be linked to preexisting chronic pain behavior and psychological distress.[13] The reliability of the self-reported "concordancy" of pain also has not been proved. In an experimental study, subjects with known nonspinal pain due to iliac crest bone graft harvesting reported pain reproduction with disk injection.[14] That is, in subjects without discogenic pain but with a known pelvic source of pain, buttock and thigh pain was reproduced by disk injection.

Treating an annular tear without disk extrusion, as diagnosed by diskography, microdiskectomy has not been clearly shown to be effective. The basic principle of microdiskectomy is to decompress the root. For an isolated annular tear without mechanical compression, the operation may not make theoretic sense. If the painful process in these instances is a chemical irritation of the root by products escaping from the annular tear, then a procedure that puts a larger hole in the disk may not be helpful.

Determining Outcomes

Lumbar diskectomy in a patient with severe incapacitating sciatica can be one of the most dramatically successful procedures in modern medicine. Near-immediate pain relief, rapid neurologic recovery, and return to high levels of function often are seen and usually are anticipated. However, a number of patients remain unimproved, rapidly relapse, have recurrent herniations, or develop disabling axial symptoms. In fact, the ineffective surgical treatment of sciatica caused by herniated lumbar intervertebral disks is a major health care problem. Depending on the series reviewed, up to 20% to 40% of diskectomies done for herniated lumbar intervertebral disks result in serious postoperative difficulties.[2,6,8,15-20]

Research has focused on the type of decompression, the demographic characteristics and psychological profile of surgical patients, and diagnostic accuracy in an effort to explain surgical failure.[1,9,17-19,21] As described above, modern imaging studies have improved to the point that negative explorations are rare, and the clinical presentation of a patient with acute sciatica usually is straightforward. Yet failures continue to occur; each year in the United States, surgical failures may occur in 40,000 to 80,000 patients with serious persistent or recurrent spinal troubles.[1,22]

Junge and associates[23] found that patient level of education, application for disability benefits, and duration and severity of preoperative symptoms, as well as preoperative work loss, depression, and the presence of other bodily pains or "back diagnoses," had predictive value in determining clinical outcome after lumbar disk surgery. Nygaard and associates[24] also found that duration of sciatica, as well as duration of sick leave, had value as predictive factors concerning postoperative results after lumbar diskectomy.

Spengler and associates,[6] in a careful clinical trial, found that abnormal scores on the Minnesota Multiphasic Personality Inventory Hypochondriasis and Hysteria scales correlated with poor outcomes. Carragee and Kim[17] reported that involvement in workers' compensation claims, concurrent medical illness, and female sex were statistically significant predictors of poor clinical outcome in surgically treated patients. More recently, Loupasis and associates[25] found that poorer final outcomes were associated with female sex, heavy labor, and level of education.

In following approximately 250 patients, Carragee and associates[26] compared the contribution to outcome variance of the most common predictive factors (Fig. 1). This analysis indicated that MRI findings of fragment type and herniation size and shape were the most consistent predictors of clinical results.

Disk Fragments and Annular Defects

Few studies to date have focused on the herniated disk itself as a predictor of clinical outcome. Faulhauer and Manicke[27] compared the frequency of recurrent herniations and the clinical outcomes for 100 patients undergoing disk fragment excision to those of 100 patients undergoing conventional diskectomy, including extensive annulotomy. They found that patients who underwent fragment "incision" had fewer recurrent herniations and postoperative instability symptoms than did patients who underwent conventional diskectomy. More recently, Vucetic and associates[28] in 1997 compared

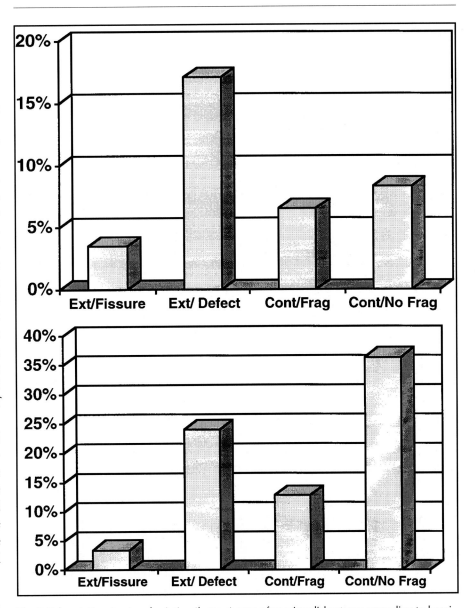

Fig. 2 Reherniation (*top*) and sciatica (*bottom*) rates after microdiskectomy according to herniation fragment type and annular defect found at surgery. Ext/Fissure = extruded or sequestrated fragments with a slit-like or minimal annular defect; Ext/Defect = extruded or sequestrated fragments resulting in large or massive annular defects; Cont/Frag = contained disks with subannular detached fragments; Cont/No Frag = contained annular prolapse without clear subannular fragments.

preoperative symptoms and postoperative outcomes in 98 patients with ruptures of the anulus fibrosus with those of 62 patients with an intact anulus fibrosus (contained disk herniations). Patients with a ruptured anulus had shorter average durations of sciatica and improved clinical outcomes compared with patients with an intact anulus.

Carragee and Kim[17] reported that patients with larger disk herniations on MRI before surgery had superior outcomes compared with patients with smaller herniations.

For the past 10 years, I have prospectively documented surgical findings regarding the type of disk herniation (contained versus extruded/sequestrated)

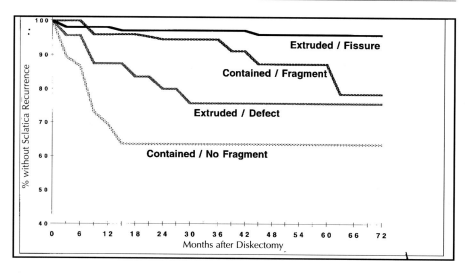

Fig. 3 Adjusted Kaplan-Meier plot of sciatica-free survival versus herniation type.

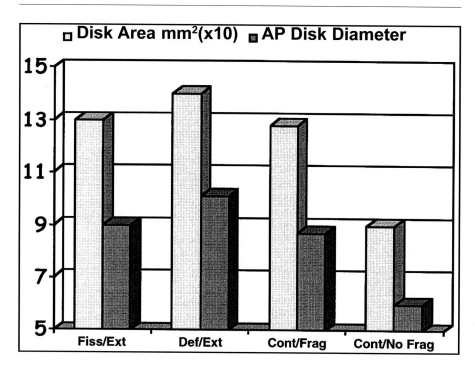

Fig. 4 The MRI measures herniation size in AP diameter (mm) and area (mm²) dimensions comparing different herniation types.

and the status of the posterior anulus fibrosus after diskectomy. An empiric classification of pathologic disk and annular findings has been developed that appears to have predictive value in clinical outcomes and rates of recurrent or persistent sciatica and revision surgery. From these observations, four catagories of disk herniations were made: (1) extruded or sequestrated fragments with a slit-like or minimal annular defect (extruded/fissure; n = 89); (2) extruded or sequestrated fragments, including the anulus fibrosus, resulting in large or massive annular defects (extruded/defect; n = 33); (3) contained disks with sub-annular detached fragments removed after oblique incision of the anulus fibrosus (minimal annular defect) (contained/fragment; n = 42); and (4) contained annular prolaspe without clear subannular fragments, "requiring" extensive annulotomy and piecemeal removal of the annular protrusion, and leaving a large or massive annular defect (contained/no fragment; n = 16).

Analysis of outcomes showed significant differences among these categories (Fig. 2). The extruded/fissure group had the best overall outcomes and the lowest incidence of reherniation (1.1%). In contrast, the extruded/defect group accounted for most of the frank reherniations and revision surgeries over time. This group also accounted for all of the multiple disk reherniations and had an 18% fusion rate. The contained/fragment group tended to do well, although the recurrence rate was slightly higher than in the extruded/fissure group.

The treatment of annular prolapse with no discrete fragment (contained/no fragment group) by conventional annulotomy and limited diskectomy was unsatisfactory. By 1 year after surgery, 30% of the group had significant recurrent sciatica. Most had no "reherniation," and aggressive conservative methods did not improve outcomes. Outcome scores reflected dramatically poorer functional, pain, and satisfaction ratings compared with the other treatment groups. It is interesting that this group had milder preoperative symptoms, a longer preoperative course, and smaller MRI measures of herniation size than did the other groups. Also noteworthy is that there were more compensation claims and psychometric abnormalities in the contained/no fragment group. This small group of patients with sciatica appears in this regard to have a clinical pro-file resembling that of chronic back pain sufferers, with atten-dant pain be-havior and social/economic factors dis-proportionate to the pathoanatomic findings.

MRI Findings

Although some authors claim that the size of disk herniation found by MRI or CT has no predictive value in sciatica,[29,30] others have reported very high success rates in a subgroup of patients with large disk herniations excised by posterior diskectomy. In studies examining preoperative MRI scans, the size and shape of the protrusion appeared to predict the success of treatment more accurately than did the clinical findings, such as compensation status, age, and gender.[17,31] Others have indicated that the integrity of the anulus fibrosus may correlate with clinical outcomes.[19,28,32,33] Specifically, in a small cohort, Carragee and Kim[17] found uniformly good results in patients with herniation AP diameters larger than 8 mm. Knop-Jergas and associates[31] noted that patients with focal as opposed to broad-based protrusions on MRI had better outcomes after diskectomy.

Carragee and associates[26] found that MRI findings predicted intraoperative findings moderately well and that intraoperative findings in turn predicted clinical outcomes (Figs. 3 and 4). These results demonstrate the clear relation of small disk size with the failure to find a subannular or extruded fragment and, consequently, poorer outcomes. Similarly, the largest disk herniations by area correlated with extruded fragments with massive annular defects, associated with increased rates of reherniation.

Summary

A very high percentage of patients coming to surgery for large disk extrusions and sciatica do very well with minimally invasive diskectomy. In most patients given relatively early surgical treatment, the primary predictor of outcome is the size of the disk herniation and the remaining competency of the anulus fibrosus. With the passage of time and with prolonged disability before surgery, psychosocial factors become increasingly important in determining outcomes. Factors such as psychological distress, depression, involvement with workers' compensation claims and disability claims, drug and alcohol abuse, and level of education appear to be secondary factors, at least initially, in subjects with large extruded fragments. In subjects with smaller disk herniation or in those with chronic disability, these factors may indicate a higher risk of treatment failure.

References

1. Frymoyer JW: Back pain and sciatica. *N Engl J Med* 1988;318:291-300.

2. Weber H: Lumbar disc herniation: A controlled, prospective study with ten years of observation. *Spine* 1983;8:131-140.

3. Saal JA, Saal JS: Nonoperative treatment of herniated lumbar intervertebral disc with radiculopathy: An outcome study. *Spine* 1989;14:431-437.

4. Carragee EJ, Han MY, Yang B, Kim DH, Kraemer H, Billys J: Activity restrictions after posterior lumbar discectomy: A prospective study of outcomes in 152 cases with no postoperative restrictions. *Spine* 1999;24:2346-2351.

5. McCulloch JA: Microdiscectomy, in Frymoyer JW, Ducker TB, Hadler NM, Kostuik JP, Weinstein JN, Whitecloud TS III (eds): *The Adult Spine: Principles and Practice.* New York, NY, Raven Press, 1991, vol 2, pp 1765-1783.

6. Spengler DM, Ouellette EA, Battie M, Zeh J: Elective discectomy for herniation of a lumbar disc: Additional experience with an objective method. *J Bone Joint Surg Am* 1990;72:230-237.

7. Goel VK, Goyal S, Clark C, Nishiyama K, Nye T: Kinematics of the whole lumbar spine: Effect of discectomy. *Spine* 1985;10:543-554.

8. Kahanovitz N, Viola K, McCulloch J: Limited surgical discectomy and microdiscectomy: A clinical comparison. *Spine* 1989;14:79-81.

9. Long DM: Decision making in lumbar disc disease. *Clin Neurosurg* 1992;39:36-51.

10. Carragee EJ, Helms E, O'Sullivan GS: Are postoperative activity restrictions necessary after posterior lumbar discectomy? A prospective study of outcomes in 50 consecutive cases. *Spine* 1996;21:1893-1897.

11. Guyer RD, Ohnmeiss DD: Lumbar discography: Position statement from the North American Spine Society Diagnostic and Therapeutic Committee. *Spine* 1995;20:2048-2059.

12. Carragee EJ, Chen Y, Tanner CM, Hayward C, Rossi M, Hagle C: Can discography cause long-term back symptoms in previously asymptomatic subjects? *Spine* 2000;25:1803-1808.

13. Carragee EJ, Tanner CM, Khurana S, et al: The rates of false-positive lumbar discography in select patients without low back symptoms. *Spine* 2000;25:1373-1381.

14. Carragee EJ, Tanner CM, Yang B, Brito JL, Truong T: False-positive findings on lumbar discography: Reliability of subjective concordance assessment during provocative disc injection. *Spine* 1999;24:2542-2547.

15. Andrews DW, Lavyne MH: Retrospective analysis of microsurgical and standard lumbar discectomy. *Spine* 1990;15:329-335.

16. Barrios C, Ahmed M, Arrotegui J, Bjornsson A, Gillstrom P: Microsurgical versus standard removal of herniated lumbar disc: A 3-year comparison in 150 cases. *Acta Orthop Scand* 1990;61:399-403.

17. Carragee EJ, Kim DH: A prospective analysis of magnetic resonance imaging findings in patients with sciatica and lumbar disc herniation: Correlation of outcomes with disc fragment and canal morphology. *Spine* 1997;22:1650-1660.

18. Dvorak J, Gauchat MH, Valach L: The outcome of surgery for lumbar disc herniation: I. A 4-17 years' followup with emphasis on somatic aspects. *Spine* 1988;13:1418-1422.

19. Eismont FJ, Currier B: Surgical management of lumbar intervertebral-disc disease. *J Bone Joint Surg Am* 1989;71:1266-1271.

20. Kotilainen E, Valtonen S: Clinical instability of the lumbar spine after microdiscectomy. *Acta Neurochir (Wien)* 1993;125:120-126.

21. Main CJ, Wood PL, Hollis S, Spanswick CC, Waddell G: The Distress and Risk Assessment Method: A simple patient classification to identify distress and evaluate the risk of poor outcome. *Spine* 1992;17:42-52.

22. Wiesel SW, Rothman RH: Lumbar disc disease and spinal stenosis, in Evarts CM (ed): *Surgery of the Musculoskeletal System.* New York, NY, Churchill Livingstone, 1983, vol 2, pp 57-84.

23. Junge A, Dvorak J, Ahrens S: Predictors of bad and good outcomes of lumbar disc surgery: A prospective clinical study with recommendations for screening to avoid bad outcomes. *Spine* 1995;20:460-468.

24. Nygaard OP, Romner B, Trumpy JH: Duration of symptoms as a predictor of outcome after lumbar disc surgery. *Acta Neurochir (Wien)* 1994;128:53-56.

25. Loupasis GA, Stamos K, Katonis PG, Sapkas G, Korres DS, Hartofilakidis G: Seven- to 20-year outcome of lumbar discectomy. *Spine* 1999;24:2323-2417.

26. Carragee E, Han M, Kim D, et al: Fragment-type and anular defect as predictive factors in lumbar discectomy, in *Proceedings of the 26th Conference of the International Society for the Study of the Lumbar Spine, Kona, HI.* Toronto, ON, Canada, ISSLS, 1999, pp 4-5.

27. Faulhauer K, Manicke C: Fragment excision versus conventional disc removal in the microsurgical treatment of herniated lumbar disc. *Acta Neurochir (Wien)* 1995;133:107-111.

28. Vucetic N, de Bri E, Svensson O: Clinical history in lumbar disc herniation: A prospective study in 160 patients. *Acta Orthop Scand* 1997; 68:116-120.

29. Deyo RA: Magnetic resonance imaging of the lumbar spine: Terrific test or tar baby? *N Engl J Med* 1994;331:115-116.

30. Enzmann DR: On low back pain. *AJNR Am J Neuroradiol* 1994;15:109-113.

31. Knop-Jergas BM, Zucherman JF, Hsu KY, DeLong B: Anatomic position of a herniated nucleus pulposus predicts the outcome of lumbar discectomy. *J Spinal Disord* 1996; 9:246-250.

32. Burton AK, Tillotson KM, Main CJ, Hollis S: Psychosocial predictors of outcome in acute and subchronic low back trouble. *Spine* 1995; 20:722-728.

33. Pople IK, Griffith HB: Prediction of an extruded fragment in lumbar disc patients from clinical presentations. *Spine* 1994;19:156-158.

Lumbar Microdiskectomy: Microsurgical Technique for Treatment of Lumbar Herniated Nucleus Pulposus

Rick B. Delamarter, MD

Introduction

Several studies published during the past decade have noted little difference in the ultimate outcomes between microsurgical diskectomy and standard laminectomy and diskectomy,[1-3] even though the microscope provides better illumination and visualization than do loops and headlights. However, patients who undergo microscopic techniques have less morbidity and are discharged earlier than are patients who undergo standard or limited diskectomies.[4-6]

With the microscope, the surgeon can limit the amount of tissue dissection by working through a small exposure directly over the pathology to be removed. Microsurgical techniques preserve the ligamentum flavum and epidural fat while minimizing postoperative epidural fibrosis. With this approach, the disk herniation can be easily removed, lateral recess stenosis can be decompressed, and nerve root manipulation is kept to a minimum. I have been using this technique since 1986 for most lumbar disk herniations and have found the approach to be safe, with fewer dural tears and nerve root injuries and less postoperative epidural fibrosis than with standard diskectomy.

Technique

The patient is positioned prone with the abdomen free, relieving pressure on the abdominal venous system and decreasing venous backflow through Batson's plexus into the spinal canal. Several frames are available that place the patient in the knee-chest position to free the abdomen.

A lumbar microdiskectomy usually is done with the patient under general anesthesia, primarily for control of the airway and sedation. Another advantage of general anesthesia is that it allows the option of hypotensive anesthesia. The procedure also can be done with the patient under epidural or local anesthesia.

Identification of Level of Surgery

Before surgical preparation and draping, the level of the disk to be removed can be localized by fluoroscopy or plain radiography. This is best done by placing a spinal needle approximately 2 cm to the side of the spinous process on the side opposite that of surgery. The spinal needle can be placed down to the level of the facet joint and the skin marked accordingly. The side of entry is generally determined by the most symptomatic side, although occasionally a midline disk herniation may be approached from both sides. Even though a radiograph, taken before the incision is made, localizes the level, a radiograph with a marker at the appropriate level always should be taken after exposure. In most cases, wrong-level surgery occurs when only a preincision radiograph is taken and is highly unlikely when an intraoperative radiograph has been taken.

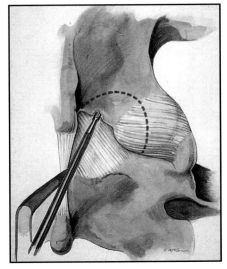

Fig. 1 Following skin exposure and subperiosteal elevation, the retractor in position reveals the interlaminar interval, with exposure of the upper and lower laminae. Several millimeters of the cephalad lamina and 2 to 3 mm of the medial edge of inferior facet are removed with the high-speed burr. This bone can be safely removed because the undersurface is protected by the ligamentum flavum.

Skin Incision and Interlaminar Space Exposure

The skin incision generally is 2 to 3 cm long and can be made in the midline or up to 1 cm lateral to the spinous process on the symptomatic side. The dorsal lumbar fascia is sharply split in line with the incision, and subperiosteal muscle dissection and elevation are done at the interlaminal level being exposed. (A

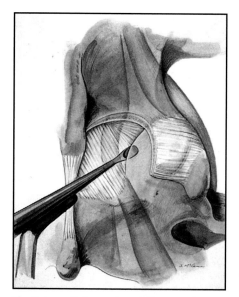

Fig. 2 A small, forward-angled curette frees the ligamentum flavum from its attachment to the medial edge of the superior facet. The ligamentum flavum also can be freed from the undersurface of the upper and lower laminae.

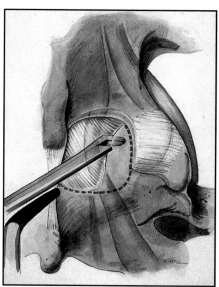

Fig. 3 A 3-mm or 4-mm Kerrison rongeur is used to remove the lateral recess (subarticular) stenosis (ie, the medial edge of the superior facet) back to the pedicle of the lower vertebra and cephalad to the top of the superior facet. This bony resection removes the lateral recess (subarticular) stenosis and allows exposure of the lateral disk space.

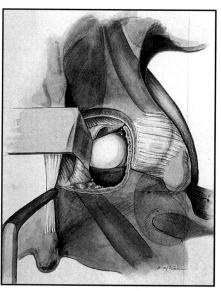

Fig. 4 A nerve root retractor is used to retract the ligamentum flavum, nerve root sleeve, and epidural fat toward midline over the herniated disk. Bipolar cautery can be used to cauterize the epidural plexus over the disk herniation.

localizing radiograph can be taken at this point by placing a forward-angle curette underneath the ligamentum flavum or lamina.) Once the interlaminar space is exposed, the retractor is positioned and the microscope is brought into position for the microdiskectomy (Fig. 1).

Spinal Canal Entry
A high-speed burr (AM-8; Midas Rex, Ft. Worth, TX) is used to remove several millimeters of the cephalad lamina and 2 to 3 mm of the medial aspect of the inferior facet (Fig. 2). Once this cephalad lamina and medial aspect of the inferior facet have been removed, the ligamentum flavum is easily seen because it attaches to the medial edge of the superior facet as well as to the upper and lower laminae. The ligamentum flavum attaches at the very cephalad edge of the lower lamina but approximately halfway up the upper lamina. Thus, up to 50% of the upper lamina as well as

the medial aspect of the inferior facet can be removed without exposure of the dural sac or nerve root because they are covered by the ligamentum flavum.

The ligamentum flavum is now released from the medial edge of the superior facet and from the upper and lower laminae with a small forward-angled curette (Fig. 2). After release of the ligamentum flavum, the medial edge of the superior facet is resected with 2-mm, 3-mm, and 4-mm Kerrison rongeurs. This resection goes from the lower pedicle to the tip of the superior facet (Fig. 3). Removal of the medial edge of the superior facet decompresses the lateral recess stenosis and allows easy exposure of the lateral disk space. If necessary, some of the lateral ligamentum flavum, particularly into the foramen, can be removed with 3-mm and 4-mm Kerrison rongeurs.

At this point, minimal bleeding can be controlled with bipolar cautery along

the lateral disk space directly cephalad to the pedicle. This allows easy visualization of the lateral disk space. The nerve root retractor is now placed on the lateral disk space, and the ligamentum flavum, epidural fat, and nerve root are retracted across the herniated disk toward the midline (Fig. 4). This maneuver provides excellent exposure of the disk herniation and, again, bipolar cautery can be used to cauterize any epidural veins over the disk herniation. Any large fragments of disk can now be removed (Fig. 5). Frequently the annulotomy created by the disk herniation is all that is necessary to allow cleaning out of any loose nucleus pulposus inside the disk space, although the annulotomy can be enlarged with a No. 11 blade.

After removal of any loose nucleus pulposus, the disk is irrigated with a long angiographic catheter, and pituitary forceps are used to free any loose fragments. The spinal canal is then palpated under-

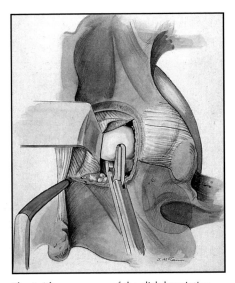

Fig. 5 After exposure of the disk herniation, large free fragments can be removed with a pituitary rongeur, and/or the natural annulotomy from the disk herniation can be enlarged with a No. 11 blade.

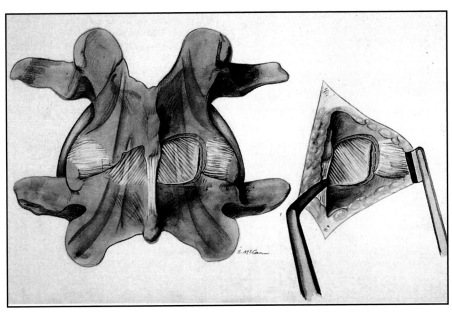

Fig. 6 After thorough irrigation, the nerve root retractor is released, allowing the ligamentum flavum and nerve root sleeve to return to their normal anatomic positions.

neath the nerve root and across the vertebral body toward the midline for any residual disk fragments. Although curettes can occasionally be used inside the disk space to remove loose nucleus pulposus, caution should be taken not to curette the end plates.

Once decompression is complete, the entire exposure is thoroughly irrigated with an antibiotic solution, and any bleeding controlled with bipolar cautery or gel foam. After complete hemostasis and removal of all gel foam, closure can proceed (Fig. 6).

The dorsal lumbar fascia is closed with No. 1 or 0 sutures, followed by the subcutaneous layer with 2-0 sutures and the skin with 3-0 subcuticular sutures. After closure, the skin can be injected with 0.5% bupivacaine with epinephrine, which provides immediate early postoperative pain relief. Sixty mg of ketorolac tromethaine (Toradol; Hoffmann-La Roche, Newark, NJ) are given 20 minutes before closure of the skin, and 30 mg are given intramuscularly or intravenously every 6 hours for the first postoperative day.

Postoperative Course

Many lumbar microdiskectomies can be done on an outpatient basis. (For example, when a patient lives within 30 to 45 minutes of the hospital and is able to urinate, the patient may be discharged from the outpatient facility.) Most patients generally are sent home within 23 hours. Most are encouraged to walk as tolerated, and many return to work within 5 to 10 days, particularly those with light-duty or desk jobs. All patients are required to participate in lumbar physical therapy, primarily stabilization and mobilization, beginning around 4 weeks after surgery. They are allowed to return to normal athletic activity when the physical therapist agrees that strength and mobilization are back to normal. Most athletes return to their normal athletic activities within 8 weeks after surgery. However, the postoperative course is variable and return to normal activities depends on the patient's overall medical condition and neurologic and overall recovery.

Discussion

In a critical analysis of 395 patients with more than 2 years of follow-up in whom lumbar microdiskectomies were performed using this ligamentum flavum-sparing microsurgical approach, all patients had symptomatic disk herniations unresolved with conservative care. Of the 395 patients, 215 had herniations at L4-5, 158 at L5-S1, and 22 at L3-4. Twenty-nine patients had herniations of two disks. Their average age was 42 years (range, 15 to 93 years). Follow-up of 2 to 12 years (average, 3.1 years) revealed excellent or good results in 93% of the patients, fair results in 6%, and poor results in 1% (three patients). Complications were minimal and included five dural tears, three instances of postoperative diskitis, and eight recurrent disk herniations. There were no nerve root or cauda equina injuries.

Compared with standard diskectomy techniques, this ligamentum flavum-sparing approach provides similar (if not better) long-term results, with decreased frequency of retained lateral recess stenosis and recurrent disk herniations. By not disturbing the ligamentum flavum, nerve root sleeve, and epidural fat, this approach is safe, with a decreased instance of dural tears, nerve root injury, and postoperative epidural fibrosis.

References

1. Abramovitz JN, Neff SR: Lumbar disc surgery: Results of the Prospective Lumbar Discectomy Study of the Joint Section on Disorders of the Spine and Peripheral Nerves of the American Association of Neurological Surgeons and the Congress of Neurological Surgeons. *Neurosurgery* 1991;29:301-308.

2. Barrios C, Ahmed M, Arrotegui J, Bjornsson A, Gillstrom P: Microsurgery versus standard removal of the herniated lumbar disc: A 3-year comparison in 150 cases. *Acta Orthop Scand* 1990;61:399-403.

3. Striffeler H, Groger U, Reulen HJ: "Standard" microsurgical lumbar discectomy vs "conservative" microsurgical discectomy: A preliminary study. *Acta Neurochir (Wien)* 1991;112:62-64.

4. Caspar W, Campbell B, Barbier DD, Kretschmmer R, Gotfried Y: The Caspar microsurgical discectomy and comparison with a conventional standard lumbar disc procedure. *Neurosurgery* 1991;28:78-87.

5. Silvers HR: Microsurgical versus standard lumbar discectomy. *Neurosurgery* 1988;22: 837-841.

6. Tullberg T, Isacson J, Weidenhielm L: Does microscopic removal of lumbar disc herniation lead to better results than the standard procedure? Results of a one-year randomized study. *Spine* 1993;18:24-27.

Microsurgery in the Lumbar Intertransverse Interval

John A. McCulloch, MD, FRCSC
Bradley K. Weiner, MD

Introduction

The interlaminar window (laminectomy) is the obvious route for lumbar decompression or diskectomy, but some lumbar encroachment pathology should be approached laterally, through the intertransverse window (Fig. 1). In addition, the most common lumbar fusion procedure still involves placing bone graft material in the intertransverse interval. It is not an anatomic area of the spine that has received much attention, except as the area lateral to the facet joint and pars interarticularis "where bone is laid at the end of the case in hope of achieving a fusion."

The intertransverse window is not easily understood without the use of the operating microscope.[1] The transverse process/intertransverse ligament complex is on the same coronal (frontal) plane as the floor of the spinal canal. When crossing the intertransverse ligament to enter the foramen, the surgical field becomes deeper than the interlaminar entry into the spinal canal. In addition, the ability to maneuver surgical instruments in the intertransverse window is more restricted. The depth of the field and the limited maneuverability of instruments require the magnification and especially the illumination of the microscope to facilitate surgery in the lumbar intertransverse interval.[2]

Anatomy of the Intertransverse Window

The superior and inferior boundaries of the intertransverse window are the respective superior and inferior borders of the transverse processes (except at L5-S1, where the ala of the sacrum forms the inferior border).[3] The lateral extent of the window is the tip of each transverse process and is the least important aspect of the anatomy. The key point of the anatomy of the window is medial, where the border is formed by the lateral margin of the respective superior facets, linked by the lateral pars interarticularis. The lateral pars interarticularis is so named to distinguish it from the isthmic pars interarticularis, where spondylolytic lesions occur. The lateral pars is simply the thickened lateral edge of the lamina, with the thickened or buttressed bone running from the base of the superior facet to the top of the inferior facet. The roof of the intertransverse window is the intertransverse ligament. It is important to maintain this ligament as a bed on which to place bone graft for intertransverse fusions.

Opening the intertransverse ligament allows entry to the foramen and the extraforaminal regions of the spinal canal (Fig. 2). The most important anatomic feature of the foramen is that its medial border is bounded by the lateral border of the lateral pars interarticularis. This is true of every level except L5, an intertransverse window that is different from all others (see below) (Fig. 3, A). Otherwise, this anatomic description applies to the intertransverse windows L4-L5, L3-L4, L2-L3, and L1-L2. Accepting that the medial border of the foramen is

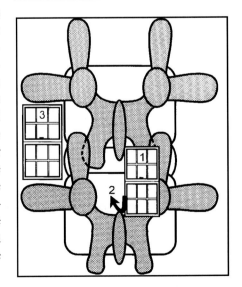

Fig. 1 There are three "windows of opportunity" into the spinal canal: (1) the interlaminar window, (2) the ipsilateral interlaminar window, to enter the contralateral side of the canal, and (3) the intertransverse window.

One or more of the authors or the departments with which they are affiliated have received something of value from a commercial or other party related directly or indirectly to the subject of this chapter.

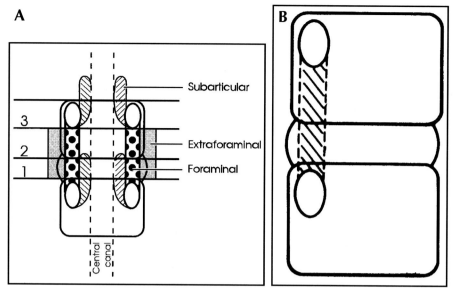

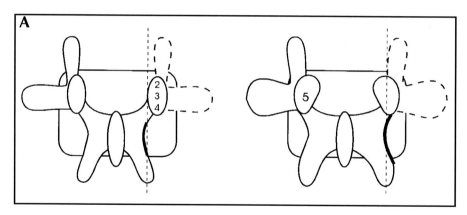

Fig. 2 A, The "grid" used to read each anatomic segment on MRI. (1) First story: disk space level. (2) Second story: foraminal level. (3) Third story: pedicle level. The lateral zone is made up of a subarticular zone, foraminal zone, and extraforaminal zone. B, The borders of the foramen are superior/inferior (pedicles), medial (medial borders of pedicle), and lateral (lateral borders of pedicle).

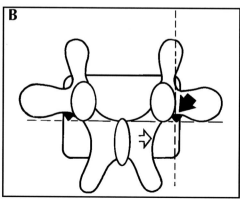

Fig. 3 A, Left, The medial border of the pedicle is on the same sagittal plane as the lateral border of the lamina (the lateral pars interarticularis, indicated by the heavy line) at L2/L3/L4. Right, The exception to this rule is L5 where the lateral pars border is on the midpedicle sagittal plane. B, The accessory process (solid arrow) marks the lateral border of the pedicle. The open arrow indicates the lateral pars interarticularis.

on the same sagittal plane as the lateral pars means that the foramen has no bony roof; its roof is the intertransverse ligament. The lateral border of the foramen is on the same sagittal plane as the accessory process (Fig. 3, B).

The L5 intertransverse window is different from the other lumbar intertransverse windows because it is smaller and much more difficult to enter surgically. It is smaller because of many factors,[3] the most important of which is the location of the lateral border of the pars interarticularis in the midsagittal plane of the pedicle (Fig. 3). The L5 foramen does have a bony roof, which is the lateral pars and lamina.

The nerve root that travels through the intertransverse window is the exiting nerve root, identified by the same number as the anatomic segmen through which it passes. Another way of stating this is that lumbar nerve roots are numbered according to the pedicle beneath which they pass to exit (or, if sensory roots, enter) the spinal canal.

The floor of the intertransverse window medially is formed by the vertebral body above and the disk space. The floor of the intertransverse window laterally is the psoas muscle that contains the extracanalicular branches of the lumbar nerves, the most important of which is the branch between L4 and L5, the furcal nerve.[2] When opening the intertransverse window to approach the foramen, it is important not to get too far laterally and damage these anastomotic branches. The furcal nerve from L4 to L5 often carries most of the motor ankle dorsiflexors, which, if damaged, may lead to a drop foot. This anatomic fact also explains that rare occasion when the L5 nerve is damaged at surgery and the patient wakes with little noticeable neurologic deficit (except for extensor hallucis longus weakness).

Pathology Deep to the Intertransverse Window

Opening the intertransverse window to enter the foramen and extraforaminal regions can provide access to various pathologies: anterior, posterior, cephalad/caudad, or combination. Anterior pathology is any pathology anterior to the nerve root; posterior pathology is any pathology posterior to the nerve root.

Anterior Pathology

Extraforaminal and/or Foraminal Lumbar Disk Herniation (E/FLDH) The most common pathology to be approached through the intertransverse window is the E/FLDH[3] (Fig. 4). Before CT was available, patients who presented with an acute radicular syndrome from an E/FLDH underwent interlaminar approaches, at which time no pathology was noted within the canal.[4] Until 1974,[5] this disk herniation location remained largely unknown. Scaglietti and Fineshi[6] in 1962 described finding this disk herniation after a negative exploration of the canal, after which they then excised the inferior facet to follow the root laterally to the disk herniation. Macnab[4] was the first to describe this disk herniation in the English literature. With the combination of sagittal and axial MRI images, this disk herniation can be clearly seen as located lateral to the lateral pars interarticularis and lying mostly in the foramen or mostly in the extraforaminal region.[3]

Most of these disk herniations occur into the L4 foramen or cephalad foramina, causing acute radicular syndromes in the lumbar plexus (anterior thigh pain). Approximately 10% occur at the L5-S1 foraminal level, affecting the exiting L5 nerve root. These herniations occur in older patients (average age, 60 years), and most come out of wide disk spaces. They are to be distinguished from the posterior foraminal root

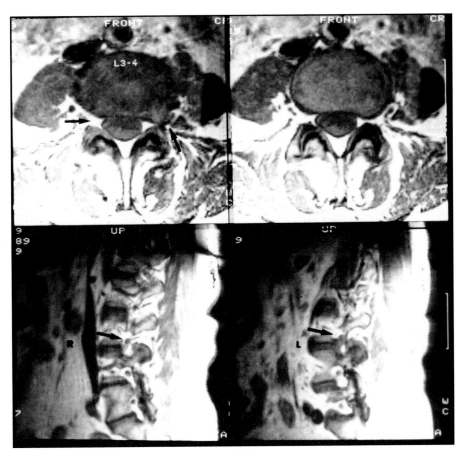

Fig. 4 *Top row*, Axial T1 MRI view with FLDH (*vertical arrow, left*). *Bottom right*, The left parasagittal T1 with FLDH (*arrow*). *Bottom left*, The right parasagittal T1 of the right foramen, which is open (*arrow*). The T1 parasagittal cut gives fat a high signal intensity and a more accurate depiction of the foramen compared with T2 parasagittal cuts.

encroachment resulting from facet subluxation and from capsular hypertrophy seen in various combinations in the degenerative spines of stenotic patients.

Uncinate Spur Originally described by Ray,[7] an uncinate spur is an osteophyte that develops on the inferior edge of the vertebral body of L5, secondary to degenerative changes in the L5-S1 motion segment (Fig. 5). Along with disk space narrowing, annular bulging, and facet subluxation, it contributes to narrowing of the L5 foramen. The uncinate spur alone usually does not cause radicular pain.

Posterior Pathology

Superior Facet Subluxation/Capsular Hypertrophy Degenerative changes in a motion segment are many and variable. One of these changes is disk space narrowing. If facet joint degeneration is also present, osteophyte enlargement of the joint (especially the superior facet) and superior migration of the tip of the superior facet (or inferior migration of the pedicle/nerve root complex), along with capsular hypertrophy, can close down from behind the foraminal space available for the nerve root (Fig. 6). A retrospondylolisthesis of the cephalad vertebral segment or on the concavity of a degenerative scoliosis further

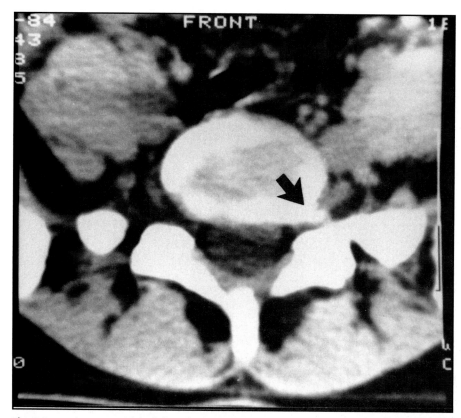

Fig. 5 An uncinate spur of the left L5 foramen (*arrow*).

Table 1
Comparison of Surgical Probing of Foramina With Radiologists' Reporting of "Foraminal Stenosis" on MRI

Foramen	Surgical Probing (%)	Radiologists' Report
Fully patent	66	32%
Stenosis		
Partial	20	68%*
Complete	14	—

*When we determined that the foramen was open to surgical probing, the radiologists reported "foraminal narrowing or stenosis" 68% of the time

narrows the nerve root foramen. The syndrome that may result is chronic radicular pain.

Cephalad/Caudad Pathology
Symmetric narrowing of a disk space without osteophytic lipping or annular bulging is a common normal aging process. With this reaction there is no (or little) reduction in the space available for the nerve root in the foramen. A forward vertebral slip (spondylolisthesis) or asymmetric narrowing of the disk space can result in a pedicular kinking of a nerve root and radicular pain (Fig. 7). The associated clinical syndrome is chronic radicular pain.

Combination Pathology
Segmental degenerative changes in the lumbar spine may combine to narrow the foramen. It is not unusual to see anterior pathology (uncinate spur) in association with facet subluxation and capsular hypertrophy, complicated by pedicular kinking, all combining to compress the nerve root in the foramen. It is unusual to see an E/FLDH (acute radicular syndrome) in conjunction with chronic radicular syndromes from facet subluxation/capsular hypertrophy and/or pedicular kinking.

Radiologic Examination of the Foramen
It is a radiologic principle that when looking at a tubular structure for encroachment pathology, the most information is gained from a slice tangential to the tubular structure. Thecal sac encroachment is best detected on axial cuts; parasagittal cuts are best to determine if there is foraminal stenosis (Figs. 4 and 6). This is one of the many reasons why MRI is superior to CT in the assessment of symptomatic degenerative lumbar disk disease.

Overreporting of Foraminal Stenosis by Radiologists
The lumbar foraminal area was not easily seen until CT became available in the past 3 decades. Before CT, foraminal pathology was not seen on myelography, and patients undergoing surgery for an acute radicular syndrome from an E/FLDH usually had negative disk explorations. After the discovery of E/FLDH on CT,[5] it became the custom to report foraminal pathology, including stenosis, on the basis of axial CT cuts. Since the advent of MRI (and routine sagittal slices) a little over a decade ago, the foramen can be seen much better on parasagittal cuts (Figs. 4 and 6).

There is still a tendency by radiologists to report any "narrowing" of the foramen on axial cuts as foraminal stenosis, when in fact the foramen is open on parasagittal slices. To test our

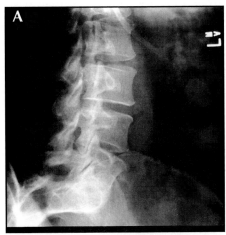

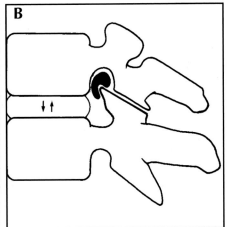

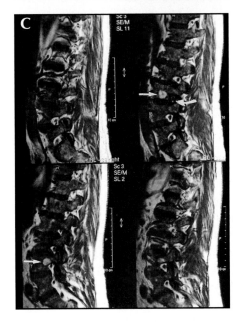

Fig. 6 A, Plain radiograph showing L5 facet subluxation. B, Schematic of superior facet subluxation secondary to disk space narrowing (*arrows*) compressing the exiting nerve root. C, T1 parasagittal MRI scan. *Top,* A full L3 foramen (right) from facet subluxation and capsular hypertrophy (*curved arrow*). Note the high signal intensity from fat forming a bright (white) halo around the foramen above and below L3. *Bottom,* Open foramen (*left*). The arrows identify marrow fatty necrosis (L3, *right*).

tific study. For a patient who has, in addition to radicular symptoms, severe back pain (especially with a degenerative scoliosis), decompression with instrumentation is the appropriate choice. For a patient who has radicular symptoms caused by foraminal stenosis but no back pain, the principles discussed here are a viable option. It is assumed that in this latter patient group, nature has stabilized the segment but in doing so has narrowed the foramen. It is also likely that in the decompression/stabilization group of patients, multiple levels need surgical redress, whereas in the patient needing decompression of the foramen for dominant radicular pain, one, and rarely two, levels need to be approached surgically.

Principles of Surgery in the Intertransverse Window

There are two surgical approaches to the intertransverse window. The first is the paraspinal approach, splitting the paraspinal muscles to approach the interval directly (Fig. 8). This is a nonexpansile approach that allows surgery in the foraminal and extraforaminal zones only. If surgery is required inside the spinal canal, this approach will not expand to meet that need. The paraspinal approach is an approach for E/FLDH excision and foraminal stenosis decompression when no spinal canal stenosis is present.

The second approach is the standard midline approach, expanding into the intertransverse interval without excising the pars interarticularis and the inferior facet to expose the foramen and extraforaminal zone. In accordance with the principles of least-invasive spine surgery, excising the inferior facet (and potentially destabilizing the segment) is not an acceptable option.

One caution in regard to the paraspinal approach is that it is very easy for the surgeon to get too far laterally and become lost. Our experience from teaching this approach is that this is the most common mistake made. The surgeon

impression that foraminal stenosis is overreported by radiologists, we passed a 3.5-mm probe through 100 foramina at the time of spinal canal stenosis surgery. Each foramen was classified at surgery as fully patent, partially stenotic, or completely stenotic (Table 1). The surgical findings were then compared with the readings of our radiologists (who were unaware of the study). A high false-positive rate (68%) on radiologic reporting was noted (Table 1). We also found an 80% agreement of our surgical probing conclusion and parasagittal MRI interpretation of foraminal stenosis. It was concluded that

radiologists routinely overreport foraminal stenosis by misinterpretation of axial MRI slices.

Microsurgical Approach to the Intertransverse Window

Three surgical procedures can be done in the intertransverse window: excision of an E/FLDH, decompression of foraminal stenosis, and uninstrumented intertransverse fusion. Determining whether microsurgical decompression of a narrowed foramen or restoration of foraminal patency with instrumentation and/or interbody procedures is more appropriate will require a long, multicentered, scien-

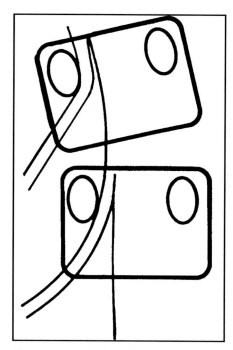

Fig. 7 Pedicular kinking of nerve root from asymmetric disk space narrowing.

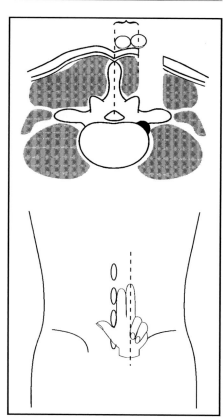

Fig. 8 The paraspinal muscle–splitting approach, starting a finger and a half's breadth off the midline.

winds up in the body of the psoas muscle, where extracanalicular branches of the lumbar plexus can be damaged. To avoid this error, it is best to adhere to the fundamental principle of never beginning to open the intertransverse window until a direct line of vision to the lateral border of the pars interarticularis is available. This border is on the same sagittal plane as the medial border of the pedicle and, therefore, is in the path of the exiting nerve root, which is the structure requiring decompression.

One other word of caution is necessary in regard to staying medial in the intertransverse window. On the rare occasion when it is necessary to approach an L1-2 foraminal disk herniation, it is easy to damage the common dural sac in the foramen because the pars interarticularis border lies more medial than any other level. Stated another way, the lateral border of the pars is medial to the medial border of the foramen at L1. At L2-3 (the L2 foramen), the relationship between the lateral border of the pars is

neutral relative to the common dural sac. Most foraminal approaches for E/FLDH are at the L4 and L3 levels and, for stenosis, at the L4 and L5 levels. It is to these cases (those except L1) that the previously stated principle applies: the surgeon should not start to open the intertransverse window until there is a direct line of vision to the lateral border of the pars interarticularis.

If facet subluxation and capsular hypertrophy have closed the intertransverse window, this is excised to open the window (Fig. 9). If facet subluxation and capsular hypertrophy have not occurred, a "safe haven" should be chosen to start opening the window (Fig. 10).

The operating depth in the intertransverse (extracanalicular) window is greater than in the interlaminar (canalicular) window. There is less neurologic

tissue to damage in the intertransverse window (one root versus the entire thecal sac), but there is not a lot of room to maneuver in the intertransverse interval. It is often common to have three instruments in the interlaminar exposure (nerve root retractor, suction, and the operating tool). Because of the narrowness of the intertransverse window, only two instruments fit comfortably and the suction by necessity becomes the nerve root retractor. For all of these reasons, the magnification and illumination of the surgical microscope are integral parts of surgery in the intertransverse window.

Surgical Procedures in the Intertransverse Window

Excision of an E/FLDH A disk herniation lateral to the lateral pars interarticularis lies in a foraminal or extraforaminal location (Figs. 2 and 4), and the best approach for excision is the paraspinal approach. It allows direct observation of the fragment without sacrificing the inferior facet. Trying to remove this disk herniation from within the canal does not provide sufficient exposure to ensure that all of the ruptured fragments of disk material have been removed. By trying to see "all of the pathology" and assure its total removal, the inferior facet often has to be sacrificed, to the detriment of future segmental stability. If the disk rupture lies even farther lateral in the extraforaminal zone (Fig. 11), it will not be seen even through an interlaminar approach, thus almost certainly leading to sacrifice of the inferior facet to find the fragment. Starting off in the intertransverse interval gives the surgeon a direct view of the foraminal and extraforaminal zones and significantly reduces the struggle of excising E/FLDH while preserving the integrity of the facet joint.

Excision of an L5 foraminal disk herniation is a special situation. Fortunately, these herniations are rare, because operating for anterior foraminal path-

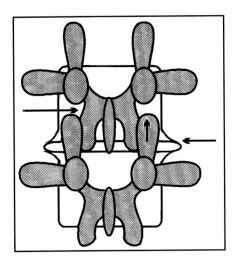

Fig. 9 With disk space narrowing (*right arrow*) and facet subluxation (*vertical arrow*), it is necessary to remove the capsule and tip of the superior facet (*left arrow*) to open the intertransverse interval.

ology is very difficult in the L5-S1 intertransverse window. After trying both the intertransverse (extracanalicular) approach and the interlaminar (canalicular) approach to the L5 foramen, we recommend the interlaminar approach to remove anterior pathology (E/FLDH) from the L5 foramen. This is done by completing a fairly wide L5 hemilaminectomy to view the medial and lateral borders of the fifth lumbar root beside the L5 pedicle. This can easily be done without sacrificing the inferior facet of L5. Following the medial border of the L5 root leads to the foraminal disk herniation.[2] For L5 posterior foraminal pathology, the intertransverse approach, discussed below, is easier.

Decompression of Foraminal Stenosis The most common cause of foraminal stenosis is superior facet subluxation, with or without capsular hypertrophy. It can be compounded by asymmetric disk space narrowing or the concavity of degenerative scoliosis.

Because of the unique relationship between the lateral pars interarticularis,

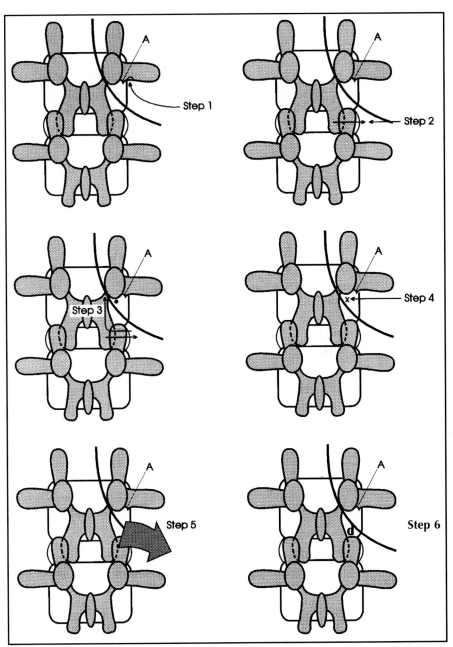

Fig. 10 Opening the intertransverse ligament to excise an FLDH. Step 1, A safe place to start is immediately lateral to the accessory process to find the lateral border of the pars interarticularis (away from the nerve root) and establish perception of depth of nerve root. Step 2, Open the capsule. Step 3, Remove the tip of the superior facet (*single arrow*) and then dissect the intertransverse ligament off the anterior aspect of the lateral pars. Step 4, Join steps 1 and 3 to free the intertransverse ligament. Step 5, Reflect the intertransverse ligament laterally. Step 6, Find the FLDH (d).

the pedicle, and the posterior position of the superior facet, the foramen cannot be decompressed from within the spinal canal. This is not a serious problem when instrumentation is used, but it is not acceptable when least-invasive spine surgery is done. Without direct observation, one cannot be certain that an ade-

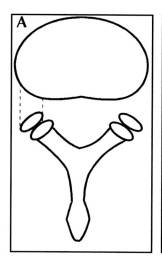 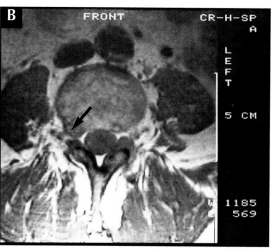 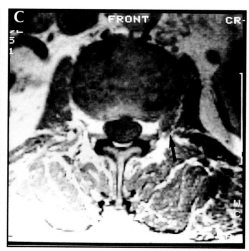

Fig. 11 A, On axial cut, the foraminal zone is between the dotted lines, which mark the medial and lateral borders of the superior facet. B, A fragment that is largely within this zone (*arrow*) is an FLDH. C, A fragment that is lateral to this zone is an E/FLDH (*arrow*).

quate decompression has been achieved. Working lateral to the pars, on the other hand, one has a direct view of the facet joint and capsule and can be sure that a complete decompression of the exiting nerve root has been accomplished.

Isolated foraminal stenosis that can be approached paraspinally is rare (Fig. 8). More common is foraminal stenosis in association with spinal canal stenosis (SCS). In this situation, a midline exposure is necessary to decompress the SCS (and the usual accompanying subarticular stenosis). Rather than reach out from within the canal to try a foraminal decompression, it is simpler and more effective to expand the exposure laterally by first going posterior to the pars interarticularis and facet joint, then lateral into the inter-trans-verse window. It is then a simple operation to open the capsule of the facet joint laterally (Fig. 10, step 2) and remove the tip of the superior facet and the capsule.

If there is a component of cephalad or caudad stenosis with pedicular kinking of the nerve root, the pedicle can be easily removed from outside the canal. This can be done with the egg-shell technique.[8] If the nerve root is still not free (a

rare occurrence), the uncinate spur and annular bulging should be excised.

Uninstrumented Intertransverse Fusion
For single- or two-level fusions, the "soft-tissue envelope" technique of uninstrumented intertransverse fusion is a viable operation.[9] Performing it least invasively and with the aid of the microscope at the time of SCS decompression for the stabilization of a degenerative spondylolisthesis has been successful. In addition, with the anticipated development of bone morphogenic protein,[10] which will abrogate the need for autologous bone graft harvest, the soft-tissue envelope technique will become even more viable. (The bilateral paraspinal approach was originally described by Wiltse and Spencer[11] for intertransverse fusion. Because it does not allow for creation of the soft-tissue envelope, the senior author [J.A.M.] has given up this approach to fusion, although it is still a good approach for a simple intertransverse fusion with pedicle screws.)

Summary
The intertransverse interval has long been known as a place to lay bone graft in hope of achieving a solid arthrodesis.

Opening it to use the interval to gain access into the foraminal and extraforaminal regions of the spinal canal has only recently been done. The anatomy is simple and embodies a common lumbar spine principle, which is to find a pedicle, because medial to it will be a nerve root. In the intertransverse interval, the lateral border of the pars interarticularis is on the same sagittal plane as the medial border of the pedicle (except for L5). Once through the interlaminar window, the anatomy is very simple—there is only one nerve root to find. The limited ability to manipulate instruments and the increased depth of the exposure make the use of the operating microscope very important.

More so than axial MRI cuts and far more so than axial CT cuts, parasagittal MRI cuts reveal a true picture of the openness of the foramen. The type of pathology, whether E/FLDH or foraminal stenosis, can be clearly delineated on parasagittal MRI. It is important, however, that radiologists not overcall foraminal stenosis on axial cuts, either CT or MRI.

Foraminal stenosis is easily decompressed by a lateral approach and is very difficult to completely decompress from within the spinal canal. If foraminal stenosis has been left behind from a previous midline SCS decompression, and if the patient has continuing leg pain, then it is easy to avoid the previous midline surgical route and take a paraspinal muscle–splitting approach to complete the foraminal decompression.

Other, as yet undiscovered uses for the intertransverse window approach likely exist. The senior author has used this approach to remove a third- or fourth-time recurrent canalicular disk herniation where the fragment is opposite the disk space (the usual situation). By avoiding the previous scarred-in canal and nerve root, it has been possible to remove the ruptured disk. Visualization, however, is not good with this approach.

Acknowledgment

The authors wish to thank Melanie Morscher, PT, for putting this manuscript together and bringing it to a successful conclusion.

References

1. McCulloch JA, Young PH: The microscope as a surgical aid, in *Essentials of Spinal Microsurgery*. Philadelphia, PA, Lippincott-Raven, 1998, pp 3-17.

2. McCulloch JA, Young PH: Foraminal and extraforaminal lumbar disc herniation, in *Essentials of Spinal Microsurgery*. Philadelphia, PA, Lippincott-Raven, 1998, pp 383-428.

3. McCulloch JA, Young PH: Musculoskeletal and neuroanatomy of the lumbar spine, in *Essentials of Spinal Microsurgery*. Philadelphia, PA, Lippincott-Raven, 1998, pp 249-292.

4. Macnab I: Negative disc exploration: An analysis of the causes of nerve-root involvement in sixty-eight patients. *J Bone Joint Surg Am* 1971; 53:891-903.

5. Abdullah AF, Ditto EW III, Byrd EB, Williams R: Extreme-lateral lumbar disc herniations: Clinical syndrome and special problems of diagnosis. *J Neurosurg* 1974;41:229-234.

6. Scaglietti O, Fineschi G: Post-foraminal discal hernias in the spinal column. *Arch Putti* 1962; 17:556-565.

7. Ray CD: Far lateral decompressions for stenosis: The paralateral approach to the lumbar spine, in White AH, Rothman RH, Ray CD (eds): *Lumbar Spine Surgery: Techniques and Complications*. St Louis, MO, CV Mosby, 1987, pp 175-186.

8. Weiner BK, McCulloch JA: Microdecompression without fusion for radiculopathy associated with lytic spondylolisthesis. *J Neurosurg* 1996;85:582-585.

9. McCulloch JA, Young PH: Posterolateral uninstrumented lumbar fusion, in *Essentials of Spinal Microsurgery*. Philadelphia, PA, Lippincott-Raven, 1998, pp 531-552.

10. Cook SD, Rueger DC: Osteogenic protein-1: Biology and applications. *Clin Orthop* 1996; 324:29-38.

11. Wiltse LL, Spencer CW: New uses and refinements of the paraspinal approach to the lumbar spine. *Spine* 1988;13:696-706.

Advantages of the Operating Microscope in Lumbar Spine Surgery

John A. McCulloch, MD, FRCSC
Derek Snook, MD
Cyril F. Kruse, MD

Introduction

The use of the operating microscope as an aid in degenerative spine surgery is standard for most neurosurgeons, although a few may not use it routinely for lumbar disk excision.[1] In contrast, few orthopaedic surgeons use the operating microscope despite the large number of spinal surgeries being done for degenerative orthopaedic conditions. The main reason for this difference is that the use of the operating microscope is widespread throughout neurosurgical training programs, whereas its use is infrequent in orthopaedic training programs. The orthopaedic surgeon who decides to become a spine surgeon is unlikely to have seen the operating microscope used in spine surgery and may be reluctant to learn a new technique because of anticipated higher complication rates, longer surgical time, and difficulty in handling the microscope. The orthopaedic surgeon is more familiar with the use of loupes, and this is the preferred method of achieving magnification for orthopaedic spine surgeons. As more

emphasis is placed on increasing precision and decreasing utilization of hospital resources, however, the use of the operating microscope as an aid in degenerative spine surgery will become more common.[2]

The Operating Microscope

Using a microscope is analogous to using binoculars to look through a magnifying glass.[2] Between the binoculars and the magnifying glass is a magnification chamber (Fig. 1). These elements are represented in the magnification equation (Fig. 2).

Also part of the microscope is a strong illumination system that provides bright, white, Xenon illumination parallel (coaxial) to the viewer's line of vision. In addition, photographic documentation equipment can be added to the microscope.

Characteristics of the Operating Microscope

The use of the operating microscope during spine surgery is advantageous because of three important factors.[3] First, there is

no direct hand-eye coordination because the microscope is positioned between the surgeon's eyes and most of the shaft of the operating instrument. The operating end of the surgical instrument is all that can be seen when looking through the microscope into the depth of the surgical wound. Arthroscopic surgery is similar in concept.

Second, the operating microscope has a limited field of vision. The average field of vision is slightly less than 4 cm, and even less if the wound opening is 2 cm. The magnification and illumination of the operating microscope enhance visibility. Nothing can be seen outside of the field of vision. Therefore, the surgeon must have detailed knowledge of spinal anatomy and know the exact location of the pathology to be approached so that surgical invasion and wound opening are at the correct spine level. The most common mistake associated with spinal microsurgery is wrong-level exploration, which is less likely to happen with a larger, nonmicrosurgical exposure to the sacrum and then "counting up" from the sacrum to the desired level of exposure.

Third, the line of vision is such that, with a small, deep wound, it is easy to

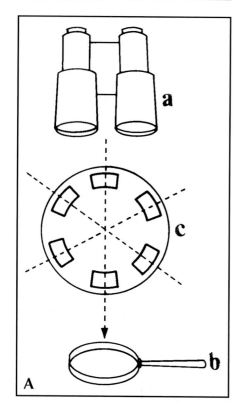

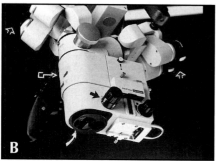

Fig. 1 A, A surgical microscope is equivalent to binoculars (a) looking through a magnifying glass (b) with a magnification chamber (c) in between. B, A Zeiss microscope head (Carl Zeiss, Thornwood, NY). Open arrows = binoculars set at 180° to each other for spine surgery. Curved arrow = magnifying glass, otherwise known as the objective. In this model, the objective has an adjustable focal distance (solid arrow), known as a varioscope. Box arrow = the magnification chamber.

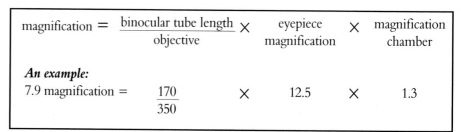

$$\text{magnification} = \frac{\text{binocular tube length}}{\text{objective}} \times \frac{\text{eyepiece}}{\text{magnification}} \times \frac{\text{magnification}}{\text{chamber}}$$

An example:

$$7.9 \text{ magnification} = \frac{170}{350} \times 12.5 \times 1.3$$

Fig. 2 Magnification Equation

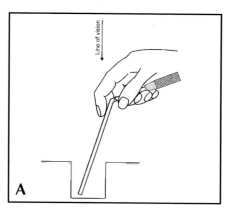

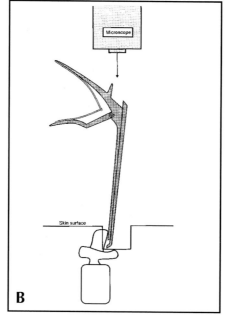

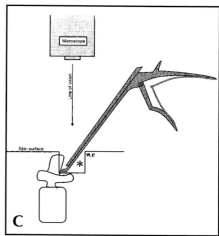

Fig. 3 A, An assistant's hand and suction in the line of vision. B, A Kerrison rongeur can also get into the line of vision. C, To avoid interference in the line of vision while operating in the "microsurgical tunnel" (*), a long instrument such as an 8" Kerrison rongeur should be used, with the narrow shaft braced on the "biologic plasticity" of the wound edge (w,e).

look down the tunnel and see an instrument or an assistant's hand (Fig. 3). Positioning of the operating microscope and the microsurgical instruments, and discipline of the assistant are easy to manage.

The Operating Microscope Compared With Loupes

Many orthopaedic surgeons believe that loupe magnification works just as well as the operating microscope. However, the use of loupes has several disadvantages. Magnification with loupes is fixed, usually at ×2.5, and cannot go above ×3.5 without a change in the prism system and much additional weight. The magnification of the operating microscope ranges from ×1 to ×20 and, on the newer microscopes, can be altered by hand or foot switches.

Although they are less expensive than the operating microscope, loupes are custom-measured and built for the individual surgeon, whereas the operating microscope can be used by several surgeons across multiple disciplines. Because loupes are custom-built, the surgeon must keep the neck in a fixed, flexed position to maintain focus, a feat unnecessary with the operating microscope. Over time, the surgeon who uses loupes will likely develop a sore neck which is less apt to occur with the use of the operating microscope.

The optics of the operating microscope compress the interpupillary distance to about 22 mm, which means that through a small, 22-mm (1 inch) skin incision, three-dimensional (3-D) vision in any depth of wound can be maintained. With loupes, the human interpupillary distance starts at approximately 60 to 65 mm, and the loupe telescopes must be angled to obtain focused 3-D visibility deep in the wound. The deeper the wound, the wider the incision needed to maintain 3-D visual depth.

Although the light source for loupes is said to be perfectly coaxial to the line of vision, fine adjustments are necessary to achieve this, and the lighting is not always perfect. The light source in the microscope is perfectly coaxial to the line of vision and routinely is a stronger, whiter light (Xenon bulb) than are the light systems generally available with loupes.

A final drawback of loupes is that observation of the surgical procedure is limited to the surgeon; the assistant and operating room personnel see little or nothing. In contrast, the operating microscope allows the assistant to see what the operating surgeon sees. Furthermore, photographic aids that can be attached to the operating microscope allow the procedure to be seen by operating room personnel and make videotaping possible.

Retrospective Study
A review of 500 consecutive lumbar microsurgical procedures, including diskectomy, decompression, and uninstrumented fusion, found results comparable to standard open procedures, with the advantages of shorter hospital stays (most were outpatient procedures), faster return to normal activity, and fewer complications.

Complications in the diskectomy group included one dural tear but no other intraoperative complications, such as root injury. No major complication of anterior disk perforation, penetrating great vessels, or other abdominal structures occurred in this group. No hospital complications, such as urinary tract infection, deep vein thrombosis, pulmonary emboli, or atelectasis, occurred in the diskectomy patients.

One diskectomy patient developed a superficial wound infection, but no patients developed diskitis. One diskectomy patient underwent repeat surgery within 30 days for a sudden recurrence of sciatica, at which time another large fragment of disk tissue was removed.

Acknowledgment
The authors wish to thank Melanie Morscher, PT, for manuscript preparation.

References
1. Fager CA: Progress, reason, and fallacy in today's world of neurosurgery. *Cleve Clin J Med* 1987;54:261-270.

2. McCulloch JA, Young PH (eds): The microscope as a surgical aid, in *Essentials of Spinal Microsurgery*. Philadelphia, PA, Lippincott-Raven, 1998, pp 3-17.

3. McCulloch JA, Young PH (eds): Complications (adverse effects) in lumbar microsurgery, in *Essentials of Spinal Microsurgery*. Philadelphia, PA, Lippincott-Raven, 1998, pp 503-529.

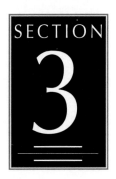

SECTION

3

Lumbar Spinal Stenosis

Lumbar Spinal Stenosis

Lumbar spinal stenosis is a common condition encountered by orthopaedic spine surgeons. In this section, four chapters written by a group of renowned spine specialists are presented regarding the pathoanatomy, clinical features, diagnostic evaluation, and nonsurgical and surgical treatment options of this condition. These chapters provide a thorough overview of lumbar spinal stenosis and also serve as an excellent introduction for medical students, residents, fellows, or general orthopaedic surgeons while also providing an excellent reference source for active orthopaedic spine surgeons.

Drs. Steven Garfin and Wolfgang Raushning introduce the concept of spinal stenosis in their chapter, defining it as "a narrowing of the spinal canal as a result of aging." The pathoanatomy of spinal stenosis as it relates to the degenerative cascade described by Kirkaldy-Willis is discussed next. Well-detailed and informative illustrations of cryotome sections of the degenerative lumbar spine accompany a descriptive analysis of the pathogenesis of canal narrowing. The various aspects of central canal and lateral recess and foraminal stenosis are also described. After additional analysis of the pathoanatomy, the following question is posed: "Why don't all patients with spinal stenosis have symptoms?" The pathophysiology of canal stenosis as it relates to nerve mechanical compression, inflammation, vascular compromise, and nutritional deficiencies are investigated in the context of clinical features. Finally, a brief review of the signs and symptoms of spinal stenosis is presented.

Dr. Richard Herzog reviews the role of imaging modalities in the diagnosis of lumbar spinal stenosis, including plain radiographs, CT with and without myelography, and MRI. Dr. Herzog stresses that the various degenerative findings noted on advanced imaging studies do not necessarily correlate with the clinical symptoms of spinal stenosis. Plain radiographs serve as a global evaluation of the degenerative process but typically do not provide information regarding the specific location of pain.

The merits of CT and MRI are then compared and contrasted. CT provides the best detail given the bony etiology of stenosis from vertebral end plate ridging or facet joint hypertrophy. MRI best shows how stenosis affects soft-tissue structures. Dynamic testing such as lumbar myelography provides a means to detect stenosis in both the supine and standing positions, although it remains unclear if the additional information provided by this modality ultimately affects treatment decisions. The use of supine and standing MRI, a relatively new dynamic modality, is also discussed. As a final point, the anatomic dilemma of lumbar foraminal stenosis is addressed, and although it is not stressed enough in this chapter, this problem must be considered in any patient who does not improve following surgical intervention.

Drs. Eric Truumees and Harry Herkowitz supply an informative chapter on the treatment of spinal stenosis, including both nonsurgical and surgical options. Nonsurgical management is typically effective, and numerous modalities are presented. However, several treatments, especially epidural steroid injections, although variably clinically effective, have not been shown with scientific reliability to have significant long-term effects. Notwithstanding, nonsurgical treatments remain the mainstay for spinal stenosis.

The indications for surgical treatment are also presented and include progressive neurologic deficit, intractable pain, or persistent functional limitations. A well-conceived section on the principles of surgical management is provided, including the goals and techniques of laminectomy and laminotomy. The controversial subject of lumbar fusion for spinal stenosis is also discussed. The main indications for arthrodesis include the presence of preoperative instability (degenerative spondylolisthesis or scoliosis) or intraoperative changes in stability (excessive facet removal). Arthrodesis for mechanical back pain is a less-well accepted indication for fusion in the presence of spinal stenosis.

Finally, Drs. Dan Riew and John Rhee address the innovative topic of microsurgery and how it relates to the management of lumbar spinal stenosis. The perceived advantages of microsurgery include adequate neural decompression in the absence of significant resection of host bone or destruction of soft tissues, perhaps improving on postoperative recovery. The indications for microdecompression are described, including the requirements that the stenosis be at the level of the disk space as opposed to diffuse or congenital and that significant spondylolisthesis be absent.

The most informative aspect of this chapter is the emphasis placed on the importance of preoperative and intraoperative planning. The "three-floor concept" described by McCullough and Young is reviewed and stresses the critical understanding of the anatomy and pathoanatomy of stenosis to ensure a reasonable clinical outcome. The technique of microsurgical lumbar laminaplasty is thoroughly reviewed from patient positioning to landmark identification to the intricacies of the decompression itself. A contralateral laminar approach on the side of the majority of leg symptoms is recommended. This approach allows for greater undercutting of the lateral recess and for nerve root decompression.

Louis G. Jenis, MD
Clinical Assistant Professor, Orthopaedic Surgery
Tufts University School of Medicine
Boston, Massachusetts

Spinal Stenosis

Steven R. Garfin, MD
Wolfgang Rauschning, MD, PhD

Introduction

Spinal stenosis by definition is a narrowing of the spinal canal, which is a common finding in an aging or degenerative spine.[1,2] Clinically, it describes a condition, usually found in older individuals, of leg pain, leg weakness, and difficulty ambulating, that may or may not be associated with a neurologic deficit. Although the imaging and pathoanatomic findings are fairly ubiquitous (and might be universal if everyone lived long enough), symptoms do not occur in all people despite similar radiographic findings.

The stenosis can occur centrally across the cauda equina, or more laterally.[3-5] The degenerative changes include disk bulging, thickening and overriding of laminae and ligamentum flavum, and arthritic changes with hypertrophy of the facets and facet capsules (Figs. 1 through 7). The stenosis may be associated with degenerative spondylolisthesis, frequently at the L4-5 segmental level.

Laterally, the nerve roots may be compressed within three areas around the facet joints. This lateral compression can occur subarticularly, in the foramen, or extraforaminally. It may involve the dorsal root ganglion (DRG).[6]

Congenital stenosis occurs in individuals with small pedicles, such as in achondroplastic dwarfs. It also may occur in normal-sized individuals with large vertebral bodies; short, round pedicles; and protruding disks. This stenosis frequently becomes symptomatic in the 30- to 45-year age range.

Acquired stenosis occurs over time. It can be associated with normal degenerative changes, or with posttraumatically or iatrogenically induced pars defects. The latter can occur during surgery when the pars and/or facet joints are removed, or thinned, excessively.

The symptoms of stenosis may be related to local changes involving one root as a result of a hypertrophic facet, degenerative disk, or facet cyst (ganglion). The latter usually occurs at the L4-5 level. There can be segmental changes, which often clinically involve one motion segment. This usually is L4-5 and often is associated with degenerative spondylolisthesis at that level. Frequently, however, the symptoms are related to generalized, multilevel involvement.

With our current level of knowledge, normal, age-related disk degeneration is difficult to separate from pathologic changes leading to symptoms.[7-10] The degenerative process usually begins at age 20 years in men and age 30 years in women. By age 50 years, 95% of the population have imaging and/or pathologic changes that demonstrate degenerative changes.[11] The degenerative cascade, as described by Kirkaldy-Willis and associates,[3] occurs relatively concurrently in the disk and the facet joints. The disk changes proceed from small tears to circumferential or radial tears. In young individuals this may lead to herniated disks. The early changes of degeneration are followed by decreased disk height, possible instability, and

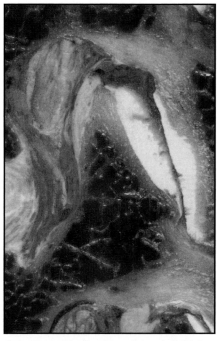

Fig. 1 Sagittal high-power photograph of the L4-5 facet joint and foramen in a spine that had been positioned in extension. Extension induces a posterior translation of L4 on L5. The tip of the inferior articular process contacts the pars interarticularis of L5 which also contacts, from inferiorly, the superior articular process of S1. The joint capsules also elongate. The ligamentum flavum and a joint capsule attach broadly to the anterior surface of the superior articular process, which is pushed into the subpedicular notch and compresses and flattens the dorsal root ganglion posteriorly.

osteophyte formation, all of which can lead to compromise of the space available for the cauda equina or nerve roots. At the same time, facet degeneration

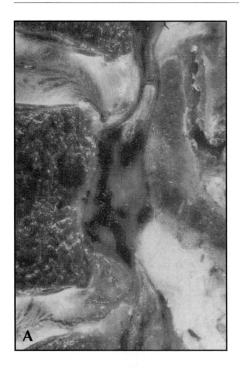

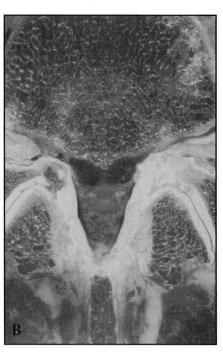

Fig. 2 A, Sagittal section, and **B,** Cross section showing pronounced disk degenerations L4-5 and L5-S1. The intact torso had been frozen in axial rotation. At L4-5 the root traversing the lateral recess is severely compressed. Anteriorly there is a motion-induced (functional) retrolisthesis of L4 on L5 that also causes the disk to move posteriorly. Posteriorly the lateral portion of the lamina and the most medial portion of the superior articular process of L5 have moved anteriorly. Note the gaping (vacuum phenomenon) in the joint. At L5-S1, disk material pushes the outermost anulus posteriorly and has caused detachment of periosteum from the vertebral body (contained disk herniation). At the lower insertion of the anulus a spondylophyte projects posteriorly, compressing the S1 root against the infolding ligamentum flavum.

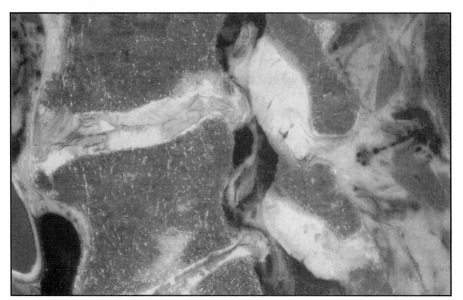

Fig. 3 Sagittal section through a moderately degenerated lower lumbar spine of a 77-year-old man who had a history of intermittent claudication. This section is carried through the lateral recesses of L4-5 and L5-S1. The L4-5 disk is grossly disrupted and protrudes both anteriorly (underneath the anterior longitudinal ligament) and posteriorly into the lateral recess, abutting the markedly thickened and infolding ligamentum flavum, thereby completely blocking the epidural veins, which are engorged both above and below this obstruction level. The L5-S1 disk is completely resorbed with total loss of disk height. Focal end-plate sclerosis and erosions of the end plates are obvious. A (probably still contained) disk herniation tracks inferiorly and reaches the ligamentum flavum, again obstructing the epidural veins at this level.

occurs, including synovial reactions followed by cartilage erosion, osteophyte formation, perhaps some "slippage," and associated bone and capsular thickening. In general, disk degeneration precedes visible facet changes, although in 20% of individuals, facet degeneration can be found without disk degeneration.[12]

The primary biochemical constituents of a disk include collagen, proteoglycans, and water.[13,14] Collagen provides connectivity and stability. Type I collagen is found primarily in the anulus and type II in the nucleus.[14,15] The absolute amount of collagen increases with age. This particularly reflects an increase in type I collagen. Proteoglycans help retain water within their intertwined structures, thereby providing an ability to enhance swelling pressure and turgor.[16-20] Over time there is a loss of water content, from 90% in children decreasing to 70% in adults. There also is an associated decrease in proteoglycans, with increased link proteins and increased proteolysis.

Facet joint arthritis occurs in a process similar to that found in other major joints. Cartilage degeneration is followed by increased, or altered, bone contact stresses with localized sclerosis and adjacent osteoporosis as weight bearing across the joint is redistributed. These abnormal forces can lead to osteophyte formation, further joint deterioration, and associated facet capsule buckling. As the joint narrows, instability, including progressive anterior subluxation, can occur with an alteration of the configuration of the joint, particularly in those that start with a more sagittal orientation.[21]

If there is increased lordosis across the degenerative section with more weight bearing posteriorly, hypertrophy of the laminae and spinous processes can occur. This hypertrophy, coupled with disk protrusion and osteophytes, can lead to circumferential bony as well as ligamentous and disk related stenosis.

Instability across a motion segment can occur by translation (anterolisthesis or retrolisthesis) or rotation. Retrolisthesis occurs when facets allow the segment to settle posteriorly; this usually occurs at L5-S1. Anterolisthesis usually is associated with facet erosion or alignment alteration, particularly when there is a preexisting sagittal configuration of the joint;[21-23] this usually occurs at L4-5 and to a lesser extent at L3-4. Rotational changes are often associated with degenerative scoliosis. These changes also occur with some facet laxity; they may create narrowing across the neuroforamen and impingement of the nerve by the joint, particularly when there is associated disk settling and facet and capsular hypertrophy.

The changes seen in spinal stenosis are also seen in normal disk degeneration. These changes include progressive loss of disk height, posterior disk bulging, gradual increase of lordosis, degenerative changes in the facet joint, osteophyte formation, and, occasionally, degenerative spondylolisthesis. The unanswered question, therefore, is why

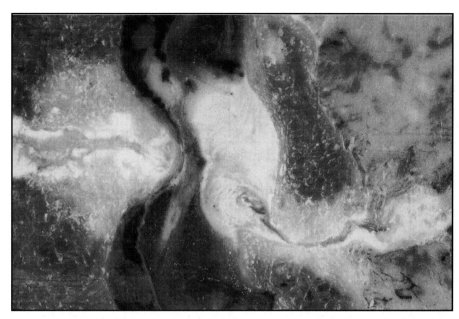

Fig. 4 Close-up view of the midlumbar spinal canal in a severely degenerated and stenotic specimen from an elderly male adult who had a history of prolonged low back pain with radicular symptoms. The intervertebral disk is completely reabsorbed. Posterior to the vertebra, the ventral internal veins are engorged. At the posterior aspect of the disk a beak-shaped spondylotic ridge projects into the spinal canal. The bone of this projecting osteophyte has a light color (sclerotic); note that the outermost anulus fibrosus (darker color) is still present. Posteriorly the loss of segmental height leads to an approximation of the spinous processes and laminae (kissing spines). The interlaminar ligamentum flavum is probably only thickened by retraction due to the redundance; it mushrooms into the spinal canal and compresses the traversing intrathecal root against the hard spondylophytic beak.

some people have back and/or leg pain related to these processes and the majority do not.

Pain usually occurs with a combination of compression and inflammation. Compression alone usually does not lead to pain. The pain from a herniated disk, which tends to be an excruciating, lancinating pain, is often different than the more diffuse, difficult to describe leg pains related to spinal stenosis. This difference may be related to the asymmetric, rapid compression related to a sudden onset of disk herniation and associated chemical irritation (inflammation), as opposed to the more gradual, global, circumferential type of compression associated with spinal stenosis. The latter occurs slowly and gives the neural elements time to adjust to their altered state and environment.

Compression, however, is important in the clinical symptoms related to spinal stenosis.[24,25] The degree, as well as the duration, of compression is important.[26] Schonstrom and associates[27] have demonstrated that many patients develop symptoms when the amount of cauda equina compression compromises over two thirds of the space available for the cauda equina. This compression leads to an increase in the pressure within the cauda equina to 100 mm Hg. When the narrowing is to 63% of normal, the intrathecal pressure raises to 50 mm Hg. The same pressures have been shown to have significant effects.[24,28-33] At a pressure of 50 mm Hg there is decreased capillary flow, decreased electrophysiologic conduction, and increased edema formation within and along the nerve roots. Pressures greater than this lead to

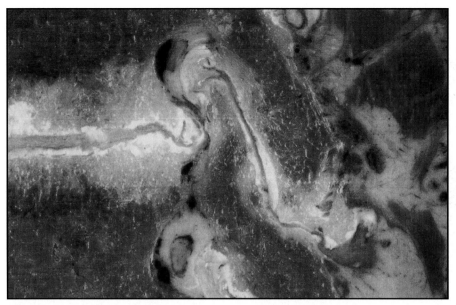

Fig. 5 Sagittal section through the L4-5 neuroforamen illustrates the five components that contribute to the extremely severe stenosis of the foramina in this specimen. The almost complete loss of intervertebral disk height causes the pedicle of L4 to "fall down" on or compress the root like a guillotine, thereby also kinking it (up-down stenosis). The second component is a front-back stenosis that is caused by the slight retrolisthesis of L4 on L5 induced by the obliquity of the facet joint in the sagittal plane. The mass effect is caused by the superior articular process of L5 intruding into the neuroforamen from below; the outermost anulus fibrosus is partially ossified and extruded, obliterating the lower portion of the foramen; and the ligamentum flavum is redundant and thickened.

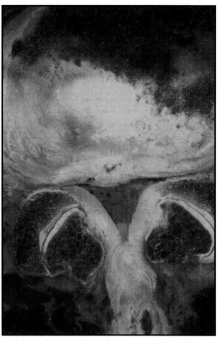

Fig. 6 Severe degenerative spinal stenosis at the L4-5 level in a 70-year-old patient with a history of intermittent claudication and occasional radicular leg pain. The central and lateral stenosis is most pronounced at this motion segment level and is almost exclusively caused by soft tissues. Anteriorly, the circumferentially ballooning disk narrows the thecal sac anteriorly and also completely obliterated the retrodiscal portion of the root canals (neuroforamina). The facet joints, especially the superior articular processes are moderately hypertophied. The thecal sac is severely compressed posterolaterally by the thick ligamentum flavum and assumes a triangular slit-shaped configuration.

arteriolar compromise and more dramatic electrophysiologic and pathophysiologic changes.

Although not measuring pain per se, findings in animal models are consistent with cadaveric and, more significantly, human anatomic cross-sectional area studies in individuals with symptoms of spinal stenosis. Delamarter and associates[34] also demonstrated the clinical significance of 50% to 75% canal compromise in terms of loss of cauda equina function and ability to functionally improve if the decompression is relieved. Other authors have shown that the magnitude and duration of compression affect the sensory components of spinal nerve roots and the cauda equina more than motor function or motor root conduction.[26,35-37] Pressures above systolic, maintained for over 2 hours, can lead to irreversible nerve conduction changes,

whereas lesser pressures for shorter periods of time are less significant. There is more rapid resolution of electrophysiologic changes in the sensory nerves than in the motor nerves, which is consistent with resolution of pain more often than motor deficits following surgical decompression in patients being treated for symptomatic spinal stenosis. These studies also suggest there is more occurring than just mechanical compression. Ischemia also is created with arterial occlusion, compounded by venous pooling and stasis, further compromising nerve root function.[38-41]

Compression, besides the mechanical effect on the neural tissue and compression of the vasculature, also leads to nutritional alterations.[42-48] Cerebrospinal fluid (CSF) normally is a conduit of nutritional components to, and metabolic breakdown products from, the cauda

equina. However, the percolation of the CSF around the neural elements is compromised by stenosis. The compression and lack of CSF alters the diffusion capabilities from the cells and axons. This alteration, coupled with the ischemia and lack of normal nutritional support and toxin removal, affects cell membrane permeability. The greater the level of compression, the longer the duration of compression, and the more levels involved (multisegmental), the greater the negative effect on the nerve roots of the cauda equina.

In the clinical setting Takahashi and associates[49] have introduced epidural catheters to measure pressure in asymptomatic and symptomatic individuals. Alterations in posture have a significant affect on cauda equina pressure. These pressures tend to increase when people stand or extend their spine, as well as with walking. These maneuvers also tend to increase leg symptoms in patients with spinal stenosis.

Anatomic and biomechanical effects can also jeopardize the nerve root. As the stenosis increases, particularly laterally, there can be tethering of the nerve roots as normal fluid nerve root motion is restrained.[50-52] Internal nerve root disruption can occur, altering the electrophysiologic function. A spinal nerve root normally moves 2 to 5 mm within a foramen. If the root is tethered or compromised, internal disruption can occur before failure is noted externally.

Perhaps the most important component leading to pain relates to inflammation.[53-55] A number of authors have shown that compression alone does not lead to pain unless it also is associated with an inflammatory reaction. Biochemical pain enhancers are produced with compression.[28,34,44] In animals, pain response such as increased foot (paw) hypersensitivity in the distribution of sensory nerves has been demonstrated when the neural elements are irritated. With compression across the DRG there is an associated increase in vasoactive proteins and an alteration in microvasculature with increased permeability, all leading to a further release of chemicals that can enhance the inflammatory reactions and, therefore, pain.[56-58]

The anatomy itself can help explain some of the variability of symptoms and signs noted in patients with spinal stenosis. Cadaveric and imaging studies have demonstrated the organized alignment of nerve fibers within the thecal sac.[59-61] In the cauda equina, the proximally numbered segments are layered

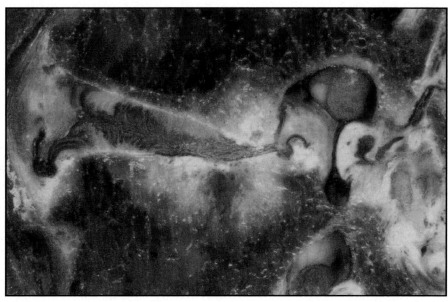

Fig. 7 Isthmic spondylolisthesis at L4-5 in a 44-year-old man. No clinical data were available in this case. This sagittal section runs through the medial border of the pedicle. At this level the beak of the pars interarticularis is displayed as it plunges into the interlaminar ligamentum flavum, causing it to mushroom anteriorly and into the lateral recess. The body of L4 is markedly rotated posteriorly, which appears to be facilitated by the severe internal disruption of the L4 disk. Its posterior anulus is partially detached superiorly from the apophyseal rim and allows the posterior anulus fibrosus to project posteriorly, virtually closing the lateral recess inferiorly. The extension-rotation of L4 causes the sharp lower rim of the pedicle to compress the ganglion.

more ventrally with the sacral roots the most dorsally situated as they course through the cauda equina. In addition, the motor components of the roots are anteromedial, and the larger sensory components more posterolateral at each segmental level within the thecal sac, as well as within the neuroforamen. Asymmetric compression may, therefore, lead to an irregularity in symptoms, depending on which neural components are affected.

The primary treatment of spinal stenosis, once symptoms start, is directed at attempting to decrease inflammation. In many cases the symptoms do improve, even though the compression itself is not altered. Surgery addresses the compression, reducing the pressure on the nerves and improving vascular flow. This indirectly decreases the progressive inflammatory effects. The latter are

related to and/or compounded by mechanical compression, altered vascularity, decreased permeability with loss of localized nutritional support, release of local chemical constituents that further irritate the nerve root, increased edema and swelling, and, therefore, further compromise of the space available for the nerve roots and cauda equina.

Clinical Presentation

The important part of treatment, particularly surgical treatment, is patient selection. Because most humans eventually will have imaging studies consistent with spinal stenosis, the correct treatment (particularly if surgery is chosen) depends on identifying patients whose symptoms are consistent with their lumbar spine pathoanatomy.[62-70]

In spinal stenosis, women develop symptoms more often than do men.

This tends to occur in the age range of 65 to 70 years. A combination of congenital with degenerative changes occurs in a younger age group and is more difficult to treat (surgically, as well as nonsurgically).

Back pain tends to occur insidiously. Initially, it is often described as an ache or stiffness, and tends not to be disabling.

The leg pain is inconsistent and may be asymmetric. The symptoms may change in any one individual, depending on the activity, duration of symptoms, and so forth. The leg complaints may be described as numbness, tingling, cramping, weakness, or severe pain. The pain may be in the buttock and/or down the leg. It may involve any of a number of lumbar roots and vary from time to time. This inconsistency in symptoms may have led in previous eras to a diagnosis of a psychologic disorder or depression. In fact, it is consistent with the multilevel, often slightly asymmetric involvement from stenosis. The leg pains (occasionally back symptoms can be similar) tend to increase with walking and spine extension. They decrease somewhat with flexion. These individuals tend to do well using a shopping cart or squatting, as necessary, to relieve symptoms. They tend to do worse standing erect, and climbing stairs or inclines.

The neurologic symptoms may be sparse. There may be an alteration in deep tendon reflexes. Symmetric loss of ankle reflexes is common in older individuals. Asymmetric loss of either the ankle, knee, or posterior tibial tendon reflexes may suggest a spinal origin for patients' complaints. Frequently the only motor deficit is in the extensor hallicus longus or hip abductors (positive Trendelenburg test). This may only be noted with a stress-induced neurologic examination, which is performed by having patients walk repetitively in the hall until their symptoms occur, and then reexamining them. Marked weaknesses are rarely noted. Bowel and bladder loss is relatively rare.

Because this is a gradual, symmetric narrowing, straight leg raising tests and tension signs usually are negative. Gait, at least in the initial phase, is usually normal. However, with walking and the beginning of pain and perhaps weakness, there may be an antalgic, or shuffling component to the gait pattern.

The differential diagnoses from spinal stenosis include vascular claudication and peripheral neuropathy. For leg pain related to vascular claudication, there tend to be symmetric reflexes (often bilaterally absent). The leg pain usually is described more as cramping with ambulation. Atrophic signs of the skin, including lower extremity hair loss, and most significantly, pulse asymmetry or loss of peripheral pulses can be noted. With neurogenic claudication (spinal stenosis) on the other hand, the pain tends to be related to back position. Pulses are symmetric and there usually is normal hair distribution on the lower extremities.

Individuals with peripheral neuropathy tend to have a stocking type of sensory deficit. They also may have other signs of systemic neurologic disorders. They may have a slap foot or steppage gait. A diagnosis frequently is made clinically and on electromyography and nerve conduction velocity studies. Occasionally, nerve (neural) or muscle biopsies are necessary.

The back pain complaints must be differentiated from pain caused by a tumor or infection. These pain complaints tend to increase over time, and are not relieved with rest. In addition, systemic signs may be noted. Patients with osteoporotic compression fractures may have back pain and some leg pain, consistent with stenosis. Radiographs, however, will help separate that diagnosis.

References

1. Arnoldi CC, Brodsky AE, Cauchoix J, et al: Lumbar spinal stenosis and nerve root entrapment syndromes: Definitions and classification. Clin Orthop 1976;115:4-5.

2. Kirkaldy-Willis WH, Paine KW, Cauchoix J, McIvor G: Lumbar spinal stenosis. Clin Orthop 1974;99:30-50.

3. Kirkaldy-Willis WH, Wedge JH, Yong-Hing K, et al: Pathology and pathogenesis of lumbar spondylosis and stenosis. Spine 1978;3:319-328.

4. Kirkaldy-Willis WH: The relationship of structural pathology to the nerve root. Spine 1984;9:49-52.

5. Verbiest H: A radicular syndrome from developmental narrowing of the lumbar vertebral canal. J Bone Joint Surg Br 1954;36:230-237.

6. Lindblom K, Rexed B: Spinal nerve injury in dorso-lateral protrusions of the lumbar disks. J Neurosurg 1948;5:413-432.

7. Coventry MB, Ghormley RK, Kernohan JW: The intervertebral disc: Its microscopic anatomy and pathology. Part III: Pathological changes in the intervertebral disc. J Bone Joint Surg Am 1945;27:460-474.

8. Naylor A: The biophysical and biochemical aspects of intervertebral disc herniation and degeneration. Ann R Coll Surg Engl 1962;31:91-114.

9. Pearce RH, Grimmer BJ, Adams ME: Degeneration and the chemical composition of the human lumbar intevertebral disc. J Orthop Res 1987;5:198-205.

10. Coventry MB, Ghormley RK, Kernohan JW: The intervertebral disc: Its mircroscopic anatomy and pathology. Part II: Changes in the intervertebral disc concomitant with age. J Bone Joint Surg Br 1945;27:233-247.

11. Miller JA, Schmatz C, Schultz AB: Lumbar disc degeneration: Correlation with age, sex, and spine level in 600 autopsy specimens. Spine 1988;13:173-178.

12. Videman T, Malmivaara A, Mooney V: The value of the axial view in assessing discograms: An experimental study with cadavers. Spine 1987;12:299-304.

13. Eyre DR: Biochemistry of the intervertebral disc. Int Rev Connect Tissue Res 1979;8:227-291.

14. Eyring EJ: The biochemistry and physiology of the intervertebral disk. Clin Orthop 1969;67:16-28.

15. Eyre DR, Muir H: Types I and II collagens in intervertebral disc: Interchanging radial distributions in annulus fibrosis. Biochem J 1976;157:267-270.

16. Buckwalter JA, Pedrini-Mille A, Pedrini V, Tudisco C: Proteoglycans of human infant intervertebral disc: Electron microscopic and biochemical studies. J Bone Joint Surg Am 1985;67:284-294.

17. Gower WE, Pedrini V: Age-related variarion in protein-polysaccharides from human nucleus pulposus, annulus fibrosus, and costal cartilage. J Bone Joint Surg Am 1969;51:1154-1162.

18. Lipson SJ, Muir H: Experimental intervertebral disc degeneration: Morphologic and proteoglycan changes over time. Arthritis Rheum 1981;24:12-21.

19. Naylor A, Horton WG: The hydrophilic properties of the nucleus pulposus of the intervertebral disc. *Rheumatism* 1955;11:32-35.

20. Urban JP, McMullin JF: Swelling pressure of the lumbar intervetebral discs: Influence of age, spinal level, composition, and degeneration. *Spine* 1988;13:179-187.

21. Groebler LJ, Anderson PA, Novotny JE, et al: Etiology of spondylolisthesis: Assessment of the role played by lumbar facet joint morphology. *Spine* 1993;18:80-91.

22. Newman PH: Stenosis of the lumbar spine in spondylolisthesis. *Clin Orthop* 1976;115:116-121.

23. Rosenberg NJ: Degenerative spondylolisthesis: Predisposing factors. *J Bone Joint Surg Am* 1975;57:467-474.

24. Garfin SR, Rydevik BL, Brown RA: Compressive neuropathy of spinal nerve roots: A mechanical or biological problem? *Spine* 1991;16:162-166.

25. Rydevik B, Brown MD, Lundborg G: Pathoanatomy and pathophysiology of nerve root compression. *Spine* 1984;9:7-15.

26. Pedowitz RA, Garfin SR, Massie JB, et al: Effects of magnitude and duration of compression on spinal nerve root conduction. *Spine* 1992;17:194-199.

27. Schonstrom N, Hansson T: Pressure changes following constriction of the cauda equina: An experimental study in situ. *Spine* 1988;13:385-388.

28. Olmarker K: Spinal nerve root compression: Nutrition and function of the porcine cauda equina compressed in vivo. *Acta Orthop Scand* 1991;242(suppl):1-27.

29. Olmarker K, Rydevik B, Holm S, Bagge U: Effects of experimental graded compression on blood flow in spinal nerve roots: A vital microscopic study on the porcine cauda equina. *J Orthop Res* 1989;7:817-823.

30. Rydevik B, Lundborg G: Permeability of intraneural microvessels and perineurium following acute, graded experimental nerve compression. *Scan J Plast Reconstr Surg* 1977;11:179-187.

31. Rydevik B, Lundborg G, Bagge U: Effects of graded compression on intraneural blood flow: An in vivo study on rabbit tibial nerve. *J Hand Surg Am* 1981;6:3-12.

32. Rydevik B, Nordborg G: Changes in nerve function and nerve fibre structure induced by acute, graded compression. *J Neurol Neurosurg Psychiatry* 1980;43:1070-1082.

33. Rydevik BL, Pedowitz RA, Hargens AR, Swenson MR, Myers RR, Garfin SR: Effects of acute, graded compression on spinal nerve root function and structure: An experimental study of the pig cauda equina. *Spine* 1991;16:487-493.

34. Delamarter RB, Bohlman HH, Dodge LD, Biro C: Experimental lumbar spinal stenosis: Analysis of the cortical evoked potentials, microvasculature, and histopathology. *J Bone Joint Surg Am* 1990;72:110-120.

35. Olmarker K, Holm S, Rydevik B: Importance of compression onset rate for the degree of impairment of impulse propagation in experimental compression injury of the porcine cauda equina. *Spine* 1990;15:416-419.

36. Olmarker K, Rydevik B, Holms S: Edema formation in spinal nerve roots induced by experimental, graded compression: An experimental study on the pig cauda equina with special reference to differences in effects between rapid and slow onset of compression. *Spine* 1989;14:579-563.

37. Olmarker K, Lind B, Holm S, Rydevik B: Continued compression increases impairment of impulse porpagation in experimental compression of the porcine cauda equina. *Neuro Orthop* 1991;11:75-81.

38. Parke WW, Gammell K, Rothman RH: Arterial vascularization of the cauda equina. *J Bone Joint Surg Am* 1981;63:53-62.

39. Parke WW, Watanabe R: The intrinsic vasculature of the lumbosacral spinal nerve roots. *Spine* 1985;10:508-515.

40. Watanabe R, Parke WW: Vascular and neural pathology of lumbosacral spinal stenosis. *J Neurosurg* 1986;64:64-70.

41. Yoshizawa H, Kobayashi S, Hachiya Y: Blood supply of nerve roots and dorsal root ganglia. *Orthop Clin North Am* 1991;22:195-211.

42. Olmarker K, Rydevik B: Single- versus double-level nerve root compression: An experimental study on the porcine cauda equina with analyses of nerve impulse conduction properties. *Clin Orthop* 1992;279:35-39.

43. Cornefjord M, Takahashi K, Matsui H, Olmarker K, Holms S, Rydevik B: Impairment of nutritional transport at double level cauda equina compression: An experimental study. *Neuro Orthop* 1992;13:107-112.

44. Olmarker K, Rydevik B, Hansson T, Holm S: Compression-induced changes of the nutritional supply to the porcine cauda equina. *J Spinal Disord* 1990;3:25-29.

45. Rydevik B, Holm S, Brown MD, Lundborg G: Diffusion from the cerebrospinal fluid as a nutritional pathway for spinal nerve roots. *Acta Physiol Scand* 1990;138:247-248.

46. Garfin SR, Cohen MS, Massie JB, et al: Nerve-roots of the cauda equina: The effects of hypotension and acute graded compression on function. *J Bone Joint Surg Am* 1990;72:1185-1192.

47. Lind B, Massie JB, Lincoln T, Myers RR, Swenson MR, Garfin SR: The effects of induced hypertension and acute graded compression on impulse progagation in the spinal nerve roots of the pig. *Spine* 1993;18:1550-1555.

48. Takahashi K, Olmarker K, Holm S, Porter RW, Rydevik B: Double-level cauda equina compression: An experimental study with continuous monitoring of intraneural blood flow in the porcine cauda equina. *J Orthop Res* 1993;11:104-109.

49. Takahashi K, Miyazaki T, Takino T, Matsui T, Tomita K: Epidural pressure measurements: Relationship between epidural pressure and posture in patients with lumbar spinal stenosis. *Spine* 1995;20:650-653.

50. Kwan MK, Rydevik B, Myers RR, Triggs K, Woo LY-Y, Garfin S: Biomechanical and histological assessment of human lumbosacral spinal nerve roots. *Trans Orthop Res Soc* 1989;14:348.

51. Smith SA, Massie JB, Chestnut R, Garfin SR: Straight leg raising: Anatomical effects on the spinal nerve root without and with fusion. *Spine* 1993;18:992-999.

52. Spencer DL, Irwin GS, Miller JA: Anatomy and significance of fixation of the lumbosacral nerve roots in sciatica. *Spine* 1983;8:672-679.

53. Cornefjord M, Olmarker K, Farley DB, Weinstein JN, Rydevik B: Neuropeptide changes in compressed spinal nerve roots. *Spine* 1995;20:670-673.

54. Olmarker K, Blomquist J, Stromberg J, Nannmark U, Thomsen P, Rydevik B: Inflammatogenic properties of nucleus pulosus. *Spine* 1995;20:665-669.

55. Olmarker K, Rydevik B, Nordborg C: Autologous nucleus pulposus induces neurophysiologic and histologic changes in porcine cauda equina nerve roots. *Spine* 1993;18:1425-1432.

56. McLain RF, Weinstein JN: Ultrastructural changes in the dorsal root ganglion associated with whole body vibration. *J Spinal Disord* 1991;4:142-148.

57. Wall PD, Devor M: Sensory afferent impulses originate from dorsal root ganglia as well as from the periphery in normal and nerve injured rats. *Pain* 1983;17:321-339.

58. Weinstein J, Pope M, Schmidt R, Seroussi R: Neuropharmacologic effects of vibration on the dorsal root ganglion: An animal model. *Spine* 1988;13:521-525.

59. Cohen MS, Wall EJ, Brown RA, Rydevik B, Garfin SR: Cauda equina anatomy: II. Extrathecal nerve roots and dorsal root ganglia. Spine 1990;15:1248-1251.

60. Cohen MS, Wall EJ, Kerber CW, Abitbol JJ, Garfin SR: The anatomy of the cauda equina on CT scans and MRI. *J Bone Joint Surg Br* 1991;73:381-384.

61. Wall EJ, Cohen MS, Massie JB, Rydevik B, Garfin SR: Cauda equina anatomy: I. Intrathecal nerve root organization. *Spine* 1990;15:1244-1247.

62. Boden SD, Davis DO, Dina TS, Patronas NJ, Wiesel SW: Abnormal magnetic-resonance imaging scans of the lumbar spine in asymptomatic subjects: A prospective investigation. *J Bone Joint Surg Am* 1990;72:403-408.

63. Jensen MC, Brant-Zawadzki MN, Obuchowski N, Modic MT, Malkasian D, Ross JS: Magnetic resonance imaging of the lumbar spine in people without back pain. *N Engl J Med* 1994;331:69-73.

64. Modic MT, Masaryk T, Boumphrey F, Goormastic M, Bell G: Lumbar herniated disk disease and canal stenosis: Prospective evaluation by surface coil MR, CT, and myelography. *Am J Neuroradial* 1986;7:709-717.

65. Jonsson B, Stromqvist B: Symptoms and signs in degeneration of the lumbar spine: A prospective, consecutive study of 300 operated patients. *J Bone Joint Surg Br* 1993;75:381-385.

66. Johnsson K-E, Rosen I, Uden A: The natural course of lumbar spinal stenosis. *Clin Orthop* 1992;279:82-86.

67. Jonsson B, Stromqvist B: Symptoms and signs in degeneration of the lumbar spine: A prospective, consecutive study of 300 operated patients. *J Bone Joint Surg Br* 1993;75:381-385.

68. Katz JN, Dalgas M, Stucki G, et al: Degenerative lumbar spinal stenosis: Diagnostic value of the history and physical examination. *Arthritis Rheum* 1995;38:1236-1241.

69. Kirkaldy-Willis WH, Farfan HF: Instability of the lumbar spine. *Clin Orthop* 1982;165: 110-123.

70. Lipson S: Clinical diagnosis of spinal stenosis. *Semin Spine Surg* 1989;1:143-144.

Radiologic Imaging in Spinal Stenosis

Richard J. Herzog, MD

Introduction

Lumbar spinal stenosis has been defined as any type of narrowing of the central spinal canal, nerve root canals (lateral recess), or the neural foramina.[1] The narrowing may be due to osseous or soft-tissue elements. When stenosis causes intractable pain, weakness, or functional disability, it may be necessary to order a diagnostic imaging test to assess the nature and extent of the pathoanatomic changes of the spine to select the optimal form of therapy. Radiologic imaging studies provide a snapshot in time of the degenerative process affecting many patients with stenotic symptoms. These studies provide morphologic information, the significance of which can be determined only by precise correlation to the patient's clinical condition. The radiologic studies currently used for the evaluation of patients with stenotic symptoms include plain films, myelography, CT, CT-myelography, and MRI. The value of these tests depends on their sensitivity, specificity, precision, reliability, accuracy, risk, cost, and availability.

Prior to 1970, plain film radiography was the primary radiologic study available to evaluate patients with symptoms of spinal stenosis. Plain films only provide direct information on the morphology and alignment of the osseous components of the spinal motion segments. Any pathologic process that causes osseous destruction, degeneration, or remodeling can be detected on plain films if a sufficient amount of bone is affected. Plain film findings that may be associated with symptomatic spinal stenosis include end plate proliferation and remodeling, facet arthrosis, malalignment in the sagittal or coronal plane, a developmentally small spinal canal, postoperative or posttraumatic spinal deformity, and any pathologic condition that may cause enlargement of the osseous structures, for example, Paget's disease.

Plain Radiographs

To determine the value of plain radiographs in the workup of patients with symptoms of spinal stenosis, it is necessary to know the spectrum of findings detected on plain films obtained on asymptomatic patients. Frymoyer and associates[2] evaluated the plain films of 292 patients, including 96 with no history of back pain, 134 with a history of previous or current moderate back pain, and

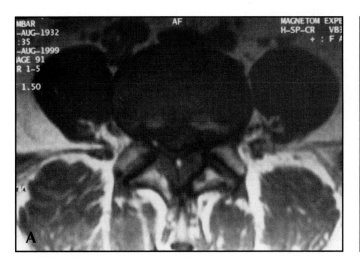
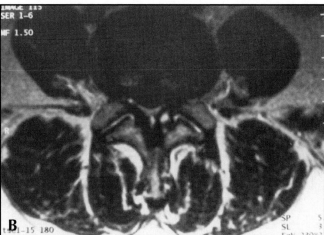

Fig. 1 At the L4-5 level, on the T1-weighted (**A**) and T2-weighted (**B**) axial images, there is severe compression of the thecal sac by a posterior midline disk protrusion and hypertrophied ligamenta flava. The left ligamentum flavum contains a small synovial cyst.

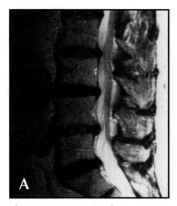
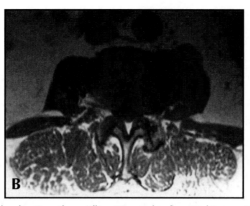
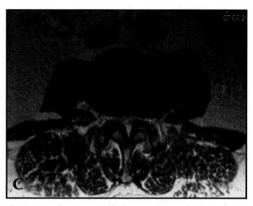

Fig. 2 In a patient with neurogenic claudication, the midline T2-weighted sagittal image (**A**) depicts multisegmental degenerative changes along with a posterior midline disk protrusion at the L4-5 level. Axial images orthogonal to the disk space are obtained to assess the degree of thecal sac deformation. On the T1-weighted (**B**) and T2-weighted (**C**) axial images at the L2-3 level, mild/moderate right and moderate/severe left facet arthrosis along with posterior bulge of the disk results in severe constriction of the thecal sac. Only a minimal amount of cerebrospinal fluid surrounds the cauda equina.

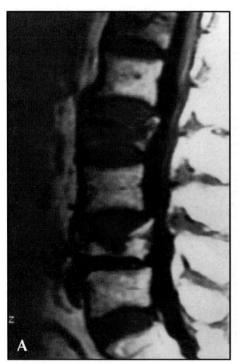
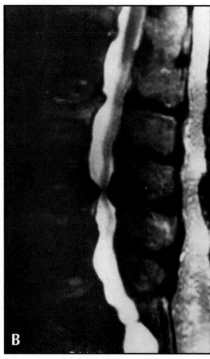

Fig. 3 In an elderly patient with a history of a fall and who is currently experiencing neurogenic claudication, the T1-weighted (**A**) and T2-weighted fat saturated (**B**) sagittal images depict severe central canal stenosis at the L1-2 and L3-4 levels due to osteopenic compression fractures. There are changes of Kummel's disease in the L2 vertebral body.

62 with a history of prior or current severe back pain. In the three groups, the frequency of transitional vertebrae, Schmorl's nodes, disk vacuum phenomenon, claw spurs, and disk-space narrowing at the L3-4 and L5-S1 disk levels were similar. Traction spurs and disk-space narrowing at the L4-5 level had a positive correlation to severe low back pain. Witt and associates[3] compared the plain film findings in patients with and without back pain. There was no difference in the prevalence of disk degeneration or spondylosis when comparing the 238 patients with low back pain and sciatica to 68 asymptomatic patients. The prevalence of disk degeneration and spondylosis increased with age in the two groups. Torgerson and Dotter[4] evaluated 217 asymptomatic patients between the ages of 40 and 70 years, and 387 symptomatic patients with back pain in the same age range. They found a higher incidence of spondylolysis and spondylolisthesis in the symptomatic patients

Plain films provide a global depiction of the severity of degenerative spinal disease, but they are extremely limited in determining the precise location of neural entrapment. When interpreting plain films, each spinal motion segment should be scrutinized for the presence of disk degeneration, facet arthrosis, and central canal or neural foraminal stenosis. Spinal alignment in the sagittal and coronal planes must be assessed as well as any rotatory deformity. The routine plain film evaluation of the lumbar spine includes an erect anteroposterior (AP) view, a lateral view that includes the spine from the thoracolumbar junction to the upper sacrum, and a cone-downed lateral view of the lumbosacral junction. Flexion and extension and lateral bending views may be warranted in the initial assessment of a patient if dynamic instability is clinically suspected, or if there is evidence of malalignment on the routine radiographs. Erect films are needed for the assessment of spinal balance. In patients with scoliosis, specific supine stress views may be obtained to determine the structural versus the functional component of the deformity. After the initial examination of the spine, repeat plain films should be limited to the assessment of new symptoms or evaluation of the stability of spinal alignment.

Computed Tomography and Magnetic Resonance Imaging

With the development and implementation of radiologic cross-sectional imaging studies, for example, MRI and CT with multiplanar reformations (CT/MPR), it became possible to directly evaluate all the osseous components of each spinal motion segment in the three anatomic planes of the body, as well as to assess the soft-tissue structures. With CT, it also is possible to create a three-dimensional model of the spine that may facilitate the comprehension of complex anatomic relationships. With CT's excellent delineation of osseous structures, it is the optimal modality to characterize the nature and degree of osseous stenosis, whether related to the vertebral end plates or facet joint. The advantage of MRI is its ability to depict the soft-tissue structures that may precipitate stenotic symptoms, for example, thickened ligamenta flava, hypertrophied facet capsules, prominent epidural fat, and herniated disk material (Fig. 1). MRI provides direct information concerning nerve root entrapment and the degree of thecal sac deformation. Another advantage of MRI compared with CT is the greater length of the spine that can be evaluated on a standard MRI examination.

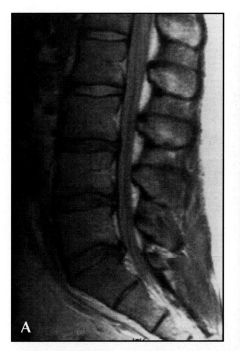
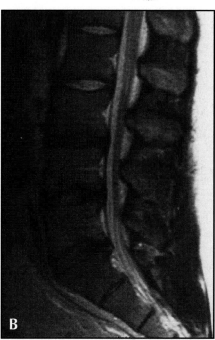
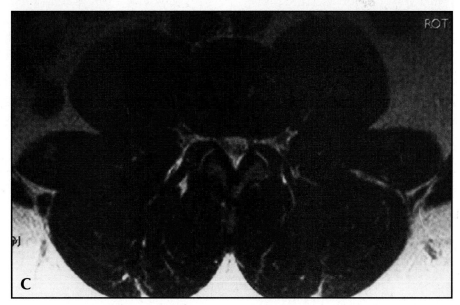

Fig. 4 On the proton-density-weighted (**A**) and T2-weighted (**B**) sagittal images there is mild/moderate developmental stenosis of the lumbar central spinal canal from L3 to L5, along with changes of disk degeneration at the L3-5 and L5-S1 levels. On the T2-weighted axial image (**C**) at the L3-4 level, there is developmental central canal stenosis and mild thecal sac deformation.

To achieve the maximum amount of information on a CT or MRI study it is necessary to perform the optimal imaging examination. A routine CT examination of the lumbar spine includes sequential axial 3 mm-thick sections from the pedicle of L3 through the L5-S1 disk level. Thin axial sections are needed for optimal spatial resolution and to create the computer-generated sagittal reformations that should be obtained for every patient. Coronal reformations

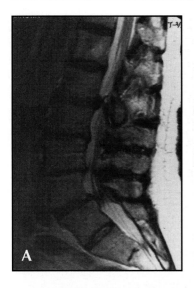

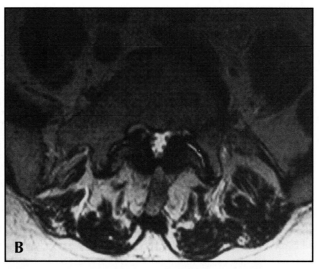

Fig. 5 In a patient with back and leg pain, on the T2-weighted sagittal image (**A**), there is multisegmental central canal stenosis along with a degenerative anterolisthesis at the L4-5 level. On the T2-weighted axial image (**B**), at the L4-5 level, moderate/severe facet arthrosis is causing moderate central canal stenosis along with stenosis of the subarticular lateral recesses and entrapment of the L5 nerve roots.

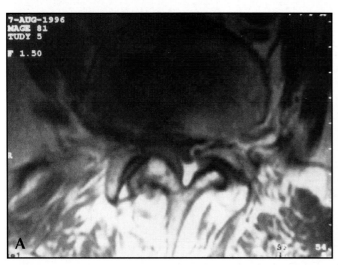

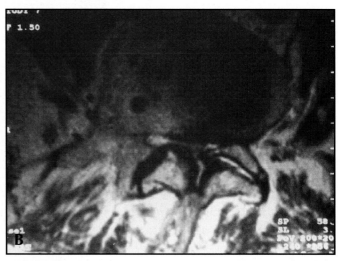

Fig. 6 At the L4-5 level, on the T1-weighted (**A**) and T2-weighted (**B**) axial images, there is severe central canal stenosis predominantly due to facet arthrosis and hypertrophy of the right ligamentum flavum. Facet tropism is present with the right facet joint oriented more sagittally than the left. Only the more sagittally oriented right facet joint is anteriorly subluxated.

are needed to assess spinal alignment in patients with scoliosis or in patients with a segmental lateral listhesis. All CT images should be evaluated in both soft-tissue and bone windows.

When possible, MRI examinations of the lumbar spine should be performed on a high field strength MRI system (1.0 to 1.5 Tesla) to achieve rapid high-resolution imaging. Low field strength (0.1 to 0.3 Tesla) MRI systems are indicated for obese patients or patients with claustrophobia who can not undergo an examination in a high field strength system. Almost all open MRI scanners are low field strength systems. The routine MRI examination of the lumbar spine performed on a patient with back or leg pain will include: a T1 or proton-density-weighted sagittal sequence and a fast spin-echo T2-weighted sagittal sequence (typically fat saturated), using a section thickness of 4 mm and an interslice gap of 0.5 mm; a T1 or proton-density-weighted axial sequence with a section thickness of 4 mm and an interslice gap of 0.5 mm; and a fast spin echo T2-weighted axial sequence with a section thickness of 3 to 4 mm and an interslice gap of 0.5 mm. At least one axial sequence should have contiguous sections from the pedicle of L2 or L3 through the L5-S1 disk level and not merely angled sections through the disk spaces.

Disk degeneration may induce segmental instability and secondary hypertrophy and hyperplasia of the connective tissue elements. The degenerative tissue may encroach into the central spinal canal,

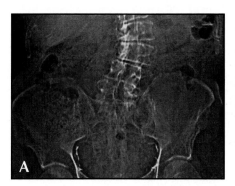 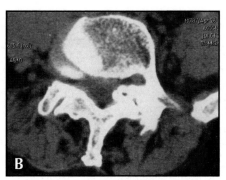 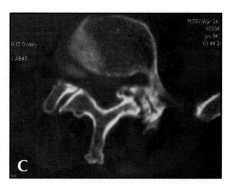

Fig. 7 On a patient with a mild/moderate lumbar rotatory levoscoliosis and a left lateral listhesis at the L3-4 level (**A**), CT demonstrates asymmetrical facet arthrosis and moderate/severe central canal stenosis at the L3-4 level depicted on the axial images photographed for soft-tissue (**B**) and bone (**C**) resolution.

the subarticular lateral recess, or the neural foramina and impinge, entrap, or compress the neural structures. The central canal narrowing may involve the bony canal alone or the dural sac, or both.[1] The degenerative changes most often associated with central canal stenosis include posterior bulging of the disk, osteophytes projecting off the vertebral body end plates, hypertrophy and bony proliferation of the facet joints, and hypertrophy of the ligamenta flava and anterior facet capsules.[5,6] The goal of both MRI and CT/MPR in the evaluation of patients presenting with back pain, radiculopathy, or intermittent claudication is not just to demonstrate the presence of stenosis, but to define that spinal components are causing the stenosis (Fig. 2).

Degenerative spinal disease is a continuous subclinical process which may not evoke symptoms. Abnormalities are frequently detected on CT and MRI studies performed on asymptomatic individuals.[7] The spondylotic changes do not represent false positive findings, but true pathologic changes of spinal structures that are not evoking symptoms. In addition to degenerative osseous changes that may lead to stenosis of the central spinal canal, other osseous abnormalities that may cause stenosis include posttraumatic deformities (Fig. 3), overgrowth of a spinal fusion, Paget's disease, fluorosis

and vertebral hemangiomas. Intraspinal masses, for example, synovial cysts and epidural lipomatosis, may also precipitate symptoms of neurogenic claudication.

In order to obtain a true AP diameter of the lumbar central spinal canal, axial images orthogonal to the long axis of the spinal canal or midline sagittal images must be obtained. With the excellent spatial resolution of osseous structures, CT/MPR is the best examination to ascertain precise osseous spinal measurements. The classification of spinal stenosis as congenital, developmental, and acquired is helpful when evaluating a small spinal canal.[8,9] Congenital stenosis is a result of disturbed fetal development and may occur as one element of a congenital malformation of the lumbar spine. Developmental stenosis is a growth disturbance of the posterior elements, involving the pedicles, lamina, or articular processes, resulting in decreased volume of the spinal canal. In the lumbar spine, a true midline osseous sagittal diameter measuring less than 12 mm is considered relative stenosis, and a diameter of less than 10 mm is considered absolute stenosis.[10] This diameter is measured from the middle of the posterior surface of the vertebral body to the point of junction of its spinous process and laminae. With developmental stenosis, the

reserve capacity of the spinal canal is reduced, thus predisposing the neural elements to impingement or compression by any material encroaching into the central canal (Fig. 4). Developmental central canal stenosis may be associated with developmental narrowing of the neural foramina. Acquired stenosis is the narrowing of the central spinal canal, the subarticular lateral recess, or the neural foramina by degenerative changes of the discovertebral joint, facet joints, and ligamenta flava. Acquired stenosis may be superimposed on developmental stenosis. Central and neural foraminal stenosis frequently coexist in the same patient.

Spinal degeneration may be associated with altered spinal alignment, scoliosis, or spondylolisthesis. Spondylolisthesis is defined as a slip of the spine, and depending on the relationship of the vertebral bodies at the involved motion segment, the displacement will be an anterolisthesis, a retrolisthesis, or a lateral listhesis. Degenerative spondylolisthesis is an important cause of central canal stenosis and most frequently involves the L4-5 disk level (Fig. 5). Disk degeneration along with degenerative changes of sagittally-oriented facet joints predispose the motion segment to an anterolisthesis, which rarely progresses beyond a grade I slip because there is an

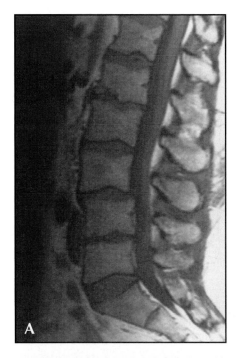

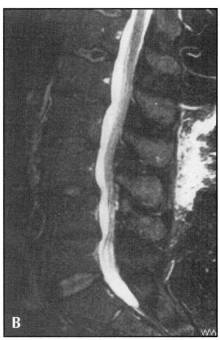

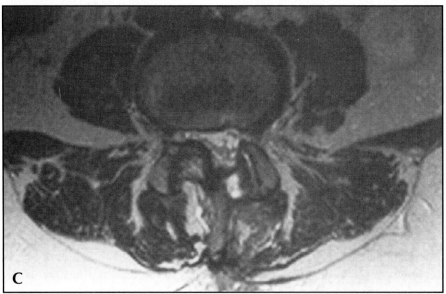

Fig. 8 In a patient who developed a new anterolisthesis at the L3-4 level and new right leg radicular symptoms after an L3-4 left laminectomy, on the T1-weighted (**A**) and T2-weighted (**B**) sagittal images, there is a grade I anterolisthesis at the L3-4 level along with changes of multisegmental disk degeneration. On the T2-weighted axial image (**C**) anterior subluxation of the right inferior articular process of L3 results in compression of the right L4 axillary pouch. A left laminectomy defect is present.

ponent and asymmetrical stenosis of the subarticular lateral recesses (Fig. 6). Asymmetrical central canal stenosis is also seen in adult patients with scoliosis and a degenerative lateral listhesis (Fig. 7). In postoperative patients who develop new radicular symptoms, MRI is excellent for detecting nerve root entrapment resulting from spinal instability (Fig. 8).

Myelography

Myelography provides opacification of the thecal sac and a means to assess its dimensions in both the supine and erect positions, including stress views with flexion and extension. Many clinicians prefer myelography and CT-myelography for the assessment of patients with stenosis. Erect myelography provides the opportunity to assess the size of the thecal sac in various stressful positions that may provoke the patient's symptoms. Although erect myelography provides a more provocative stress examination than a supine MRI, CT, or myelographic study, its is still unclear whether the information provided on an erect myelogram is unique in predicting patient outcome or needed in selecting the optimal mode of therapy. Some studies have shown no relationship between preoperative myelograms and postoperative outcome; however, Herno and associates[11] reported that the severity of myelographic findings was significantly related to the outcome of patients who underwent surgery for spinal stenosis. Seventy-six percent of patients with a complete or subtotal block on nonfunctional myelography (not erect or stressed) had a good or excellent outcome after spinal surgery.

Because there is potential morbidity with myelography, the question arises whether the same information can be achieved with CT or MRI. Wildermuth and associates[12] recently reported on the comparison of supine and erect MRI (with the patient seated in flexion or extension) to supine and erect myelography in a group of 30 patients, most of

intact neural arch. The combination of osseous ridges projecting off the anteromedial margin of the facet joints, hypertrophy of the ligamenta flava, posterior bulge of the disk, and an anterolisthesis

may result in severe central canal and subarticular lateral recess stenosis. If there is asymmetry in the orientation of the facet joints (facet tropism), the anterolisthesis may have a rotatory com-

whom were being evaluated for stenotic symptoms. They demonstrated a high ($r = 0.81$ to 0.97) correlation between MRIs and myelographic measurements. They demonstrated only a small positional difference in dural sac diameters from the supine to the erect position, and they concluded that the additional information gained on the erect MRI study when compared to that obtained on the standard supine MRI examination is limited.

Neural foraminal stenosis should always be considered as a possible etiology for radicular symptoms. Considering that all neural foramina in the spinal column have a vertical and horizontal dimension as well as a length, the foramen is truly a three-dimensional structure, that is, a canal. Pathologic changes of any structure that borders the neural foramen may impinge or compress the exiting nerve root or dorsal root ganglion. The most common etiology of neural foraminal stenosis are osteophytes projecting off the vertebral end plates[5,13] (Fig. 9).

Degenerative changes of the superior articular process may lead to decreased volume of the posterosuperior compartment of the neural foramen, potentially causing neural compression. Decreased disk height results in cephalocaudal stenosis of the neural foramen, which may be amplified with an anterolisthesis (Fig. 10). Sagittal imaging is mandatory with both MRI and CT to evaluate the neural foramina for the presence of stenosis. Extraforaminal (far-out) stenosis[14] may occur at the L5-S1 disk level because of the apposition of the base of the transverse process of L5 to the adjacent sacral ala.

Evaluation and Diagnosis

While plain films, CT, MRI, and myelography are currently used to evaluate patients with stenotic symptoms, there are few controlled studies documenting the relative value of these tests for the evalu-

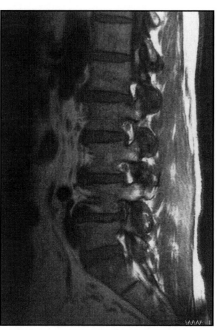

Fig. 9 Bulging of the disk and end plate proliferation results in mild neural foraminal stenosis at the L2-3 and L3-4 levels and moderate stenosis at the L4-5 level. There is impingement of the left L4 nerve root in the neural foramen on the T1-weighted sagittal image.

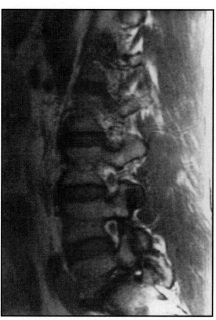

Fig. 10 In a patient with a grade II isthmic spondylolisthesis at the L5-S1 disk level, there is severe cephalocaudal stenosis of the neural foramen and compression of the L5 nerve root between the base of the L5 pars interarticularis and the superior end plate of S1 on the proton density-weighted sagittal image.

ation of these patients. Amundsen and associates[15] reported on 100 patients with symptomatic lumbar spinal stenosis who were evaluated with plain films, myelography, and CT. As emphasized by the authors, this cohort group was a selected group of patients who were hospitalized for sciatica, but workup determined that lumbar stenosis and not a disk herniation, neoplasm, or inflammatory process was the cause of their symptoms. The radiologic studies were used to determine the type and degree of stenosis. As stated by the authors, the criteria for diagnosing central and lateral (lateral recess and neural foramina) stenosis are difficult to define. Stenosis was determined by evaluating the shape of the spinal canal, the appearance of the facet joints, and the measured dimensions of pedicle length, interpedicular width, and sagittal diameter of the thecal sac.

The diagnosis of stenosis was based on the combination of visual impression by the radiologists and direct measurements, which makes the results of this study difficult to validate by other investigators. In their cohort group, 95% had back pain in addition to sciatica. Lateral stenosis was demonstrated in 51 patients and central canal stenosis in 49. A degenerative spondylolisthesis was present in 12 patients. There was no difference in the symptoms of patients with lateral and central stenosis. Claudication was present in both groups and at all degrees of stenosis. There was no significant correlation between the severity of pain and the degree of stenosis. The radiologic changes were more extensive than expected by the clinical findings, and multilevel changes were detected in patients with lateral and central canal stenosis. The number of the clinically symptomatic nerve roots could not be predicted from the radiologic findings. The authors concluded that clinical and radiologic assessment together are necessary to determine the diagnosis of symptomatic lumbar spinal stenosis. They also stated that perhaps the determination of the cross-sectional area of the spinal canal may provide useful information in the evaluation of patients with stenosis. While CT is the best method to measure the cross-sectional area of the osseous central canal, MRI is optimal to measure the cross-sectional area of the thecal sac.

Herno and associates[16] reported on the lack of correlation between CT findings and patients' symptoms after laminectomy for lumbar spinal stenosis. The structural changes identified on the postoperative CT study did not correlate significantly with the patients' pain patterns, walking capacity, or subjective disability. Herno and associates[17] also recently reported on a long-term (10-year) postoperative follow-up study of patients with lumbar spinal stenosis. MRI was used for the evaluation of these patients, and the authors found no significant difference in patient symptoms whether or not they had stenosis diagnosed on the MRI study. They did find that evidence of disk degeneration had a significant effect on patient walking capacity. The poor correlation of MRI to patient symptoms may have been affected by the lack of quantitative measurements used in the study to characterize the degree of stenosis.

An important question, which to date has not been resolved, is which study, myelography, CT, CT-myelography, or MRI, should be ordered when additional information is needed in the evaluation of a patient with spinal stenotic symptoms. Considering the rapid evolution of MRI and CT technology, a study on their effectiveness may be difficult to complete and still provide relevant information on the appropriate application of these diagnostic tests. The recent Cochrane review reported that there is no scientific evidence on the effectiveness of any form of surgical decompression or fusion for degenerative lumbar spondylosis compared with natural history, placebo, or conservative management.[18] Perhaps using the optimal imaging study in the assessment of these patients may improve surgical management and patient outcome.

References

1. Arnoldi CC, et al: Lumbar spinal stenosis and nerve root entrapment syndromes: Definition and classification. *Clin Orthop* 1976;115:4-5.

2. Frymoyer JW, Newberg A, Pope MA, Wilder DG, Clements J, MacPherson B: Spine radiographs in patients with low-back pain: An epidemiological study in men. *J Bone Joint Surg Am* 1984;66:1048-1053.

3. Witt I, Vestergaard A, Rosenklint A: A comparative analysis of x-ray findings of the lumbar spine in patients with and without lumbar pain. *Spine* 1984;9:299-300.

4. Torgerson WR, Dotter WE: Comparative roentgenographic study of the asymptomatic and symptomatic lumbar spine. *J Bone Joint Surg Am* 1976;58:850-853.

5. Rauschning W: Normal and pathologic anatomy of the lumbar root canals. *Spine* 1987;12:1008-1019.

6. Schneck CD: The anatomy of lumbar spondylosis. *Clin Orthop* 1985;193:20-37.

7. Boden SD, David DO, Dina TS, Patronas NJ, Wiesel SW: Abnormal magnetic-resonance scans of the lumbar spine asymptomatic subjects. *J Bone Joint Surg Am* 1990;72:403-408.

8. Verbiest H: Fallacies of the present definition, nomenclature, and classification of the stenosis of the lumbar vertebral canal. *Spine* 1976;1: 217-225.

9. Verbiest H: Words, images, knowledge, and reality: Some reflections from the neurosurgical perspective. *Acta Neurochirugica* 1983;69:163-193.

10. Verbiest H: Results of surgical treatment of idiopathic development stenosis of the lumbar vertebral canal. *J Bone Joint Surg Br* 1977;59:181-188.

11. Herno A, Airaksinen O, Saari T, Miettinen H: The predictive value of preoperative myelography in lumbar spinal stenosis. *Spine* 1994;19:1335-1338.

12. Wildermuth S, Zanetti M, Duewell S, et al: Lumbar spine: Quant itative and qualitative assessment of positional (upright flexion and extension) MR imaging and myelography. *Radiology* 1998;207:391-398.

13. Bohatirchuk F: The aging vertebral column (macro- and historadiographical study). *Br J Radiol* 1955;28:389-404.

14. Wiltse L: Far-out syndrome, in Rothman LG, Glenn WVJ (eds): *Multiplanar CT of the Spine.* Baltimore, MD, University Park Press, 1985, pp 384-393.

15. Amundsen T: Lumbar spinal stenosis: Clinical and radiologic features. *Spine* 1995;20: 1178-1186.

16. Herno A, Airaksinen O, Saari T: Computed tomography after laminectomy for lumbar stenosis. *Spine* 1994;19:1975-1978.

17. Herno A, Partanen K, Talaslahti T, et al: Long-term clinical and magnetic resonance imaging follow-up assessment of patients with lumbar spinal stenosis after laminectomy. *Spine* 1999;24:1533-1537.

18. Gibson JNA, Grant IC, Waddell G: The Cochrane review of surgery for lumbar disc prolapse and degenerative lumbar spondylosis. *Spine* 1999;24:1820-1832.

Lumbar Spinal Stenosis: Treatment Options

Eeric Truumees, MD
Harry N. Herkowitz, MD

Nonsurgical Treatment Options

Because rapid symptomatic or functional decline is rare in patients with lumbar spinal stenosis, a course of nonsurgical management is recommended. Various nonsurgical modalities are often sufficient to control symptoms, and surgery may be deferred.[1,2] Regardless of the modalities ultimately selected, the patient should be actively involved in decision making and symptom management. Reassurance and education by way of books and videotapes are recommended.

Activity modification, including decreased lifting, twisting, and forward bending, is a mainstay in nonsurgical management. A period of relative rest may be advised for symptom flare-ups.[2] Although rest may temporarily control symptoms, exercise is another crucial element of management.[3] Exercise offers many benefits, including weight reduction, cardiopulmonary fitness, and release of endorphins. Stationary bicycle riding (while partially forward flexed), aquatic exercises, and partially unloaded treadmill exercises are well tolerated.[4]

A formal physical therapy program may pave the way for earlier recovery, decreased recurrence, and decreased disability and pain.[2,5] Hyperextension regimens should be avoided;[2,4,6,7] flexion exercises are preferred.[8,9] These exercises increase flexibility of lumbar soft tissues and hamstrings, provide for truncal stabilization, and help strengthen abdominal muscles, thereby helping to maintain a position of slight flexion.

A lumbar corset may decrease motion and at the same time reduce pain. Bracing may lead to weakness and is therefore controversial.[10,11] Muscle deconditioning must be carefully avoided with a concomitant exercise program.

Various medications such as acetaminophen and nonsteroidal anti-inflammatory drugs (NSAIDs) are frequently recommended in the treatment of lumbar spinal stenosis. However, in the elderly population, particular care must be taken relative to potential systemic complications such as gastrointestinal ulceration or impaired renal function. The newer class of COX-2 specific NSAIDs are not free of complications. Narcotics are occasionally prescribed for flare-ups; however, long-term narcotic use is to be avoided because it can lead to constipation, dependence, and impaired mental function.[10] Antidepressants used in low doses are occasionally helpful in promoting sleep and decreasing neurogenic and back pain.[12] Nasal calcitonin has been found to be helpful in mild cases.[13] Muscle relaxants and oral steroids are not recommended.[10,14]

Injection therapies are variably recommended in the sacroiliac joints, trigger points, and nerve root sleeves.[15] Epidural steroid injections are more common, yet also remain controversial.[16,17] Such injections may be helpful in the face of acute flare-ups, with significant radicular complaints, to allow institution of a nonsurgical treatment regimen including physical therapy, or in those for whom surgery is not an option.[18] Typically, three weekly injections of 80 mg Depo-Medrol and 0.5% xylocaine are given through the sacral hiatus. This approach avoids the technical difficulty of inserting a needle through the arthritic posterior elements of the spine, but may then miss symptoms from levels about the level of tightest stenosis. In two retrospective evaluations of the effectiveness of epidural steroid injections for lumbar spinal stenosis, 50% of patients experienced short-term pain relief.[19,20] Two reviews used meta-analysis, with differing conclusions. In one, a 14% improvement over the natural history of degenerative spinal disease was noted.[21] Another review of the use of epidural steroid injections in multiple trials found little support for the practice.[22] Epidural steroid injections may predict results of decompressive surgery.[23]

Other modalities of nonsurgical treatment of spinal stenosis include manipulation, acupuncture, stress reduction, ultrasound, transcutaneous electrical nerve stimulation units, thermal modalities, and traction. These modalities cannot be recommended based on available data.[24-28] In 1987, the Quebec Task Force on Spinal Disorders found no evidence for any nonsurgical approach in the treatment of lumbar spinal stenosis.[26] They did recommend orthoses, activity modification, traction, and exercise based on practice patterns and empirical evidence.

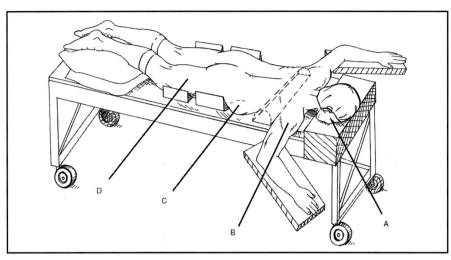

Fig. 1 Patient positioning is critical. Because these procedures are often lengthy, all bony prominences must be well padded. The eyes must be carefully padded (**A**). Careful attention to arm position will decrease the likelihood of postoperative brachial plexus palsy (**B**). Abdominal contents are allowed to hang free to decrease back pressure on the epidural venous plexus (**C**). The legs may be extended for a more normal lumbar lordosis (**D**). Here the final decompression will more closely mimic the standing position. (© William Beaumont Hospital, Royal Oak, MI)

Results of Nonsurgical Treatment

Very little objective evaluation of the various nonsurgical modalities has been done. In one series of 145 patients treated nonsurgically, 70% had significant symptomatic improvement, whereas 23% had mild improvement.[29] Johnsson and associates[30] followed 32 patients with lumbar spinal stenosis treated nonsurgically for a mean of 49 months. The pain was unchanged in 70%, improved in 15%, and worse in 15%. Atlas and associates[31] reported better results with surgery at 1 year in a prospective cohort study of surgically and nonsurgically treated patients with lumbar spinal stenosis. At 1 year, 15% of the nonsurgical group reported worse leg pain, while 20% had worse back pain.

Indications for Surgical Treatment

Except in the rare case of rapidly progressive neurologic deficits, surgery in patients with lumbar spinal stenosis is elective.[32,33] Indications include progressive neurologic deficit, intractable pain, and persistent impairment/functional limitations.[34-36] Because low back pain alone is not reliably alleviated, it alone is not an indication for surgery.[37-39] There is significant geographic variation in how these indications are applied.[40-43] Larequi-Lauber and associates[44] evaluated the appropriateness of surgical indications in 328 consecutive patients undergoing laminectomy for lumbar spinal stenosis. They found that in 38% of patients, surgical indications were inappropriate, particularly because of an inadequate trial of nonsurgical treatment.

There are no absolute contraindications to surgery. Although medical comorbidities significantly influence outcomes, age alone is not a contraindication.[36,45-47] However, patients without concordance of history, physical examination, and imaging data should be managed nonsurgically.

Principles of Surgical Management

The goals of surgery are increased function, decreased pain, and prevention of neurologic deficit progression. Central to achieving these goals is complete decompression of the neural elements. The extent of the decompression required is determined by the patient's pathoanatomy. Even with unilaterally symptomatic patients, unilateral surgery should be avoided in patients with radiographic evidence of bilateral stenosis. These patients will soon present with contralateral symptoms. Further, the number of levels involved should not be underestimated. Physical examination will often not allow localization to singular levels.[48]

Within the larger goal of obtaining a complete decompression, preservation of spinal stability is critical to the prevention of late failure. First, facet integrity may be maintained by undercutting with angled instruments. Second, protection of the pars will obviate postoperative fractures and incipient back pain and instability.[49] Third, unforeseen difficulties in decompression may require fusion in any patient undergoing a decompression. Therefore, all patients should be prepared for this possibility.

Before surgery, a complete medical and nutritional evaluation is recommended. For more extensive procedures, it remains our practice to encourage autologous blood donation. There are several other issues outside of the transmission of infectious viral diseases that make autologous blood transfusion preferable. These include the risk of unsuspected antibodies. In the operating room, a headlight and loupes or an operating microscope are valuable. Some authors use intraoperative monitoring to determine adequacy of decompression.[50] Others find that return of cerebrospinal fluid pulsation signals adequacy of decompression.[51] The patient is positioned prone or kneeling with the abdomen hanging free to decrease central venous pressure[52] (Fig. 1). Some authors recommend maintaining lumbar

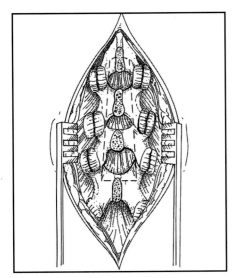

Fig. 2 Once the exposure has been completed, a radiograph is obtained to confirm spinal level. Then, the spinous processes from the inferior half of the superiormost and the superior half of the inferiormost levels to be decompressed are removed with double-action rongeurs. The entire spinous process of each intermediate level is removed. (© William Beaumont Hospital, Royal Oak, MI)

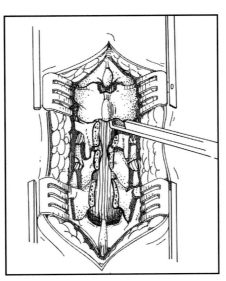

Fig. 3 Posteroanterior view demonstrating completed central decompression. The hypertrophic ligamentum flavum laterally causing continued compression is noted. (© William Beaumont Hospital, Royal Oak, MI)

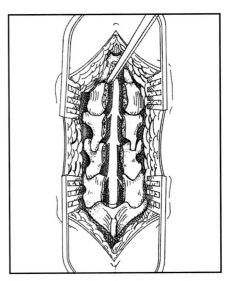

Fig 4 Posteroanterior view demonstrating lateral recess decompression. (© William Beaumont Hospital, Royal Oak, MI)

lordosis in that this positioning more closely emulates the symptomatic, standing position. Moreover, a fusion may then be undertaken in a more physiologically appropriate position. The disadvantage of this position is laminar shingling, which increases the difficulty of entering the canal.

Techniques of Surgical Decompression

Laminectomy remains the standard procedure for surgical decompression in lumbar spinal stenosis. Laminectomy begins with a central decompression. Herein, the inferior half of the superior spinous process and the superior half of the inferior spinous process are removed (along with all intermediate spinous processes) with a double-action rongeur (Fig. 2). A Leksell rongeur is then used to remove additional bone and soft tissue and to thin the laminae.

A Kerrison rongeur is used to remove the remainder of the central laminae and flavum in a caudad to cephalad direction (Fig. 3).

Next, a decompression of the lateral recesses is undertaken by partial medial facetectomy (Fig. 4). To prevent destabilization, an undercutting technique with a 45° upbiting Kerrison rongeur is used. The decompression is taken out laterally to the pedicles (Fig. 5). Finally, the foramina are decompressed after the nerve roots are identified. The Kerrison rongeur is inserted dorsal to the roots and overlying spurs are removed. An angled dural separator or a ball-tip probe may be used to assess the adequacy of decompression. A 4-mm probe should pass without difficulty (Fig. 6). Finally, the root, when retracted with a Penfield dissector, should demonstrate 1 cm of medial displacement. Disk herniation is occasionally seen in conjunction with lumbar spinal stenosis. These herniations, if lateral or foraminal, may require removal. Central bulges alone are adequately decompressed with a laminectomy.[53]

Another common method of decompression is the laminotomy. Unilateral laminotomy has been advocated in certain patients with localized lateral recess stenosis and monoradicular complaints.[54] More often, however, a bilateral laminotomy is recommended as a spinous process- and ligament-sparing alternative to a complete laminectomy. This procedure is indicated if stenosis is limited to disk/facet joint level. It is contraindicated in patients with congenital stenosis and global narrowing. The role of laminotomy in patients with scoliosis and spondylolisthesis remains to be defined; however, posterior element preservation may minimize the risk of progression.[51] Disadvantages include increased technical difficulty, duration of surgery, and neurologic risk.

A patient undergoing laminotomy is positioned in the same manner as a laminectomy patient.[55] During the surgical approach to the spine, the supraspinous ligaments and spinous processes should be preserved. The inferior laminotomy is extended laterally to the base of the inferior facet. Then, a medial facetectomy of the inferior facet, including

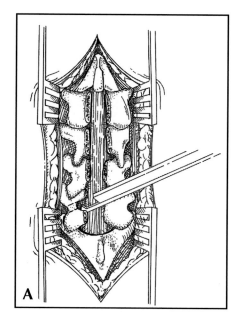

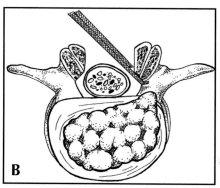

Fig. 5 A, Posteroanterior view demonstrating technique for foraminotomy. The Kerrison rongeur is passed over the nerve root into the foramen to allow decompression. Caution should be taken to prevent excessive pressure over the root. **B,** The axial view demonstrates a Kerrison rongeur used to perform an undercutting maneuver from the opposite side. (© William Beaumont Hospital, Royal Oak, MI)

undercutting of the laminae, is performed with a sharp osteotome. This maneuver exposes the underlying superior facet so that its medial portion can be removed using Kerrison rongeurs (Fig. 7). Others have described a similar procedure using high-speed burrs for facetectomies and undercutting of facet joints.[56]

Other, less commonly applied methods of decompression include the Ipsi-

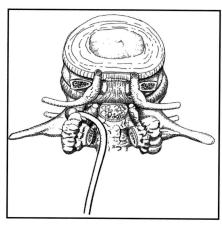

Fig. 6 Axial view of the completed decompression. Note that the probe passes easily out into the foramen. The undersurfaces of the facets and their associated osteophytes have been removed with an undercutting technique, thereby preserving the bulk of the facet itself. (© William Beaumont Hospital, Royal Oak, MI)

Contra procedure and lumbar canal expansive laminoplasty.[57,58]

Results of Lumbar Canal Decompression

Most case series report greater than 85% good-to-excellent results after lumbar decompression for stenosis.[53,59-64] Verbiest[65] reviewed 91 of his patients with up to 20 years follow-up and noted complete relief of preoperative symptoms in 62 (68%); 29 had residual symptoms of which lumbago was the most frequent (47%). Herron and Mangelsdorf[66] reported on 140 patients of whom 80% had major improvement in leg pain. Another 11% had some improvement and 67% had major improvement in back pain. Female sex, compensation or litigation factors, no relief of symptoms from prior surgical procedures, or an objective postoperative sensory deficit predicted a poor outcome. Outcomes in patients with coexisting illnesses (osteoarthritis, cardiac disease, rheumatoid arthritis, chronic obstructive pulmonary disease) are less favorable.[39,40,67-69] Katz and associates[67] and later Jonsson and associates[70] have noted

some deterioration of the early results of decompressive surgery over time. In Katz and associates' series, 17% of patients ultimately underwent a second procedure for instability or recurrent stenosis.

There are fewer series reporting outcomes of laminotomy procedures. However, most have reported 82% to 91% good-to-excellent results.[56,64,71] Postacchini and associates[72] assigned 67 patients with central lumbar stenosis to either multiple laminotomy or total laminectomy groups. In this series, some patients with severe stenosis were converted from laminotomy to laminectomy if inadequate decompression was performed, risk of neural injury was high, or too much bone was taken. After a 3.7-year follow-up, there were 78% good-to-excellent results reported in the laminectomy group and 81% in the multiple laminotomy group. The authors noted that the amount of blood loss was the same; however, duration of surgery and neurologic complications were increased with laminotomy. On the other hand, laminotomy patients had increased relief of back pain and no postoperative instability.

Fusion in the Treatment of Lumbar Spinal Stenosis

Although there appears to be a consensus that patients with lumbar spinal stenosis benefit from decompression if nonsurgical treatment fails, recommendations for fusion are less clearly established. The goals of fusion in these patients are elimination of motion at a painful degenerated segment, elimination of instability, prevention of progression of olisthesis, kyphosis, or scoliosis, or prevention of recurrent stenosis.

Ultimately, the decision to fuse is based on two factors: the preoperative condition of the spine and changes in the stability of the spine stemming from the decompression. Fusion has occcasionally been suggested for all patients undergoing decompression because of the difficulties in identifying unstable spines.[73,74]

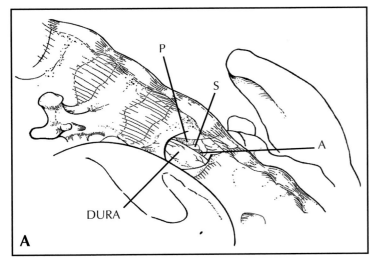
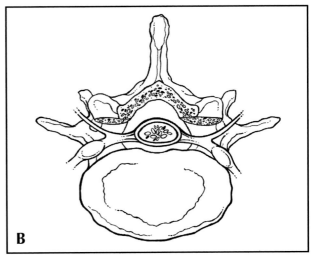

Fig. 7 A, An oblique view of a standard hemilaminotomy for decompression of central and lateral recess stenosis. Here, the ligamentum flavum and leading and trailing edges of the laminae have been removed. A dural retractor is used to protect the dura while a Kerrison rongeur is used to remove facet spurs. P = pedicle (nerve root may be compressed in this area); S = end plate spur; A = disk anulus (bulge may contribute to stenosis). **B,** The axial view demonstrates a sublaminar decompression performed from a laminotomy approach. Note that the medial aspects of the inferior facet of the superior level and the superior facet of the inferior level are removed. (© William Beaumont Hospital, Royal Oak, MI)

On the other hand, in one large series of patients undergoing wide decompression for stenosis, only 2% developed enough instability to require late fusion.[51]

Others argue that fusion increases morbidity with little added benefit and should rarely be required. Deyo and associates[75] reviewed 13,622 Medicare patients treated for lumbar spinal stenosis. Six percent of these patients underwent fusion after wide laminectomy. In fusion patients, complication rates were 1.9 times higher, transfusion rates were 5.8 times higher, nursing home placement was required 2.2 times more often, and the 6-week postoperative mortality was two times higher than in those undergoing decompression alone. Grob and associates[60] performed a randomized study of 45 patients with lumbar spinal stenosis without obvious signs of instability. They found no statistically significant difference in pain relief an average of 28 months of follow-up.

There is more support for routine fusion in patients with preoperative evidence of instability such as a degenerative spondylolisthesis or scoliosis. Here,

decompression may accelerate deformity progression.[76] Yet, Herron and Trippi[77] argued that, with careful decompression, slips did not progress in their series of 24 patients. Even if the slip progresses, its effect on ultimate outcome was occasionally disputed.[66,77,78]

The emerging consensus, however, is to fuse spondylolisthetic segments in patients undergoing decompression for lumbar spinal stenosis.[79-85] Katz and associates[68] studied 105 patients with at least a 5 mm slip or 15° of scoliosis and found superior back pain relief at both 6 and 24 months in patients undergoing uninstrumented fusions versus patients undergoing either no fusion or instrumented fusions. Johnsson and associates[86] found that postoperative increases in listhesis were twice as common in patients with poor results. Herkowitz and Kurz[87] published a prospective study comparing decompressive laminectomy alone with decompressive laminectomy and intertransverse arthrodesis in 50 patients with single level spinal stenosis associated with degenerative spondylolisthesis. In their series the 90% good-to-excellent results

in the fused group was a statistically significant improvement compared with the 44% good-to-excellent results in the nonfusion group.

When performing fusion on a patient who has degenerative spondylolisthesis, attempts to reduce the slip have been advocated. Such reduction is appealing in that restoration of the normal alignment may relieve anterior compression of the nerve roots, shorten the course of the nerve roots, and decrease the tension under which the fusion mass is placed. On the other hand, active, forceful reduction may increase the possibility of an intraoperative neurologic injury. Various techniques to achieve reduction have been described, including use of a sacral bar and Harrington distraction instrumentation[88] or a transpedicle screw and plate method.[89] Often, a two-level extension of the instrumentation to increase biomechanical stability of the construct is required.[90] Montgomery and Fischgrund[90] prospectively evaluated passive reduction in a series of patients undergoing decompressive laminectomy and fusion for degenerative spondylolisthesis. They found an average decrease in slip of 24% from the preoperative flexion view to the intraoperative prone lateral view. In many cases this passive reduction obviates the need for multilevel reconstructions of single-level slips and the danger of intraoperative reduction maneuvers in many cases.

Indications for fusion are even less clearly defined in patients with lumbar spinal stenosis and degenerative scoliosis.[91] Moreover, the additional surgery required to stabilize these multilevel deformities adds significant potential morbidity to the procedure. Most reports have focused on retrospective analysis of surgical technique without comparative reviews of the various options.[65]

It appears that not all degenerative scoliosis patients require fusion for stenosis symptoms. Decompression alone may suffice in patients with single root involvement when the facets can be preserved.[92] Indications for fusion include a large or progressive curve (> 35°), pain in the curve, loss of lumbar lordosis to the extent that it causes sagittal imbalance, and cardiopulmonary complications related to the curve (rare). In patients with radicular symptoms within the concavity of a curve, partial correction of the deformity with an instrumented fusion may be needed to reduce pedicular kinking.[93] Moreover, a curve demonstrating correctability on side bending will likely progress with laminectomy alone.[93] Careful consideration to fusion should be given in the presence of asymmetric tilt of single interspace (especially L4-5), lateral spondylolisthesis, or multiplanar instability.

Fusion may be required as a function of the decompression. The exact degree of instability engendered by a given decompression is difficult to predict. However, the prevailing wisdom has held that removal of one third to one half of both or all of one facet at a given level is tolerated.[71,94,95] Hazlett and Kinnard[96] reported on 33 patients undergoing unilateral or bilateral complete facet joint excision, many with concomitant disk excision. Only four showed signs of late instability and only two of these four had poor results. Grobler and associates[97] reported that progression of spondylolisthesis was more likely caused by facet joint orientation and dimensions than absolute amount of bone removed.

Recurrent stenosis at the same level or stenosis adjacent to a previously decompressed and fused segment also warrants fusion in that further compromise of the facet joints is usually needed for adequate decompression of restenotic patients.

Posterolateral fusion is sufficient in most patients with lumbar spinal stenosis. In addition, 360° fusions, via anteroposterior surgery or posterior lumbar interbody fusion, may be useful to increase correction and fusion rates in certain complex reconstruction situations. Whether instrumentation is required also remains controversial. The goals of instrumentation include deformity correction, spinal stabilization, improved rates of fusion, and reduced rehabilitation time. In patients with hyperlordosis or hyperkyphosis, improvement in the sagittal alignment through instrumented reduction and stabilization may improve outcome. On the other hand, instrumentation confers increased potential for complications, surgery time, and expense.

A pseudarthrosis may not represent a clinical failure.[98,99] Fischgrund and associates[100] reported the results of 68 patients with spinal stenosis and degenerative spondylolisthesis in a prospective study. The authors noted a significantly higher fusion rate (83%) in the instrumented group versus the noninstrumented group (45%). However, the clinical outcome was similar whether instrumentation was used or not. Bridwell and associates[101] found that uninstrumented fusion patients had significantly increased progression of their slips compared with instrumented patients.

The present indications for instrumented fusion include correction of a supple progressive scoliosis or kyphosis; or arthrodesis of two or more motion segments with a decompressive laminectomy; recurrent spinal stenosis with iatrogenic spondylolisthesis; transitional motion greater than 4 mm in flexion and extension and angular motion > 10° compared with adjacent levels; and revision for symptomatic pseudarthrosis.

Postoperative Care

The postoperative regimen is similar for all of the various surgical interventions described. The patient is mobilized to a chair the evening of surgery. Then, ambulation begins the next morning. Braces are typically not used. The patient should refrain from bending, lifting, or twisting for 6 to 12 weeks. Drains are removed on the first or second postoperative day. Most patients go home in 2 to 4 days as a function of extent of their procedure and medical comorbidities. Some elderly patients require inpatient rehabilitation. An office visit is undertaken at 2 weeks for wound check and staple removal. The occasional patient returns to physical therapy at 4 to 6 weeks for a two- to three-visit course to reinforce stretching and strengthening principles. NSAIDs are restricted in all fusion patients.

Complications

Ciol and associates[61] analyzed the data on 30,000 patients undergoing surgical treatment for lumbar spinal stenosis. Complications were divided into four groups: infectious, vascular, cardiopulmonary, and death. Mortality rates were related to age and the presence of comorbidities. In patients younger than age 75 years, the mortality rate was < 1%. In patients older than age 80 years, mortality rose to 2.3%. Complications were twice as frequent as well.

Another potential source of clinical failure is recurrent stenosis by way of laminar regrowth. Postachinni and Cinotti[102] reported on laminar regrowth after decompressive laminectomy for spinal stenosis. They reviewed 40 patients with average 8.6-year follow-up. A preoperative spondylolisthesis was present preoperatively in 16. Of these 16, 6 underwent laminectomy alone; 10 had an added arthrodesis. The authors found that those without arthrodesis had significantly poorer clinical outcome.

There are many potential causes for late-term failure of surgical decompression in lumbar spinal stenosis patients. Among these are recurrent stenosis at the decompressed level and degeneration with stenosis at segments adjacent to that previously treated.[103] In patients undergoing spinal fusion, changes in segmental stiffness may increase forces applied to adjacent segments, thereby accelerating degeneration. Alternatively, proprioceptive changes and postoperative weakness in the lumbar extensors may adversely influence the natural history of spinal stenosis. Both recurrent and adjacent segment stenosis may lead to recurrence of leg pain and pseudo-claudicatory symptoms.

References

1. Johnsson KE, Uden A, Rosen I: The effect of decompression on the natural course of spinal stenosis: A comparison of surgically treated and untreated patients. Spine 1991;16:615-619.
2. LaBan MM, Taylor RS: Conservative management of lumbar spinal stenosis, in Herkowitz HN, Garfin SR, Balderston RA, Eismont FJ, Bell GR, Wiesel SW (eds): Rothman-Simeone: The Spine, ed 4. Philadelphia, PA, WB Saunders, 1999, pp 806A-806F.
3. Davies JE, Gibson T, Tester L: The value of exercises in the treatment of low back pain. Rheumatol Rehabil 1979;18:243-247.
4. Fritz JM, Erhard RE, Vignovic M: A nonsurgical treatment approach for patients with lumbar spinal stenosis. Phys Ther 1997;77:962-973.
5. Mayer GT: Spine functional restoration, in Rothman RH, Simeone FA (eds): The Spine, ed 3. Philadelphia, PA, WB Saunders, 1992, vol 2, pp 1929-1944.
6. Cailliet R (ed): Low Back Pain Syndrome, ed 5. Philadelphia, PA, FA Davis, 1995.
7. Sikorski JM: A rationalized approach to physiotherapy for low-back pain. Spine 1985;10:571-579.
8. Williams PC: Lesions of the lumbosacral spine: Acute traumatic destruction of the lumbosacral intervertebral disc. J Bone Joint Surg Am 1937;19:343-363.
9. Paine KW: Clinical features of lumbar spinal stenosis. Clin Orthop 1976;115:77-82.
10. Zdeblick TA: The treatment of degenerative lumbar disorders: A critical review of the literature. Spine 1995;20(suppl 24):126S-137S.
11. Frymoyer JW: Back pain and sciatica. N Engl J Med 1988;318:291-300.
12. Ward NG: Tricyclic antidepressants for chronic low-back pain: Mechanisms of action and predictors of response. Spine 1986;11:661-665.
13. Eskola A, Pohjolainen T, Alaranta H, Soini J, Tallroth K, Slatis P: Calcitonin treatment in lumbar spinal stenosis: A randomized, placebo-controlled, double-blind, cross-over study with one-year follow-up. Calcif Tissue Int 1992;50:400-403.
14. Basmajian JV: Acute back pain and spasm: A controlled multicenter trial of combined analgesic and antispasm agents. Spine 1989;14:438-439.
15. Schwarzer AC, Aprill CN, Bogduk N: The sacroiliac joint in chronic low back pain. Spine 1995;20:31-37.
16. Cuckler JM, Bernini PA, Wiesel SW, Booth RE Jr, Rothman RH, Pickens GT: The use of epidural steroids in the treatment of lumbar radicular pain: A prospective, randomized, double-blind study. J Bone Joint Surg Am 1985;67:63-66.
17. Ferrante FM: Epidural steroids in the management of spinal stenosis. Semin Spine Surg 1989;1:177.
18. Benzon HT: Epidural steroid injections for low back pain and lumbosacral radiculopathy. Pain 1986;24:277-295.
19. Hoogmartens M, Morelle P: Epidural injection in the treatment of spinal stenosis. Acta Orthop Belg 1987;53:409-411.
20. Rosen CD, Kahanovitz N, Bernstein R, Viola K: A retrospective analysis of the efficacy of epidural steroid injections. Clin Orthop 1988;228:270-272.
21. Rapp SE, Haselkorn JK, Elam K, Deyo RA, Ciol MA: Abstract: Epidural injection in the treatment of low back pain: A meta-analysis. Anesthesiology 1994;(suppl A923):81.
22. Bigos SJ, Bower O, Braen G, Brown KC, Deyo RA, Haldeman S, et al: Acute low back problems in adults, in Clinical Practice Guideline No 14: AHCPR Publication No: 95-0642. Rockville, MD, Department of Health and Human Services, 1995.
23. Derby R, Kine G, Saal JA, et al: Response to steroid and duration of radicular pain as predictors of surgical outcome. Spine 1992;17(suppl 6):S176-S183.
24. Curtis P: Spinal manipulation: Does it work? Occup Med 1988;3:31-44.
25. Grieve GP (ed): Mobilisation of the Spine: Notes on Examination, Assessment, and Clinical Method, ed 4. Edinburgh, Scotland, Churchill Livingstone, 1984.
26. Scientific approach to the assessment and management of activity-related spinal disorders: A monograph for clinicians: Report of the Quebec Task Force on Spinal Disorders. Spine 1987;12(suppl 7):S1-S59.
27. Dimaggio A, Mooney V: Conservative care for LBP, What works? J Musculoskeletal Med 1987;4:27.
28. Pal B, Mangion P, Hossain MA, Diffey BL: A controlled trial of continuous lumbar traction in the treatment of back pain and sciatica. Br J Rheumatol 1986;25:181-183.
29. Onel D, Sari H, Donmez C: Lumbar spinal stenosis: Clinical/radiologic therapeutic evaluation in 145 patients: Conservative treatment or surgical intervention? Spine 1993;18:291-298.
30. Johnsson KE, Rosen I, Uden A: The natural course of lumbar spinal stenosis. Clin Orthop 1992;279:82-86.
31. Atlas SJ, Deyo RA, Keller RB, et al: The Maine Lumbar Spine Study: 1-year outcomes of surgical and nonsurgical management of lumbar spinal stenosis. Spine 1996;21:1787-1795.
32. Kirkaldy-Willis WH (ed): Managing Low Back Pain. New York, NY, Churchill Livingstone, 1983.
33. Van Akkerveeken P: Classification and treatment of spinal stenosis: History and classification on spinal stenosis, in Wiesel SW, Weinstein JN, Herkowitz HN, Dvorak J, Bell GR (eds): The Lumbar Spine, ed 2. Philadelphia, PA, WB Saunders, 1996, vol 2, pp 724-731.
34. Hanley EN Jr, Eskay ML: Degenerative lumbar spinal stenosis. Adv Orthop Surg 1985;8:396-403.
35. Selby DK: When to operate and what to operate upon. Orthop Clin North Am 1983;14:577-588.
36. Wiltse LL, Kirkaldy-Willis WH, Mclvor GW: The treatment of spinal stenosis. Clin Orthop 1976;115:83-91.
37. Grabias S: The treatment of spinal stenosis. J Bone Joint Surg Am 1980;62:308-313.
38. Hall S, Bartleson JD, Onofrio BM, Baker HL Jr, Okazaki H, O'Duffy JD: Lumbar spinal stenosis: Clinical features, diagnostic procedures, and results of surgical treatment in 68 patients. Ann Intern Med 1985;103:271-275.
39. Katz JN, Lipson SJ, Brick GW, et al: Clinical correlates of patient satisfaction after laminectomy for degenerative lumbar spinal stenosis. Spine 1995;20:1155-1160.
40. Ciol MA, Deyo RA, Howell E, Kreif S: An assessment of surgery for spinal stenosis: Time trends, geographic variations, complications and reoperations. J Am Geriatr Soc 1996;44:285-290.

41. Katz JN: Lumbar spinal fusion: Surgical rates, costs, and complications. *Spine* 1995;20(suppl 24):78S-83S.

42. Taylor VM, Deyo RA, Cherkin DC, Kreuter W: Low back pain hospitalization: Recent United States trends and regional variations. *Spine* 1994;19:1207-1213.

43. Volinn E, Mayer J, Diehr P, Van Koevering D, Connell FA, Loeser JD: Small area analysis of surgery for low-back pain. *Spine* 1992;17: 575-581.

44. Larequi-Lauber T, Vader JP, Burnand B, et al: Appropriateness of indications for surgery of lumbar disc hernia and spinal stenosis. *Spine* 1997;22:203-209.

45. Fellrath RF Jr, Hanley EN Jr: The causes and management of pseudarthrosis following anterior cervical arthrodesis. *Semin Spine Surg* 1995;7:43-51.

46. Sanderson PL, Wood PL: Surgery for lumbar spinal stenosis in old people. *J Bone Joint Surg Br* 1993;75:393-397.

47. Spengler DM: Lumbar decompression for spinal stenosis: Surgical indications and technique, in Frymoyer JW, Ducker TB, Hadler NM, Kostuik JP, Weinstein JN, Whitecloud TS III (eds): *The Adult Spine: Principles and Practice.* New York, NY, Raven Press, 1991, vol 2, pp 1811-1819.

48. Katz JN, Dalgas M, Stucki G, Lipson SG: Degenerative lumbar spinal stenosis: Diagnostic value of the history and physical examination. *Arthritis Rheum* 1995;38: 1236-1241.

49. Rosen C, Rothman S, Zigler J, Capen D: Lumbar facet fracture as a possible source of pain after lumbar laminectomy. *Spine* 1991;16(suppl 6):S234-S238.

50. Herron LD, Trippi AC, Gonyeau M: Intraoperative use of dermatomal somatosensory-evoked potentials in lumbar stenosis surgery. *Spine* 1987;12:379-383.

51. Whiffen JR, Neuwirth MG: Spinal stenosis, in Bridwell KH, DeWald RL, Hammerberg KW, et al (eds): *The Textbook of Spinal Surgery,* ed 2. Philadelphia, PA, Lippincott-Raven, 1997, vol 2, pp 1561-1580.

52. DiStefano VJ, Klein KS, Nixon JE, Andrews ET: Intra-operative analysis of the effects of position and body habitus on surgery of the low back: A preliminary report. *Clin Orthop* 1974;99:51-56.

53. Garfin SR, Glover M, Booth RE, Simeone FA, Rothman RH: Laminectomy: A review of the Pennsylvania hospital experience. *J Spinal Disord* 1988;1:116-133.

54. Lee CK, Rauschning W, Glenn W: Lateral lumbar spinal canal stenosis: Classification, pathologic anatomy and surgical decompression. *Spine* 1988;13:313-320.

55. Lin PM: Internal decompression for multiple levels of lumbar spinal stenosis: A technical note. *Neurosurgery* 1982;11:546-549.

56. Young S, Veerapen R, O'Laoire SA: Relief of lumbar canal stenosis using multilevel subarticular fenestrations as an alternative to wide laminectomy: Preliminary report. *Neurosurgery* 1988;23:628-633.

57. diPierro CG, Helm GA, Shaffrey CI, et al: Treatment of lumbar spinal stenosis by extensive unilateral decompression and contralateral autologous bone fusion: Operative technique and results. *J Neurosurg* 1996;84:166-173.

58. Matsui H, Tsuji H, Sekido H, Hirano N, Katoh Y, Makiyama N: Results of expansive laminoplasty for lumbar spinal stenosis in active manual workers. *Spine* 1992;17 (suppl 3):S37-S40.

59. Getty CJ: Lumbar spinal stenosis: The clinical spectrum and the results of operation. *J Bone Joint Surg Br* 1980;62:481-485.

60. Grob D, Hunke T, Dvorak J: Degenerative lumbar spinal stenosis: Decompression with and without arthrodesis. *J Bone Joint Surg Am* 1995;77:1036-1041.

61. Ciol MA, Deyo RA, Howell E, Kreif S: An assessment of surgery for spinal stenosis: Time, trends, geographic variation, complications, and reoperations. *J Am Geriatr Soc* 1996;44:285-290.

62. Herkowitz HN, Garfin SR, Bell GR, Bumphrey F, Rothman RH: The use of computerized tomography in evaluating nonvisualized vertebral levels caudad to a complete block on a lumbar myelogram: A review of thirty-two cases. *J Bone Joint Surg Am* 1987;69:218-224.

63. McNulty SE, Weiss J, Azad SS, Schaefer DM, Osterholm JL, Seltzer JL: The effect of the prone position on venous pressure and blood loss during lumbar laminectomy. *J Clin Anesth* 1992;4:220-225.

64. Nakai O, Ookawa A, Yamaura I: Long-term roentgenographic and functional changes in patients who were treated with wide fenestration for central lumbar stenosis. *J Bone Joint Surg Am* 1991;73:1184-1191.

65. Verbiest H: Results of surgical treatment of idiopathic developmental stenosis of the lumbar vertebral canal: A review of twenty-seven years' experience. *J Bone Joint Surg Br* 1977;59:181-188.

66. Herron LD, Mangelsdorf C: Lumbar spinal stenosis: Results of surgical treatment. *J Spinal Disord* 1991;4:26-33.

67. Katz JN, Lipson SJ, Larson MG, McInnes JM, Fossel AH, Liang MH: The outcome of decompressive laminectomy for degenerative lumbar stenosis. *J Bone Joint Surg Am* 1991;73:809-816.

68. Katz JN, Lipson SJ, Lew RA, et al: Lumbar laminectomy alone or with instrumented or noninstrumented arthrodesis in degenerative lumbar spinal stenosis: Patient selection, costs, and surgical outcomes. *Spine* 1997;22: 1123-1131.

69. Thalgott JS, Cotler HB, Sasso RC, LaRocca H, Gardner V: Postoperative infections in spinal implants: Classification and analysis. A multicenter study. *Spine* 1991;16:981-984.

70. Jonsson B, Annertz M, Sjoberg C, Stromqvist B: A prospective and consecutive study of surgically treated lumbar spinal stenosis: Part I. Clinical features related to radiographic findings. *Spine* 1997;22:2932-2937.

71. Aryanpur J, Ducker T: Multilevel lumbar laminotomies: An alternative to laminectomy in the treatment of lumbar stenosis. *Neurosurgery* 1990;26:429-433.

72. Postacchini F, Cinotti G, Perugia D, Gumina S: The surgical treatment of central lumbar stenosis: Multiple laminotomy compared with total laminectomy. *J Bone Joint Surg Br* 1993;75: 386-392.

73. Chen Q, Baba H, Kamitani K, Furusawa N, Imura S: Postoperative bone re-growth in lumbar spinal stenosis: A multivariate analysis of 48 patients. *Spine* 1994;19:2144-2149.

74. Hopp E, Tsou PM: Postdecompression lumbar instability. *Clin Orthop* 1988;227:143-151.

75. Deyo RA, Ciol MA, Cherkin DC, Loeser JD, Bigos SJ: Lumbar spinal fusion: A cohort study of complications, reoperations, and resource use in the Medicare population. *Spine* 1993;18:1463-1470.

76. Lombardi JS, Wiltse LL, Reynolds J, Widell EH, Spencer C III: Treatment of degenerative spondylolisthesis. *Spine* 1985;10:821-827.

77. Herron LD, Trippi AC: L4-5 degenerative spondylolisthesis: The results of treatment by decompressive laminectomy without fusion. *Spine* 1989;14:534-538.

78. Fitzgerald JA, Newman PH: Degenerative spondylolisthesis. *J Bone Joint Surg Br* 1976;58:184-192.

79. Caputy AJ, Luessenhop AJ: Long-term evaluation of decompressive surgery for degenerative lumbar stenosis. *J Neurosurg* 1992;77:669-676.

80. Dall BE, Rowe DE: Degenerative spondylolisthesis: Its surgical management. *Spine* 1985;10:668-672.

81. Feffer HL, Wiesel SW, Cuckler JM, Rothman RH: Degenerative spondylolisthesis: To fuse or not to fuse. *Spine* 1985;10:287-289.

82. Katz JN, Lipson SJ, Chang LC, Levine SA, Fossel AH, Liang MH: Seven- to 10-year outcome of decompressive surgery for degenerative lumbar spinal stenosis. *Spine* 1996;21:92-98.

83. Lehmann TR, Spratt KF, Tozzi JE, et al: Long-term follow-up of lower lumbar fusion patients. *Spine* 1987;12:97-104.

84. Smith DW, Lawrence BD: Vascular complications of lumbar decompression laminectomy and foraminotomy: A unique case and review of the literature. *Spine* 1991;16:387-390.

85. Farfan HF, Kirkaldy-Willis WH: The present status of spinal fusion in the treatment of lumbar intervertebral joint disorders. *Clin Orthop* 1981;158:198-214.

86. Johnsson KE, Redlund-Johnell I, Uden A, Willner S: Preoperative and postoperative instability in lumbar spinal stenosis. *Spine* 1989;14:591-593.

87. Herkowitz HN, Kurz LT: Degenerative lumbar spondylolisthesis with spinal stenosis: A prospective study comparing decompression with decompression and intertransverse process arthrodesis. *J Bone Joint Surg Am* 1991;73:802-808.

88. Zielke K, Strempel AV: Posterior lateral distraction spondylodesis using the two-fold sacral bar. *Clin Orthop* 1986;203:151-158.

89. Roy-Camille R, Saillant G, Mazel C: Internal fixation of the lumbar spine with pedicle screw plating. *Clin Orthop* 1986;203:7-17.

90. Montgomery DM, Fischgrund JS: Passive reduction of spondylolisthesis on the operating room table: A prospective study. *J Spinal Disord* 1994;7:167-172.

91. Nash CL Jr, Moe JH: A study of vertebral rotation. *J Bone Joint Surg Am* 1969;51:223-229.

92. Abitbol JJ, Dowling TJ, Benz RJ, Kostuik JP: Adult scoliosis, in Herkowitz HN, Garfin SR, Balderston RA, Eismont FJ, Bell GR, Wiesel SW (eds): *Rothman-Simeone: The Spine,* ed 4. Philadelphia, PA, WB Saunders, 1999, pp 809-834.

93. Garfin SR, Rydevik BL, Lipson SJ, et al: Spinal stenosis, in Rothman RH, Simeone FA (eds): *The Spine,* ed 3. Philadelphia, PA, WB Saunders, 1992, pp 791-857.

94. White AH, Wiltse LL: Postoperative spondylolisthesis, in Weinstein PR, Ehni G, Wilson CB (eds): *Lumbar Spondylolysis: Diagnosis, Management, and Surgical Treatment.* Chicago, IL, Year Book Medical Publishers, 1977, pp 184-194.

95. Boden SD, Martin C, Rudolph R, Kirkpatrick JS, Moeini SM, Hutton WC: Increase of motion between lumbar vertebrae after excision of the capsule and cartilage of the facets: A cadaver study. *J Bone Joint Surg Am* 1994;76:1847-1853.

96. Hazlett JW, Kinnard P: Lumbar apophyseal process excision and spinal instability. *Spine* 1982;7:171-176.

97. Grobler LJ, Robertson PA, Novotny JE, Ahern JW: Decompression for degenerative spondylolisthesis and spinal stenosis at L4-5: The effects on facet joint morphology. *Spine* 1993;18:1475-1482.

98. DePalma AF, Rothman RH: The nature of pseudarthrosis. *Clin Orthop* 1968;59:113-118.

99. Garfin SR, Herkowitz HN: Surgical management of spinal stenosis: Part II. Indications and surgical results of arthrodesis following spinal stenosis decompression, in Herkowitz HN, Garfin SR, Balderston RA, Eismont FJ, Bell GR, Wiesel SW (eds): *Rothman-Simeone: The Spine,* ed 4. Philadelphia, PA, WB Saunders, 1999, p 806M.

100. Fischgrund JS, Mackay M, Herkowitz HN, Brower R, Montgomery DM, Kurz LT: Degenerative lumbar spondylolisthesis with spinal stenosis: A prospective, randomized study comparing decompressive laminectomy and arthrodesis with and without spinal instrumentation. *Spine* 1997;22:2807-2812.

101. Bridwell KH, Sedgewick TA, O'Brien MF, Lenke LG, Baldus C: The role of fusion and instrumentation in the treatment of degenerative spondylolisthesis with spinal stenosis. *J Spinal Disord* 1993;6:461-472.

102. Postacchini F, Cinotti G: Bone regrowth after surgical decompression for lumbar spinal stenosis. *J Bone Joint Surg Br* 1992;74:862-869.

103. Truumees E, Fischgrund J, Herkowitz HN: Management of spinal stenosis adjacent to a previously treated segment. *Semin Spine Surg* 1999;11:282-291.

Microsurgical Techniques in Lumbar Spinal Stenosis

K. Daniel Riew, MD
John Rhee, MD

Introduction

The traditional surgical approach to degenerative lumbar spinal stenosis is an extensive, wide decompression. Although this method can be useful in relieving neural compression, potential problems include iatrogenic instability as well as prolonged postoperative recovery because of extensive muscle, ligament, and bone resection. Thus, microsurgical techniques for decompression have been advocated as alternatives to the traditional technique. The advantage of the microsurgical approach is that it allows maximal neural decompression while simultaneously minimizing resection of the stabilizing and supportive structures of the spine. Most degenerative spinal stenosis can be treated with microsurgical decompression because the pathologic neural compression tends to occur at discrete points in the spine (ie, at the level of the disk spaces), making the global removal of "nonoffending" bony and soft-tissue elements not only unnecessary but also counterproductive. In this chapter, we review the indications for microsurgical lumbar decompression and present our technique of microlumbar laminoplasty.

Clinical Presentation

Degenerative lumbar spinal stenosis is an acquired condition that affects middle-aged and older patients. Progressive degeneration of the three-joint complex leads to loss of disk height, arthritic changes in the facet joints, and hypertrophy of the ligamentum flavum. These changes cause narrowing of the spinal canal, leading most often to lateral recess stenosis but also to central canal and foraminal stenosis. Patients generally complain of an insidious onset of symptoms and relate a history consistent with slowly progressive neurogenic claudication. Physical findings are variable, and many patients have no neurologic abnormalities on examination. Standing AP and lateral radiographs are essential in evaluating patients with suspected spinal stenosis. Functional tests, such as the bicycle-treadmill test, can be useful in confirming the diagnosis.[1] A vascular examination and evaluation for symp-tomatic arthritis of the hips and knees also should be done, especially when the patient's presentation is not classic for spinal stenosis or when multiple etiologies for pain are present.

Physical therapy, general aerobic conditioning, and nonsteroidal anti-inflammatory medications are the first line of nonsurgical treatment. Patients with predominantly radicular patterns of pain may benefit from selective nerve root injections, which function as both diagnostic and therapeutic maneuvers. Epidural steroids may similarly improve symptoms; long-term relief of pain has been demonstrated with both types of injections.[2,3] Surgical management can be considered to improve patient function and quality of life when the appropriate conservative measures fail.

Indications for Microsurgical Decompression

In general, microsurgical decompression can be considered when most of the neural compression occurs at the levels of the disk space and neural foramina. Patients with congenital spinal stenosis are not good candidates for a microsurgical approach because the areas of compression are continuous rather than discrete. Although compression may be most severe at the level of the disk space, a complete laminectomy usually is necessary in these patients to adequately relieve all of the pathologic compression. Similarly, patients with grade II or higher spondylolisthesis also have a more global compression of the neural elements and generally require a wider decompression. These patients may also need a fusion. Technical factors that may make microsurgical decompression inappropriate include dense midline adhesions and significant lordosis. These factors hinder visualization of the contralateral side when attempting to perform microsurgical decompression through the laminoplasty technique described below (Fig. 1), and a more traditional approach to decompression is recommended.

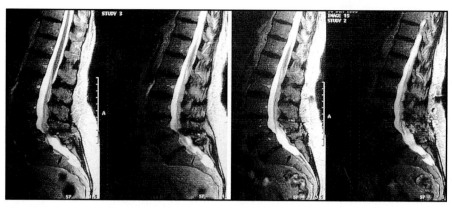

Fig. 1 Preoperative and postoperative axial MRI sections in a patient with severe stenosis at L3-4 and L4-5. A two-level microlumbar laminoplasty was done.

Table 1
Relative Indications for Fusion Associated With Lumbar Decompressions

Important stabilizing structures have been sacrificed during decompression
Recurrent stenosis
Degenerative spondylolisthesis with hypermobility on standing lateral flexion-extension views
Both coronal and sagittal listhesis at the level to be decompressed
Transition syndrome adjacent to previous fusion
Associated isthmic spondylolisthesis
Associated scoliosis

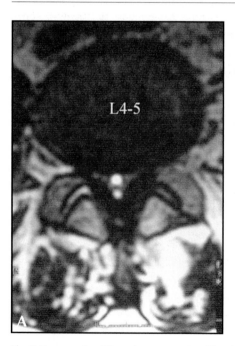
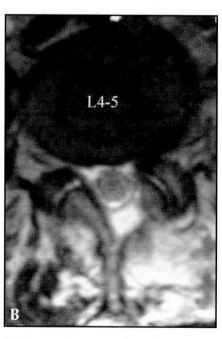

Fig. 2 Preoperative **(A)** and postoperative **(B)** axial MRI scans of a patient who underwent L4-5 microsurgical lumbar laminoplasty. Preoperatively, note that the stenosis arises focally at the level of the L4-5 disk space.

The Role of Fusion

In general, fusion has a limited role in the treatment of spinal stenosis uncomplicated by instability (Table 1). Although a detailed discussion of fusion and instrumentation is beyond the scope of this chapter, several studies have noted improved outcomes with arthrodesis in patients who have spinal stenosis and degenerative spondylolisthesis.[4-7] Caution should be exercised when considering decompression alone in these patients because progression of the slip may require subsequent fusion.[8] Exceptions to this general rule include elderly patients with spondylolisthesis and a severely degenerated disk space who demonstrate limited motion on flexion-extension films.

Preoperative Planning
The Three-Floor Spine Concept

A precise understanding of how the more ventral neural structures relate to the dorsally visible bony and soft-tissue anatomy is critical to performing microsurgical decompression. This knowledge allows the microsurgeon to perform an adequate and safe decompression through a limited exposure. To translate the pathologic findings seen on MRI or CT myelogram into a surgical road map, it is useful to have a mental model for localizing lesions within the spinal canal. McCulloch and Young[9] described the spinal segment as a "three-floor anatomical house."

The first floor of this house is the disk level. Here, multiple structures (eg, bulging and herniated disks, hypertrophied and infolded ligamentum flavum, hypertrophied and subluxated facets) commonly converge to produce most of the stenosis within the house (Fig. 2). The second floor is the foraminal level, which extends from the inferior end plate to the inferior border of the pedicle. At this level, superior capsular hypertrophy and proximal migration of the superior facet because of disk flattening can lead to

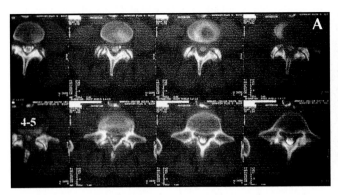
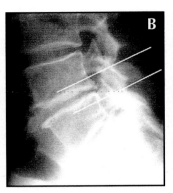
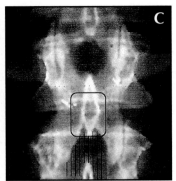

Fig. 3 Preoperative radiographs in a patient who underwent L4-L5 microsurgical lumbar laminoplasty. **A,** Postmyelogram CT scan reveals that the pathology extends from just above to just below the L4-L5 disk level (the first floor of the anatomical house). The exact location of the incision and the amount of bone requiring resection can be precisely plotted on the AP and lateral radiographs (**B** and **C**).

foraminal stenosis (Fig. 3). The third floor, the pedicle level, comprises the region from the inferior border of the pedicle to the superior end plate. Few structures cause pathologic compression here except for the inferior portion of a hypertrophied superior facet, which can compress the nerve root just before it enters the lateral recess.

The spine can be further subdivided in the coronal plane into the central, foraminal, and extraforaminal zones.[9] The central zone lies between the pedicles and includes the lateral recesses. Offending structures in this zone include the ligamentum flavum, bulging or herniated disks, hypertrophied facets, and osteophytes. Spondylolisthesis also can contribute to central stenosis. Synovial cysts can lead to significant lateral recess stenosis and often are very adherent to the underlying dura. The foraminal zone extends from the medial to the lateral border of the pedicle. The extraforaminal zone is lateral to the lateral edge of the pedicle.

Based on the CT myelogram or MRI findings, the surgeon can visualize on the three-floor model the precise locations of compression. The exact positions of pathology are then superimposed on the preoperative AP radiograph to determine the site of the skin incision and the extent of posterior bone resection required to obtain an adequate decompression. Furthermore, the model allows the surgeon to navigate intraoperatively between the neural structures to be decompressed and the pedicle, foramen, disk space, ligamentum flavum, and lamina.

Choosing the Appropriate Limited Decompression Procedure

After localizing the lesions in three dimensions, the next step is to choose the appropriate method of decompression to treat the problem without sacrificing uninvolved structures. Several methods of limited decompression have been described. Multiple hemilaminotomies preserve the midline ligaments and bone and can be used in patients with lateral recess compression but no central canal stenosis. A sublaminar decompression preserves the superior portion of the cephalad lamina and the inferior portion of the caudad lamina. However, the approach is bilateral and some spinous process as well as midline ligaments must be removed to expose the interlaminar space and allow undercutting of the adjacent laminae. This technique can be used in the presence of central stenosis that is confined to the first floor (ie, disk level). The microsurgical laminoplasty technique, popularized by McCulloch,[10] preserves midline ligaments and bone as well as contralateral bone and paraspinal mus-culature. Of the limited decompression procedures, this technique is probably the least invasive method for providing the most complete decompression of the central canal, lateral recesses, and bilateral foramina.

Technique
Patient Positioning

We prefer to do the decompression with the patient's lumbar spine flexed. This position keeps the posterior ligaments taut, which widens the interlaminar spaces and opens the neural canal, making it easier to enter the epidural space and decompress the neural elements. However, the disadvantage of the flexed position is that, because it tends to en-large certain regions (eg, the foramina), these areas may have to be "over-decompressed" to ensure that they remain adequately enlarged when the patient is upright with the spine extended (Fig. 4). A flexed position should also be avoided during instrumented fusion to avoid iatrogenic loss of lumbar lordosis.

The abdomen must be free throughout the procedure. If the abdomen is compressed, the resultant increase in intra-abdominal pressure causes epidural venous engorgement and leads to greater blood loss. To avoid peripheral nerve palsies, care must be taken to ensure that excessive

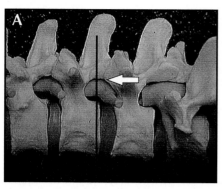
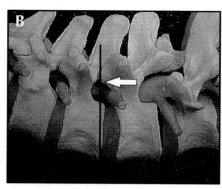

Fig. 4 Change in foraminal dimensions with position. In flexion (**A**), the foramen is relatively larger. In extension (**B**), the foramen narrows and the superior facet migrates proximally. Note also that there is more overhang of the lamina in the extended versus the flexed position. Thus, decompressions done with the spine flexed must account for this, and the appropriate amount of lamina should be undercut even though it may not appear to be impinging on the canal in flexion.

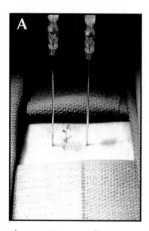
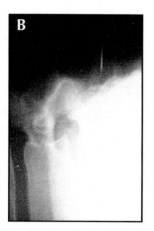
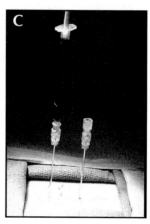

Fig. 5 A, Two needles are used to isolate the disk level. **B,** A localizing radiograph is used to determine site of skin incision. **C,** Indigo carmine is injected into proximal needle only. The dye can be readily identified after exposure of the appropriate lamina.

pressure is not placed on the elbows, axilla, and other prominences. The eyes also must be free of compression.

Anesthesia

Although posterior lumbar decompressions usually are done with general anesthesia, other options include epidural or even local anesthesia. If an epidural or local anesthesia is used, varying degrees of sedation are given based on patient or surgeon preference. The advantages of an epidural anesthetic include shorter time spent in the recovery room, faster return of orientation and alertness, and avoidance of the postoperative nausea and vomiting that occurs with general anesthesia. In addition, because the epidural anesthetic has a vasodilatory effect on the lower extremities, intraoperative bleeding is thought to be decreased.

The disadvantages of an epidural anesthetic include the possibility of hypotension secondary to peripheral vasodilatation, difficulty establishing an airway in the event of a complication, patient movement during the surgical procedure, and the possibility of compli-cations from placement of the epidural anesthetic itself, including neurologic injury and dural tears. In addition, epidural anesthetics can cause urine retention.

Localizing the Level: Plain Radiographic Technique

We prefer to obtain radiographs after the patient is positioned but before the incision is made. Two 18-gauge spinal needles are used to localize the skin incision. For the L4-L5 level, we place one spinal needle overlying the L4 lamina and the second one overlying the L5 lamina. The needles are placed on the ipsilateral side one and a half finger-breadths lateral to the midline (Fig. 5). The superior-inferior position is determined by palpating the top and bottom of the spinous process and placing the needle one third of the distance from the superior point. If these landmarks are not palpable, the needles are left shallow to prevent inadvertent perforation of the dura. Before draping, a lateral portable radiograph is obtained to confirm the positions of these needles. Two needles are used so that the distance between them can be used as a frame of reference when looking at the magnified radiograph. Once the radiograph is reviewed and the needles are on the correct laminae, 0.3 mL of indigo carmine dye is injected through one of the needles to mark its position. The dye may make the patient's urine pale blue for the first void. Methylene blue should never be used because it can cause neurotoxicity or death if inadvertently placed intradurally. Additional localizing radiographs usually are not necessary using this technique.

Alternatively, the levels can be localized once the incision has been made. Metal markers such as towel clips can be placed on the appropriate spinous processes. Regardless of the method used, it is absolutely mandatory to obtain high-quality radiographs containing the landmarks necessary to confirm the

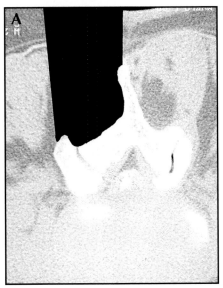
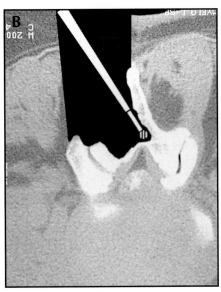
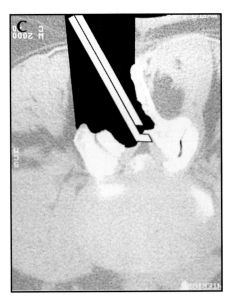

Fig. 6 Schematic of the microlumbar laminoplasty technique. **A,** A hemilaminotomy is done, generally on the side opposite the greatest lateral recess and foraminal stenosis. **B,** Kerrison rongeurs and a high-speed burr are used to undercut the midline and contralateral lamina to effect a central decompression. The contralateral ligamentum flavum is left intact at this point to protect the underlying dura. **C,** The contralateral ligamentum flavum is excised after completion of laminar work. A central decompression has been done, and attention can now be turned to the lateral recesses and foramina.

proper levels. This caveat is even more important when performing microsurgical decompressions than traditional wide decompressions because the surgeon's view of dorsal landmarks is more limited. Repeat radiographs are obtained until the surgeon is certain that the correct levels have been identified.

It is surprisingly easy to decompress the wrong levels or not decompress enough levels using a microlaminoplasty technique. It is therefore recommended that, until the surgeon is very experienced in the technique, radiographs also be obtained after decompression to document that the appropriate levels have been decompressed.

Microsurgical Lumbar Laminoplasty
Microsurgical lumbar laminoplasty is done through a unilateral exposure of either the left or the right hemilamina, depending on the pathology. The bone and muscles on the opposite side are left intact. The midline ligaments, including the interspinous and paraspin-

ous ligaments, are preserved. Although the approach is unilateral, a thorough bilateral decompression of the central canal, lateral recesses, and foramina can be achieved[9,10] (Fig. 1). This is accomplished by sculpting the undersurface of the contralateral lamina to allow visualization of the contralateral structures (Fig. 6). The microscope can be angled as necessary to see all regions. Dural elevators are used to separate the neural elements from the structures to be decompressed. A wide selection of Kerrison rongeurs, including curved ones, should be available to provide access to difficult-to-reach areas. The preservation of the midline and contralateral muscles and ligaments may help to prevent postoperative instability and permit faster recovery.

Exposure
After appropriate radiographic localization, the incision is made about 1 cm lateral to the midline on the side on which the hemilaminotomy will be done. It is preferable to perform the hemilaminoto-

my on the side opposite the greatest lateral recess and foraminal stenosis because visualization of these regions is improved from the contralateral side. If the patient's pathology does not dictate the side selected for the hemilaminotomy, a left-sided approach is generally suited to right-handed surgeons. A curvilinear incision is made in the lumbodorsal fascia and a flap is raised, with the larger portion of the flap reflected toward the midline. The paraspinal muscles are then unilaterally stripped off the spinous process and lamina. The lateral pars should be exposed so that it can be preserved.

Ipsilateral Hemilaminotomy
Self-retaining retractors are placed into the wound and the microscope is brought into position. The lamina is then thinned down with a high-speed burr and removed with Kerrison rongeurs. Generally, about one half of the inferior portion of the cephalad lamina (ie, just superior to the insertion of the ligamentum flavum) and one third of

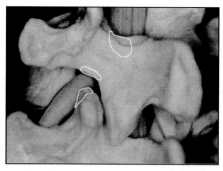

Fig. 7 Foraminal compression generally arises from superior facet hypertrophy and proximal migration because of disk space narrowing.

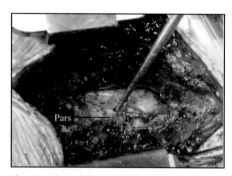

Fig. 8 Ipsilateral foraminal decompression through a combined approach. A ball-tipped probe has been placed in the foramen from inside the canal. The lateral approach was used to decompress the foramen from the outside in. The tip of the probe is seen in the foramen.

the superior portion of the caudad lamina need to be resected. Extreme care must be exercised during this maneuver to preserve the lateral pars (ie, that portion between the superior and inferior articular facets). At least 6 to 7 mm of lateral pars should be left intact to prevent an iatrogenic pars fracture.

The laminae are undercut at the proximal and distal extents of the hemilaminotomy to provide adequate central decompression without removing excess bone. The ipsilateral ligamentum flavum is then resected, thereby opening the central canal and providing access to the epidural space. Next, the base of the spinous process is thinned down to provide access to the contralateral side.

Contralateral Decompression

The microscope is tilted to view the contralateral side. The patient also can be tilted away from the surgeon if necessary. In a large individual with a deep wound, it may be more difficult to see the contralateral side. Offset lateral muscle blades can be used to move the retractor blade away from the line of vision. Using Penfield or other blunt dissectors, the dura is then separated from the overlying flavum and lamina. If dense adhesions are encountered that cannot be released, it may be prudent to abort the laminoplasty procedure and convert to a bilateral decompression. The opposite lamina is then carefully undercut from within the spinal canal using a combination of a high-speed burr and large and medium Kerrison rongeurs. The ligamentum flavum is removed only after all burr work is completed to protect the dura from injury. Decompression of the contralateral central canal proceeds in this manner until adequate space for the thecal sac is verified by direct observation and by passing a probe under the margins of the hemilaminotomy.

To decompress the contralateral lateral recess, it is helpful to identify the contralateral pedicle and facet joint early to positively verify the positions of the disk space, nerve root, and foramen. If they cannot be seen, then further undercutting of the contralateral lamina may be necessary. After palpating the contralateral pedicle and the margins of the facet joint, the contralateral nerve root is identified and gently swept toward the midline away from the bony margins in the lateral recess. Kerrison rongeurs are then used to undercut the contralateral superior facet and decompress the traversing nerve root in the lateral recess. The attachments of the ligamentum flavum to the medial border of the facet joint often contribute to lateral recess stenosis and are also removed. Adequate lateral recess decompression is verified by inspection and palpation of the nerve

root as it hugs the medial border of the pedicle.

Generally, the contralateral foramen and the traversing nerve root (eg, L5 root for an L4-L5 decompression) can be seen clearly. In contrast, access to the exiting root (eg, L4 root for an L4-L5 decompression) is much more difficult with a laminoplasty approach. A lateral approach (described below) should be considered when a foraminotomy of the exiting root is necessary or when difficulty is encountered in seeing the traversing nerve root in its foramen. Decompression of the traversing nerve root in the contralateral foramen is easier with the use of small (2 to 3 mm), curved Kerrison rongeurs. It is often possible to see this nerve root well into the foramen and even into the extraforaminal zone.

Ipsilateral Decompression

Once the decompression is completed on the contralateral side, the microscope is adjusted for the ipsilateral decompression. A medial facetectomy is done on the inferior and superior facets to the medial border of the pedicle. This can be done with a combination of Kerrison rongeurs and a high-speed burr. Medial facetectomy of the inferior facet is fairly straightforward from a direct posterior route. Medial facetectomy of the superior facet is safer if one first follows the superior border of the caudad lamina laterally to the medial wall of the pedicle. The nerve root can be identified there at the inferior border of the pedicle in an area where it is generally free. The tightest region of the lateral recess tends to be superior to this area. By knowing where the root is, a medial facetectomy of the superior facet can then be done safely from a caudal to rostral direction.

A foraminotomy on the ipsilateral side is more difficult than on the contralateral side.[9] Whereas the microscope can be canted at a low enough angle to view the foramen and the nerve root on the contralateral side, the spinous process prevents adequate visualization of the neural foramen on the ipsilateral side. To complete the decompression of the neural foramen on the ipsilateral side, it may be necessary to combine the decompression from inside the canal with a far lateral approach.

The Combination Approach

In patients with severe foraminal stenosis, often the easiest way to do a thorough foraminal decompression is to first perform a central and lateral recess decompression from within the canal, then approach the foramen from a far lateral approach. The paraspinal muscles are stripped out to the transverse processes. The facet joint inferior to the stenotic foramen is identified. Often, the foraminal stenosis is caused by a superiorly migrated and hypertrophic superior facet impinging on the ganglion of the nerve root (Fig. 7). A partial lateral capsulectomy of the facet is done, followed by resection of the overriding portion of the superior articular facet in the foramen. The foraminotomy is then continued from outside (lateral to the pars) in. Care is taken again to ensure that 6 to 7 mm of lateral pars is left intact. A Woodson or other angled elevator is used from inside the canal to separate the exiting nerve root from the structures to be decompressed. This combined technique ensures that the neural foramen is thoroughly decompressed (Fig. 8).

Complications

Microsurgical lumbar laminoplasty is generally a safe procedure with minimal complications when done by experienced surgeons. Instability is rare with this approach. Dural injury is the most common complication. Generally, the dural tears can be easily repaired at the time of the procedure, and long-term sequelae

are rare.[11] Knowledge of the anatomy and course of the nerve roots and good surgical assistance to retract the neural elements from the areas to be decompressed will help prevent neural injury. Use of a Kerrison rongeur parallel to the course of the nerve root can help limit damage to the nerve root. With proper techniques and instruments, the rate of permanent nerve injury should be far less than 1%.

Postoperative wound infections also are rare. Rates have been reported to be less than 1% of all lumbar decompressions.[12] We routinely use a short course of perioperative antibiotics. It has been our experience that there is an increased risk of epidural hematoma formation after microsurgical lumbar laminoplasty because raw bony surfaces are left exposed on the undersurfaces of the laminae, which can continue to bleed. The use of deep drains after decompression may help to prevent symptomatic postoperative epidural hematomas.

Summary

The rationale for microsurgical decompression is to maximize neural decompression while minimizing the destabilization and resection of uninvolved structures. Microsurgical decompression is appropriate for most degenerative lumbar spinal stenosis because the pathoanatomy tends to be concentrated at the levels of the disk space and foramen. Careful preoperative analysis of the imaging studies will guide the surgeon to the most appropriate method of decompression for a particular patient and help focus the decompression to the appropriate regions. Thorough knowledge of surgical spinal anatomy is mandatory because the exposure is limited with a microsurgical approach; however, visualization can be excellent with proper attention to surgical technique.

References

1. Tenhula J, Lenke LG, Bridwell KH, Gupta P, Riew KD: Prospective functional evaluation of surgical treatment of neurogenic claudication in patients with lumbar spinal stenosis. *J Spinal Disord* 2000;13:276-282.

2. Riew KD, Yin Y, Gilula L, Bridwell KH, Lenke LG, Lauryssen C, Goette K: The effect of nerve-root injections on the need for operative treatment of lumbar radicular pain: A prospective, randomized, controlled, double-blind study. *J Bone Joint Surg Am* 2000;82:1589-1593.

3. White AH: Injection techniques for the diagnosis and treatment of low back pain. *Orthop Clin North Am* 1983;14:553.

4. Bridwell KH, Sedgewick T, O'Brien M, Lenke LG, Baldus C: The role of fusion and instrumentation in the treatment of degenerative spondylolisthesis with spinal stenosis. *J Spinal Disord* 1993;6:467-472.

5. Caputy A, Lessenhop A: Long term evaluation of decompressive surgery for degenerative lumbar stenosis. *J Neurosurg* 1992;77:669-676.

6. Herkowitz HN, Kurtz LT: Degenerative lumbar spondylolisthesis with spinal stenosis: A prospective study comparing decompression with decompression and intertransverse process arthrodesis. *J Bone Joint Surg Am* 1991; 73:802-808.

7. Yuan HA, Garfin SR, Dickman CA, Mardjetko SM: A historical cohort study of pedicle screw fixation in thoracic, lumbar and sacral spinal fusions. *Spine* 1994;19:2279S-2296S.

8. Postacchini F, Cinatti G, Perugia D, Gumina S: The surgical treatment of central lumbar stenosis: Multiple laminotomy compared with total laminectomy. *J Bone Joint Surg Br* 1993;75: 386-392.

9. McCulloch JA, Young PH: *Essentials of Spinal Microsurgery*. Philadelphia, PA, Lippincott-Raven, 1998.

10. McCulloch JA: Microsurgery for spinal canal stenosis: the resculpturing or laminaplasty procedure, in McCulloch JA, Young PH (eds): *Microsurgery of the Lumbar Spine*, Rockville, MD, 1990.

11. Wang JC, Bohlman HH, Riew KD: Dural tears secondary to operations on the lumbar spine: Management and results after a two-year-minimum follow-up of eighty-eight patients. *J Bone Joint Surg Am* 1998;80:1728-1732.

12. Deyo RA, Cherkin DC: Morbidity and mortality in association with operations on the lumbar spine. *J Bone Joint Surg Am* 1992;74: 536-543.

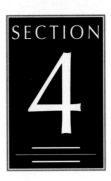

SECTION 4

Pediatric Spine

Pediatric Spine

The two articles in this section were written by true pioneers in pediatric spine surgery. Dr. Robert Winter is considered the "godfather" of congenital spine deformity, and Dr. Robert Hensinger is recognized as the "resident expert" of various pediatric spinal conditions.

The most cogent message in Dr. Winter's chapter is that allowing the relentless progression of a congenital deformity must be avoided; it is a mistake to believe that the spine should be allowed to grow for a while so that it will not be shortened by an early spinal fusion. Thus, all of us who care for children with these abnormalities must carefully and consistently measure the curves on radiographs using the same curve end points. Each time a new image is obtained, it must be consistently compared with the original image and each one thereafter. This radiographic evaluation must be coupled with a detailed physical examination each time patients are seen. Parents and patients, if they are old enough, should be asked whether they have noticed any changes in appearance, in the magnitude of the deformity, or in physical function.

Consistent application of these principles is helpful in preventing unchecked progression of a deformity. This disciplined approach must also include making tough decisions; sometimes it requires suggesting early surgical treatment when it becomes necessary, even if the patients are very young. If progression of a relatively small deformity can be arrested with fusion of part of the spine before compensatory curves or a major deformity develops, fusion is a far better option than allowing the deformity to progress until it becomes very complex and ultimately difficult and dangerous to correct later on.

Dr. Winter highlights the factors that influence the natural history of these congenital abnormalities to better predict their course and to educate parents. Frank, accurate discussions with parents and patients must be part of the "controlled observation" of these children.

Once evidence of curve progression becomes clear either from radiographs and/or physical examination, the best procedures for controlling the deformity can be considered. Through the years Dr. Winter has advocated in situ posterior spinal fusion with abundant bone graft as the procedure of choice to control congenital deformities. He also discusses other treatment options for other specific deformities, but it is clear from my own rather extensive experience that in situ posterior spinal fusion alone is not always the best choice for certain deformities. If this procedure does not control the curve, future corrective surgery may be more difficult because of the presence of a fusion mass. Procedures such as hemivertebrectomy, convex hemiepiphysiodesis/hemiarthrodesis, and combined anterior and posterior spinal fusions all supplemented with internal fixation may be better choices. In particular, hemivertebra excision under the proper conditions offers the best chance of correction (over a short segment of the spine) and curve control (because it removes the source of the deformity). This assumes, however, that the surgeon is capable of performing these procedures.

No matter what procedure is done, the spinal canal must be imaged prior to surgical treatment. A congenital spine deformity must be carefully monitored until skeletal maturity, even if carefully and correctly chosen treatment has been rendered, because of the strong and sometimes unpredictable effect of growth. Additional procedures may be indicated if the deformity progresses. Note that early, prompt, and selective treatment offers the best chance for curve control. In situ posterior spinal fusion may be the best and most appropriate option for some patients; different procedures may provide a better solution for others.

One final thought about congenital deformities is that many children have rather severely affected thoracic cages because of missing and/or fused ribs, severe spinal deformity, or other congenital anomalies. Though Dr. Winter does not address this problem, early evidence suggests that the titanium rib and thoracic enlargement as popularized by Dr. Robert Campbell may offer an alternative to other "spine shortening" procedures. Thoracic enlargement is still considered experimental; at press, the implants have not been released for general use by the US Food and Drug Administration, and the follow up is relatively short. Nonetheless, this new technique may offer another tool in our armamentarium against congenital deformities.

Dr. Hensinger's article presents a thorough overview of back pain in children. He correctly points out that persistent back pain in children is distinctly worrisome because in general children do not have secondary gain issues as adults frequently do. Therefore, these symptoms must be taken seriously. His reported series shows that most patients had readily recognizable causes for their back pain. The remaining minority also eventually had a specific diagnosis to explain their symptoms.

Because children, especially young ones, cannot describe signs or symptoms, careful observation of gait and other muscle function is required during the office visit. Examination of active and passive back motion, along with range of motion and the presence of pain on motion, is required as well. Remember that painful, limited back motion in children indicates a spinal cord tumor until proven otherwise. The presence of skin lesions may also be evidence of intraspinal lesions. Various spinal and lower extremity deformities may provide clues to intraspinal abnormalities that result in subtle muscle imbalance and weakness that can change growth of these areas and may also cause pain. Sometimes the cause of a child's lower extremity pain may actually be a spinal lesion, though a lesion may not be suspected because of the way the physical examination was performed.

Many years ago I was called to see a patient who was thought to have a septic hip. When I arrived, the resident who called me grabbed the child's legs and moved them all about while simultaneously bending the spine. The child screamed in pain. After waiting a few minutes, I gave the child a pacifier and allowed her to settle down. I then gently moved her hips while stabilizing her pelvis with one hand so that the spine did not move. I could move the hips as much as I wanted without causing the child any apparent discomfort. However, once I flexed the lumbar spine, the child shrieked in pain. Subsequent evaluation showed that the patient had diskitis in the lumbar spine, not a septic hip. This example illustrates how a careful and gentle physical examination can help pinpoint the problem.

Once the physical examination is completed, use of selective imaging modalities can make an exact anatomic diagnosis. Making a precise diagnosis is important because then the treatment can be precise as well. A number of different imaging techniques may be necessary to define the problem. MRI has proved to be very helpful in this regard because of the detailed anatomy that can be seen on the images. Radiographs also provide a significant amount of information. A number of different laboratory tests can be ordered, but aside from a complete blood count, erythrocyte sedimentation rate, C-reactive protein, and HLA-B27, the results are not usually that helpful. Once a firm diagnosis is made, a rational treatment plan can be formulated and initiated.

Dr. Hensinger reviewed some of the more common entities associated with back pain, but these will not be reviewed at this time. What he says about them certainly is reasonable in terms of the timing and type of treatment.

Back pain in children should be taken seriously because it is generally real and has an anatomic basis. However, I am beginning to see in teenagers the same types of nonspecific chronic back pain that typically occurs in adults. This development makes careful evaluation and diagnosis even more important and reinforces the importance of making as precise a diagnosis as possible.

The information presented in the following two articles is very timely, important, and practical, and it should be part of every orthopaedic surgeon's knowledge base, even though he or she may need to refer the patient for appropriate treatment.

John P. Lubicky, MD
Ronald L. DeWald, MD, Professor of Orthopaedic Surgery
Department of Orthopaedic Surgery
Rush Medical College
Rush-Presbyterian-St.Luke's Medical Center
Chief of Staff, Shriners Hospitals for Children
Chicago, Illinois

Congenital Spinal Deformity

Robert B. Winter, MD
John E. Lonstein, MD
Oheneba Boachie-Adjei, MD

Congenital spinal deformities, which are caused by congenitally anomalous vertebral development, usually are seen on conventional radiographs but may be detected on tomograms, on magnetic resonance images (MRI), or at the time of surgery. Although patients who have myelomeningocele have congenitally anomalous vertebrae, most of the spinal deformity in such patients is paralytic in nature; therefore, they will not be included in the present discussion.

The three major patterns of congenital spinal deformity are lordosis, kyphosis, and scoliosis. Although combinations such as lordoscoliosis and kyphoscoliosis are common, the natural history and methods of treatment of spinal deformity correspond to the three major subdivisions. It is important to distinguish between scoliosis with marked rotation (which should not be labeled kyphoscoliosis) and true kyphoscoliosis (in which rotation is not a major component of the deformity).

Etiology

Congenital spinal anomalies are divided into two basic groups: defects of formation and defects of segmentation. A classic example of a defect of formation is a hemivertebra that has a mobile disk both caudad and cephalad to it (a so-called free hemivertebra). A classic example of a defect of segmentation is a unilateral unsegmented bar, in which one side of the

spine has failed to segment over the length of several vertebrae while the other side has segmented normally. The cause of congenital spinal deformities usually is unknown. Embryologically, spinal anomalies must develop between the fifth and eighth weeks of gestation; however, even a detailed maternal history seldom reveals that any untoward events occurred during that time.

Most patients have mixed anomalies in which both types of defects are present. The most important step in the evaluation of these patients is to estimate whether the spine is balanced and will remain balanced during growth; the greater the potential growth discrepancy between the two sides, the greater the likelihood that the deformity will progress. In very few patients is the amount of growth discrepancy clearly predictable, so all patients must be monitored with carefully made and carefully measured radiographs.

Genetics

A positive family history of congenital spinal deformity is rare; in a review of the records of 1,250 patients managed at our center, we found that only 13 had a positive family history.[1] Wynne-Davies,[2] in a comprehensive review of the families of 337 patients, reported that an isolated anomaly such as a hemivertebra was a sporadic lesion genetically that carried no risk of a similar lesion in siblings or sub-

sequent generations, whereas multiple-level, complex anomalies carried a 5% to 10% risk of such an occurrence. Wynne-Davies observed a higher hereditary relationship than is seen in North America because the study was performed in Scotland, where there is a higher prevalence of spina bifida cystica.

Studies of twins usually have shown that if one twin has an anomaly, the other does not, even when the twins are identical.[3-5] At our center, we have seen five patients with congenital scoliosis who had an identical twin sibling; none of the twin siblings had congenital spinal deformity.

However, hereditary congenital scoliosis has been described by several investigators.[6-12] Most of the patients in those reports had extensive defects of segmentation in association with spondylocostal, costovertebral, or spondylothoracic dysplasia (Jarcho-Levin syndrome). In addition to the defects of segmentation in the spine, there are often such defects in the ribs, leading to a small, stiff thorax and frequently to pulmonary compromise. Such defects also may extend into the cervical spine as a Klippel-Feil anomaly. We examined one family in which all three siblings had an almost identical congenital scoliosis. The parents were unrelated, and neither had radiographic evidence of scoliosis or any other congenital spinal anomaly. In addition, the oldest of the three siblings had a child who was free of anomalies.

Evaluation

The evaluation of the patient who has a congenital spinal deformity is very different from that of the patient who has the more common idiopathic or neuromuscular spinal deformities, because a congenital deformity has a very high frequency of associated anomalies both within and outside the spine. The most common associated lesion is spinal dysraphism, a group of conditions currently considered to include any congenital anomaly of the neural axis. Although a number of textbooks and medical dictionaries have defined dysraphism as the failure of two halves of an organ to fuse (as seen, for example, in myelomeningocele), the current definition also includes conditions in which there is an abnormal midline structure in the neural axis. Hence, diastematomyelia, in which the midline structures have fused but a spike of bone projects anteriorly from a fused vertebral arch, is also an example of spinal dysraphism. Moreover, as the use of computed tomographic (CT) scanning and MRI has increased, other anomalies, such as a tight filum terminale, frequently have been associated with diastematomyelia. The prevalence of dysraphic lesions was approximately 40% in three independent studies: MRI demonstrated such abnormalities in 16 of 42 patients in the study by Bradford and associates[13] and in 20 of 48 patients in the study by Winter and associates.[14] Dowling[15] observed a similar prevalence of such lesions with use of CT myelography.

Various other spinal abnormalities may be seen, including Arnold-Chiari malformation, syringomyelia, diplomyelia, and intraspinal tumors. These lesions may or may not be associated with a cutaneous hairy patch, a nevus, or a detectable neurologic deficit. Because of the potential for a neurologic lesion, it is always important to perform a very careful neurologic examination.

Another frequent site of associated anomalies is the genitourinary system.[16,17]

Approximately 20% of these patients will be seen to have an anomaly on routine intravenous pyelography or ultrasound studies. Urologic abnormalities were present in 42 of 231 patients in the study by MacEwen and associates.[17] Cardiac anomalies are seen in approximately 12% of patients.[18] The reader is referred to the excellent review by Beals and associates[18] for more details concerning the many lesions associated with congenital spinal deformity.

After evaluating the patient for associated anomalies, one should study the spine carefully. We look for the anatomic area or areas of deformity, the pattern of deformity (scoliosis, kyphosis, or lordosis), the stiffness of the curvature, the presence or absence of decompensation (as measured by the degree of deviation from a plumb line), whether the shoulders are level, whether the head is tilted, the range of motion of the cervical spine, and the pattern and height of any rotational prominence of the ribs.

Congenital Lordosis

Congenital lordosis, the least common of the three major patterns of congenital spinal deformity, is caused by a defect of segmentation posteriorly in the presence of active growth anteriorly. We have not seen any patients in whom congenital lordosis was caused by a defect of formation. Most patients who have congenital lordosis also have some degree of scoliosis.

The deformity associated with congenital lordosis is usually progressive. When the deformity occurs in the thoracic spine, it inevitably produces respiratory compromise, and early death can result.[19] One patient who was seen at our center died at the age of 9 years; at autopsy, the anterior aspect of the spine was only 8 mm from the posterior aspect of the sternum. When the deformity occurs in the lumbar spine, it results in hyperlordosis, with the spine approaching the anterior abdominal wall.

The treatment of congenital lordosis is purely surgical. Bracing cannot halt the progression of the deformity. Exercises and stretching are totally useless.

There are two types of surgery, one for stabilization and the other for correction. So-called stabilizing surgery can be done when the surgeon has the opportunity to see the patient before major deformity (and loss of pulmonary function) has developed. It is then the obligation of the surgeon to perform an anterior arthrodesis of the entire involved area and one or two vertebrae cephalad and caudad to the lesion. This procedure welds the spine by eliminating the anterior growth plates, thereby preventing the development of any curvature. The anterior fusion of one or two additional levels cephalad and caudad to the lesion may create the effect of an epiphysiodesis in these areas. Over time, continued growth of the posterior elements at these levels may result in some actual improvement in the deformity.

So-called corrective surgery is done when the patient has a major deformity and, usually, a substantial loss of pulmonary function. The goal is to improve not only spinal alignment but also pulmonary function.[20] The operation is complex, as the entire area of deformity must be approached both anteriorly and posteriorly. Through the anterior approach, the disks should be completely excised, as should the wedges of bone cephalad and caudad to them. These gaps should be left open and not packed with bone graft, as they should close when the posterior stage is completed. The posterior portion of the operation consists of multiple osteotomies of the laminar synostosis, performed at the same levels from which the disks were excised anteriorly. Sublaminar wires then are passed, with care being taken to avoid the spinal cord (which lies in the posterior part of the canal). The wires are then twisted over a kyphotically contoured, stiff rod and are tightened gradually, with the surgeon working from each end toward the center, to correct the lordosis. We prefer to use 6.3-mm Luque rods. Whenever feasible, we perform both the anterior and posterior procedures during the same anesthetic session in order to gain an immediate increase in lung volume and vital capacity.

Congenital Kyphosis

Congenital kyphosis is more common than congenital lordosis but far less common than congenital scoliosis. There are two types: defects of segmentation and defects of formation. Defects of segmentation occur most often in the midthoracic or thoracolumbar regions and may involve two to eight levels. Defects of formation, which are more common, may involve only one level, but multiple consecutive defects are possible. Because posterior growth continues in the absence of anterior growth, progression of the deformity can occur; the more severe the anterior defect, the more progressive the deformity.

Congenital kyphosis due to a defect of segmentation tends to produce a round kyphosis rather than a sharp angular gibbus; thus, paraplegia is rarely a problem.[21] The main clinical symptom, apart from the visible deformity, is low-back pain caused by the necessary compensatory lumbar hyperlordosis. The deformity tends to progress slowly, and the magnitude of the deformity is related to the number of vertebrae involved as well as to the severity of the growth discrepancy.

Congenital kyphosis due to a defect of formation has a much worse prognosis. Paraplegia resulting from the natural progression of the lesion is a very real possibility, as reported in several series.[22-25] In North America, congenital kyphosis is the most common cause of paraplegia due to spinal deformity. Paralysis can occur at any age but is most common during the pubertal growth spurt, when the deformity progresses suddenly.

Congenital kyphosis must be treated surgically; all forms of nonsurgical treatment, including full-time bracing, are useless.

Defects of segmentation, if discovered early, can be treated with a prompt posterior arthrodesis, which should include the entire kyphosis and one vertebra cephalad and caudad to the lesion. This procedure can prevent further progression, but it cannot correct an existing deformity. If correction is the goal, an anterior approach is needed, with multiple osteotomies of the anterior bar of bone followed by the posterior arthrodesis. For larger patients, posterior compression instrumentation is desirable. If the patient is too small for instrumentation, hyperextension casting is needed to maintain the correction until the area of the arthrodesis has fused.

For defects of formation, the main goal is the prevention of paraplegia. All other goals are secondary. If the defect is detected early (when the patient is younger than 5 years old) and there is less than 50° of kyphosis on a radiograph made with the patient supine, posterior fusion alone will produce the desired outcome. To achieve a good result, the surgeon must perform a posterior arthrodesis, have the child wear a hyperextension cast (not a brace) for 6 months, perform a second operation to augment the arthrodesis with additional bone grafts, and return the child to the hyperextension cast for another 6 months. This approach usually (but not always) produces a solid fusion mass, and the remaining anterior growth plate produces a gradual correction of the deformity (the posterior epiphysiodesis effect).[26]

When the deformity is large or when the patient is an older child or an adult, a combined anterior and posterior arthrodesis is mandatory.[27] The anterior arthrodesis is done first, with radical excision of the shortened anterior longitudinal ligament, the disks, and the related ligaments. Removal of a bone (vertebrec-

tomy) is not necessary, because the fundamental problem is the congenital absence of an adequate amount of bone anteriorly. If possible, a distractor should be used to lengthen the anterior column, and structural autogenous grafts from the rib or fibula should be placed anteriorly to maintain the achieved height.

The anterior procedure is followed (either on the same day or a week later) by a posterior arthrodesis and compression instrumentation if the bones are large enough to accept hooks and rods. If compression instrumentation cannot be used, the patient is managed with posterior arthrodesis followed by hyperextension casting and bed rest for several months. If a pseudarthrosis occurs, both the anterior and posterior arthrodeses must be done again in order to achieve healing.

A patient who has a neurologic deficit at the time of presentation requires special consideration. If the neurologic deficit is mild-that is, spasticity manifested by hyperactive reflexes and positive Babinski signs but no loss of motor, bowel, or bladder function-a formal anterior decompression of the spinal cord is not necessary. Thorough anterior and posterior arthrodeses should be carried out, as described already, and the neurologic deficit will disappear gradually once the spinal canal has been realigned and the area has been stabilized. If the neurologic deficit is severe, the anterior and posterior arthrodeses must be combined with an anterior decompression of the spinal cord. A laminectomy is never indicated to relieve compression of the spinal cord due to congenital kyphosis.

Congenital Scoliosis

While congenital scoliosis can be caused by a defect of formation or by a defect of segmentation, combined defects are by far the most common. Deformities can occur in any area of the spine, from the cervical to the lumbosacral region.

The natural history of congenital scoliosis has been described in several ex-

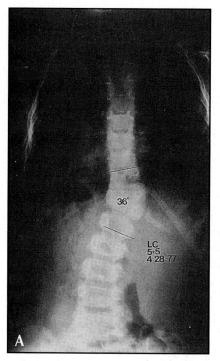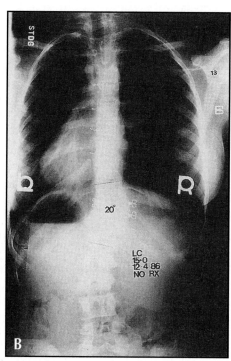

Fig. 1 Radiographs of a patient who had scoliosis in association with an isolated hemivertebra. **A,** Radiograph made when the patient was 5 years and 5 months old, showing a hemivertebra at the thoracolumbar junction and a 36° curve. There were no kyphosis and no tethered-cord problems. **B,** Radiograph made when the patient was 15 years old, showing that the curve had spontaneously improved to 20°. The patient had had no treatment of any kind, only periodic examinations.

cellent studies.[28-34] Overall, there was remarkable consistency in those studies with regard to the frequency of progression: 25% of the curves were nonprogressive, 25% were slowly progressive, and 50% were very progressive. The propensity for progression is related especially to the type of anomaly, but also to the rate of growth of the patient. Without question, the most progressive type of scoliosis is that due to a unilateral unsegmented bar with a contralateral hemivertebra. This type of curve can progress at a rate of 10° to 12° per year. Over the 14 years that an average child grows, a deformity of 140° to 180° can occur.

Scoliosis caused by an isolated unilateral unsegmented bar is the next most severely progressive type of curve, followed by scoliosis caused by two consecutive free hemivertebrae on the convex side.

Progression of a curve caused by a single hemivertebra is extremely difficult to predict; this type of curve may progress severely, slowly, or not at all. We even have seen such a curve improve spontaneously (Fig. 1).

It is important to know whether a curve is progressing. This determination depends on accurate and precise monitoring, both clinically and radiographically. The child should be examined every 6 months to be certain that the shoulders are level, the pelvis is balanced, the curve is unchanged, and there are no signs of decompensation. The degree of curvature is best measured on detailed serial radiographs made with the patient supine; the radiographs must be of excellent quality in order to permit accurate measurements. Congenital scoliosis is more difficult to measure than either id-

iopathic or neuromuscular scoliosis, because the radiographs often do not show the vertebral endplates clearly. At every visit, the current radiograph should be compared with both the previous and the original radiograph. The most common error in the treatment of congenital spinal deformity is the failure to measure the radiographs properly. The second most common error is to document that progression is taking place but then fail to do something to stop that progression.

The primary goal in the treatment of congenital scoliosis is to prevent the development of a severe deformity; one should not wait until a severe deformity has developed (Fig. 2) and then attempt to perform a major and dangerous corrective procedure.

There are only two methods of preventing progression of the curve. The first is bracing and the second is arthrodesis. Bracing is far less successful for congenital scoliosis than it is for idiopathic scoliosis. This does not mean that bracing is totally useless as we have stated it to be for congenital lordosis and kyphosis. One major study of bracing for congenital scoliosis found it to be effective for controlling long, flexible curves (as shown on radiographs made with the patient bending) until the time of the pubertal growth spurt but not for short, rigid curves.[35] At no time should bracing be continued if progression of the curve is not being controlled.

Because a high percentage of curves in congenital scoliosis are progressive and few respond to bracing, surgical treatment is the mainstay of care. The questions are, then, what type of surgery and when. The four basic operations for the treatment of congenital scoliosis are posterior arthrodesis, combined anterior and posterior arthrodesis, convex growth arrest (epiphysiodesis), and hemivertebra excision. Instrumentation is merely an adjunct to one of these procedures.

Posterior spinal arthrodesis is the standard of care. Thousands of patients have been managed successfully with this procedure. In a long-term follow-up study of a large series of patients, we found that a solid fusion usually can be achieved safely, with little deterioration over time.[36] When performing a posterior arthrodesis, the surgeon should meticulously expose the entire curve, excise any mobile facet joints, decorticate the spine thoroughly, and add an autogenous bone graft.

Correction of the curve can be achieved with internal instrumentation or with a cast or brace externally. Congenital scolioses tend to be rather stiff, and the average correction is much less than can be achieved in patients who have idiopathic scoliosis. Arthrodesis therefore should be done earlier (that is, when the curve is smaller) than is indicated for other forms of scoliosis. However, there is no magic number of degrees that absolutely indicates the need for surgical intervention.

Arthrodesis without instrumentation but with external correction with a cast or brace is not a so-called arthrodesis in situ, as that term implies fusion without correction of the deformity. In our large series, instrumentation added 5° of correction compared with treatment with a cast, but it also was associated with the only instances of paraplegia in the study.[36] Instrumentation should never be used without a preoperative evaluation of the spinal canal (with use of MRI or CT myelography) for the presence of dysraphic lesions. An intraoperative evaluation with a wake-up test should be done whenever spinal instrumentation is used. Electronic monitoring of the spinal cord can be used, but it is not a substitute for the wake-up test.

Critics of isolated posterior arthrodesis have implied that a combined anterior and posterior arthrodesis is needed routinely in order to prevent bending of the fusion mass over time (the so-called crankshaft effect). Careful analysis of the results of isolated posterior fusion has shown that late bending does occur, but only in a small percentage of patients (14% [40 of 290 patients] in our study).[36] As pointed out by Lopez-Sosa and associates,[37] the few patients who have substantial rotation as part of the deformity will continue to have rotation even with a solid fusion when a substantial potential for growth remains. Apparently, the crankshaft effect occurs only in the presence of healthy growth plates anteriorly, as is the case in patients who have juvenile idiopathic scoliosis. The reason that so many patients who have congenital scoliosis do not demonstrate this phenomenon is that their anterior growth plates are so abnormal.

A combined anterior and posterior arthrodesis adds the potential benefit of greater correction of the deformity because the excision of disks allows for greater mobility of the segments. It also decreases the likelihood of pseudarthrosis and prevents late bending (the crankshaft effect). However, it incurs the added risks of the anterior procedure. The role of instrumentation is the same as in the isolated posterior arthrodesis. The risks of anterior surgery have been small in most patients, but the thoracotomy should be approached with great caution in patients who have major pulmonary compromise. When this approach is added, very skilled anesthetists, intensivists, and experts in pulmonary medicine are highly valuable in the postoperative management of these patients. Preoperative tracheotomies are not routinely necessary.[38]

Convex growth arrest, or epiphysiodesis on the convex side of the curve, has a definite but limited role. It is obviously appropriate only for patients with some growth potential remaining on the concave side. This procedure must be done early (before the patient is 5 years old) and before the curve has progressed beyond 50° or 60°.[39-41] The technique is not complex. A combined anterior and posterior arthrodesis is performed on the convex half of the spine only; the concave side must never be touched. Postoperatively, the child wears a corrective cast for 6 months. The patient must be followed until the end of growth, because an early good result can deteriorate during the pubertal growth spurt. The presence of any degree of kyphosis is a contraindication to this procedure, because the anterior fusion will aggravate that condition.

Hemivertebra excision was first done in 1921 by Royle[42] in Australia. More recently, especially through the pioneering work of Leatherman and Dickson,[43] the procedure has been refined so that the risks are small and the potential benefits great. Still, very few of the patients who have hemivertebrae need to have them excised. Most can be managed with the much safer procedures described already. Hemivertebra excision has higher risks than the other procedures, including greater blood loss and increased risk of neurologic injury.[44]

Hemivertebra excision is indicated for patients with a fixed decompensation in whom adequate alignment cannot be achieved with other procedures. In our experience, this problem usually has been due to a hemivertebra at the fourth or fifth lumbar level. Hemivertebra excision is safer in this area than in the thoracic region, because the cauda equina is more tolerant of manipulation than is the spinal cord.[45]

The technique initially requires a direct anterior exposure, removal of the body of the hemivertebra and its adjacent disks back to the spinal canal, and removal of the anterior half of the pedicle. The patient is then placed prone, and the posterior elements, including the hemilamina, the transverse process, and the posterior half of the pedicle, are removed. Arthrodesis of the entire curve always must be done as well. Correction can be done internally with convex compression instrumentation or externally with a cast. Immobilization must continue until the fusion is solid.

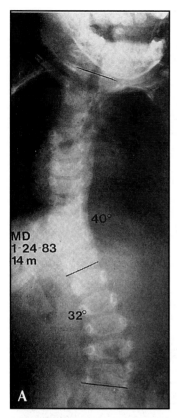

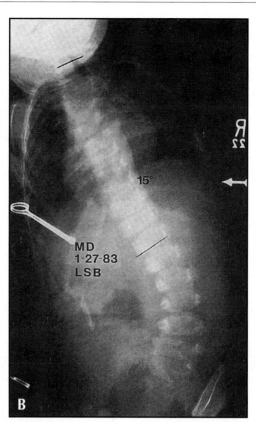

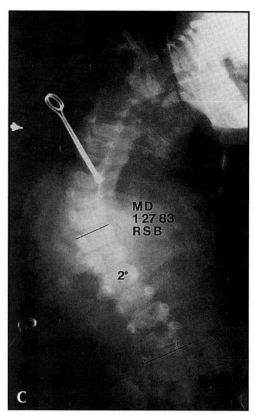

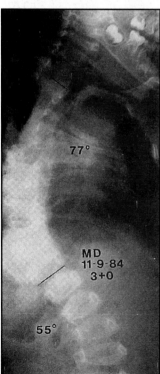

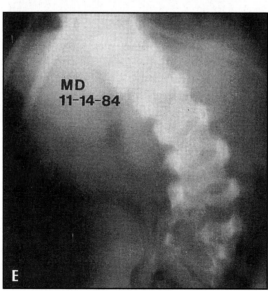

Fig. 2 Radiographs showing progression of congenital scoliosis in the absence of surgical treatment. There are minor congenital anomalies in the thoracic region and at the lumbosacral level, but the area between those two regions is free of anomalies. **A,** Radiograph made when the patient was 14 months old, showing a 40° thoracic curve and a 32° lumbar curve. **B,** Radiograph made with the patient bending to the left, showing the thoracic curve to be correctable to 15°. The minor anomalies in the upper thoracic region can be seen clearly. **C,** Radiograph made with the patient bending to the right, showing the lumbar curve to be correctable to 2°. Again, no anomalies can be seen other than at the fifth lumbar and first sacral levels. No treatment was given. **D,** Radiograph made at the time of a routine check-up when the patient was 3 years old. The thoracic curve had progressed to 77° and the lumbar curve to 55°. In hindsight, bracing should have been instituted earlier. **E,** Tomogram made when the patient was 3 years old, showing a hemivertebra at the fifth lumbar level.

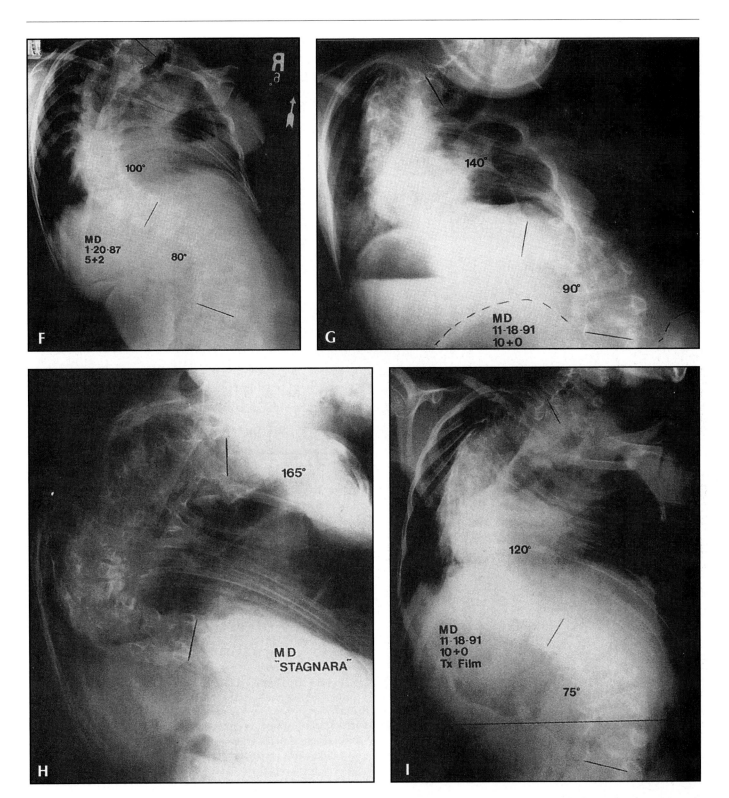

Fig. 2 (cont.) F, Radiograph made when the patient was 5 years and 2 months old, showing that the thoracic curve had progressed to 100° and the lumbar curve to 80°. No treatment was given. **G,** Radiograph made when the patient was 10 years old, showing that the thoracic curve had progressed to 140° and the lumbar curve to 90°. The patient had severe respiratory compromise. **H,** The rotational thoracic deformity is better analyzed with this Stagnara projection, which shows that the true curve measured 165°. **I,** A traction radiograph, made to evaluate flexibility, showed the deformity to be very stiff, the thoracic curve was corrected only to 120° and the lumbar curve to 75°.

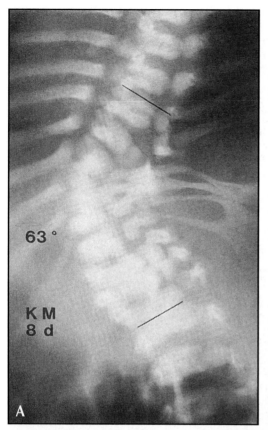

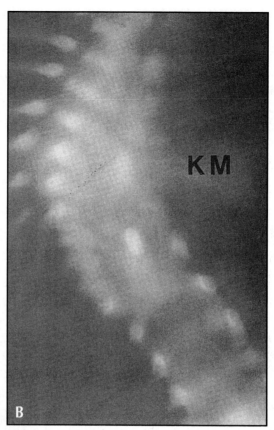

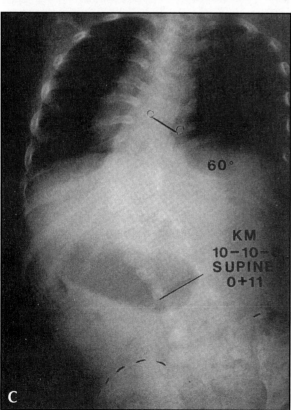

Fig. 3 Radiographs and photographs of a patient who was managed with bracing after surgical treatment of severe congenital scoliosis. **A,** Radiograph made when the patient was 8 days old, showing a 63° curve and severe congenital anomalies, including a unilateral unsegmented bar with fused ribs in the lower thoracic spine, multiple convex hemivertebrae, interpedicular widening, and a midline osseous spur in the upper lumbar spine. The patient was intact neurologically and quite healthy otherwise. **B,** Posterolateral tomogram showing the midline osseous spur of the diastematomyelia. **C,** Radiograph made when the patient was 11 months old, at which time the curve measured 60°. The patient was managed at this time with neurosurgical removal of the osseous spur of the diastematomyelia, followed 1 week later by a combined anterior and posterior convex hemiepiphysiodesis of the entire curve. Postoperatively, the patient was placed in a Milwaukee brace with correction of the curve to 40°. She was kept supine for 6 months until the fusion was solid radiographically and then was allowed to walk in the brace.

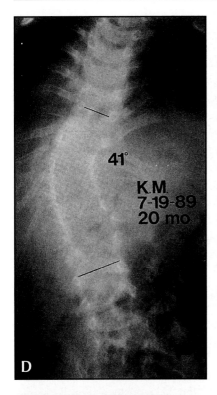

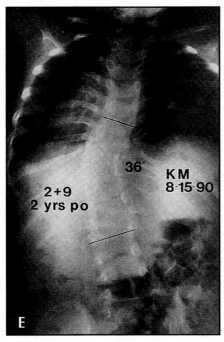

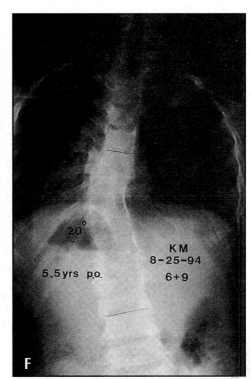

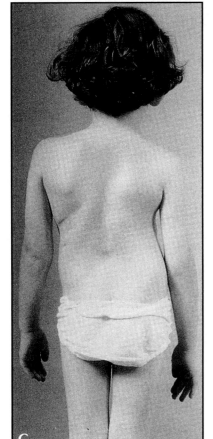

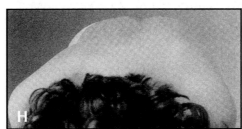

Fig. 3 (cont.) D, Radiograph made 9 months after surgery, when the patient was 20 months old, at which time the curve measured 41°. The fusion was solid. The inlaid rib graft can be seen readily at the convexity of the curvature. **E,** Radiograph made nearly 2 years after the operation, when the patient was 2 years and 9 months old. She had been out of the brace for more than 1 year. The curve measured 36°. **F,** Radiograph made 5.5 years after the operation, when the patient was 6 years and 9 months old, showing that the curve had improved to 20° because of the epiphysiodesis effect on the convex side, both cephalad and caudad to the area of the unilateral unsegmented bar. The patient remained neurologically intact at this time. **G,** Posterior photograph made when the patient was 6 years and 9 months old. **H,** Photograph made with the patient bending forward, showing the complete absence of any rotational deformity.

The timing of spinal arthrodesis has been of great concern to both surgeons and patients. A dilemma exists because there is a strong desire to perform the arthrodesis in order to prevent progression and, at the same time, a strong desire to delay the arthrodesis in order to permit spinal growth. It is important to remember that a patient who has congenital scoliosis typically has no growth potential on the concave part of the curve. Unfortunately, there is growth potential only on the convex side, and this growth is not productive of vertical height but only of deformity. Actually, the child will be taller if arthrodesis is done earlier, because increasing deformity shortens the trunk. We believe that it is better to be short and relatively straight than to be shorter and more crooked. Increasing deformity cannot be tolerated. If it is occurring, then it must be stopped either by bracing or by surgery. This very simple fact is the essence of treatment of congenital spinal deformity. Unfortunately, it has been ignored all too often.

Treatment of a spinal deformity that is associated with spinal dysraphism requires close cooperation between the orthopaedic surgeon and the neurosurgeon. The simple presence of a dysraphic lesion does not necessarily mean that the patient needs surgery. Many patients have lived their entire life with such a lesion and never have had a problem. However, anyone who has a progressive neurologic deficit should have appropriate neurosurgical management. The most serious problem arises in the patient with a dysraphic lesion but no neurologic deficit for whom the orthopaedic surgeon wishes to perform a corrective spinal procedure. A study by the Scoliosis Research Society showed that, in the surgical treatment of spinal deformity, the highest rate of paralysis is in patients who have a congenital spinal deformity.[46] The main cause of paralysis appears to be the use of distraction instrumentation or strong traction, such as the halo-pelvic device or

halo-femoral traction. We have been able to avoid neurologic problems in the past few years by completing a careful and thorough preoperative evaluation, performing appropriate neurosurgical releases before correcting the deformity, avoiding the use of distraction instrumentation, shortening the convexity (by means of hemivertebra excision) rather than lengthening the concavity, and carefully monitoring the patient both intraoperatively and postoperatively. At our center, we have continued to manage a large number of patients with casts or a brace rather than following the modern trend and using lots of instrumentation (Fig. 3).

Conclusion

The diagnosis, evaluation, and treatment of the patient with congenital spinal deformity are considerably different from the approach used for the more common types of scoliosis. Patients who have congenital scoliosis have a high frequency of associated anomalies, both within and outside the spine, which makes a thorough evaluation essential. The natural history ranges from no progression or clinical symptoms to extremely severe deformity, pulmonary compromise, early death, or paraplegia. The challenge to the medical profession is to prevent these dire problems from ever occurring.

Appropriate management involves careful evaluation of the patient, very careful and precise monitoring for progression of the deformity, and prompt action when progression is observed. Bracing is useless for the treatment of congenital kyphosis, congenital lordosis, and congenital scoliosis with a short and stiff curve pattern. Bracing can be useful for scoliosis with a long and flexible curve pattern.

Spinal arthrodesis is the mainstay of treatment. There are four main operative procedures: (1) posterior arthrodesis, (2) combined anterior and posterior arthrodesis, (3) epiphysiodesis (convex growth

arrest), and (4) hemivertebra excision. Each has value, and the clinician must select the procedure that is best suited for a particular patient at a particular time. Instrumentation is only an adjunct to these procedures and must be used with great care since it may create a serious neurologic deficit, such as paraplegia, in these patients who are particularly vulnerable because of the congenital spinal deformity.

Finally, the timing of the arthrodesis is of great concern. Many surgeons are reluctant to perform an arthrodesis early in a child's growth, for fear of stunting the growth of the trunk. This is a foolish idea, because the concave side of the curve seldom has any capacity to grow. The child will end up taller and straighter if the arthrodesis is done early than if the curve is allowed to progress and the arthrodesis is done late. Arthrodesis never should be postponed until the end of growth.

The key to all treatment is to stop progression of deformity. Our obligation to the patient was well stated in the study by Hall and associates:[47] "Ideally, no spine with congenital scoliosis should need correction, since the deformity ought to be recognized early and fusion performed before the curve progresses to the extent that correction is necessary."

References

1. Winter R, Moe J, Lonstein J: A review of family histories in patients with congenital spinal deformities. *Orthop Trans* 1983;7:32.

2. Wynne-Davies R: Congenital vertebral anomalies: Aetiology and relationship to spina bifida cystica. *J Med Genetics* 1975;12:280-288.

3. Hattaway GL: Congenital scoliosis in one of monozygotic twins: A case report. *J Bone Joint Surg* 1977;59A:837-838.

4. Peterson HA, Peterson LF: Hemivertebrae in identical twins with dissimilar spinal columns. *J Bone Joint Surg* 1967;49A:938-942.

5. Pool RD: Congenital scoliosis in monozygotic twins: Genetically determined or acquired in utero? *J Bone Joint Surg* 1986;68B:194-196.

6. Bartsocas CS, Kiossoglou KA, Pappas CV, et al: Costovertebral dysplasia. *Birth Defects* 1974;10:221-226.

7. Beighton P, Horan FT: Spondylocostal dysostosis in South African sisters. *Clin Genet* 1981;19:23-25.

8. Fogarty EE, Beatty T, Dowling F: Spondylocostal dysplasia in identical twins. *J Pediatr Orthop* 1985;5:720-721.

9. Jarcho S, Levin PM: Hereditary malformation of the vertebral bodies. *Bull J Hopkins Hosp* 1938;62:216-226.

10. Langer LO Jr, Moe JH: A recessive form of congenital scoliosis different from spondylothoracic dysplasia. *Birth Defects* 1975;11:83-86.

11. Rimoin DL, Fletcher BD, McKusick VA: Spondylocostal dysplasia: A dominantly inherited form of short-trunked dwarfism. *Am J Med* 1968;45:948-953.

12. Roberts AP, Conner AN, Tolmie JL, et al: Spondylothoracic and spondylocostal dysostosis: Hereditary forms of spinal deformity. *J Bone Joint Surg* 1988;70B:123-126.

13. Bradford DS, Heithoff KB, Cohen M: Intraspinal abnormalities and congenital spine deformities: Radiographic and MRI study. *J Pediatr Orthop* 1991;11:36-41.

14. Winter RB, Lonstein JE, Denis F, et al: Prevalence of spinal canal or cord abnormalities in idiopathic, congenital, and neuromuscular scoliosis. *Orthop Trans* 1992;16:135.

15. Dowling FE: Spinal cord abnormalities in congenital scoliosis: Clinical and radiological evaluation. *Orthop Trans* 1987;11:103.

16. Kohler R, Dodat H, Charollais Y: Congenital vertebral and urinary malformations: Incidence of their asociation and management. *Pediatrie* 1982;37-81-100.

17. MacEwen GD, Winter RB, Hardy JH: Evaluation of kidney anomalies in congenital scoliosis. *J Bone Joint Surg* 1972;54A:1451-1454.

18. Beals RK, Robbins JR, Rolfe B: Anomalies associated with vertebral malformations. *Spine* 1993;18:1329-1332.

19. Winter RB, Moe JH, Bradford DS: Congenital thoracic lordosis. *J Bone Joint Surg* 1978;60A:806-810.

20. Winter RB, Leonard AS: Surgical correction of congenital thoracic lordosis. *J Pediatr Orthop* 1990;10:805-808.

21. Mayfield JK, Winter RB, Bradford DS, et al: Congenital kyphosis due to defects of anterior segmentation. *J Bone Joint Surg* 1980;62A:1291-1301.

22. Rougerie J: *Les Compressions Medullaires Nontraumatiques de L'enfant.* Paris, France, Masson, 1973, p 186.

23. James JIP: Kyphoscoliosis. *J Bone Joint Surg* 1955;37B:414-426.

24. Montgomery SP, Hall JE: Congenital kyphosis. *Spine* 1982;7:360-364.

25. Savini R, Cervallati, Cioni A, et al: Congenital kyphosis: Natural history and treatment, in Gaggi A (ed): *Proceedings of the Italian Group for Scoliosis.* Bologna, Italy, 1982, pp 195-217.

26. Winter RB, Moe JH: The results of spinal arthrodesis for congenital spinal deformity in patients younger than five years old. *J Bone Joint Surg* 1982;64A:419-432.

27. Winter RB, Moe JH, Lonstein JE: The surgical treatment of congenital kyphosis: A review of 94 patients age 5 years or older, with 2 years or more follow-up in 77 patients. *Spine* 1985;10:224-231.

28. Kuhns JG, Hormell RS: Management of congenital scoliosis: Review of one hundred seventy cases. *Arch Surg* 1952;65:250-263.

29. MacEwen GD, Conway JJ, Miller WT: Congenital scoliosis with a unilateral bar. *Radiology* 1968;90:711-715.

30. McMaster MJ, Ohtsuka K: The natural history of congenital scoliosis: A study of two hundred and fifty-one patients. *J Bone Joint Surg* 1982;64A:1128-1147.

31. Nasa RJ, Stelling FH III, Steel HH: Progression of congenital scoliosis due to hemivertebrae and hemivertebrae with bars. *J Bone Joint Surg* 1975;57A:456-466.

32. Rathke FW, Sun HY. Investigations of scoliosis caused by malformations. *Zeit Orthop* 1963;97:173-188.

33. Winter RB, Moe JH, Eilers VE: Congenital scoliosis: A study of 234 patients treated and untreated. Part I: Natural history. *J Bone Joint Surg* 1968;50A:1-47.

34. Winter RB, Moe JH, Eilers VE: Congenital scoliosis: A study of 234 patients treated and untreated. Part II: Treatment. *J Bone Joint Surg* 1968;50A:15-47.

35. Winter RB, Moe JH, MacEwen GD, et al: The Milwaukee brace in the nonoperative treatment of congenital scoliosis. *Spine* 1976;1:85-96.

36. Winter RB, Moe JH, Lonstein JE: Posterior spinal arthrodesis for congenital scoliosis: An analysis of the cases of two hundred and ninety patients, five to nineteen years old. *J Bone Joint Surg* 1984;66A:1188-1197.

37. Lopez-Sosa FH, Guille JT, Bowen JR: Curve progression and spinal rotation in congenital scoliosis. *Orthop Trans* 1993;17:382.

38. Rawlins BA, Winter RB, Lonstein JE, et al: Reconstructive spine surgery in pediatric patients with major loss in vital capacity. *Orthop Trans* 1994;18:95-96.

39. Andrew T, Piggott H: Growth arrest for progressive scoliosis: Combined anterior and posterior fusion of the convexity. *J Bone Joint Surg* 1985;67B:193-197.

40. Dubousset J, Katti E, Seringe R: Epiphysiodesis of the spine in young children for congenital spinal deformations. *J Pediatr Orthop* 1993;1B:123-130.

41. Winter RB, Lonstein JE, Denis F, et al: Convex growth arrest for progressive congenital scoliosis due to hemivertebrae. *J Pediatr Orthop* 1988;8:633-638.

42. Royle ND: The operative removal of an accessory vertebra. *Med J Australia* 1928;1:467.

43. Leatherman KD, Dickson RA: Two-stage corrective surgery for congenital deformities of the spine. *J Bone Joint Surg* 1979;61B:324-328.

44. Bradford DS, Boachie-Adjei O: One-stage anterior and posterior hemivertebral resection and arthrodesis for congenital scoliosis. *J Bone Joint Surg* 1990;72A:536-540.

45. Holte DC, Winter RB, Lonstein JE, et al: Excision of hemivertebrae and wedge resection in the treatment of congenital scoliosis. *J Bone Joint Surg* 1995;77A:159-171.

46. MacEwen GD, Bunnell WP, Sriram K: Acute neurological complications in the treatment of scoliosis: A report of the Scoliosis Research Society. *J Bone Joint Surg* 1975;57A:404-408.

47. Hall JE, Herndon WA, Levine CR: Surgical treatment of congenital scoliosis with or without Harrington instrumentation. *J Bone Joint Surg* 1981;63A:608-619.

16

Acute Back Pain in Children

Robert N. Hensinger, MD

It is uncommon for a child to complain of pain in the back. Unlike the adult population, in whom back pain seems to be part of everyday life, relatively few children have symptoms serious enough to warrant a visit to a physician. For most of those who do seek care, the problems respond to simple measures. Several years ago, we reviewed 100 children who were presented to the pediatric orthopaedic clinic with the complaint of back pain.[1] The children's problems were divided into three categories: (1) developmental (35%), predominantly caused by kyphosis or, to a lesser extent, scoliosis; (2) traumatic (35%), the majority of which were spondylolysis of L5-S1; and (3) spontaneous onset (15%), usually caused by tumor or infection. The remaining 15% were originally undetermined, but the etiology for several of these was determined later. Thus, nearly 90% had objective problems, and, importantly, the vast majority of these problems could be successfully diagnosed and managed with a very satisfactory outcome.

Clinical Findings

The fact that children are not very specific in their complaints can be disconcerting to the examining physician. Children are poor at localizing pain and tend to be more global in their description. They usually complain of pain in the entire back rather than a more discreet complaint limited to the lumbosacral or dorsal lumbar junction. The complaint of leg pain may represent simple hamstring tightness and night cramps, or it may be the radicular pain of a herniated disk. These are very typical complaints of children which in an adult might suggest a strong emotional overlay.

Because children are less familiar with the glossary of terms associated with illness, such as numbness, tingling, and weakness, they find it difficult to express these complaints. Similarly, the fact that children have difficulty remembering and describing the specifics of their activity or injury mechanisms can be frustrating and confusing to the examiner.

The mechanism or circumstance of injury is often an important clue to the diagnosis. A spondylolysis should be suspected if the onset of the pain is during athletics such as diving, during a back walkover in gymnastics, or while performing a racing turn or the butterfly stroke in swimming.[2,3] Similarly, increasing pain with repetition may indicate the onset of a stress reaction in the pars interarticularis.[3,4] The high rate of occurrence of spondylolysis among family members and certain ethnic groups is often an important clue to the correct diagnosis.[5] Night pain and the relief of symptoms with aspirin (or Naprosyn) should lead one to suspect an osteoid osteoma or osteoblastoma (Fig. 1).[6-8] Morning stiffness may represent the beginning of juvenile ankylosing spondylitis.

The dangerous signs of childhood back pain are persistent pain unrelieved by rest or immobilization, increasing pain, unexplained fever, and symptoms of systemic illness, weight loss, general malaise or simply "not feeling well" (Fig. 2). Neurologic signs, complaints of nerve root irritation, radicular pain, numbness, and tingling are uncommon accompaniments to childhood back pain and, when found, suggest that a serious problem is in progress, which demands immediate evaluation. Similarly, bladder and bowel dysfunction or perineal hypoesthesia would justify extensive investigation.

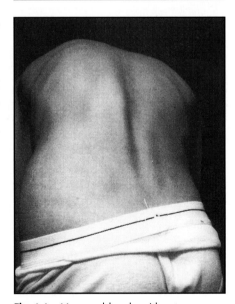

Fig. 1 An 11-year-old male with extreme back pain and guarding caused by an osteoid osteoma of L4. Forward bending demonstrates a curvature of the spine, which resolved with removal of the tumor.

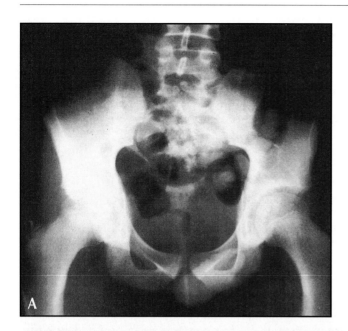

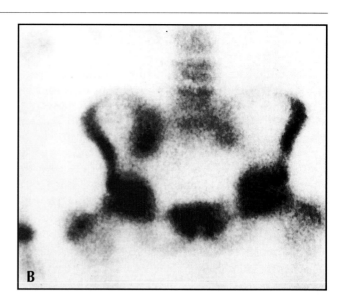

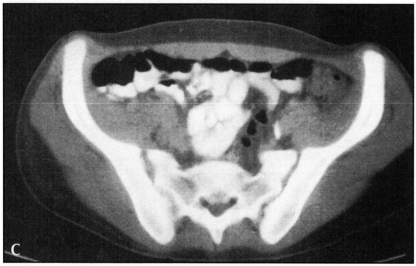

Fig. 2 A 14-year-old with a pyogenic infection of the right sacral iliac joint. **A,** Plain radiographs of the pelvis do not reveal the lesion. **B,** Bone scan demonstrates increased uptake in the region of the right sacral iliac joint. **C,** CT scan demonstrates destructive and erosive changes in the sacral iliac joint suggesting an infection.

An intraspinal tumor must be considered in young children (commonly, those younger than 4 years of age) who complain of recurrent back pain. The differential is extensive, including a malignant astrocytoma, benign tumors such as dermoid cysts, lipomas, intramedullary cysts, diastematomyelia and syringomyelia.[9-11] Cutaneous abnormalities, such as a hairy patch, nevi, or dermal sinus, suggest the presence of an intraspinal anomaly. The examiner should search carefully for a subtle gait alteration, limp, leg or arm weakness, and such neurologic findings

as hyperreflexia or a positive Babinski.[12] These findings usually precede the onset of back pain. Bowel and bladder dysfunction are frequent, but these can be difficult to evaluate in a young child who has only been recently trained in toileting.

It is uncommon for a child with idiopathic scoliosis to complain of back pain. If the pain is persistent, one should exclude other causes, such as tumor, infection, or spondylolysis.[8] Spondylolysis occurs with the same frequency (5%) in children with idiopathic scoliosis as in the general population. Conversely, a

spondylolisthesis may be the cause of a lumbar scoliosis. One should be particularly sensitive to a spine curvature that does not follow the typical right thoracic left lumbar pattern of idiopathic scoliosis (Fig. 3). If the family history is negative or the curvature progresses rapidly (particularly in the male), a careful search for another etiology should be conducted.[13]

Physical examination should include routine inspection of the spine with forward bending to examine for scoliosis. Stiffness and guarding can be extreme and forward bending at the hips may be severely limited by hamstring tightness. Because the child's spine is much more flexible than an adult's, severe posturing and spine curvature is a common finding (Fig. 1).[8,14] Movements of the spine such as hyperextension or side-to-side bending may point to the etiology of the problem. Spondylolysis can be particularly uncomfortable with backward extension. Children with Scheuermann's dorsal lumbar kyphosis find forward bending accentuates the problem. The neurologic examination should include a careful search for muscle weakness and nerve root impingement. Limitation of straight leg raising is very common in children with low back complaints, particularly spondylolysis and spondylolisthesis.[15]

Radiologic Investigation

The most important radiographs are a standing anteroposterior (AP) and a lateral of the entire spine. As children are not precise in localizing the area of discomfort, the long (36-in) films used for scoliosis and kyphosis are very helpful. The study should show the spine well above and below the area of the suspected problem. The standing film often accentuates scoliosis, lordosis, or spondylolysis.[16] If the history or physical exam suggests a spondylolysis, oblique films should be obtained, because 20% of the defects will be missed if only AP and lateral films are used. [17] The flexion-extension views, particularly of the lumbosacral and dorsolumbar junctions, can be helpful in the young child to demonstrate instability or highlight a small defect in the pars interarticularis or to document the restricted motion and stiffness caused by an inflammatory lesion. The vertebral canal should be examined for widening of the interpedicular distance, which suggests an intraspinal mass or the bone spike of a diastematomyelia.

When plain films do not provide the information needed for diagnosis, bone scans are recommended as a second level of testing.[3,18,19] The bone scan is not rec-

ommended as a routine study unless the problem has been persistent or the child exhibits findings suggesting a tumor or infection (Fig. 2). A bone scan is excellent for detecting the reactive process associated with recent trauma, repetitive stress, tumor, and inflammatory conditions that involve the spine and/or pelvis. Single photon emission computed tomography (SPECT) is a more sensitive imaging technique when a stress reaction of bone is suspected.[20]

Newer imaging techniques such as computed tomography (CT) can be helpful once the anatomic location of the problem has been identified. Magnetic resonance imaging (MRI) is an important aid in evaluating disk problems, lesions contained within the spinal canal, and the relationship between the neural structures and bony vertebral elements.

Spondylolysis/Spondylolisthesis

Spondylolysis is a common cause of acute back pain in children,[1] particularly those involved in sports, such as gymnastics, weight-lifting, and tennis, that emphasize hyperextension of the spine.[21] Spondylolysis is found after walking age but rarely before the age of 5. It gradually increases to age 20, when it reaches the adult incidence of 5%.[22,23] Because there is a genetic predisposition, many children will have a positive family history.[5]

The origin of spondylolysis as a stress or fatigue fracture of the pars interarticularis has been substantially documented.[4,23,24] It has been postulated that lumbar lordosis is accentuated by the normal flexion contractures of the hip in childhood, and that this posture focuses the force of weightbearing on the pars interarticularis.[4,23] Anatomic studies have suggested that shear stresses on the pars interarticularis are greater when the lumbar spine is extended.[4] In young people, the pars interarticularis is thin, the neural arch has not reached its maximum strength, and the intervertebral disk is less resistant to shear.[25] A fatigue fracture

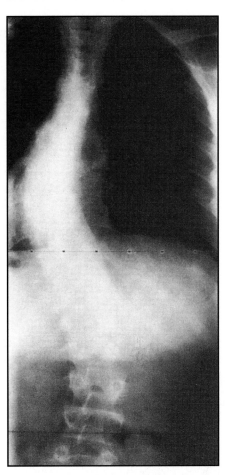

Fig. 3 A 12-year-old with a left thoracic right lumbar curvature caused by a spinal cord tumor. This pattern is the reverse of that associated with typical idiopathic scoliosis. In addition, the patient had a negative family history for scoliosis and the curvature had progressed rapidly, which would support another etiology.

of the pars interarticularis can occur at physiologic loads during cyclic flexion-extension motion of the lumbar spine.[4] These stresses may be further accentuated by lateral flexion movements on the extended spine, as can occur during a back walk-over in gymnastics, when the weight of the lower limb causes extreme hyperextension of the lumbar spine.[2,26,27] Jackson and associates[2] noted that the incidence of spondylolysis was 11% (4 times higher than normal) in female gymnasts. An increased incidence of acute spondylolysis has also been noted

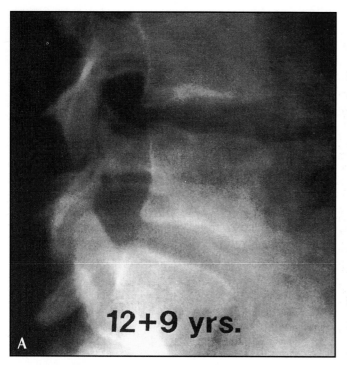 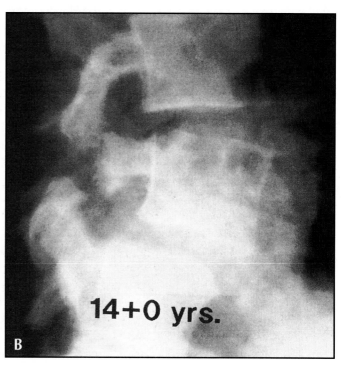

Fig. 4 Spondylolysis. **A,** At 12 years, 9 months, a small break is seen in the pars interarticularis. **B,** At age 14, radiographs of the same patient now demonstrate a widening of the defect in the pars interarticularis and grade I spondylolisthesis. The patient is asymptomatic.

in young people such as weightlifters and football linemen who engage in strenuous physical activity.[21]

An increased incidence (from 32% to 50%) has been noted in adolescents who have thoracolumbar Scheuermann's disease.[28,29] In this condition, which is now believed to be caused by excessive and repetitive mechanical loading on the immature spine, thoracolumbar kyphosis is often associated with a compensatory increase in lumbar lordosis.[28,29]

Clinical Findings

Most children first develop symptoms during the adolescent growth spurt, at approximately 11 to 14 years of age. The pain, which is very characteristic, is usually in the low back and radiates to the posterior thighs. Pain is seldom noted below the knees or in the foot.[30] Symptoms are usually initiated or aggravated by strenuous activity, particularly repetitive flexion-extension of the spine. Symptoms are decreased by rest or limi-

tation of activity.[3,4] Unlike adults, children seldom have objective signs of nerve root compression, such as motor weakness, decreased reflexes, or a sensory deficit.[30] Physical examination, however, should include a careful search for sacral anesthesia and dysfunction of the bladder, which suggests a cauda equina syndrome.

The results of physical examination may be normal in a child who has spondylolysis or mild (grade I or II) spondylolisthesis. If the posture or gait is abnormal, restricted flexion of the hips, caused by tight hamstrings, may be the only finding.[31] Eighty percent of symptomatic patients have tight hamstrings; some have considered this to be a sign of nerve root irritation, but there is no objective evidence to support that opinion.[21] Tightness of the hamstrings, which may be found in patients who have spondylolysis or any grade of spondylolisthesis, is seldom accompanied by neurologic signs.[21,30] The tightness may be so extreme that the child cannot bend forward

at the hips or that, during the straight leg-raising test, the examiner is unable to lift the foot more than a few centimeters from the examining table.

Radiologic Findings

The term spondylolysis refers to a radiolucent defect of the pars interarticularis. If the defect is large, it can be seen on nearly all views of the lumbar spine (Fig. 4). However, if it is unilateral, as it is in 20% to 25% of patients, or if it is not accompanied by spondylolisthesis, it can be a very subtle finding.[17] Oblique radiographs of the lumbar spine are often necessary to view this area in relief, apart from the overlying osseous elements (Fig. 5). It has been found that the diagnosis will be missed in 20% of young symptomatic patients if oblique radiographs are not made.[17] The so-called Scotty-dog sign of Lachapele, with the defect appearing as a collar around the dog's neck, is a helpful visual aid for those who are inexperienced in interpret-

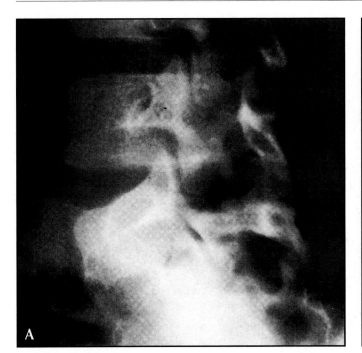
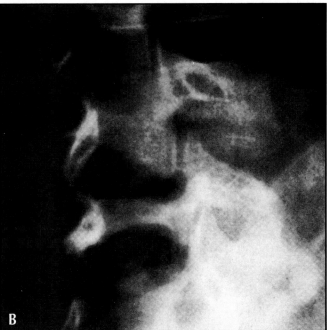

Fig. 5 A, A 9-year old male with low back pain demonstrates a unilateral spondylolysis. Oblique views demonstrate spondylolysis in the left pars interarticularis. If obliques are not obtained, the lesion could be missed in 20%. The narrow, irregular appearance suggests a recent injury. **B,** This patient can expect with time that the opposite pars interarticularis will fracture.

ing oblique radiographs. In a patient who has an acute injury, the gap is narrow and has irregular edges, whereas in a patient who has a long-standing lesion, the edges are smooth and rounded, suggesting a pseudarthrosis. The width of the gap depends on the amount of resorption of bone after the fracture and on the degree of spondylolisthesis. Confusion can occur when spondylolisthesis develops without spondylolysis, as dysplastic (Type 1) spondylolisthesis does.[21] About a third of symptomatic patients have spondylolisthesis without spondylolysis.[30] In this condition, in which there is no gap or defect in the pars interarticularis, the fifth lumbar facets appear to subluxate ventrally on the sacral facets. If the slip continues, the pars interarticularis may become attenuated, like pulled taffy (the so-called greyhound sign of Hensinger).[30]

Sherman and associates[32] described the unusual occurrence of reactive sclerosis and hypertrophy of one pedicle and lamina as well as contralateral spondylolysis in the same vertebral segment (Fig. 6). They suggested that this finding is a physiologic response to the stress of repeated trauma in the presence of an unstable neural arch and that the problem will respond satisfactorily to symptomatic treatment.[4,32] Radiographically, the appearance may be confused with the reactive sclerosis that is associated with osteoid osteoma. This becomes an important concern, because excision of the sclerotic pars interarticularis and/or pedicle associated with a contralateral spondylolysis may increase the instability of L5/S1. The presence of a nidus on CT should confirm the diagnosis of an osteoid osteoma. A bone scan may not be helpful in differentiating between the two lesions, because in both increased bone activity causes uptake of the isotope.

Bone Scans
Spondylolysis that is suspected clinically but cannot be confirmed radiographically, or that is seen early in the stress-reaction stage before fracture (prespondylolytic), may be detected by radioactive bone-scanning (Fig. 7).[3,18] Single photon emission computed tomography (SPECT) is a very sensitive method of confirming the diagnosis when a stress reaction is suspected.[20] Bone scans can demonstrate increased uptake in patients who have had symptoms for only 5 to 7 days.[3,20] Small or partial fractures may be overlooked on radiographs, but scintigrams can demonstrate the areas of increased bone turnover at the site of healing fractures.[3] Later, bone scans are helpful in distinguishing between patients who have an established nonunion and those in whom healing is still progressing and who thus may benefit from immobilization.[17,19] Bone scans are not recommended for patients who have had symptoms for more than a year or for those who are asymptomatic.[19]

Bone scans are particularly helpful in the treatment of young athletes whose activities, such as gymnastics, are known to

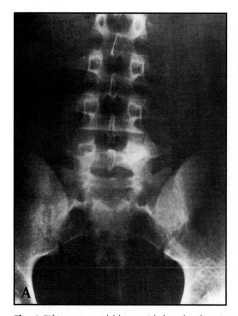
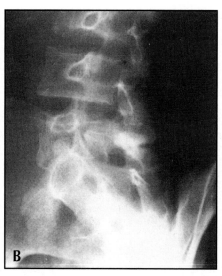
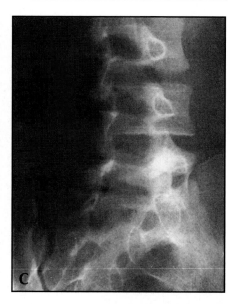

Fig. 6 Fifteen-year-old boy with low back pain. **A,** An anteroposterior radiograph demonstrates reactive sclerosis and hypertrophy of one pedicle and lamina (arrow) and contralateral spondylolysis of same vertebral segment. **B,** An oblique radiographic view shows a break in the pars interarticularis. **C,** An oblique view demonstrates reactive sclerosis. The reactive sclerosis is a physiologic response to stress resulting from repeated trauma in the presence of an unstable neural arch. Radiologically, this may be confused with reactive sclerosis associated with osteoid osteoma. (Reproduced with permission from Hensinger RN: Back pain in children, in Bradford DS, Hensinger RN (eds): *The Pediatric Spine*. New York, NY, Thieme Medical Publishers, 1985, pp 41-60.)

be associated with spondylolysis.[16] Early detection of the stress reaction can lead to appropriate treatment and, as a consequence, may shorten the recovery period. Similarly, bone scans can be used to assess recovery and to determine when an athlete can return to competition.[26]

Treatment of Spondylolysis

Several authors have reported healing of a spondylolytic defect in children and young adults after treatment with a cast or a thoracolumbosacral orthosis (TLSO).[3,4,23,33] Typically, the children in these studies had had an acute onset of symptoms and the episode of injury was clearly documented.[17,33] Unilateral defects are more likely to heal than are bilateral ones.[17] Unfortunately, not all defects heal after treatment with immobilization, but such treatment should be considered if the injury can be proved to have been recent.[23] A bone scan may be helpful to determine whether osseous repair is continuing and is likely to result in healing, or if pseudarthrosis has been established.[4]

Although, in children and teen-agers, spondylolysis of long duration is not likely to heal, a clinical response to simple nonsurgical measures can be expected.[21,30] Restriction of vigorous activities and strengthening exercises for the muscles of the back and abdomen are usually successful in controlling symptoms in patients who have mild backache and tight hamstrings.[26] Tightness of the hamstrings is an excellent clinical guide to the success or failure of treatment. Patients who have more severe or persistent complaints may need bed rest, immobilization in a cast or thoracolumbosacral orthosis, and nonnarcotic analgesics.[33] Most children will have excellent relief of symptoms and can expect to return to unrestricted activities.[26] A small percentage of young people who have spondylolysis do not respond to nonsurgical measures or are unwilling to curtail their activities, and they may require surgical stabilization.[34]

Children who, in addition, have spondylolisthesis grade I or II usually will respond to symptomatic treatment but will need continued follow-up during the growth years to observe for progression.[35,36] This is especially true for children who are younger than 10 years of age. I do not advise children or adolescents who have asymptomatic spondylolysis or minimal symptoms to restrict their activities. As 5% of the adult population reportedly have a defect of the pars interarticularis, and relatively few of them have persistent symptoms, it does not seem justified to limit the activity of an asymptomatic child or adolescent.[21,35,37]

Disk Problems
Diskitis of Childhood

Of the causes of acute back pain in children, perhaps the most unsettling is that of the vertebral diskitis. This is usually of sudden onset, often accompanied by systemic signs of sepsis, fever, and elevated sedimentation rate. Many of these patients will have a history of a recent febrile illness such as a sore throat or earache.[13,38-40] Usually any motion of the spine is extremely painful and weight-bearing, including sitting, may be uncomfortable. The young child (younger than 3 years of age) will refuse to walk or stand.[40] The lumbar spine is usually involved and paravertebral muscle spasm and limited back motion are characteristic. This condition is believed to be caused by a bacterial infection, with the inflammatory response starting at the vertebral end plate and spreading to the disk space.

Plain radiographs of the spine early in the course of the disease are typically not diagnostic (Fig. 8). If the problem is longstanding (2 to 4 weeks), the radiographs will demonstrate disk space narrowing and irregularity of the vertebral end plates. The bone scan is very helpful and usually demonstrates increased uptake early in the course of the illness.[40] Szalay and associates[41] reported that magnetic resonance imaging studies were more sensitive than bone scans in demonstrating early development of the process (Fig. 8).

In the young child, aspiration of the disk space and needle biopsy of the vertebrae, blood cultures, and other measures to document a bacterial infection are usually unsuccessful.[38,39,42,43] However, aspiration or biopsy is indicated for children who fail to respond to nonsurgical management and for the older child and adolescent in whom organisms are more typically identified (Fig. 9).[44]

Most children respond to bed rest and antibiotics. Immobilization in a cast or orthosis can be very helpful in controlling back pain. Crawford and associates[45] recommended that antibiotics be used only after failure of symptomatic treatment, such as immobilization. In-

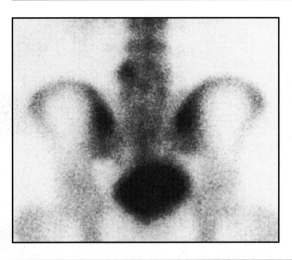

Fig. 7 A positive bone scan from a 16-year-old male with a unilateral spondylolysis. Such scans are positive by approximately 1 week after fracture and continue so for 1 year.

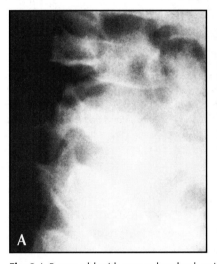
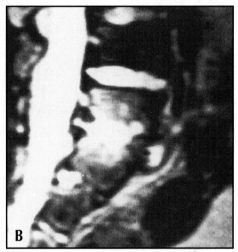

Fig. 8 A 5-year-old with severe low back pain. **A,** Radiograph of the lumbosacral junction demonstrates mild erosive changes of L5. **B,** MRI demonstrates extensive involvement of the disk space and edema in the vertebral bodies. This inflammatory process is suggestive of diskitis of childhood.

terestingly, the authors found that in 36 consecutive children with diskitis, the infection healed satisfactorily regardless of treatment.[45]

Disk Herniation
Although it is not as common as in the adult, disk herniation can occur in children as young as 12 years of age, with similar signs and symptoms.[46-51] The onset of symptoms is usually less dramatic in children, and not as frequently associated with trauma (36%).[47] DeOrio[48] suggests that disk herniation in children

is more likely to be related to cumulative trauma than to a single event. In the adolescent, back pain is a predominant finding, and symptoms are typically increased with activity and relieved by recumbency.[48,49,52] Coughing and sneezing may increase the pain, and local tenderness is inconsistent. A high percentage (85%) have positive straight leg raising, and 85% to 90% have sciatica.[47,51] The incidence of decreased deep tendon reflexes (22%) and decrease in sensation (21%) and muscle weakness (40%) is less than what would be expected in a similar adult population.[53]

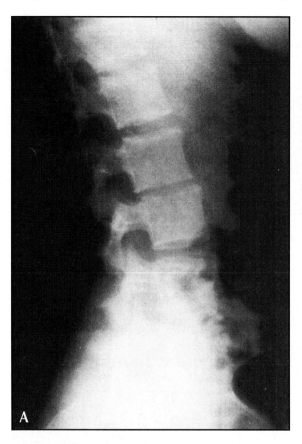

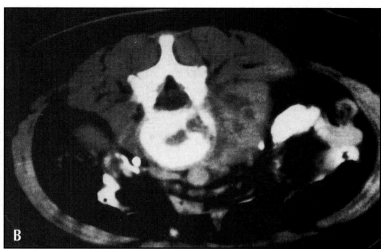

Fig. 9 A 13-year-old female with a 2-month history of back pain following a urinary tract infection. **A,** A plain lateral radiograph of the lumbar spine shows some decrease in the disk height of L3 and L4. **B,** A CT reveals a marked erosive change in vertebral body and disk space, suggesting a pyogenic vertebral osteomyelitis.

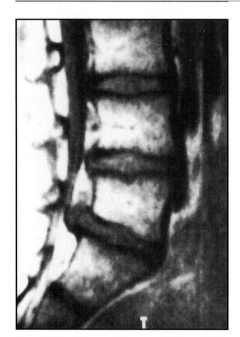

Fig. 10 This MRI of a 12-year-old female with back pain demonstrates a herniated disk at L5-S1, with almost complete extrusion of the disk.

The muscle spasm commonly causes splinting, scoliosis, and gait disturbances.[47,49,51,53] As in the adult, herniation at the L4-5 and L5-S1 levels is by far the most common.[49,51] Disk space narrowing is uncommon and plain films are typically normal in appearance, thus, diagnosis will frequently require confirmation by CT or MRI (Fig. 10).[52,53] Children with documented disk herniation usually require surgical removal.[53] Those who underwent surgical excision had a 91% good to excellent result. The nonsurgical group had 25% good to excellent and 75% poor results.[53]

Slipped Vertebral Apophysis
Slipped vertebral apophysis was previously believed to be uncommon, but, with new imaging techniques, the problem has been more frequently recognized.[54-58] The growth plate of the vertebral body, apophysis, is similar to the epiphysis in the long bone. Just as one can displace the proximal femoral epiphysis, the same problem can occur with the apophysis of the vertebral body. This typically involves the inferior rim of L4, but it can occur at any location. Clinically, the signs and symptoms are similar to those of a herniated disk. However, with this injury, both the bony rim and disk project into and narrow the spinal canal and lead to symptoms of spinal stenosis. On plain films this injury is seen as a very small fleck of calcification adjacent to the disk, but CT and MRI can successfully delineate its extent (Fig. 11).

Disk Space Calcification
This rare clinical syndrome of uncertain etiology usually involves the cervical spine, but it can also occur in the thoracic and lumbar region.[59-61] Boys are affected twice as often as girls, commonly around 7 years of age. The child presents with

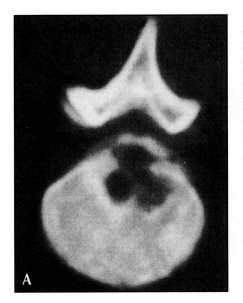

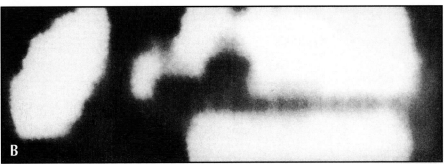

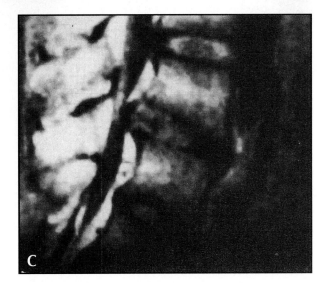

Fig. 11 A 15-year-old male with a slipped vertebral apophysis had a 1-year history of back pain, radiating into the lower extremities. **A,** This CT demonstrates a posterior defect of the vertebral body at the point of a Schmorl's node. **B,** A CT reconstruction again demonstrates the Schmorl's node and the bony projection into the spinal canal. **C,** MRI demonstrates extrusion of disk and bone into the canal.

pain, stiffness, and local tenderness. There may be signs of inflammation, with an elevated temperature, increased sedimentation rate, and leukocytosis. The condition is self-limited and usually responds quickly to symptomatic treatment. Occasionally, the involved disk is weakened by the process and can herniate into the spinal canal, in which case plain radiographs will usually reveal a hazy calcification of the disk.[62,63]

Kyphosis

A frequent cause of back complaints in children is Scheuermann's dorsal lumbar kyphosis.[64] Scheuermann, in his original article, described two forms of kyphosis. The first of these, kyphosis involving a long segment of the thoracic spine, is usually painless in onset. Scheuermann's description was further refined by Sorenson, who noted a familial tendency

and described the classic radiographic findings of three consecutive vertebrae wedged 5° or greater.[65] End plate irregularity, Schmorl's node formation, and narrowing of the disk space were common accompaniments but were not in themselves diagnostic.[65,66] The second type of kyphosis described by Scheuermann is localized to the dorsal lumbar junction and involves fewer vertebrae and more acute angulation. This kyphosis is always associated with vertebral wedging, end plate irregularity, and Schmorl's node formation. This condition is painful and is commonly found in children who perform heavy physical activity, such as shoveling clay or lifting weights (Fig. 12).[3,67,68]

There is strong clinical and experimental evidence to suggest a traumatic origin of Scheuermann's dorsal lumbar kyphosis.[3,69,70] The apophyseal ring is

thinner in its center than at the periphery and increased pressure may force the intervertebral disk through the end plate and into cancellous bone, with narrowing of the disk space.[70] End plate rupture, which has been reproduced in the laboratory by increasing the force on the spine, is believed to be analogous to the mechanism that leads to Schmorl's nodes.[69] Heavy lifting, especially when seated or bending forward, can double interdiskal pressure.[69] Micheli[3] noted that the force of flexion-extension seen with rowers, weightlifters, and gymnasts approaches the lower end of the range demonstrated experimentally to induce vertebral end plate fractures in normal vertebral specimens.[69]

In some children, the disk material passes peripherally (usually anterior), submarginally beneath the apophyseal ring (Fig. 13).[28] Radiologically there will

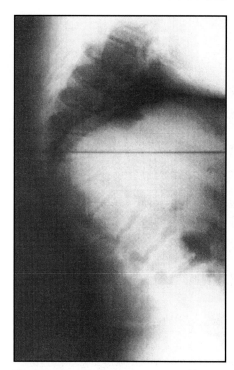

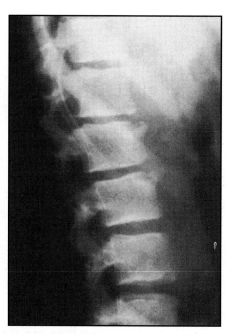

Fig. 12 This radiograph of a 14-year-old demonstrates severe kyphosis centered at the dorsolumbar junction secondary to lumbar Scheuermann's disease. Note the end plate changes, wedging, and narrowing of the disk spaces. Schmorl's node formation can be seen as well in adjacent lumbar vertebrae.

Fig. 13 This 15-year-old recreational weight lifter had persistent back pain at the dorsolumbar junction. The routine lateral film demonstrates anterior Schmorl's node formation and disk space narrowing at T11-12 and T12-L1.

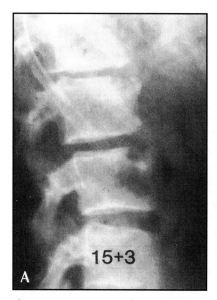

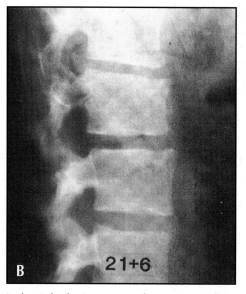

Fig. 14 A, At 15 years and 3 months, back pain due to kyphosis was treated symptomatically. **B,** Note healing changes in vertebrae at age 21. (Reproduced with permission from Green TL, Hensinger RN, Hunter LY: Back pain and vertebral changes simulating Scheuermann's disease. *J Pediatr Orthop* 1985;5:1-7.)

be separation of a triangular, smooth bone fragment from the vertebral body, which represents the ring apophysis.[28] The vertebral changes progress slowly toward healing during the time of remaining growth. However, the Schmorl's node formation and disk space narrowing generally persist and the fragment of the ring apophysis typically remains separate from the vertebral body.[71]

Symptoms may be of sudden onset, associated with a specific activity. They gradually become more persistent over time and are accentuated with forward bending. The acute phase involves sudden herniation of the disk into the vertebral body, or there can be gradual repetitive injury to the spine with a refractive process leading to the disk expulsion. This kyphosis is often accompanied by spondylolysis. The close association of the two conditions suggests that hyperlordosis, compensating for the kyphosis, increases the likelihood of stress on the pars interarticularis and that the two conditions may be related to the repetitive nature of particular sports.[28]

This condition can be managed quite successfully by simple symptomatic treatment, including immobilization and rest, which allows the vertebrae to heal. When the child is comfortable, gradual resumption of activities is permitted along with physical therapy to strengthen the back musculature. Until rehabilitation is completed, the patient must learn to avoid the specific activities that initiated the problem (Fig. 14).[28,71] Typically, these activities involve repetitive forceful flexion of the dorsal lumbar spine, such as occur during weight lifting, rowing, and gymnastics.

Benign Neoplasm

Osteoid osteoma and osteoblastoma are the most common benign tumors of the spine. Children with these tumors usually present with back pain and scoliosis. The osteoid osteoma usually involves the pedicles and posterior elements. Typ-

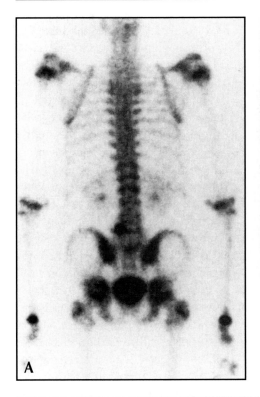

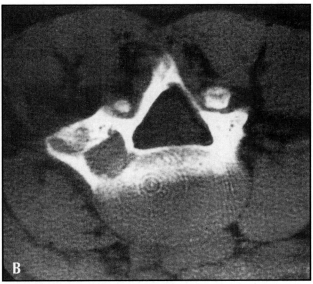

Fig.15 A 13-year-old male with back pain. **A,** Bone scan reveals an increased uptake in the region of L4 **B,** CT demonstrates an osteoid osteoma in the pedicle of L4. (Reproduced with permission from Hensinger RN: Back pain in children, in Andersson GBJ, McNeill TW (eds): *Lumbar Spine Syndromes: Evaluation and Treatment.* Berlin, Springer-Verlag, 1989, pp 126-152.)

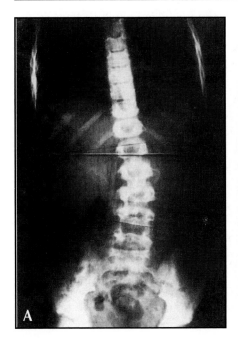

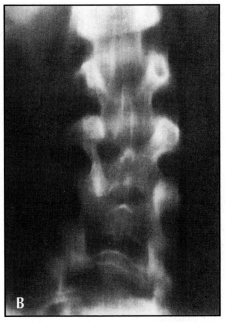

Fig. 16 A 7-year-old with an osteoblastoma. **A,** Routine radiographs demonstrate a significant lumbar scoliosis, but the lesion could not be identified on this view. **B,** A laminagram demonstrates erosion of the lamina of L3. (Reproduced with permission from Hensinger RN: Back pain in children, in Bradford DS, Hensinger RN: *The Pediatric Spine.* New York, NY, Thieme Medical Publishers, 1985, pp 41-60.)

ically, there is a large sclerotic bone response to a small nidus, best seen on the CT scan (Fig. 15).[7,72] Osteoblastomas usually cause the same clinical findings, but they are typically larger and more destructive (Fig. 16). Osteoblastomas can compress the spinal cord, particularly in the cervical and thoracic spine. The tumors are usually symptomatic and the pain is quite characteristic; it is often nocturnal and is relieved by aspirin or Naprosyn. The tumors are best localized with the bone scan, followed by definitive identification of the nidus with CT (Figs. 15 and 16).

Eosinophilic granuloma leads to a gradual replacement of the vertebral body and gradual weakening. A trivial injury

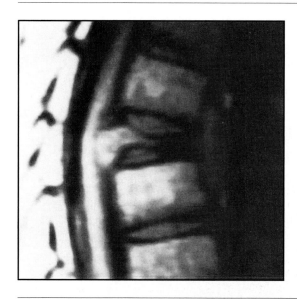

Fig. 17 A 14-year-old male with an eosinophilic granuloma. MRI demonstrates protrusion into the canal posteriorly. The patient was hyperreflexic and the lesion was removed and bone grafted.

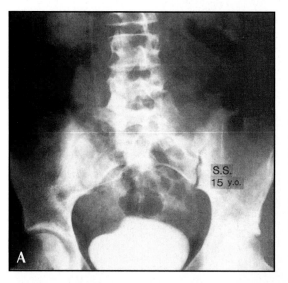

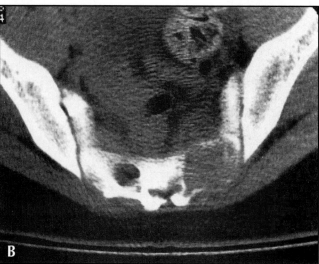

Fig. 18 Aneurysmal bone cyst in the sacrum of a 15-year-old girl. **A,** An anteroposterior radiograph of the pelvis. Overlying gas shadows and material in the bowel prevent complete examination of the sacrum. **B,** CT reveals a large aneurysmal bone cyst in the sacrum. (Reproduced with permission from Hensinger RN: Back pain in children, in Bradford DS, Hensinger RN (eds): *The Pediatric Spine*. New York, NY, Thieme Medical Publishers, 1985, pp 41-60.)

can precipitate a sudden collapse and bleeding initiating the onset of pain (Fig. 17).[73] Plain films usually reveal the classic radiographic findings of vertebral plana. MRI can confirm the diagnosis. However, in some patients, the radiographic appearance may be confused with Ewing's sarcoma. In such cases, definitive diagnosis requires biopsy. Occasionally, the tumor herniates posteriorly into the spinal canal, causing spinal cord compression, but paraplegia is a rare complication.

The aneurysmal bone cyst may be present for a long period without causing symptoms. The onset of symptoms and discovery is triggered by a fracture through the weakened bone, collapse, and spontaneous hemorrhage. These cysts generally occur in the thoracic or lumbar vertebral body and sacrum but are occasionally found in posterior structures (Fig. 18). Exploration and bone grafting usually resolves the problem.

Malignant Neoplasms

Primary malignant tumors are rare in the spine, the most common being Ewing's sarcoma, leukemia, and lymphoma.[74] More commonly, such lesions are metastatic and represent spread from a distant primary site, usually from bone or bone marrow. In children, the most common skeletal metastases to the spine are neuroblastomas and rhabdomyosarcomas. Less common are teratoma, teratocarcinoma, Wilm's tumor, and osteogenic sarcoma.[74-76] Depending on the series reported, up to 70% of patients with neuroblastoma will have metastatic skeletal disease at the time of their initial diagnosis or during the course of their treatment.[75,77] The spine is typically involved. The diffuse permeative destruction of bone resembles the changes seen in the metaphyseal areas of long bones, with cortical destruction and variable amounts of periosteal reaction.[77] Rhabdomyosarcoma is the most common soft-tissue malignancy in children, and spine metastases occur in 30% to 50% of patients.[78] The abnormal cells displace the normal bone-forming elements, and the vertebra becomes structurally weak and collapses with minor trauma.[76,79] Back pain is a common initial complaint, usually in the region of the collapse, and neurologic complications can occur.[9,75] The bone scan is the most sensitive method for diagnosis of a metastasis or primary bone tumor, and in children is more sensitive than skeletal surveys.[75,80] Many children with a leukemia or lymphoma will have involvement of the viscera, as well as the skeleton at other sites in addition to the spine (Fig. 19).

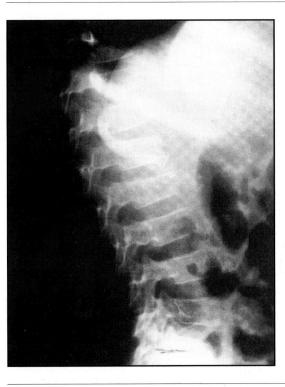

Fig. 19 Radiograph of a 4-year-old with acute lymphatic leukemia and no history of injury demonstrates multiple compression fractures of the lumbar spine. The presenting symptom was back pain. (Reproduced with permission from Hensinger RN: Back pain in children, in Bradford DS, Hensinger RN (eds): *The Pediatric Spine*. New York, NY, Thiemc Medical Publishers, 1985, pp 41-60.)

Conclusion

Back pain in children is serious. It is uncommon, and children who have this complaint should be evaluated promptly. Most conditions can be diagnosed with simple measures, such as routine radiographs and bone scan. A few may require more extensive measures, such as CT and MRI. A vast majority will be found to have an objective disease that can be managed quite successfully.

Physicians evaluating acute back pain in children should be particularly alert for those who have persistent pain. Most problems during childhood are relieved with rest and decrease in activity. If there is persistent pain and/or increasing pain, fever, or such neurologic signs as bladder incontinence or nerve root compression, the evaluation should be swift and persistent until the etiology has been determined.

References

1. Hensinger RN: Back pain in children, in Bradford DS, Hensinger RN (eds): *The Pediatric Spine*. New York, NY, Thieme, 1985, pp 41-60.

2. Jackson DW, Wiltse LL, Cirincione RJ: Spondylolysis in the female gymnast. *Clin Orthop* 1976;117:68-73.

3. Micheli LJ: Low back pain in the adolescent: Differential diagnosis. *Am J Sports Med* 1979;7:362-364.

4. Letts M, Smallman T, Afanasiev R, et al: Fracture of the pars interarticularis in adolescent athletes: A clinical-biomechanical analysis. *J Pediatr Orthop* 1986;6:40-46.

5. Wynne-Davies R, Scott JHS: Inheritance and spondylolisthesis: A radiographic family survey. *J Bone Joint Surg* 1979;61B:301-305.

6. Keim HA, Reina EG: Osteoid-osteoma as a cause of scoliosis. *J Bone Joint Surg* 1975;57A:159-163.

7. Kirwan EO, Hutton PAN, Pozo JL, et al: Osteoid osteoma and benign osteoblastoma of the spine: Clinical presentation and treatment. *J Bone Joint Surg* 1984;66B:21-26.

8. Mehta MH Murray RO: Scoliosis provoked by painful vertebral lesions. *Skelelal Radiology* 1977;1:223-230.

9. Conrad EU III, Olszewski AD, Berger M, et al: Pediatric spine tumors with spinal cord compromise. *J Pediatr Orthop* 1992;12:454-460.

10. Hood RW, Riseborough EJ, Nehme AM, et al: Diastematomyelia and structural spinal deformities. *J Bone Joint Surg* 1980;62A:520-528.

11. McMaster MJ: Occult intraspinal anomalies and congenital scoliosis. *J Bone Joint Surg* 1984;66A:588-601.

12. Rasool MN, Govender S, Naidoo KS, et al: Foot deformities and occult spinal abnormalities in children: A review of 16 cases. *J Pediatr Orthop* 1992; 12:94-99.

13. Coonrad RW, Richardson WJ, Oakes WJ: Left thoracic curves can be different. *Orthop Trans* 1985;9:126-127.

14. Winter RB, Lipscomb PR Jr.: Back pain in children. *Minnesota Med* 1978;61:141-147.

15. Turner PG, Green JH, Galasko CSB: Back pain in childhood. *Spine* 1989;14:812-814.

16. Lowe RW, Hayes TD, Kaye J, et al: Standing roentgenograms in spondylolisthesis. *Clin Orthop* 1976; 117:80-84.

17. Libson E, Bloom RA, Dinari G: Symptomatic and asymptomatic spondylolysis and spondylolisthesis in young adults. *Internat Orthop* 1982;6:259-261.

18. Papanicolaou N, Wilkinson RH, Emans JB, et al: Bone scintigraphy and radiography in young athletes with low back pain. *Am J Roentgenol* 1985;145:1039-1044.

19. van den Oever M, Merrick MV, Scott JHS: Bone scintigraphy in symptomatic spondylolysis. *J Bone Joint Surg* 1987;69B:453.

20. Bodner RJ, Heyman S, Drummond DS, et al: The use of single photon emission computed tomography (SPECT) in the diagnosis of low-back pain in young patients. *Spine* 1988;13:1155-1160.

21. Hensinger RN: Spondylolysis and spondylolisthesis in children and adolescents. *J Bone Joint Surg* 1989;71A:1098-1107.

22. Baker DR, McHollick W: Spondyloschisis and spondylolisthesis in children. *J Bone Joint Surg* 1956;38A:933-934.

23. Wiltse LL, Widell EH Jr, Jackson DW: Fatigue fracture: The basic lesion in isthmic spondylolisthesis. *J Bone Joint Surg* 1975;57A:17-22.

24. Krenz J, Troup JD: The structure of the pars interarticularis of the lower lumbar vertebrae and its relation to the etiology of spondylolysis, with a report of a healing fracture in the neural arch of a fourth lumbar vertebra. *J Bone Joint Surg* 1973;55B:735-741.

25. Cyron BM, Hutton WC: Variations in the amount and distribution of cortical bone across the partes interarticulares of L5: A predisposing factor in spondylolysis? *Spine* 1979;4:163-167.

26. Jackson DW: Low back pain in young athletes: Evaluation of stress reaction and discogenic problems. *Am J Sports Med* 1979;7:364-366.

27. Micheli LJ: Back injuries in dancers. *Clin Sports Med* 1983;2:473-484.

28. Greene TL, Hensinger RN, Hunter LY: Back pain and vertebral changes simulating Scheuermann's disease. *J Pediatr Orthop* 1985;5:1-7.

29. Ogilvie JW, Sherman J: Spondylolysis in Scheuermann's disease. *Spine* 1987;12:251-253.

30. Hensinger RN, Lang JR, MacEwen GD: Surgical management of spondylolisthesis in children and adolescents. *Spine* 1976;1:207-216.

31. Phalen GS, Dickson JA: Spondylolisthesis and tight hamstrings. *J Bone Joint Surg* 1961;43A:505-512.

32. Sherman FC, Wilkinson RH, Hall JE: Reactive sclerosis of a pedicle and spondylolysis in the lumbar spine. *J Bone Joint Surg* 1977;59A:49-54.

33. Steiner ME, Micheli LJ: Treatment of symptomatic spondylolysis and spondylolisthesis with the modified Boston brace. *Spine* 1985;10:937-943.

34. Seitsalo S, Osterman K, Poussa M, et al: Spondylolisthesis in children under 12 years of age: Long-term results of 56 patients treated conservatively or operatively. *J Pediatr Orthop* 1988;8:516-521.

35. Pizzutillo PD, Hummer CD III: Nonoperative treatment for painful adolescent spondylolysis or spondylolisthesis. *J Pediatr Orthop* 1989;9:538-540.

36. Seitsalo S, Osterman K, Hyvarinen H, et al: Progression of spondylolisthesis in children and adolescents: A long-term follow-up of 272 patients. *Spine* 1991;16:417-421.

37. Frennered AK, Danielson BI, Nachemson AL: Natural history of symptomatic isthmic low-grade spondylolisthesis in children and adolescents: A seven-year follow-up study. *J Pediatr Orthop* 1991;11:209-213.

38. Menelaus MB: Discitis: An inflammation affecting the intervertebral discs in children. *J Bone Joint Surg* 1964;46B:16-23.

39. Spiegel PG, Kengla KW, Isaacson AS, et al: Intervertebral disc-space inflammation in children. *J Bone Joint Surg* 1972;54A:284-296.

40. Wenger DR, Bobechko WP, Gilday DL: The spectrum of intervertebral disc-space infection in children. *J Bone Joint Surg* 1978;60A:100-108.

41. Szalay EA, Green NE, Heller RM, et al: Magnetic resonance imaging in the diagnosis of childhood discitis. *J Pediatr Orthop* 1987;7:164-167.

42. Boston HC Jr, Bianco AJ Jr, Rhodes KH: Disk space infections in children. *Orthop Clin North Am* 1975;6:953-964.

43. Smith RF, Taylor TKF: Inflammatory lesions of intervertebral discs in children. *J Bone Joint Surg* 1967;49A:1508-1520.

44. McNeill TW: Spinal infections, in Greene WB (ed): *Instructional Course Lectures, Volume XXXIX.* Park Ridge, Illinois, The American Academy of Orthopaedic Surgeons, 1990, pp 515-524.

45. Crawford AH, Kucharzyk DW, Ruda R, et al: Diskitis in children. *Clin Orthop* 1991;266:70-79.

46. Borgesen SE, Vang PS: Herniation of the lumbar intervertebral disk in children and adolescents. *Acta Orthop Scand* 1974;45:540-549.

47. Bradford DS, Garcia A: Herniations of the lumbar intervertebral disk in children and adolescents: A review of 30 surgically treated cases. *JAMA* 1969;210:2045-2051.

48. DeOrio JK, Bianco AJ Jr: Lumbar disc excision in children and adolescents. *J Bone Joint Surg* 1982;64A:991-996.

49. Epstein JA, Epstein NE, Marc J, et al: Lumbar intervertebral disk herniation in teenage children: Recognition and management of associated anomalies. *Spine* 1984;9:427-432.

50. Garrido E, Humphreys RP, Hendrick EB, et al: Lumbar disc disease in children. *Neurosurgery* 1978;2:22-26.

51. Kurihara A, Kataoka O: Lumbar disc herniation in children and adolescents: A review of 70 operated cases and their minimum 5-year follow-up studies. *Spine* 1980;5:443-451.

52. Takata K, Takahashi K: Hamstring tightness and sciatica in young patients with disc herniation. *J Bone Joint Surg* 1994;76B:220-224.

53. DeLuca PF, Mason DE, Weiand R, et al: Excision of herniated nucleus pulposus in children and adolescents. *J Pediatr Orthop* 1994;14:318-322.

54. Handel SF, Twiford TW Jr, Reigel DH, et al: Posterior lumbar apophyseal fractures. *Radiology* 1979;130:629-633.

55. Keller RH: Traumatic displacement of the cartilagenous vertebral rim: A sign of intervertebral disc prolapse. *Radiology* 1974;110:21-24.

56. Lippitt AB: Fracture of a vertebral body end plate and disk protrusion causing subarachnoid block in an adolescent. *Clin Orthop* 1976;116:112-115.

57. Lowrey JJ: Dislocated lumbar vertebral epiphysis in adolescent children: Report of three cases. *J Neurosurg* 1973;38:232-234.

58. Techakapuch S: Rupture of the lumbar cartilage plate into the spinal canal in an adolescent: A case report. *J Bone Joint Surg* 1981;63A:481-482.

59. Melnick JC, Silverman FN: Intervertebral disk calcification in childhood. *Radiology* 1963;80:399-408.

60. Schechter LS, Smith A, Pearl M: Intervertebral disk calcification in childhood. *Am J Dis Child* 1972;123:608-611.

61. Sonnabend DH, Taylor TKF, Chapman GK: Intervertebral disc calcification syndromes in children. *J Bone Joint Surg* 1982;64B:25-31.

62. McCartee CC Jr, Griffin PP, Byrd EB: Ruptured calcified thoracic disc in a child: Report of a case. *J Bone Joint Surg* 1972;54A:1272-1274.

63. Peck FC Jr: A calcified thoracic intervertebral disk with herniation and spinal cord compression in a child: Case report. *J Neurosurgery* 1957;14:105-109.

64. Scheuermann H: Kyphosis dorsalis juvenilis. *Ztschr Orthop Chir* 1921;41:305-317.

65. Sorenson KH: Scheuermann's juvenile kyphosis: Clinical appearances, radiography, aetiology and prognosis. Copenhagen, Munksgaard, 1964.

66. Bradford DS, Moe JH, Montalvo FJ, et al: Scheuermann's kyphosis and roundback deformity: Results of Milwaukee brace treatment. *J Bone Joint Surg* 1974;56A:740-758.

67. Edgren W, Vainio S: Osteochondrosis juvenilis lumbalis. *Acta Chir Scand* 1957;227(suppl):1-47.

68. Wassmann K: Kyphosis juvenilis Scheuermann: An occupational disorder. *Acta Orthop Scand* 1951;21:65-74.

69. Jayson MIV, Herbert CM, Barks JS: Intervertebral discs: Nuclear morphology and bursting pressures. *Ann Rheum Dis* 1973;32:308-315.

70. Resnick D, Niwayama G: Intravertebral disk herniations: Cartilaginous (Schmorl's) nodes. *Radiology* 1978;126:57-65.

71. Lowe TG: Scheuermann's disease. *J Bone Joint Surg* 1990;72A:940-945.

72. Gitelis S, Schajowicz F: Osteoid osteoma and osteoblastoma. *Orthop Clin North Am* 1989;20:313-325.

73. Nesbit ME, Kieffer S, D'Angio GJ: Reconstitution of vertebral height in histiocytosis X: A long-term follow-up. *J Bone Joint Surg* 1969;51A:1360-1368.

74. Young JL Jr, Miller RW: Incidence of malignant tumors in U.S. children. *J Pediatr* 1975;86:254-258.

75. Leeson MC, Makley JT, Carter JR: Metastatic skeletal disease in the pediatric population. *J Pediatr Orthop* 1985;5:261-267.

76. Ogden JA, Ogden DA: Skeletal metastasis: The effect on the immature skeleton. *Skeletal Radiology* 1982;9:73-82.

77. Fernbach DJ, Williams TE, Donaldson MH: Neuroblastoma, in Sutow WW, Vietti TJ, Fernbach DJ (eds): *Clinical Pediatric Oncology*, ed 2. St Louis, MO, CV Mosby, 1977, pp 506-537.

78. Maroteaux P: Malignant tumors, in Maroteaux P (ed): *Bone Diseases of Children*. Philadelphia, PA, JB Lippincott, 1979, pp 397-420.

79. Rogalsky RJ, Black GB, Reed MH: Orthopaedic manifestations of leukemia in children. *J Bone Joint Surg* 1986;68A:494-501.

80. Gilday DL, Ash JM, Reilly BJ: Radionuclide skeletal survey for pediatric neoplasms. *Radiology* 1977;123:399-406.

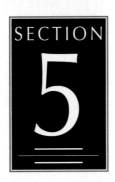

SECTION 5

Spondylolisthesis

Spondylolisthesis

The two articles in this section describe the diagnosis, classification, pathoanatomy, and surgical treatment of low- and high-grade spondylolisthesis. Both articles supply superb descriptions of relevant surgical and nonsurgical treatments. Spondylolisthesis is defined as the "forward slippage of one particular segment of the spine onto the next lower segment." However, understanding spondylolisthesis is difficult because many types of slips are prevalent within the population, and the literature often "mixes" the types when reporting results.

Dr. Michael O'Brien's article on low-grade spondylolisthesis describes the different classification schemes that have led to this persistent confusion. The principal issue arises from the use of the term "isthmic lesion," as described by Wiltse. This term has been used indiscriminately to describe spondylolistheses whenever a discontinuation of the pars interarticularis is present, regardless of whether the cause is dysplasia or repetitive stresses. Clearly, these two entities require separate discussion and management. The 1963 Newman classification and later the 1994 Marchetti and Bartolozzi classification attempted to distinguish the difference between these entities; this distinction should continue to be stressed, as is briefly mentioned by Drs. Lawrence Lenke and Keith Bridwell in their article on high-grade spondylolisthesis.

Dr. O'Brien's article eloquently describes the epidemiology of low-grade spondylolisthesis. Its prevalence has been reported to be between 3.5% and 6% but can vary across racial lines, with a lower prevalence among blacks and a higher prevalence (up to 50%) in specific Eskimo populations. Spondylolisthesis is not a congenital lesion but rather a developmental one, most commonly occurring at L5-S1 (87%) secondary to spondylolysis. It is rarely identified in patients younger than age 5, but it occurs in up to 6% of individuals younger than age 18 years. The etiology remains unclear but appears to be a combination of genetic, biomechanical, anatomic, and traumatic factors.

Imaging should include thin-slice CT and standing radiographs in addition to the standard AP, lateral, and oblique views of the lumbosacral spine. Bone scans are most useful for adolescents who have back pain from spondylolysis; these scans can identify the reparative ability of the lytic defect of the pars interarticularis. The presence of increased uptake on a bone scan may suggest that the lytic defect is of recent origin and could benefit from a period of immobilization, whereas a "cold" scan may imply that the defect is long standing and inactive and therefore not likely to be amenable to nonsurgical treatment.

In his discussion of the clinical presentation and treatment options, Dr. O'Brien cites low back pain and/or radicular symptoms as the most common on presentation.

The radicular complaints can occur as a result of hypermobility, foraminal narrowing, or the fibrocartilaginous scar that forms around the lytic defect within the pars interarticularis. However, the presence of radicular pain in patients with a spondylolysis should not exclude other possible etiologies such as disk herniation, especially far lateral disk herniation at adjacent vertebral levels.

Low back pain in patients with spondylolisthesis must be distinguished from pain secondary to other causes. The mere presence of a spondylolisthesis does not mean that it has caused the patient's symptoms. In fact, patients with low-grade spondylolisthesis often are asymptomatic or have minimal symptoms. Progression of low-grade spondylolisthesis in the adult is uncommon. An adult with a spondylolisthesis usually has had the slippage for many years and is typically stable. In a medical-legal context, the presence of low back pain following a traumatic event in individuals with previously asymptomatic spondylolistheses may be the result of aggravation of spondylolisthesis or some other cause such as herniated disk or lumbar strain.

Nonsurgical treatment of symptomatic spondylolisthesis consists of physical therapy, including passive modalities, isometric and isokinetic exercises, and aerobic conditioning. Bracing is appropriate for symptomatic adolescents with a "hot" bone scan. Surgical treatment includes pars repair, arthrodesis across the pars interarticularis lytic lesion, or decompression or fusion between the adjacent vertebrae. Decompression may be necessary if the symptoms are radicular or stenotic. Although the initial results of decompression alone (ie, Gill laminectomy) were encouraging, longer follow-up and later studies have reported poorer results with this approach. Thus, Dr. O'Brien suggests that given the current instrumentation systems available for stabilization, the Gill laminectomy alone is probably not advisable; he recommends decompression with fusion for symptomatic low-grade spondylolisthesis. He also suggests anterior column support when there is a large or hypermobile disk or when patients are at increased risk for pseudarthrosis. Anterior column support can be performed from a formal anterior, posterolateral, or transforaminal interbody approach. Whether the anterior column support in low-grade spondylolisthesis improves the technical success and clinical outcome is not clear in the current literature.

The second article in this section, authored by Drs. Lawrence Lenke and Keith Bridwell, describes the evaluation and treatment of high-grade spondylolisthesis. Their focused discussion offers recommendations regarding the surgical treatment of high-grade slips. The article begins by describing the dysplasia involved in this deformity; it succinctly outlines the Marchetti and Bartolozzi classification but lacks a detailed explanation of the continued misuse of the term isthmic lesion, as described previously.

The authors cite the two most important radiographic parameters to evaluate in high-grade slips—the Meyerding grading of the L5 translation and the slip angle. The slip angle measures the amount of lumbosacral kyphosis between L5 and the sacrum and is used as a guide to determine not only the severity of the spondylolisthesis but also the main corrective parameter during surgical treatment. As stated in Dr. O'Brien's article, standing AP and lateral radiographs are strongly recommended as part of the preoperative workup. A standing lateral view taken with a long cassette demonstrates the overall sagittal profile and the C7 plumb line. Pelvic incidence, which was first described by Legaye and associates,[1] is defined by the angle perpendicular to the superior sacral end plate at its midpoint and the line connecting this midpoint to the middle axis of the femoral heads.[2] The normal pelvic incidence is around 50°. This has been shown to be an independent radiographic parameter that influences sagittal spinal balance, pelvic orientation, and risk of progression.

On occasion, sciatic scoliosis may develop in high-grade spondylolisthesis as a result of pressure on the cauda equina. A lumbosacral MRI is recommended for all patients undergoing surgery to evaluate the neuroanatomy and the health of the adjacent disks. As described for low-grade spondylolisthesis, patients with high-grade slips typically have surprisingly mild low back pain despite the severity of the slip. Most patients have some neurologic symptoms. Of these, L5 radiculopathy is the most common; most often it is unilateral, but it also can be bilateral. Nearly all patients will have tight hamstrings on a straight leg raising test, which according to the authors is considered a neurologic sign to the lower extremities. Neurologic examination should include a careful evaluation of anal sphincter tone and sensation and the L5 motor function (foot dorsiflexion and the extensor hallucis longus), as the L5 nerve is at the highest risk for postoperative weakness and diminished function.

The authors conclude their article with the assertion that surgical treatment is indicated for all patients with high-grade spondylolistheses, even in those rare situations in which a patient is relatively asymptomatic, despite a grade III or more slip and a fair degree of dysplasia to the lumbosacral region. The authors mention many different surgical techniques but clearly recommend posterior decompression and instrumentation with posterior and anterior arthrodesis.

In the past, in situ arthrodesis was indicated for high-grade spondylolisthesis primarily because appropriate instrumentation was lacking. Pseudarthrosis rates approached 50% with this technique; the greatest risk was in patients with the following characteristics: excessive L5-S1 mobility, dysplastic anatomy, small lumbar transverse processes, a marked kyphotic slip angle, signs of sacral root stretch, and overall global anterior sagittal imbalance. Reduction of the slip places the L5 nerve root at risk for subsequent dorsiflexion weakness or even complete drop foot.

The authors emphasize that the risk of pseudarthrosis is higher in patients who are in a biomechanically unstable position, with marked residual forward translation and especially angulation in the sagittal plane with a kyphotic slip angle. For these patients, the authors recommend partial reduction to improve both the slip angle and ultimately the biomechanics of the spine while improving the opportunity for osteosynthesis and limiting the risk of neurologic injury.

The authors conclude with a description of the way they treat high-grade spondylolisthesis, specifically emphasizing wide decompression, partial reduction, and correction of the lumbosacral kyphotic slip angle. Careful neurologic monitoring of the L5 nerve is essential during the surgical reduction of high-grade spondylolisthesis, with direct nerve stimulation before and after the reduction. A single pantaloon brace is typically used, and patients may begin ambulation soon after surgery depending on the security of fixation obtained.

In summary, these articles cover a large topic quite succinctly. Dr. O'Brien provides a good general approach to the issues regarding low-grade slips. Drs. Lenke and Bridwell discuss the more precarious evaluation and treatment of high-grade dysplastic spondylolisthesis, including the neurologic risks and their surgical approach to the problem of partial reduction and correction of the lumbosacral kyphosis.

Christopher J. DeWald, MD
Assistant Professor
Department of Orthopaedic Surgery
Rush Medical College
Rush-Presbyterian-St. Luke's Medical Center
Chicago, Illinois

References
1. Legaye DB, Hecquet M: Pelvic incidence: A fundamental pelvic parameter for three-dimensional regulation of spinal sagittal curves. *Eur Spine J* 1998; 7:99-103.
2. Curylo LJ, Edwards C, DeWald RW: Radiographic markers in spondyloptosis: Implications for spondylolisthesis progression. *Spine* 2002;27:2021-2025.

Low-Grade Isthmic/Lytic Spondylolisthesis in Adults

Michael F. O'Brien, MD

Abstract

Three basic classification schemes have been developed to categorize spondylolisthesis, the slippage or forward displacement of one vertebra over another. Two rely on radiographic appearance, and the third stresses the developmental aspect of the pathology. The pathology is relatively rare in individuals younger than 18 years, appears to be influenced by race, and is found more frequently in males than females and in patients with symptomatic low back pain. Lytic spondylolisthesis occurs more frequently at certain spinal levels, and certain sports activities have been implicated in its development. The etiology remains unclear, but hereditary factors are unlikely with no evidence of the lytic defect in newborns. Recent research indicates that the architecture of the pelvis may be an important parameter. Some have postulated that the underlying pathomechanical event is a fracture, either acute or secondary to fatigue. Once the pars defect has been created, anatomic and biomechanical forces conspire to prevent healing of the fracture and create a spondylolisthesis. Although mechanical considerations are likely most significant, genetic considerations have also been discussed. All the imaging modalities play useful roles in defining the pathoanatomy, including diskography. Patients typically report symptoms as back pain and/or neurologic symptoms; however, these symptoms can have other causes even though a spondylolisthesis is present. A thorough history and physical examination, along with the radiographic investigations, are essential to determining proper treatment. Nonsurgical options are activity modification, bracing, physical therapy, and intervention in the form of medications or injections. Use of muscle relaxers and narcotics may be appropriate for managing initial acute pain. Surgical options are direct repair of the pars defect, decompression, fusion, or a combination of these procedures. The various techniques of pars repair are recommended only for patients younger than 30 years. Although decompression alone may be suitable in some situations, decompression with fusion is more standard, certainly when instability and low back pain exist.

Nazarian generalized the concept of spondylolisthesis in 1992, describing it as "slippage of a portion of the spine on the underlying portion."[1] Other authors have discussed the etiology, symptoms, and means of treatment for symptomatic spondylolisthesis.[2-6] More sophisticated radiographic tools, including MRI and CT, have demonstrated a wide diversity of pathoanatomy. Attempts have been made to categorize or classify spondylolisthesis based on radiographic appearance and presumed pathologic biomechanics. Recently, several groups[7-10] have pointed out the importance of various lumbosacral and pelvic anatomic alignments in the development of spondylolisthesis. In unpublished data presented at the Scoliosis Research Society Annual Meeting in 2001, Labelle showed a direct correlation between the increasing grade of spondylolisthesis and the increasing pelvic incidence.

Classification

In 1963, Newman and Stone[11] reviewed 319 patients with a follow-up of 15 years. They attempted to describe spondylolisthesis both in terms of radiographic appearance and potential causality (Fig. 1). They believed that the slippage in group I (congenital, n = 66) resulted from attenuation of the pars interarticularis allowing slippage of one vertebra on the next. Patients in group II (spondylotic, n = 164) were believed to have normal L5-S1 articulations but with a lytic lesion in the pars interarticularis that allowed L5 to slip forward onto S1. Patients in group III (traumatic, n = 3) also were believed to have normal L5-S1 facet joints but like the spondylotic group had a fracture of the pars interarticularis. The patients in group IV (n = 80) were classified as degenerative. The authors believed that arthritic changes in the L5-S1 joint

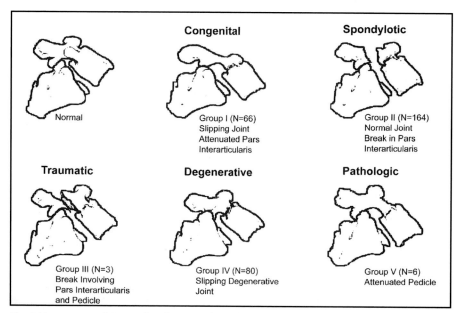

Fig. 1 Newsman and Stone classification of spondylolisthesis in 319 patients. (Reproduced with permission from Newman PH, Stone KH: The etiology of spondylolisthesis. *J Bone Joint Surg Br* 1963;45:39-59.)

Table 1
Classification of Spondylolisthesis by Wiltse and Associates[12]

Type	Description
I	Congenital (dysplastic)
II	Isthmic—defect in the pars interarticularis
IIA	Spondylolytic—stress fracture of the pars region
IIB	Pars elongation
IIC	Acute pars traumatic fracture
III	Degenerative—resulting from long-standing intersegmental instability
IV	Posttraumatic—acute fractures in the posterior elements beside the pars region
V	Pathologic—destruction of the posterior elements from generalized or localized bone pathology

(Adapted with permission from Wiltse LL, Newman PH, Macnab I: Classification of spondylolysis and spondylolisthesis. *Clin Orthop* 1976;117:23-29.)

allowed slippage of the degenerative facet joint and, therefore, a spondylolisthesis of L5 on S1. The patients in group V (n = 6) were termed pathologic; their L5-S1 spondylolisthesis was believed to be the result of an attenuated pedicle. Wiltse and associates[12-14] later refined and reorganized Newman and Stone's classification (Table 1).

In 1982, Marchetti and Bartolozzi[15] proposed a new classification (Table 2) that relied on primarily developmental components rather than observed anatomic pathology. The initial version of their classification divided all spondylolisthesis into either developmental or acquired pathology. Developmental pathology included lytic lesions, spondylolisthesis caused by elongation of the pars interarticularis, and spondylolisthesis secondary to traumatic events such as acute fractures or stress fractures. The acquired group consisted of iatrogenic, pathologic, and degenerative conditions. Marchetti and Bartolozzi[16] later refined their classification to include high and low dysplastic groups within the developmental category. Each of these groups could have interarticular lysis or elongation of the pars interarticularis. The acquired group was expanded to include traumatic, postsurgical, pathologic, and degenerative conditions.

The other two classification systems rely on the radiographic appearance of the anatomy to classify the spondylolisthesis, making no attempt at being predictive. Marchetti and Bartolozzi, however, stress the importance of the developmental aspect of the pathology, highlighting dysplasia of the posterior elements as a significant factor in the development and progression of spondylolisthesis. This is the first classification that suggests a possible etiology and provides a predictive quality.

The remainder of this chapter will deal with spondylolisthesis classified by Wiltse and associates as type II: isthmic spondylolytic spondylolisthesis (IIA), isthmic pars defects (IIC), and posttraumatic spondylolisthesis (type IV). The corresponding groups in Marchetti and Bartolozzi's classification are low dysplastic spondylolisthesis with lysis, traumatic, and postsurgical spondylolisthesis.

Prevalence
Although it was once suggested that the spondylolytic defect might be congenital, no newborn or neonatal specimens have ever been identified with a true spondylolysis. In fact, the pathology seems to be rare in patients younger than 5 years. In Stewart's[17] review of spondylolisthesis, he identified the pathology in only 3% to 4% of his population younger than 6 years. In patients between ages 6 and 18 years, the incidence was 4.4%, whereas in patients older than 18 years, a 6% incidence was identified. Stewart showed that by age 40 years, the incidence had

stabilized between 10% and 33%. Virta and associates[18] identified a 2:1 occurrence in males versus females. In their review of 1,100 individuals in Finland ranging in age from 45 to 64 years, Virta and associates reported a 7% incidence of spondylolisthesis in a population of individuals who had radiographic evaluation because of back pain.

The prevalence of spondylolisthesis appears to be influenced by the racial or genetic background of the population studied. African-Americans have the lowest rate of spondylolisthesis at 1.8%, and the Inuit Eskimos may have a prevalence rate of 50%.[12,17] South Africans and Caucasians fall in an intermediate range, with 3.5%[20] and 5.6%,[12] respectively. Spondylolisthesis is also found two to five times more frequently in patients with low back pain. Patients with symptomatic low back pain have a spondylolisthesis rate of 5.3% to 11%, while asymptomatic patients may have a rate of occult spondylolisthesis of 2.2%.[17]

Lytic spondylolisthesis also occurs more frequently at certain spinal levels identified at L5 in 87% of patients, L4 in 10%, and L3 in 3%.[19,20] There is also an increasing prevalence of spondylolisthesis in active sports enthusiasts. Gymnasts have long been identified as an at-risk group for development of spondylolisthesis. Jackson and associates[21] noted an 11% incidence of bilateral pars defects in 100 female gymnasts. An even higher rate of spondylolysis or spondylolisthesis has been identified in a similar population of Oriental female gymnasts. Other sports involving chronic repetitive hyperextension, including football and rugby, also have been implicated in the development of spondylolysis. Other less obvious sports implicated in the development of spondylolisthesis include pole vaulting and volleyball.[13,22-24] Generally, the course of this pathology is relatively benign.[25]

Etiology

The etiology of this deformity/pathology

remains unclear. A truly congenital etiology seems unlikely because no evidence exists for the presence of the lytic defect in the newborn. Work by Vaz and associates,[8] Legaye and associates,[10] and Labelle's presentation at the Scoliosis Research Society Annual Meeting suggest that the intrinsic architecture of the pelvis may be an important parameter, modulating the mechanical stresses experienced by the lumbosacral junction. This finding, along with the increased prevalence of spondylolysis and spondylolisthesis among athletes in certain sports, suggests a mechanical etiology.[11,23,24,26-28] The trauma sustained to the low lumbar spine during the hyperextension activities involved in many of these sports has been implicated in the development of spondylolisthesis. Several authors[24,29-32] have postulated that the underlying pathomechanical event in the development of a lytic spondylolisthesis is a fracture.[33] This may be either an acute event or secondary to fatigue during repetitive stress.[34]

Biomechanical studies have suggested that the pars interarticularis is the weakest part of the posterior neural arch.[21,30-32] During flexion and extension, the pars interarticularis is cycled through alternating compressive and tensile loads. During extension, the pars experiences posterior compressive forces and anterior tensile forces (Fig. 2). Krenz and Troup[35] have suggested that because the pars is primarily of cortical bone,[36] its ability to resist the compressive and tensile forces during flexion and extension is related to the thickness of the bone. Although the ultimate strength is undoubtedly high, as evidenced by the generally low prevalence of spondylolisthesis in the population, Hutton and associates[32,37] have suggested that fatigue fractures can be precipitated during biomechanical testing. Using 507 N of force at 100 cycles per minute, pars fractures could be created with as few as 1,500 cycles. Other specimens were able to tolerate 54,000 cycles before developing a fracture.

Once the pars defect has been creat-

1982 Group	Pathology	1994 Type	Form	Condition
Developmental		Developmental		
	Lysis		High dysplastic	Interarticular lysis
	Elongation of the pars interarticularis			Elongation of the pars interarticularis
	Traumatic		Low dysplastic	Interarticular lysis
	Acute fracture			Elongation of the
	Stress fracture			pars interarticularis
Acquired		Acquired		
	Iatrogenic		Traumatic	Acute fracture
	Pathologic			Stress fracture
	Degenerative		Postsurgical	Direct surgery
				Indirect surgery
			Pathologic	Local pathology
				Systemic pathology
			Degenerative	Primary
				Secondary

Table 2
Classification of Spondylolisthesis by Marchetti and Bartolozzi[16]

(Adapted with permission from Marchetti PC, Bartolozzi P: Classification of spondylolisthesis as a guideline for treatment, in Bridwell KH, DeWald RL, Hammerberg KW, et al (eds): *The Textbook of Spinal Surgery*, ed 2. Philadelphia, PA. Lippincott-Raven, 1997, vol 2, pp 1211-1254.)

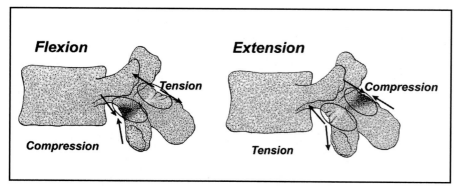

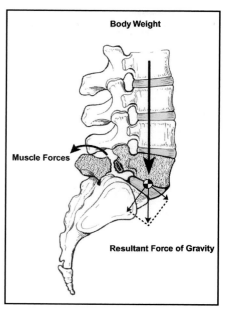

Fig. 2 Compressive and tensile forces experienced in the region of the pars interarticularis during flexion and extension. (Reproduced with permission from Marchetti PC, Bartolozzi P: Classification of spondylolisthesis as a guideline for treatment, in Bridwell KH, DeWald RL, Hammerberg, et al (eds): *The Textbook of Spinal Surgery*, ed 2. Philadelphia, PA, Lippincott-Raven, 1997, pp 1211-1254.)

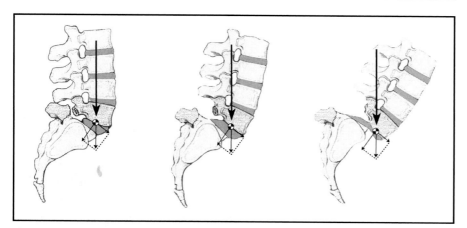

Fig. 4 The alteration in pathomechanics as a spondylolysis proceeds from a low-grade to a high-grade spondylolisthesis. (Adapted with permission from Marchetti PC, Bartolozzi P: Classification of spondylolisthesis as a guideline for treatment, in Bridwell KH, DeWald RL, Hammerberg, et al (eds): *Textbook of Spinal Surgery*, ed 2. Philadelphia, PA, Lippincott-Raven, 1997, pp 1211-1254.)

Fig. 3 Forces affecting distraction of the spondylolytic defect at L5. (Reproduced with permission from Marchetti PC, Bartolozzi P: Classification of spondylolisthesis as a guideline for treatment, in Bridwell KH, DeWald RL, Hammerberg, et al (eds): *The Textbook of Spinal Surgery*, ed 2. Philadelphia, PA, Lippincott-Raven, 1997, pp 1211-1254.)

ed, anatomic and biomechanical forces conspire to prevent healing of the fracture and create a spondylolisthesis. Shear forces created by the center of gravity tend to cause anterior displacement of L5 on the sacrum (Fig. 3) while posterior muscular forces tend to extend the posterior elements, thus opening the spondylolysis. This motion tends to distract the fracture site, preventing spontaneous healing. These initial events tend to precipitate a cascade of worsening biomechanics as the center of gravity moves progressively anterior, causing the resultant vector to increase the shear forces across the lumbosacral junction (Fig. 4). The worsening biomechanical scenario may be exacerbated by a low intercristal line and small transverse process of L5, which may provide less muscular and ligamentous connections to the pelvis that could assist in restraining the forward slippage of L5 on S1.

Although mechanical considerations probably are the most significant in the development of lytic spondylolisthesis, genetic considerations have been discussed by some authors.[38] Wynne-Davies and Scott[39] have suggested an autosomal dominant genetic predisposition with reduced penetrance that may be multifactorial. Wiltse[28] on the other hand, suggested that a cartilaginous defect in a vertebral model may be an autosomal recessive characteristic with varying expressivity.

The mechanical or underlying genetic components involved in the etiology of spondylolysis and spondylolisthesis may be exacerbated by anatomic considerations that could be important in the development of spondylolisthesis. The human bipedal gait causes L5 to be precariously balanced on the sacrum. In the best scenario, the anterior and posterior opposing forces are neutralized so that L5 remains stably placed on the sacrum in spite of its inclined position. However, unbalancing of these forces may precipitate a spondylolisthesis. Posterior elements

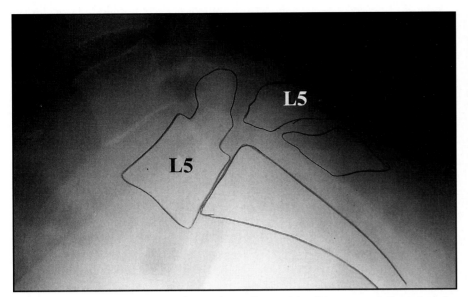

Fig. 5 A grade I spondylolisthesis with complete collapse of the disk space and distraction of the spondylolytic defect at L5.

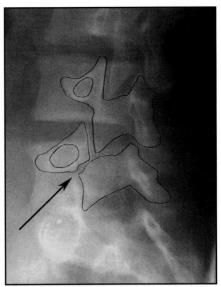

Fig. 6 An oblique view of the lumbar spine showing the collar of the scottish terrier (Scottie dog).

already compromised by spina bifida or dysplastic lumbosacral facet joints may not withstand even normal daily activities for the life of a patient. A high-riding L5 vertebral body with short transverse processes may be insufficiently protected because it has fewer ligamentous attachments to the pelvis and therefore may be at risk for the development of L5 spondylolisthesis. Undoubtedly, the etiology for spondylolisthesis is multifactorial; however, at this time, mechanical forces are highly implicated in both the development of lytic pars interarticularis defects and the resulting spondylolisthesis.

Imaging

All the imaging modalities are important for complete definition of the three-dimensional pathoanatomy in spondylolysis and spondylolisthesis.[40] Each modality contributes a unique view of the various aspects of the pathology. Plain radiographs are typically obtained first. These films must be obtained with the patient in an upright standing position. Supine films may not show subtle instability. A complete plain radiographic investigation of a potential pars interarticularis defect

or spondylolisthesis includes AP, lateral, right and left oblique, Ferguson AP, and possibly flexion-extension lateral views to identify instability. In addition, long cassette (scoliosis) AP and lateral radiographs may be useful to document overall coronal alignment if a significant spondylolisthesis or segmental instability is present.

Each of these radiographic views is useful in identifying certain aspects of the pathology. The AP projection may show spina bifida occulta,[41] pars defects, or dysplastic posterior elements. Lateral views often allow identification of a pars defect when spondylolisthesis is present (Fig. 5) and even when there is no spondylolisthesis. Oblique (scottie dog) views often will define the pars defect more clearly (Fig. 6). The Ferguson AP provides an enface view of L5 that may improve the visualization of the transverse process and the sacrum and identify more clearly a high-riding L5 vertebral body. Flexion-extension views may uncover subtle instabilities not apparent on static standing views. Instability will certainly be overlooked if only supine views are obtained. Other important anatomic fea-

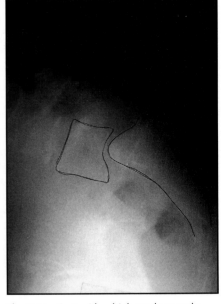

Fig. 7 A patient with a high-grade spondylolisthesis (III-IV) with remodeling of both the anterior lip of the sacrum and the inferior surface of L5. In flexion-extension radiographs, this patient also shows a high degree of mobility of this unstable spondylolisthesis.

tures that can be identified on plain radiographs are rounding off of the sacrum, wedging or erosion of L5 in high-grade

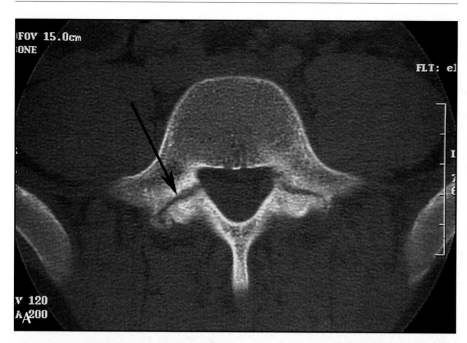

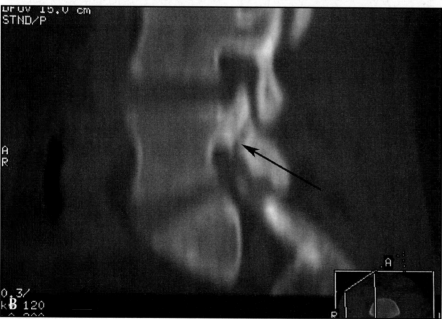

Fig. 8 Axial and sagittal-reconstructed CT views of the lytic spondylolysis (*arrows*).

tinuous scale of 0 to 20 to be applied to each spondylolisthesis.[11,46,47]

CT scans are useful to clearly identify the bony architecture of the posterior elements.[48] They can clearly define pars defects even when no spondylolisthesis is present (Fig. 8). They allow excellent definition of complex anatomy in both the axial and the coronal and sagittal planes when reformatted images are obtained. When combined with myelography, they may give excellent definition to subtle neurologic compression within complex osseous deformities. On CT scan axial images, the spondylolytic defect is typically identified as a linear lesion with sclerotic bone and hypertrophic osteophytes in the vicinity of the lesion. The osteophytes are typically identified at or immediately adjacent to the axial image containing the pedicles of that vertebral body.

Plain myelograms may be obtained at the time a CT myelogram is ordered. Plain myelography is useful in identifying the longitudinal effect of either the spondylolisthesis or the intercanal compromise secondary to hypertrophic bone and cicatrix formed as a result of the instability. MRI is excellent for evaluating the soft-tissue component of the spondylolisthesis[49,50] and can also help define the degenerative changes associated with the instability. The ability of MRI to differentiate and clearly distinguish the neural elements from the surrounding soft tissue and osseous elements is excellent, but the definition may not be as precise as that of CT myelography. However, this small drawback is offset by the fact that MRI studies do not involve ionizing radiation, myelographic dye that could precipitate an anaphylactic reaction, or invasive techniques. MRI studies can be used to identify both central and foraminal stenosis and provide a good view of the degree of neural compression. A consistent finding on MRI scans is a large, bulging disk at the level of the spondylolisthesis, trapping the exiting nerve root

spondylolisthesis (Fig. 7), flexion at the S1-2 disk, or bending of the sacrum.[42] In addition, the plain radiographs will be used to grade the degree of the deformity using either the Meyerding, Boxall, or modified Newman technique classification.[43-45] A limitation of the Meyerding classification is its inability to describe the important rotational component in the sagittal plane of the subluxating vertebral body. The modified Newman classification takes this into account. In this classification system, measurements are taken of both the anterior displacement and the vertical/downward displacement of the vertebral body in relation to the sacrum. Although somewhat tedious, this classification allows a con-

between the bulging anulus fibrosus and the pedicle of the involved level (Fig. 9). Moreover, the MRI scan can show the degree of encroachment on the neural elements by exuberant hypertrophic scar tissue caused by the unhealed spondylolytic defect (Fig. 10). The involvement of adjacent disks can also be discerned by reviewing the MRI scan. Often, in spite of a relatively normal-appearing plain radiograph or CT scan, the MRI scan of adjacent disks may show evidence of premature degeneration. The significance of or the etiologic cause for degeneration of these adjacent disks is difficult to ascertain. It is believed that abnormal biomechanics at the affected level may induce increased biomechanical stress at adjacent levels, which may precipitate degenerative disk disease at an accelerated rate. MRI and CT are also useful in identifying facet joint hypertrophy and facet joint degeneration at the level of the slip and adjacent levels. Together, these three imaging techniques can provide an excellent description of pathologic anatomy and its effect on the adjacent levels.

Additional tests that may be helpful in deciding on the treatment of spondylolisthesis are bone scans, diskography, and pars interarticularis injections. Bone scans provide information about the possible reparative ability of the lytic defect. An intensely hot single-photon emission computed tomography (SPECT) scan may suggest that the lytic defect is of recent origin and could benefit from a period of immobilization or, failing this, osteosynthesis. A cold SPECT scan, on the other hand, may imply that a lytic defect is longstanding and inactive. These defects are not likely to be amenable to nonsurgical treatment if they are symptomatic. Symptomatic lytic lesions of the pars that respond to local anesthetic injections may be amenable to fusion or repair.[46]

Although it is not used uniformly by spine surgeons, diskography may be use-

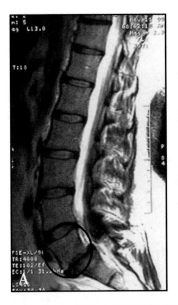
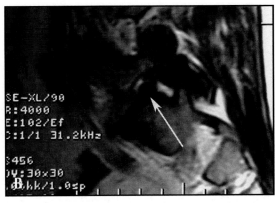

Fig. 9 Neural foraminal entrapment of an L5 nerve root caused by bulging disk and subluxated pedicle of L5.

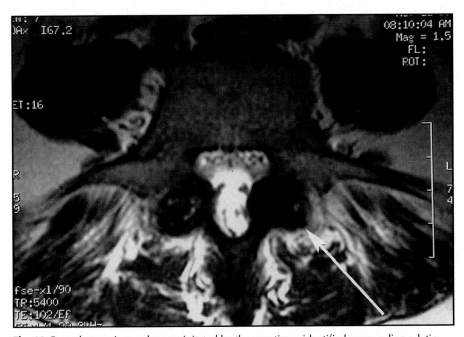

Fig. 10 Central stenosis may be precipitated by the scar tissue identified surrounding a lytic pars defect.

ful when considering surgical intervention. When pars repair is contemplated and the health of the involved disk is not certain, diskography may provide useful information about the functional quality of that disk. If a segmental fusion is required because of severe disk degeneration at the level of a pars defect and degenerative changes at the adjacent level

are evident on the MRI scan, diskography may be helpful in deciding whether a fusion of the slip level alone or inclusion of its degenerative neighbor is necessary to treat the patient's symptoms.

Several radiographic parameters have been used to grade the degree of spondylolisthesis. The Meyerding classification,[43] which grades spondylolisthesis

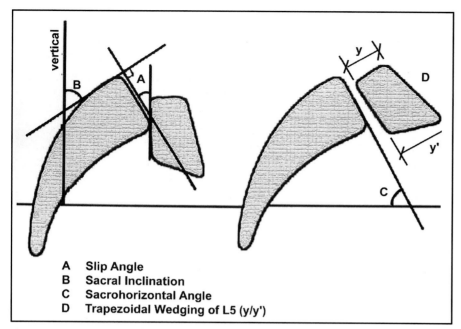

A   **Slip Angle**
B   **Sacral Inclination**
C   **Sacrohorizontal Angle**
D   **Trapezoidal Wedging of L5 (y/y')**

Fig. 11 Radiographic parameters for angular measurements in the description of spondylolisthesis. (Reproduced with permission from Lenke LG, Bridwell KH: Adult spondylolisthesis with lysis, in Bridwell KH, DeWald RL (eds): *The Textbook of Spinal Surgery*, ed 2. Philadelphia, PA, Lippincott-Raven, 1997, pp 1269-1298.)

from grade 0 (spondylolysis) through grades I, II, III, and IV (spondylolisthesis), is probably the most functional and widely used technique. Boxall and associates'[44] percentage slip is more specific but requires more precise measurement. Other important parameters used to describe spondylolisthesis, particularly in the higher grades, are slip angle, sacral inclination, and sacrohorizontal angle (Fig. 11). In addition, with high-grade slips, the wedging of the vertebral body is important for defining the degree of adaptive changes undergone by the slipping vertebral body. Defining vertebral wedging involves rostral to caudal measurements of the anterior versus the posterior vertebral body.

Clinical Presentation

Symptoms of spondylolisthesis typically are reported as back pain and/or neurologic symptoms. Although radiographic investigations are important to define the anatomy, treatment is based on history,

physical examination, and the patient's symptoms. The neurologic symptoms that accompany spondylolisthesis are typically unilateral or bilateral radiculopathy and may be intermittent or chronic. In high-grade slips with significant degenerative disease, the resulting neuroforaminal compression may cause chronic radiculopathy. However, even mild slips with significant hypermobility may be accompanied by radiculopathy. Radiculopathy may be provoked by chronic compression from severely collapsed neuroforaminal spaces or may be secondary to traction by osteophytic spurs provoked by hypermobility. A significant component of the neuroforaminal compression may result from the fibrocartilaginous scar that forms around the lytic defect posteriorly. Anteriorly, annular bulging resulting from the vertical collapse of the disk space and the anterior translation of the L5 vertebral body may cause a significant disk bulge that compresses the nerve root against the under-

surface of the adjacent pedicle (Fig. 10). Although the radiculopathy is usually caused by either central or neuroforaminal stenosis at the level adjacent to the lytic defect, more proximal spondylolisthesis may cause compression of traversing nerve roots, clinically suggesting a more distal nerve root irritation when the osseous defect and instability may be more proximal. For this reason, careful review of the radiographic studies and the clinical history and physical examination are important. Because of the predominance of spondylolysis and spondylolisthesis at L4 and L5, the nerve roots most typically involved are L5 and S1, followed by L4. However, the presence of radiculopathy in a radiographically documented spondylolysis should not cause the clinician to exclude other possible etiologies such as disk herniation, especially far lateral disk herniation.

In those patients who have central stenosis with or without neuroforaminal narrowing and in older patients with long-standing spondylolisthesis, neurogenic claudication is sometimes the presenting neurologic symptom. This is also common in patients with larger slips or slips that are hypermobile and worsen from standing. The neuroforaminal narrowing centrally may be exacerbated by severely degenerated disks. Although uncommon, patients with severe high-grade stenosis and hypermobile spondylolisthesis may have intermittent or acute cauda equina syndrome.

Although back pain is often a presenting symptom in spondylolisthesis, many spondylolytic defects are identified incidentally. Spondylolisthesis incidentally discovered in adults during screening for low back pain after trauma is typically a stable, chronic entity and not the result of the trauma.[51] There is little, if any, risk of a catastrophic structural instability that could result in either segmental structural damage or neurologic sequela. As a result, restrictions other than those needed for pain relief are typically unnecessary. Mild to moderate spondylolisthesis does not necessarily predispose the adult to low back pain. In spite of this, Libson and associates[52] have documented the chance of discovering a spondylolytic defect in symptomatic low back pain patients to be twice that of asymptomatic patients. Wiltse and Rothman[14] identified 11% of 1,124 patients undergoing lumbosacral radiographic examination for back pain as having either unilateral or bilateral pars defects.

There are many possible causes for low back pain that must be distinguished from pain secondary to a spondylolisthesis. The most common of these unrelated causes is muscle strain. The spondylolisthesis that is identified on plain radiographs during an evaluation for low back pain in an adult has usually been present for many years. However, the acute onset of low back pain in a pediatric or adolescent patient may represent an acute injury or fracture. The simple presence of a spondylolisthesis should not be presumed to be the cause of the patient's symptoms when muscular strain could have triggered the pain.[53] When a spondylolisthesis is discovered after a motor vehicle accident or lifting injury, it is often blamed for the patient's symptoms. Degenerative disk disease at, above, or below the slip level may be the cause of the patient's pain because of nuclear degeneration or annular injury. Muscular strain induced by poor sagittal alignment and poor muscular tone could also be the cause of a patient's low back pain. Although the pain may be related to hypermobility at the site of the listhetic segment, facet joint arthrosis may also be the instigator of low back pain. It is important to differentiate whether the pain is acute, chronic, or an acute exacerbation superimposed on a chronic condition. Progression of these low-grade slips is uncommon, and it will be difficult on first analysis to decide if the symptoms are a direct result of the spondylolysis or spondylolisthesis. Restrictions in activity

or physical therapy are unwarranted. Because radiculopathy is often the presenting complaint, aggressive treatment for the radiculopathy should be addressed along with managing the low back pain. Although low-grade slips and spondylolysis are probably not associated with increased incidence of low back pain, Saraste and associates[40,54] documented an elevated risk factor for back pain in patients with slippage greater than 25%. They also identified increased wedging of L5, early degenerative disk disease at L5-S1, and spondylolisthesis at L4-5 as increased risk factors for the development of back pain in the presence of spondylolisthesis.

Physical examination and patient history are essential in determining the etiology of the back pain or radiculopathy. The mere presence of a spondylolisthesis does not mean that it has caused the patient's symptoms. Important parameters in the physical examination include body habitus, coronal and sagittal alignment, and spinal mobility. Both static and dynamic examinations are important to elicit pertinent symptoms. Pain on flexion and extension may suggest hypermobility and the cause of mechanical pain. Likewise, the provocation of neurologic symptoms, particularly radiculopathy in a particular position, may also imply the presence of hypermobility. Neurologic symptoms that correlate the dermatome and myotome level with the level of stenosis or lytic instability is also corroborative of the contribution of the spondylolisthesis to the development of symptoms. Care should be taken to rule out vascular insufficiency of the lower extremities as the possible cause of pseudoneurologic symptoms in elderly patients.

The patient's history is also important. The location and duration of the symptoms and their association with various activities can be instrumental in connecting the radiographic pathology with the patient's symptoms. The patient's

exercise history and the quality and severity of pain provoked by that exercise should be noted. Discerning how much the patient is complaining of low back pain versus radiculopathy is important to assess the pertinence of the radiographics and to determine whether a nonsurgical or surgical treatment is indicated. The patient's overall health is a factor in evaluating the primary presenting symptoms and treatment options, as are specific issues such as smoking, previous surgery, previous low back pain, occupation, lifestyle, and expectations.

Treatment Options

Treatment options for symptomatic spondylolisthesis fall into two categories, nonsurgical and surgical. The nonsurgical options consist primarily of activity modification, bracing, physical therapy, and intervention in the form of medications or injections.[55] Activity modification may involve the institution of proper bending and lifting activities and development of aerobic activities. This should result in decreasing recumbent and sitting activities to facilitate a more appropriate body weight. Smoking cessation would help in decrease environmental physiologic stresses. Physical therapy activities may be active or passive. Although passive modalities may be useful in the initial periods, when acute pain is experienced, active physical therapy techniques are probably more important in the long run. Examples of passive techniques are hot and cold therapy, muscle massage, phonophoresis, ultrasound, immobilization, acupuncture, traction, and transcutaneous electrical nerve stimulation. These are useful in the early stages of symptomatic low back pain to facilitate patient involvement with active physical therapy programs. Active physical therapy includes spinal flexibility exercises and muscle strengthening, especially the abdominal and the lumbar hyperextension muscles. Pelvic stabilization techniques are also important. These

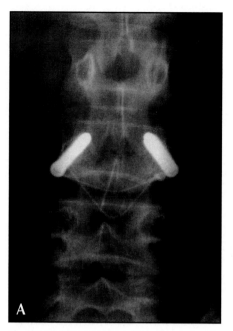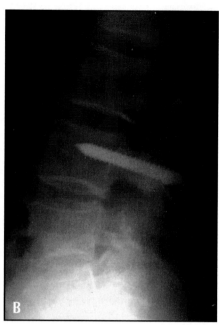

Fig. 12 AP **(A)** and lateral **(B)** radiographs of a spondylolysis treated with pedicle screws and transverse process/spinous process wiring.

may involve isometric and isokinetic exercises as well as aerobic conditioning. For those injured in the workplace, a work hardening program to specifically strengthen them against possible re-injury may be useful.

In the early phases of pain management, it may be necessary to rely on medications to some extent. Certainly non-steroidal anti-inflammatory drugs should be instituted early in the course of low back pain. Although the use of muscle relaxers and narcotics remains controversial, early liberal but temporary use of muscle relaxers and narcotics may significantly decrease the initial acute pain associated with specific injury. Long-acting, slow-release narcotics such as oxycodone may be useful in this regard, preventing the cycling from euphoria to pain often associated with the short-acting narcotics. The patient must be informed that the narcotics will not be prescribed beyond several weeks and their purpose is to facilitate the transition to physical therapy for managing the low back pain. Muscle relaxants may likewise be useful

in the early, acute period to deal with muscle spasms secondary to injury. Depending on the patient's symptoms and their severity, diagnostic and/or therapeutic injections are sometimes helpful to treat acute pain. More typically, injections will be used as a second line of treatment when the usual noninvasive approaches have failed or because symptoms have reached a plateau. Injections may include epidural steroids, selective nerve root blocks, pars injections, and facet joint injections. These may be administered for therapeutic as well as diagnostic reasons.

Surgical treatment options for symptomatic spondylolysis and spondylolisthesis include direct repair of the defect,[56,57] decompression, fusion, or a combination. Pars repairs are particularly useful in young adults who have pars defects—ideally a spondylolysis or no worse than a grade I slip, with no degenerative disk disease at the slip level. Patients best suited for this technique have a hot SPECT scan-documented lysis on CT scans and have not had suc-

cess with immobilization for treatment of their symptoms. Because of these restrictive criteria, this technique should be used cautiously in patients beyond the adolescent years.

Buck[58,59] described a translaminar screw osteosynthesis technique for direct repair in 1970. He reported on 16 patients; 15 were fused with the technique, and one required salvage with a posterolateral fusion because of failure of the pars repair. Pedersen and Hagen[60] reviewed 18 patients treated with Buck's technique and reported 83% satisfactory results. Like Buck, they recommend pars repair only in young patients with no degenerative disk disease. Bradford and Iza[61,62] presented a technique of transverse process wiring bilaterally to fix the loose posterior element and to facilitate pars interarticularis osteosynthesis. This technique has been modified with placement of pedicle screws as an anchor point for the wiring rather than the transverse processes (Fig. 12). Of the 21 (of 22) cases available for follow-up, 90% obtained solid fusion of the pars defect, and 80% had a good or excellent result. Bradford and Iza also believed the technique was best suited for patients younger than 30 years. Their presumption was that patients without degenerative disk disease do better.[62] Newer techniques include replacing the posterior wire with sublaminar hooks attached to short rods connected to the pedicle screws, allowing compressive osteosynthesis across the laminar defect (Fig. 13). Advocates of this technique suggest that improved immobilization may be achieved by allowing direct compression across the lytic defect with improved control of the loose posterior elements; the compressive effects of wires are less easily controlled.

Decompression alone or in combination with fusion may be necessary if radicular or neurogenic claudication symptoms are present. Decompression alone may be a useful technique in patients with spondylolysis or a low-grade (grade II or less) spondylolisthesis when the symptoms are primarily neurologic and there is little evidence of instability. This is a reasonable treatment for patients with little or no degenerative disease, disk space collapse, or instability. However, even in the face of presumed stability and no back pain, care must be taken to inform the patient that decompression in the face of a lytic defect or a low-grade spondylolisthesis may instigate low back pain by increasing instability. Intuitively, one would consider foraminotomies either unilaterally or bilaterally rather than a significant midline decompression in this case. In 1955, Gill and associates[63] reviewed 18 patients treated with complete removal of the loose posterior element (Gill laminectomy), reporting good results.[64] A long-term follow-up study of 43 patients published in 1965 revealed an increased slip in 14% of patients but a 90% satisfactory result in the group overall.[65] These results, however, are not universally documented. Osterman and associates[66] reported on 75 patients with long-term follow-up averaging 12 years. Although the initial results at 1-year follow-up showed 83% of patients to have fair, good, or excellent results, these results did not hold up over time. When these same patients were evaluated 5 years after surgery, satisfaction ratings had dropped to 75%, and the spondylolisthesis had progressed in 27% of patients. Marmor and Bechtol,[67] reported a patient who progressed from a grade II slip to a spondyloptosis after a Gill laminectomy. In a more dismal review on 33 patients with a 7-year follow-up, Amuso and associates[68] reported 36% poor results with Gill laminectomy. However, these authors did not identify any significant increase in progression of spondylolisthesis and believed there was no correlation between the progression of slip and poor results. With the currently available options for stabilization, Gill laminectomy alone is probably not a reasonable procedure. However, decom-

pression is often an important part of the surgical treatment of spondylolisthesis.

Decompression with fusion is the standard surgical technique for treatment of symptomatic spondylolisthesis. Fusion is necessary when instability and low back pain exist. Fusion is probably also reasonable when performing primarily decompressive surgery in patients whose main complaint is lower extremity radiculopathy and who have spondylolisthesis greater than grade II, especially in the presence of degenerative disk disease. The particular techniques used to establish stability and accomplish fusion are probably irrelevant, but they may include anterior and posterior procedures, either in combination or alone. Posterior procedures may involve posterior lumbar interbody fusions, transforaminal lumbar interbody fusions, or posterolateral fusions with instrumentation. Numerous studies extol the benefits of posterolateral uninstrumented fusions. In these historical studies, fusion rates have ranged from 67% to 96%, with outcomes ranging from 60% to 93%.[3,69-71] On the other hand, Schoenecker and associates[72] have reported significant neural complications following in situ fusion of high-grade slips. Recent studies by Bridwell and associates[73] highlight the benefit of instrumentation in achieving improved fusion rates and improved outcome. Other groups have reported high fusion rates (90% to 95%) and 90% excellent or good outcome with instrumented fusions for spondylolisthesis.[62,74]

Treatment options should also take into account the grade of the spondylolisthesis and the patient's age. For example, symptomatic spondylolysis in the pediatric and adolescent patient may be treated with immobilization only. For spondylolisthesis ≤ grade I in adolescents and perhaps young adults, pars repair is a reasonable option if the caveats previously mentioned are followed. In particular, the disk at the slip level should be lordotic and without degenerative changes. For

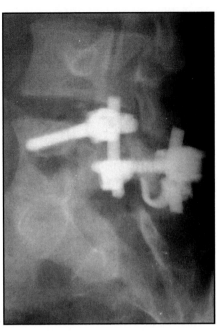

Fig. 13 An oblique radiograph showing the technique of treating a spondylolysis with pedicle screws and sublaminar claw along with autologous bone grafting to achieve osteosynthesis of a lytic defect in an adolescent male.

low-grade slips in patients requiring fusions, pedicle screw and rod constructs provide ample support, particularly when anterior interbody support is used. In the face of a mild or moderately degenerated disk without significant collapse, perhaps a posterolateral instrumented fusion alone will be sufficient if a wide decompression is not necessary and a large posterior surface area remains available for fusion. However, if an extensive decompression is required and an anterior interbody support is not provided, then fixation distal to S1 may be required. Anterior interbody support with fusion (anterior lumbar interbody fusion, transforaminal lumbar interbody fusion, posterior lumbar interbody fusion) may allow monosegmental fixation with a high degree of success. This has been advocated by Harms and associates[75] for many years. In older adults with spondylolisthesis ≤ grade I, decompression alone for treatment of primary radiculopathy may be appropriate. This may be effective treatment if there is no radiographic evidence of instability likely to progress to a higher grade of spondylolisthesis. Posterior instrumented fusions alone may be sufficient in these patients, especially if there is significant disk collapse at the slip level. This will result in less stress on the screw and rod constructs. In patients with either a large or hypermobile disk, however, anterior column support may be necessary for an effective reconstruction.

In young adolescents and adults with spondylolisthesis ≥ grade II, instrumentation and fusion in addition to decompression will likely be required. Anterior column support should be provided to ensure long-term stability of the construct and to allow for maximum correction of segmental sagittal alignment. This will protect adjacent levels. Depending on the overall sagittal alignment preoperatively and the degree of the slip, additional fixation above or below the slip level may be required. Because the majority of spondylolytic defects occur at L5, fixation to the ilium or the sacrum may be required to provide sufficient structural stability. In older patients or in those with many comorbidities with spondylolisthesis ≥ grade II, decompression alone for complaints of isolated radiculopathy may still be an option. Care must be taken to ensure that the spondylolisthesis is stable. A posterolateral instrumented fusion may be sufficient in those with collapsed disks, but in those with large or hypermobile disks or in patients with predisposing physiologic factors that may increase the possibility of pseudarthrosis, some sort of anterior column support and fusion is necessary, either through a formal anterior approach or one of the available posterior or posterolateral techniques.

Summary

Spondylolisthesis spans a diverse spectrum of osseous and neurologic pathology with a wide range of symptoms. The extremes range from the pediatric or adolescent patient with a symptomatic lysis requiring temporary external immobilization to spondyloptosis requiring resection of the entire L5 vertebral body with fusion and instrumentation to the pelvis. Even within the low-grade spondylolisthesis classification, there is a wide spectrum of presenting osseous and neurologic pathology. Many factors should be considered when developing an appropriate treatment plan.[71,76] Is the spondylolisthesis developmental or acquired? Does it have low or high dysplastic characteristics? Is there accompanying degenerative disease of the disk or the facets? What is the age and general health of the patient? What is the segmental alignment—lordotic or kyphotic? How does it relate to the center of gravity line? Is there evidence of anatomic remodeling or hypermobility? What are the patient's primary symptoms—low back pain, radiculopathy, or both? If nonsurgical treatment has failed, is the patient a reasonable candidate for surgical intervention? If surgery is to be performed, clear goals must be identified—relief of back pain, neurologic symptoms, or both. The surgeon should strive to fuse as few segments as possible while restoring segmental sagittal alignment and achieving a stable biomechanical construct to facilitate a good fusion environment. Ideally, anterior column support would be part of that biomechanical construct. Reduction as necessary to achieve good segmental sagittal balance should be attempted.

References

1. Nazarian S: Spondylolysis and spondylolytic spondylolisthesis: A review of current concepts on pathogenesis, history, clinical symptoms, imaging and therapeutic management. *Eur Spine J* 1992;1:62.

2. Jenkins JA: Spondylolisthesis. *Br J Surg* 1936;24:80-85.

3. Johnson LP, Nasca RJ, Dunham WK: Surgical management of isthmic spondylolisthesis. *Spine* 1988;13:93-97.

4. Lenke LG, Bridwell KH: Adult spondylolisthesis with lysis, in Bridwell KH, DeWald RL, Hammerberg KW, et al (eds): *The Textbook of Spinal Surgery*, ed 2. Philadelphia, PA, Lippincott-Raven, 1997, vol 2, pp 1269-1298.

5. Wiesel SW, Garfin SR, Boden SD: *Spondylolisthesis: Part I*. Philadelphia, PA, WB Saunders, 1993.

6. Wiesel SW, Garfin SR, Boden SD: *Spondylolisthesis: Part II*. Philadelphia, PA, WB Saunders, 1994.

7. Wright JG, Bell D: Lumbosacral joint angles in children. *J Pediatr Orthop* 1991;11:748-751.

8. Vaz G, Roussouly P, Berthonnaud E, Dimnet J: Sagittal morphology and balance of the spine and pelvis. *Eur Spine J* 2002;1:80-88.

9. Berthonnaud E, Roussouly P, Dimnet J: The parameters describing the shape and the equilibrium of the set back pelvis and femurs in sagittal view. *Innov Techn Biol Med* 1998;19:411-426.

10. Legaye J, Duval-Beaupere G, Hecquet J, Marty C: Pelvic incidence: A fundamental pelvic parameter for three-dimensional regulation of spinal sagittal curves. *Eur Spine J* 1998;7:99-103.

11. Newman PH, Stone KH: The etiology of spondylolisthesis: With a special investigation. *J Bone Joint Surg Br* 1963;45:39-59.

12. Wiltse LL, Newman PH, Macnab I: Classification of spondylolysis and spondylolisthesis. *Clin Orthop* 1976;117:23-29.

13. Wiltse LL, Rothman LG: Spondylolisthesis: Classification, diagnosis, and natural history. *Semin Spine Surg* 1989;1:78.

14. Wiltse LL, Rothman SLG: Spondylolisthesis: Classification, diagnosis, and natural history. *Semin Spine Surg* 1993;5:264-280.

15. Marchetti PG, Bartolozzi P: Spondylolisthesis, in Gaggi A (ed): *Modern Trends in Orthopaedic Surgery*. Bologna, Italy, 1982.

16. Marchetti PC, Bartolozzi P: Classification of spondylolisthesis as a guideline for treatment, in Bridwell KH, DeWald RL, Hammerberg KW, et al (eds): *The Textbook of Spinal Surgery*, ed 2. Philadelphia, PA. Lippincott-Raven, 1997, vol 2, pp 1211-1254.

17. Stewart TD: The age incidence of neural-arch defects in Alaskan natives, considered from the standpoint of etiology. *J Bone Joint Surg Am* 1953;35:937-950.

18. Virta L, Ronnemaa T, Osterman K, Aalto T, Laasko M: Prevalence of isthmic lumbar spondylolisthesis in middle-aged subjects from eastern and western Finland. *J Clin Epidemiol* 1992;45:917-922.

19. Rowe G, Roache M: Etiology of the separate neural arch. *J Bone Joint Surg Am* 1953;35:102.

20. Eisenstein S: Spondylolysis: A skeletal investigation of two population groups. *J Bone Joint Surg Br* 1978;60:488-494.

21. Jackson DW, Wiltse LL, Cirincoine RJ: Spondylolysis in the female gymnast. *Clin Orthop* 1976;117:68-73.

22. Monticelli G, Ascani E: Spondylolysis and spondylolisthesis. *Acta Orthop Scand* 1975;46:498-506.

23. Troup JD: Mechanical factors in spondylolisthesis and spondylolysis. *Clin Orthop* 1976;117: 59-67.

24. Wiltse LL, Widell EH Jr, Jackson DW: Fatigue fracture: The basic lesion in isthmic spondylolisthesis. *J Bone Joint Surg Am* 1975;57:17-22.

25. Fredrickson BE, Baker D, McHolick WJ, Yuan HA, Lubicky JP: The natural history of spondylolysis and spondylolisthesis. *J Bone Joint Surg Am* 1984;66:699-707.

26. Dietrich M, Kurowski P: The importance of mechanical factors in the etiology of spondylolysis: A model analysis of loads and stresses in human lumbar spine. *Spine* 1985;10:532-542.

27. Wiltse LL: Etiology of spondylolisthesis. *Clin Orthop* 1957;10:48-60.

28. Wiltse LL: The etiology of spondylolisthesis. *J Bone Joint Surg Am* 1962;44:539-560.

29. Chandler FA: Lesions of the isthmus (pars interarticularis) of the laminae of the lower lumbar vertebrae and their relation to spondylolisthesis. *Surg Gynecol Obstet* 1931;53:273-306.

30. Farfan HF, Osteria V, Lamy C: The mechanical etiology of spondylolysis and spondylolisthesis. *Clin Orthop* 1976;117:40-55.

31. Lafferty JF, Winter WG, Gambaro SA: Fatigue characteristics of posterior elements of vertebrae. *J Bone Joint Surg Am* 1977;59:154-158.

32. Hutton WC, Stott JR, Cyron BM: Is spondylolysis a fatigue fracture? *Spine* 1977;2:202-209.

33. O'Neill DB, Micheli LJ: Postoperative radiographic evidence for fatigue fracture as the etiology in spondylolysis. *Spine* 1989;14:1342-1355.

34. Pennell RG, Maurer AH, Bonakdarpour A: Stress injuries of the pars interarticularis: Radiologic classification and indications for scintigraphy. *AJR Am J Roentgenol* 1985;145: 763-766.

35. Krenz J, Troup JD: The structure of the pars interarticularis of the lower lumbar vertebrae and its relation to the etiology of spondylolysis: With a report of a healing fracture in the neural arch of a fourth lumbar vertebra. *J Bone Joint Surg Br* 1973;55:735-741.

36. Cyron BM, Hutton WC: Variations in the amount and distribution of cortical bone across the pars interarticularis of L5: A predisposing factor in spondylolysis? *Spine* 1979;4:163-167.

37. Hutton WC, Cyron BM: Spondylolysis: The role of the posterior elements in resisting the intervertebral compressive force. *Acta Orthop Scand* 1978;49:604-609.

38. Miki T, Tamura T, Senzoku F, Kotani H, Hara T, Masuda T: Congenital laminar defect of the upper lumbar spine associated with pars defect: A report of eleven cases. *Spine* 1991;16:353-355.

39. Wynne-Davies R, Scott JH: Inheritance and spondylolisthesis: A radiographic family survey. *J Bone Joint Surg Br* 1979;61:301-305.

40. Saraste H, Brostrom LA, Aparisi T: Prognostic radiographic aspects of spondylolisthesis. *Acta Radio Diagn* 1984;25:427-432.

41. Burkus JK: Unilateral spondylolysis associated with spina bifida occulta and nerve root compression. *Spine* 1990;15:555-559.

42. Antoniades SB, Hammerberg KW, DeWald RL: Sagittal plane configuration of the sacrum in spondylolisthesis. *Spine* 2000;25:1085-1091.

43. Meyerding HW: Spondylolisthesis. *Surg Gynecol Obstet* 1932;54:371-377.

44. Boxall D, Bradford DS, Winter RB, Moe JH: Management of severe spondylolisthesis in children and adolescents. *J Bone Joint Surg Am* 1979;61:479-495.

45. Bradford DS: Management of spondylolysis and spondylolisthesis. *Inst Course Lect* 1983;32: 151-162.

46. Suh PB, Esses SI, Kostuik JP: Repair of pars interarticularis defect: The prognostic value of pars infiltration. *Spine* 1991;16:(suppl 8): S445-S448.

47. Newman PH: A clinical syndrome associated with severe lumbo-sacral subluxation. *J Bone Joint Surg Br* 1965;47:472-481.

48. Grogan JP, Hemminghytt S, Williams AL, Carrera GF, Haughton VM: Spondylolysis studied with computed tomography. *Radiology* 1982;145:737-742.

49. Gibson MJ, Buckley J, Mawhinney R, Mulholland RC, Worthington BS: Magnetic resonance imaging and discography in the diagnosis of disc degeneration: A comparative study of 50 discs. *J Bone Joint Surg Br* 1986;68:369-373.

50. Szypryt EP, Twining P, Mulholland RC, Worthington BS: The prevalence of disc degeneration associated with neural arch defects of the lumbar spine assessed by magnetic resonance imaging. *Spine* 1989;14:977-981.

51. Floman Y, Margulies JY, Nyska M, Chisin R, Libergall M: Effect of major axial skeleton trauma on preexisting lumbosacral spondylolisthesis. *J Spinal Disord* 1991;4:353-358.

52. Libson E, Bloom RA, Dinari G: Symptomatic and asymptomatic spondylolysis and spondylolisthesis in young adults. *Int Orthop* 1982;6:259-261.

53. Virta L, Ronnemaa T: The association of mild-moderate isthmic lumbar spondylolisthesis and low back pain in middle-aged patients is weak and it only occurs in women. *Spine* 1993;18:1496-1503.

54. Saraste H: Long-term clinical and radiological follow-up of spondylolysis and spondylolisthesis. *J Pediatr Orthop* 1987;7:631-638.

55. Daniel JN, Polly DW Jr, Van Dam BE: A study of the efficacy of nonoperative treatment of presumed traumatic spondylolysis in a young patient population. *Mil Med* 1995;160:553-555.

56. Vathana P, Prasartritha T: A biomechanic study of the surgical repair technique of pars defect in spondylolysis. *J Med Assoc Thai* 1998;81:824-829.

57. Tonino A, van der Werf G: Direct repair of lumbar spondylolysis: 10-year follow-up of 12 previously reported cases. *Acta Orthop Scand* 1994;65:91-93.

58. Buck JE: Direct repair of the defect in spondylolisthesis: Preliminary report. *J Bone Joint Surg Br* 1970;52:432-437.

59. Buck JE: Abstract: Further thoughts on direct repair of the defect in spondylolysis. *J Bone Joint Surg Br* 1979;61:123.

60. Pedersen AK, Hagen R: Spondylolysis and spondylolisthesis: Treatment by internal fixation and bone-grafting of the defect. *J Bone Joint Surg Am* 1988;70:15-24.

61. Bradford DS: Treatment of severe spondylolisthesis: A combined approach for reduction and stabilization. *Spine* 1979;4:423-429.

62. Bradford DS, Iza J: Repair of the defect in spondylolysis or minimal degrees of spondylolisthesis by segmental wire fixation and bone grafting. *Spine* 1985;10:673-679.

63. Gill GG, Manning JG, White HL: Surgical treatment of spondylolisthesis without spine fusion: Excision of the loose lamina with decompression of the nerve roots. *J Bone Joint Surg Am* 1955;37:493-520.

64. Gill GG: Long-term follow-up evaluation of a few patients with spondylolisthesis treated by excision of the loose lamina with decompression of the nerve roots without spinal fusion. *Clin Orthop* 1984;182:215-219.

65. Gill GG, White HL: Surgical treatment of spondylolisthesis without spine fusion: A long-term follow-up of operated cases. *Acta Orthop Scand Suppl* 1965;85:5-99.

66. Osterman K, Lindholm TS, Laurent LE: Late results of removal of the loose posterior element (Gill's operation) in the treatment of lytic lumbar spondylolisthesis. *Clin Orthop* 1976;117: 121-128.

67. Marmor L, Bechtol CO: Spondylolisthesis: Complete slip following the Gill procedure: A case report. *J Bone Joint Surg Am* 1961;43: 1068-1069.

68. Amuso SJ, Neff RS, Coulson DB, Laing PG: The surgical treatment of spondylolisthesis by posterior element resection: A long-term follow-up study. *J Bone Joint Surg Am* 1970;52: 529-536.

69. Rombold C: Treatment of spondylolisthesis by posterolateral fusion, resection of the pars interarticularis, and prompt mobilization of the patient: An end-result study of seventy-three patients. *J Bone Joint Surg Am* 1966;48: 1282-1300.

70. Stauffer RN, Coventry MB: Anterior interbody lumbar spine fusion: Analysis of Mayo Clinic series. *J Bone Joint Surg Am* 1972;54:756-768.

71. Hanley EN Jr, Levy JA: Surgical treatment of isthmic lumbosacral spondylolisthesis: Analysis of variables influencing results. *Spine* 1989;14:48-50.

72. Schoenecker PL, Cole HO, Herring JA, Capelli AM, Bradford DS: Cauda equina syndrome after in situ arthrodesis for severe spondylolisthesis at the lumbosacral junction. *J Bone Joint Surg Am* 1990;72:369-377.

73. Bridwell KH, Sedgewick TA, O'Brien MF, Lenke LG, Baldus C: The role of fusion and instrumentation in the treatment of degenerative spondylolisthesis with spinal stenosis. *J Spinal Disord* 1993;6:461-472.

74. Ricciardi JE, Pflueger PC, Isaza JE, Whitecloud TS III: Transpedicular fixation for the treatment of isthmic spondylolisthesis in adults. *Spine* 1995;20:1917-1922.

75. Harms J, Jeszenszky D, Stoltze D, Böhm H: True spondylolisthesis reduction and monosegmental fusion in spondylolisthesis, in Bridwell KH, DeWald RL, Hammerberg KW, et al (eds): *The Textbook of Spinal Surgery*, ed 2. Philadelphia, PA, Lippincott-Raven, 1997, vol 2, pp 1337-1347.

76. Haraldsson S, Willner S: A comparative study of spondylolisthesis in operations on adolescents and adults. *Arch Orthop Trauma Surg* 1983;101:101-105.

Evaluation and Surgical Treatment of High-Grade Isthmic Dysplastic Spondylolisthesis

Lawrence G. Lenke, MD
Keith H. Bridwell, MD

Abstract

In children and young adults who seek medical treatment for high-grade isthmic dysplastic spondylolisthesis, common clinical symptoms are referable to the lumbosacral spine and/or the lower extremities. Pain in the lumbosacral spine may be secondary to altered lumbosacral alignment and biomechanics. It also may be caused by malalignment of the entire spinal-pelvic axis as a result of anterior sagittal imbalance. Lower extremity radiculopathies involving the L5 nerve root(s) may be present, and in severe forms of spondylolisthesis crisis, marked entrapment of the cauda equina at L5-S1 may occur.

High-grade isthmic dysplastic spondylolisthesis are treated surgically and should include appropriate central and foraminal decompressions at the L5-S1 level, followed by lumbosacral fusion. Partial reduction aiming at improving the slip angle (lumbosacral kyphosis) is more beneficial and provides less risk to the L5 nerve roots than complete reduction of the translational component of the slip. Solid anterior and posterior spinal fusion at L5-S1 appears to provide the best long-term results.

Spondylolisthesis, or the forward slippage of one particular segment of the spine onto the next lower segment, comes in many forms and levels of severity. When discussing the higher-grade forms (Meyerding translation grade III, IV, and V),[1] the traditional classification of Wiltse and Winter[2] does not always fully represent the pathoanatomy involved.

Patients with high-grade spondylolisthesis, especially those in the pediatric age range, invariably have a dysplastic component to their lumbosacral bony anatomy.[3-5] They also may or may not have actual defects of the pars interarticularis. The pars area may be stretched or elongated, with cracks developing later. The L5-S1 facet joints are almost universally dysplastic, as well as the posterior arch at L5 and, often, the proximal sacrum. Spina bifida occulta is a common finding.[4]

Marchetti and Bartolozzi[6] developed a classification system for spondylolisthesis that places the dysplastic form in a completely separate category. They further subdivided this category into low and high dysplastic forms that occur either with or without an intact pars interarticularis. Patients with high-grade dysplastic spondylolisthesis invariably have a high slip angle or high degree of lumbosacral kyphosis, which further alters the lumbosacral alignment and makes achievement of surgical success more challenging.

Radiographic Evaluation

The two most important radiographic parameters are the Meyerding grading of L5 translation on the sacrum and the slip angle.[1-3] Meyerding[1] divided the position of L5 on the sacrum into quarters (I through IV) with the high grade slips present in grades III, IV, and V. Grade V is unique in that it represents the position of L5 completely below the top of the sacrum, which is termed spondyloptosis. The slip angle, or measurement of lumbosacral kyphosis, is measured as perpendicular from the back edge of the sacrum to the angle subtended by a line drawn along the inferior or superior edge of the L5 vertebral end plate (Fig. 1). The normal slip angle in a patient without spondylolisthesis should be a lordotic value because the L5-S1 disk is normally in 20° to 25° of lordosis. However, with a high-grade spondylolisthesis, this number

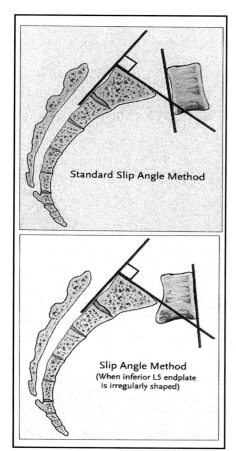

Fig. 1 Schematic representation of slip angle or kyphotic malalignment of the lumbosacral junction present in high-grade isthmic dysplastic spondylolisthesis.

is neutral or, more commonly, kyphotic. The degree of kyphosis may become quite large, representing a severe form of segmental kyphosis present at L5-S1.[4]

The standard radiographic series for evaluation of patients with a presumed or known high-grade isthmic spondylolisthesis includes a spot lateral view of the lumbosacral region that provides an optimal profile of the translational and angular measurements of L5-S1. In addition, a Ferguson coronal view should be obtained; this view is taken in an attempt to place the angle of the x-ray beam parallel with the L5-S1 disk. The profile of the L5 pedicles, transverse processes, and the sacral ala should be seen easily, and the surgeon should be able to note whether

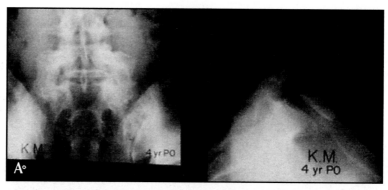

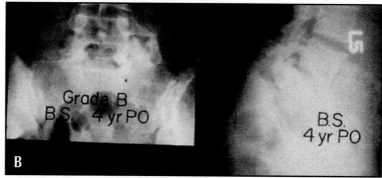

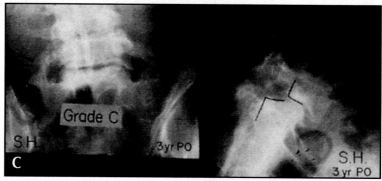

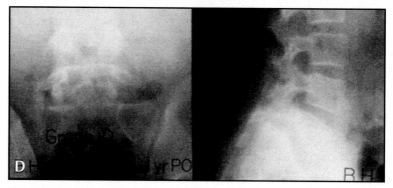

Fig. 2 The Ferguson coronal view provides a means of categorically analyzing the posterolateral fusion mass after fusion for spondylolisthesis. Fusions can be categorized into grade A, bilaterally, definitely solid (**A**); grade B, unilaterally solid with questionable fusion on the contralateral side (**B**); grade C, questionable solid fusion masses bilaterally (**C**); and grade D, definite pseudarthrosis bilaterally with possible graft resorption (**D**).

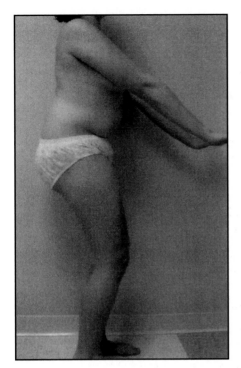

Fig. 3 The clinical deformity of a patient with high-grade isthmic dysplastic spondylolisthesis. Note the forward posture, prominent buttocks, and knee flexion present in this patient.

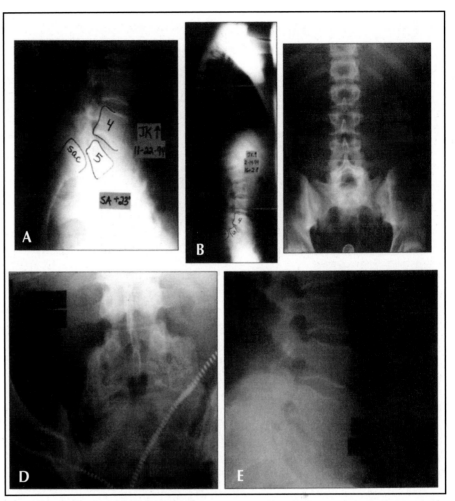

Fig. 4 A through **C,** Radiographs of a 16-year-old boy with a grade III isthmic dysplastic spondylolisthesis. Overall sagittal balance is good and L5 transverse processes are quite large. **D** and **E,** Radiographs show posterolateral fusion in situ at L4 to the sacrum with postoperative cast immobilization. At 5 years after surgery, grade A fusion bilaterally is solid with a stable slip. The patient has no clinical symptoms.

spina bifida occulta is present in the L5 segment and sacrum. The Ferguson view also has been reported to be a helpful way to determine the presence or absence of a solid lumbosacral fusion following surgical intervention[7,8] (Fig. 2).

To check the patient's overall coronal and sagittal balance, long cassette upright frontal and lateral radiographs should be obtained. The C7 plumb line should be evaluated with reference to the anterior and/or posterior edge of the sacrum. The degree of thoracolumbar and lumbar lordosis above the lumbosacral kyphotic segment should be noted because this lordosis is a common compensatory response. Any degree of associated scoliosis above the lumbosacral region should also be noted on the frontal view. This scoliosis may be secondary to a slippage that is somewhat angled in the frontal plane, or it may be an actual idiopathic scoliosis that may be associated with the spondy-

lolisthesis. In addition, patients with high-grade spondylolisthesis and nerve root tension may develop a sciatic scoliosis as a result of pressure on the lumbosacral cauda equina and/or nerve roots. A hyperextension view of the lumbosacral region with that area positioned over a bolster also will show any mobility in either the translational or sagittal rotational deformity. This mobility also can be noted on formal flexion-extension lateral radiographs taken with the patient in the supine position and showing the lumbosacral region.

A lumbosacral MRI study should be obtained on all patients being prepared for surgery in order to further define the lumbosacral alignment with the patient in a supine position. The health of disk spaces above L5 should be noted, especially that of L4-5.[8] This level often begins to degenerate in the second and third decades of life because of its proximity to the altered L5-S1 malalignment, which results in retrolisthetic forces on the L4-L5 segment. The MRI study also details the neuroanatomy quite well. Of the two most common findings, one will

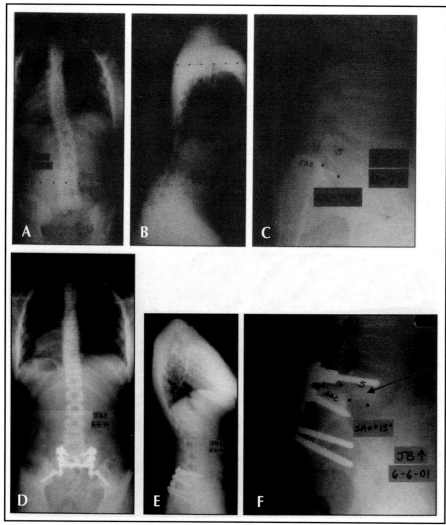

Fig. 5 Radiographs of a 12-year-old girl with a high-grade IV isthmic dysplastic spondylolisthesis. The patient has a small amount of sciatic scoliosis on the coronal view (**A** and **B**). Her sacrum is quite vertical on the sagittal radiograph (**C**), and she is positioned with her trunk anterior to her pelvis, demonstrating anterior sagittal imbalance. The patient underwent posterior decompression, partial reduction, sacral dome osteotomy, and posterolateral fusion with instrumentation from L5 to the sacrum. One week later, she underwent an anterior fibular dowel graft placement from L5 to the sacrum. Radiographs in **D** through **F** demonstrate the improved position of L5 on the sacrum and excellent alignment in her overall coronal (**D**) and sagittal (**E**) radiographs (**F**). The arrow points to the anterior edge of the fibular graft.

the facet dysplasia and possible central stenosis, especially when the arch at L5 remains intact and is being dragged forward into the canal.

Clinical Evaluation

In most patients who come to a spinal specialist with a high-grade spondylolisthesis,[5,10,11] low lumbosacral pain often is present but usually is not severe. This pain seems to correlate somewhat with the degree of postural malalignment that may be present from the overall spinal deformity. Specific areas of leg pain, numbness, and any bowel or bladder symptomatology, especially in those patients who have high-grade spondylolisthesis with central canal stenosis that can impinge on the cauda equina, should be noted.[5,10-13] It is fairly common for patients to have an L5 radiculopathy with posterior lateral thigh, anterior calf, and foot pain and/or numbness. Unilateral pain is more common than bilateral pain in our experience. The pain usually prevents athletic activity and is often the reason for initial evaluation.

Clinical examination focuses on the overall clinical deformity, postural alignment, spinal mobility, and neurologic examination. Patients with a high-grade spondylolisthesis often have a fairly marked clinical deformity involving a foreshortened trunk, a protruding abdomen, and a lower rib cage[4] (Fig. 3). They often flex their hips and knees in an attempt to counterbalance the forward position of the entire trunk on the pelvis. Patients have flattened buttocks and, occasionally, a scoliosis deformity caused by their altered spinal malalignment and tight spinal canal. Spinal mobility is usually restricted, and patients have marked limited flexion as well as severely limited extension of the spine. Patients invariably have tight hamstrings, which is a neurologic sign to their lower extremities. This is caused by tension on the L5 nerve roots by the slippage.[8] The straight-leg raising test is usually positive in these patients,

be central stenosis present at L5-S1, which usually is caused by a pincer effect from the posterior elements of L5, with an intact pars interarticularis being dragged forward into the spinal canal, thus narrowing it centrally. In addition, it is quite common to have L5 foraminal stenosis with high-grade dysplastic spondylolisthesis at L5-S1, which opti-

mally is evaluated by parasagittal MRI slices that can detail the foramina nicely.[9] This area is not evaluated very well on CT myelography because the nerve root sleeve does not extend into the foramen; thus, the myelographic dye is not present in that region. For those patients obtaining a CT myelogram, the axial view of the lumbosacral junction often displays

although the examiner must be sure that the trunk is not extended when a sitting straight-leg raise is performed. Gait often is altered, with hip and knee flexion posture continuing during forward gait.

A lower extremity neurologic examination should evaluate the motor, sensory, and reflex functions. The most common motor level involved will be L5, with weakness to the extensor hallucis longus as well as possibly to the anterior tibialis (ankle extensors) unilaterally and/or bilaterally. Dynamic assessment includes asking the patient to stand on tiptoe and back on the heels as well as ambulation. Sensory function is tested with a light touch over the L4, L5, and S1 dermatomes. In addition, patients with very high-grade spondylolisthesis, who are at risk for a cauda equina syndrome, should have sacral sensory testing as well as a rectal examination both preoperatively and postoperatively when sacral nerve root function is of concern. Lower extremity reflex function should not be altered in this condition, except for diminished ankle jerks. It is extremely important to get a good sense of motor function in the L5 distribution because this is the nerve root at highest risk for postoperative weakness and diminished function.[9]

Treatment Options

The treatment of high-grade isthmic dysplastic spondylolisthesis in the pediatric and young adult population is with surgery.[4,14-17] Even in those rare patients who are relatively asymptomatic with a grade III or more slip along with a fair degree of dysplasia to their lumbosacral region, surgical treatment is recommended. Many options for posterior treatment are available, including posterior in situ fusion with or without a decompression;[7,8,16,17] adding instrumentation to an in situ fusion;[8] posterior decompression, partial reduction, instrumentation, and fusion;[8,15,17] posterior decompression, complete reduction, instrumentation, and posterior fusion;[14,15,18,19] and for those

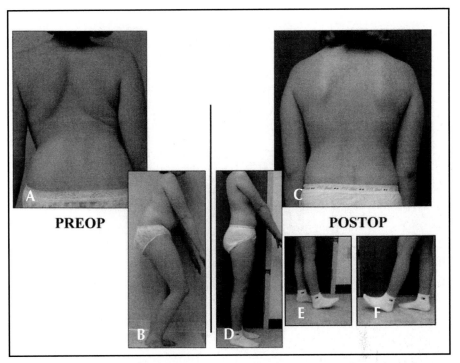

Fig. 6 Preoperative (**A** and **B**) and postoperative (**C** through **F**) clinical photographs of the patient whose radiographs are shown in Figure 5. Note the postoperative improvement in the coronal and sagittal alignment and also the excellent foot dorsiflexion function bilaterally.

patients with a true spondyloptosis, an L5 spondylolectomy with L4-sacrum fusion as popularized by Gaines[20,21] Additional posterior treatment options that can address the anterior spine include a posterior lumbar interbody fusion or a transforaminal interbody fusion using either nonstructural or structural bone graft or metallic cages. In addition, for higher-grade spondylolisthesis with a kyphotic slip angle, a posterior fibular dowel graft can be placed from posterior on the sacrum into the body of L5, through the L5-S1 disk as popularized by Smith and Bohlman.[22]

Various options for anterior treatment include anterior anulus and disk release in preparation for a posterior reduction. The technique of performing an anterior spinal fusion following a posterior reduction with either an intradiskal graft or structural cage is popular. However, the use of anterior instrumentation in the form of threaded screws compressing the bone graft is possible. For those patients with only a partial posterior reduction, sparing the L5 segment through the disk space into S1 with a fibular dowel graft is also an option for solidifying the anterior column.[23,24]

So how does a surgeon decide the approach for a specific patient with a high-grade isthmic dysplastic spondylolisthesis? The first step is to determine exactly how much reduction should be obtained. The risk of surgery, especially neurologic risk to the L5 root with subsequent dorsiflexion weakness or complete foot drop, is highest in those patients who undergo a more aggressive reduction procedure.[9,15] However, the pseudarthrosis risks are higher for patients who are left in a biomechanically unstable position with marked residual forward translation and, especially, angulation in the sagittal plane with a kyphotic slip angle[7,8] One attractive option appears to be a partial reduction aimed at improve-

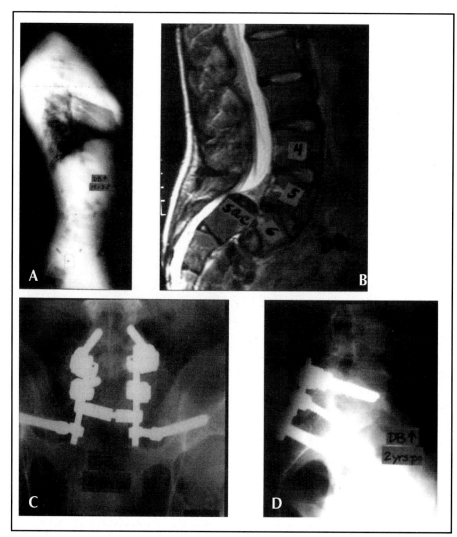

Fig. 7 **A** and **B,** Imaging studies of a teenager with a severe spondyloptosis of L6 on the sacrum. **C** and **D,** The patient underwent a L6 spondylolectomy and anterior and posterior spinal fusion with instrumentation placing L5 onto the sacrum. Radiographs at 2 years after surgery demonstrate a solid fusion between L5 and the sacrum, with near normal alignment.

ment of the slip angle, which will improve the biomechanics of the slipped segment while limiting the neurologic risk to the L5 nerve root. Postural reduction using a cast postoperatively is also an option for children, although its use seems to be declining with the advent of more versatile spinal instrumentation systems that can accommodate smaller children.[8] Each surgeon needs to form a risk/benefit ratio for each patient based on many factors, including patient presentation, the exact type of pathology, the

tolerance of the parents and the patient to accepting the risks associated with a partial reduction, and the subsequent risks of pseudarthrosis if less aggressive treatment is planned. In addition, the experience of the surgeon in these various techniques is also important in deciding the best approach.

In situ fusions with postoperative cast immobilizations were initially performed on patients with high-grade isthmic dysplastic spondylolisthesis[7] (Fig. 4); however, the pseudarthrosis rate approached

50%. Risk factors for pseudarthrosis with these in situ fusions included female gender with excessive L5-S1 mobility, a dysplastic lumbosacral region and small lumbar transverse processes, a markedly kyphotic slip angle, and signs of sacral root stretch and overall global anterior sagittal imbalance. In one group of in situ fusion patients, the size of the transverse processes in cm^2 was a statistically significant predictor of successful in situ fusion.[8] Patients with transverse process surface areas that averaged 3.59 cm^2 had successful fusions, whereas those with a surface area of only 1.59 cm^2 had pseudarthroses. A patient having only L5-S1 fusion had a higher pseudarthrosis risk than those patients having fusions from L4 to the sacrum. It is important to critically assess the fusion using a good quality Ferguson coronal view of the lumbosacral region[7] (Fig. 2).

The Authors' Preferred Treatment

Our current approach to patients with high-grade isthmic dysplastic spondylolisthesis with a kyphotic slip angle, with or without trunk imbalance, and signs of L5 and/or sacral nerve root impingement includes a wide decompression, posterior instrumentation with partial reduction, sacroplasty if required, and posteralateral fusion of L4 or L5 to the sacrum.[8] An anterior fusion by the posterior route is always planned; when adequate access cannot be obtained to the L5-S1 disk posteriorly, it is done by a formal anterior route on a different day.[23] Patients are positioned flexed at the hips and knees prior to the decompression. A Gill laminectomy and bilateral L5 and S1 nerve root decompressions are performed. It is extremely important to decompress the L5 nerve roots widely past the tips of the L5 transverse processes. Pedicle screws are placed at L5 and S1, and we also recommend an additional point of sacral pelvic fixation that includes bilateral distal iliac wing screws.[25] After placing mild distraction on the

L5-S1 segment, a sacroplasty may be performed to shorten the sacrum and decrease the stretch of the L5 nerve roots. Next, the patient is placed with the hips and knees in an extension that will secondarily flex the pelvis to meet the L5 segment. Rods are contoured, placed into the distal fixation (S1 and iliac screws), and flexed to meet the L5 segment. An attempt is made to gain access to the L5-S1 disk to place morcellized graft and/or structural cages if the reduction is such that the disk is accessible through the posterior route. The instrumentation is then locked in place. Intraoperative AP and lateral radiographs are carefully reviewed, and the patient undergoes a formal wake-up test to assess bilateral foot and ankle movement. Iliac crest bone graft already harvested proximal to the iliac screws is then placed over the decorticated transverse processes and sacral ala bilaterally (Figs. 5 and 6).

If formal anterior spinal fusion has not been performed, the patient usually will be brought back 5 to 7 days postoperatively for the procedure. Depending on the degree of reduction obtained, a formal diskectomy with structural grafts or metallic cages is used with the anterior iliac crest graft for the fusion. If the slip angle and translation correction have not been enough to allow access to the L5-S1 disk, then an allograft fibular graft is reamed over a Kirschner wire that is placed from the midportion of the L5 body through the L5-S1 disk and into the proximal sacrum.[23,24] The patient is placed in a single pantaloon brace and may begin ambulation soon after surgery depending on the security of fixation obtained.

Careful monitoring of the L5 nerve roots during these surgeries is of paramount importance. We have found that somatosensory-evoked potential monitoring, which is a mixed nerve assessment, often does not provide the best information regarding L5 nerve root function. In addition, spontaneous electromyograms have not been very helpful

in evaluating excessive L5 nerve root stretch or dysfunction noted postoperatively by toe/ankle dorsiflexion weakness. Thus, we have been using direct nerve stimulation as an attempt to carefully monitor the L5 nerve root before decompression, after decompression, and after reduction. We have found this to be the best way to keep a close eye on L5 nerve root function along with an intraoperative postinstrumentation and postreduction wake-up test to optimize foot and ankle dorsiflexion function postoperatively.

The results of these procedures at our institution have been reported by Molinari and associates,[8] who studied 60 patients with high-grade isthmic dysplastic spondylolisthesis treated by two attending spinal surgeons. Three groups were evaluated: posterior spinal fusion in situ (n = 15); posterior spinal fusion with instrumentation and postural reduction (n = 19); and posterior spinal fusion with instrumentation, partial reduction, and formal anterior spinal fusion (n = 26). The fusion rates in these three groups were 55%, 71%, and 98%, respectively. The patients with a solid fusion had the best clinical outcomes with respect to function, pain relief, and overall satisfaction with the procedure. All seven patients with pseudarthrosis following in situ fusion were revised with instrumented posterior spinal fusion and have undergone solid fusion. Three patients in the partial reduction group had temporary L5 neurapraxia. One patient had posterior migration of bilateral intrasacral rods with loss of reduction, and we have abandoned that technique for sacral pelvic fixation. Another patient had pseudarthrosis following circumferential fusion and required a revision fusion.

For those patients with a true spondyloptosis with the last vertebral segment sitting well below the top of the sacrum, the two best options appear to be in situ fusion with fibular dowel grafts placed either from posterior to anterior or vice versa[22] and a spondylolectomy or Gaines

procedure.[20,21] In this challenging procedure, the lowest vertebral segment is resected and the supra-adjacent segment is placed back onto the sacrum and held with posterior instrumentation and fusion (Fig. 7). This procedure should be done only by those surgeons who are experienced in the surgical treatment of patients with high-grade isthmic dysplastic spondylolisthesis.

Summary

Surgical treatment of patients with high-grade isthmic dysplastic spondylolisthesis is still somewhat controversial. Our surgical approach includes wide nerve root decompression, partial reduction with improvement of the slip angle, posterior instrumentation, and posterior as well as anterior fusion. This approach has proven to provide the best fusion rates and clinical outcomes with acceptable complication rates. Using sound surgical techniques and principles, a high degree of clinical success can be achieved in this patient population.

References

1. Meyerding HW: Spondylolisthesis. *Surg Gynecol Obstet* 1932;54:371-377.

2. Wiltse LL, Winter RB: Terminology and measurement of spondylolisthesis. *J Bone Joint Surg Am* 1983;65:768-772.

3. Boxall D, Bradford DS, Winter RB, Moe JH: Management of severe spondylolisthesis in children and adolescents. *J Bone Joint Surg Am* 1979;61:479-495.

4. DeWald RL, Faut MM, Taddonio RF, Neuwirth MG: Severe lumbosacral spondylolisthesis in adolescents and children: Reduction and staged circumferential fusion. *J Bone Joint Surg Am* 1981;63:619-626.

5. Muschik M, Zippel H, Perka C: Surgical management of severe spondylolisthesis in children and adolescents: Anterior fusion in situ versus anterior spondylodesis with posterior transpedicular instrumentation and reduction. *Spine* 1997;22:2036-2043.

6. Marchetti PG, Bartolozzi P: Classification of spondylolisthesis as a guideline for treatment, in Bridwell KH, DeWald RL, Hammerberg KW, et al (eds): *The Textbook of Spinal Surgery*, ed 2. Philadelphia, PA, Lippincott-Raven, 1997, vol 2, pp 1211-1254.

7. Lenke LG, Bridwell KH, Bullis D, Betz RR, Baldus C, Schoenecker PL: Results of in-situ fusion for isthmic spondylolisthesis. *J Spinal Disord* 1992;5:433-442.

8. Molinari RW, Bridwell KH, Lenke LG, Ungacta FF, Riew KD: Complications in the surgical treatment of pediatric high-grade, isthmic dysplastic spondylolisthesis: A comparison of three surgical approaches. *Spine* 1999;24:1701-1711.

9. Petraco DM, Spivak JM, Cappadona JG, Kummer FJ, Neuwirth MG: An anatomic evaluation of L5 nerve stretch in spondylolisthesis reduction. *Spine* 1996;21:1133-1139.

10. Freeman BL III, Donati NL: Spinal arthrodesis for severe spondylolisthesis in children and adolescents: A long-term follow-up study. *J Bone Joint Surg Am* 1989;71:594-598.

11. Harris IE, Weinstein SL: Long-term follow-up of patients with grade-III and IV spondylolisthesis: Treatment with and without posterior fusion. *J Bone Joint Surg Am* 1987;69:960-969.

12. Maurice HD, Morley TR: Cauda equina lesions following fusion in situ and decompressive laminectomy for severe spondylolisthesis: Four case reports. *Spine* 1989;14:214-216.

13. Schoenecker PL, Cole HO, Herring JA, Capelli AM, Bradford DS: Cauda equina syndrome after in situ arthrodesis for severe spondylolisthesis at the lumbosacral junction. *J Bone Joint Surg Am* 1990;72:369-377.

14. Dick WT, Schnebel B: Severe spondylolisthesis: Reduction and internal fixation. *Clin Orthop* 1988;232:70-79.

15. Hu SS, Bradford DS, Transfeldt EE, Cohen M: Reduction of high-grade spondylolisthesis using Edwards instrumentation. *Spine* 1996;21:367-371.

16. Johnson JR, Kirwan EO: The long-term results of fusion in situ for severe spondylolisthesis. *J Bone Joint Surg Br* 1983;65:43-46.

17. Poussa M, Schlenzka D, Seitsalo S, Ylikoski M, Hurri H, Osterman K: Surgical treatment of severe isthmic spondylolisthesis in adolescents: Reduction or fusion in situ. *Spine* 1993;18:894-901.

18. Ani N, Keppler L, Biscup RS, Steffee AD: Reduction of high-grade slips (grades III-V) with VSP instrumentation: Report of a series of 41 cases. *Spine* 1991;16(suppl 6):S302-S310.

19. Boos N, Marchesi D, Zuber K, Aebi M: Treatment of severe spondylolisthesis by reduction and pedicular fixation: A 4-6 year follow-up study. *Spine* 1993;18:1655-1661.

20. Gaines RW, Nichols WK: Treatment of spondyloptosis by two stage L5 vertebrectomy and reduction of L4 onto S1. *Spine* 1985;10:680-686.

21. Lehmer SM, Steffee AD, Gaines RW Jr: Treatment of L5-S1 spondyloptosis by staged L5 resection with reduction and fusion of L4 onto S1 (Gaines procedure). *Spine* 1994;19:1916-1925.

22. Smith MD, Bohlman HH: Spondylolisthesis treated by a single stage operation combining decompression with in situ posterolateral and anterior fusion: An analysis of eleven patients who had long-term follow-up. *J Bone Joint Surg Am* 1990;72:415-421.

23. Hanson DS, Bridwell KH, Rhee JM, Lenke LG: Dowel fibular strut grafts for high-grade dysplastic isthmic spondylolisthesis. *Spine* 2002;27:1982-1988.

24. Smith JA, Deviren V, Berven S, Kleinstueck F, Bradford DS: Clinical outcome of trans-sacral interbody fusion after partial reduction for high-grade L5-S1 spondylolisthesis. *Spine* 2001;26:2227-2234.

25. McCord DH, Cunningham BW, Shono Y, Myers JJ, McAfee PC: Biomechanical analysis of lumbosacral fixation. *Spine* 1992;17(suppl 8):S235-S243.

Adult Spinal Deformities

Adult Spinal Deformities

The articles in this section examine three controversial topics in the treatment of adult spinal deformities. In the first article, Dr. James Ogilvie describes the contributions of combined anterior and posterior spinal surgery to the treatment armamentarium. The articles by Dr. Keith Bridwell examine two common issues in adult scoliosis fusions: (1) at what distal level to stop the fusion; and (2) the importance of providing anterior structural support to the spine.

Dr. Ogilvie lists the most common indications for combined spinal fusion, including the following: (1) rigid coronal and/or sagittal deformities; (2) patients who require a long fusion (above L1) to the sacrum; (3) congenital or iatrogenic deficient posterior elements; and (4) patients with previous failed spinal deformity fusion requiring revision surgery. In addition, any condition that decreases the patient's healing potential, such as osteoporosis, chronic steroid usage, or diabetes mellitus, may be an additional indication to consider a circumferential procedure.

Once the decision has been made to use a circumferential approach, then the sequence and timing of the procedure must be carefully planned. An anterior-first approach has the advantage of releasing rigid spinal deformities in the coronal and sagittal planes, which increases the correction posteriorly. The anterior-first approach, however, also has a disadvantage. Unless secure instrumentation can be provided in the same setting, the spine is rather unstable, and the intervertebral grafts and/or cages may loosen or migrate during prone positioning of the patient or during posterior spinal reconstruction.

When a posterior-first approach is used, the spine is more stable than with the anterior-first approach. Thus, the patient can be mobilized between planned staged circumferential reconstructions. For rigid spinal deformities, the posterior procedure must optimize coronal and sagittal balance, which may be more difficult because the deformities will not have been released anteriorly. When treating pseudarthrosis of the spine, the posterior-first approach best documents the pseudarthritic levels prior to anterior augmentation to obtain a solid spinal fusion.

If a circumferential approach is technically feasible given the patient's condition and the abilities of the surgical team, then ideally both procedures should be performed on the same day. However, with difficult complex primary and revision spinal deformities, same-day surgery is impractical. Dr. Ogilvie emphasizes that surgeons should know their own limitations when attempting long, tedious spinal deformity reconstructions.

I follow a "12-hour rule," meaning that I stage procedures that cannot be finished within a 12-hour operative time. Occasionally, simultaneous anterior and posterior spinal surgery may be indicated, especially in the treatment of short-segment kyphotic deformities. This approach has advantages and disadvantages, particularly because it requires two skilled surgeons operating simultaneously. A true simultaneous operation also requires that the surgeon performing the posterior approach place segmental spinal instrumentation with the patient in the lateral decubitus position, which obviously is not the typical position for the patient during this procedure. The simultaneous operation has been used successfully at several centers with the infrastructure to operate in this manner.

The decision to use a circumferential approach, the planning of the procedures, and the techniques required to accomplish simultaneous operations are still the subject of controversy, with many factors affecting the decision-making process. Ultimately, it is the surgeon's responsibility to understand the relevant issues and apply sound clinical, biomechanical, and technical principles to surgical planning.

Dr. Bridwell's first article highlights his approach for selective fusion levels in adult patients with idiopathic scoliosis. He first presents compelling arguments for considering only those patients who are amenable to this technique. The curve patterns amenable to selective thoracic fusion in adults are similar to those in adolescents; the thoracic curve is larger and more structural both radiographically and clinically. The lumbar spine also must be free of marked degenerative changes, especially when assessing any causes of pain. Finally, the sagittal plane must be free of kyphosis at the thoracolumbar junction, as this would necessitate instrumentation and fusion covering both the thoracic and lumbar curves.

In older adults, selective fusion is much less tenable, normally because these patients often have advanced degenerative changes in the lumbar and lumbosacral spine. In these patients, the fusion must extend to either L4 or L5 or even to the sacrum. Obviously, the goal is to fuse as little of the spine as possible. However, it must be noted that if the lowest instrumented vertebra is not ideally positioned in an adult patient, significant distal transition syndromes may develop fairly rapidly postoperatively. Thus, the preoperative assessment must include evaluation of potential disk degeneration and both coronal and sagittal alignment of the lower lumbar spine when contemplating where to stop the fusion distally.

Characteristics compatible with stopping the fusion at L4 include an L4 segment that can horizontalized, centralized, and fairly neutral following the instrumentation and fusion. Also important are L4-L5 and L5-S1 segments that lack significant degeneration and have absolutely no coronal and/or sagittal subluxations or other malalignments. Optimizing coronal and especially sagittal alignment to L4 is important to maintain the long-term health of the distal unfused segments.

Very commonly, the L4-L5 segment will show evidence of significant degeneration with rotatory subluxations, sagittal subluxations, and/or stenosis that requires the instrumentation and fusion to be extended to L5. The difficulty with stopping the fusion at L5 is that the L5 pedicles are fairly patulous, and it is often difficult to secure an excellent grip on the L5 segment in a long fusion. Also, as Dr. Bridwell mentions, only one free motion segment will remain in this scenario, and significant radiographic breakdown of the L5-S1 segment can occur over time, even if it is normal preoperatively. The rate of distal transition syndrome seems to be higher with long fusions that extend from the upper thoracic spine to L5 in contrast to shorter fusions from the thoracolumbar junction to L5. In addition, the position of L5 in relation to the intercrestal line and the size of the L5 transverse processes, and thus the ilial lumbar ligaments, probably contribute to the overall stability and long-term health of the L5-S1 segment.

In many older patients, it will be impossible to stop the fusion at L5; the instrumentation and fusion will need to be extended to the sacrum. For long fusions to the sacrum, additional anterior structural support of L4-L5 and L5-S1 and additional sacropelvic fixation in the form of bilateral S1 and iliac wing screws seem to provide the most stable foundation. A longer fusion, however, requires significantly more time in surgery, and these patients are often older and at higher risk for medical and/or surgical complications. Optimal coronal and sagittal balance is critical to the clinical success of these surgeries.

Dr. Bridwell's second article discusses the role and use of anterior structural support in the treatment of various adult spinal deformities. Approximately 80% of the biomechanical force of the spine is transferred through the anterior and middle columns; therefore, the importance of anterior structural support, especially in the thoracolumbar junction and lumbar spine, has been stressed for the last decade because of the increased use of segmental pedicle screws.

For patients with fixed kyphotic deformities, anterior structural support can be provided by intradiscal bone grafts, either autogenous or allograft, or various types of cages. Optimal load sharing occurs not only with the use of anterior structural grafts or devices but also with the judicious use of posterior osteotomies to improve the anterior directed moment arm that exists in kyphotic malalignments of the spine. With posterior closing wedge osteotomies, the sagittal vertical axis of the spine can be

moved posteriorly to favorably affect the environment for posterior instrumentation alone, leading to a successful, solid spinal fusion. With long fusions using constructs that extend deep into the lumbar spine or sacrum, additional anterior load-sharing devices are placed in the disk spaces to counteract the high loads applied to that part of the spine with sitting, stance, and/or gait.

A variety of options are available for intradiscal load sharing, including autogenous iliac crest grafts; allograft bicortical or tricortical iliac crest grafts; allograft femoral, humeral, and/or fibular pieces; and various types of metallic intervertebral cage devices. Because of the morbidity associated with harvesting autogenous structural grafts, the most commonly used anterior structural load-sharing devices are allograft wedges and titanium surgical mesh cages. The main advantage of allografts is that they ultimately incorporate into the end plates, as long as they are secured with either anterior and/or posterior instrumentation. They can be cut to size, and in the context of infection transmission, overall they are fairly safe. The advantages of a titanium surgical mesh cage include the wide variety of precut sizes, the ability to place autogenous bone inside the metal device, and the additional interdigitation that occurs between the implant and the end plates given the metallic configuration of the device.

The ultimate goal of supplying optimal load sharing to the spine requires an understanding of the biomechanical aspects of the posterior tension band versus the anterior compression forces present in the spinal column. Ideally, an optimal biomechanical environment should place axis instantaneous of rotation just posterior to the posterior longitudinal ligament, which optimizes the biomechanical environment for the entire spinal column. Surgeons who perform reconstructions of spinal deformities must understand these relationships to avoid early implant-bone and/or late implant failures with resultant pseudarthrosis.

These articles nicely summarize three extremely important topics for the orthopaedic spine surgeon who treats adult spinal deformities. The authors stress the complexity of these surgical treatments and the need for complete understanding of many issues involved in the preoperative planning and intraoperative surgical technique used for these patients.

Lawrence G. Lenke, MD
The Jerome J. Gilden Professor of Orthopaedic Surgery
Chief, Spinal Service Shriners Hospital for Children
Washington University School of Medicine
Department of Orthopaedic Surgery
St. Louis, Missouri

19

Anterior and Posterior Spinal Surgery: Same-Day, Staged, Anterior First, Posterior First, or Simultaneous?

James W. Ogilvie, MD

Anterior spinal surgery was popularized through the work of Hodgson and associates[1] in their treatment of tuberculous spondylitis and deformity. With the improvement of perioperative supportive techniques, including anesthesia, blood banking, spinal instrumentation, intensive care units and the progressive and accumulative skills of spinal surgeons, combined anterior and posterior spinal surgery has become increasingly common.

While the technical ability to perform anterior and posterior spinal surgery (APSS) has improved, the indications and applications have not always been clear.[2] In the past there were recommended limitations, one of which was the separation of the two stages by at least 2 weeks.

Once the indications and prerequisites for APSS have been met, the procedure is preferably done under the same anesthesia. The advantages are (1) earlier postoperative mobilization with the decreased likelihood of deep vein thrombosis, decubitus pneumonia, and deconditioning; (2) shorter hospitalization and decreased cost; (3) better correction of spinal deformity.[3,4] The disadvantages include (1) greater intraoperative stress on the patient; and (2) surgeon and staff fatigue.

Indications for Anterior/Posterior Spinal Surgery

The appropriate clinical situations for APSS fall into four categories.

Rigid Spinal Deformities

When posterior instrumentation alone cannot achieve satisfactory improvement of coronal and sagittal deformity, first stage mobilization of the spine by anterior diskectomy and bone graft may be helpful. When an anterior release precedes posterior instrumentation and fusion for the purpose of enhancing the Cobb correction, the question must be answered, "How many degrees of correction are worth the added surgery of anterior release?" For coronal plane deformities exceeding 130°, an anterior multiple level vertebrectomy, rather than multiple level diskectomy, may be required to achieve worthwhile correction.

Correction of a sagittal plane deformity can be enhanced following meticulous anterior diskectomy by opening the disk space and inserting a structural graft, such as a femoral ring allograft or a metallic cage containing bone graft. The serrated edges of the metallic cages may lessen their tendency to dislodge anteriorly between the anterior and posterior stages.

Pseudarthrosis

Failed attempts to achieve posterior spinal arthrodesis may be an indication for APSS. Risk factors and technical difficulties for successful spinal fusion include obesity, tobacco use, previous in-fection in the fusion site, osteopenia, and pre-existing failed fusion. In treating a pseudarthrosis, it is my strong preference to use autogenous bone whenever possible. In the thorax and thoracolumbar junction, the use of a vascularized rib may be preferable, particularly when previous surgery has exhausted the supply of iliac bone graft.

Fusion to the Pelvis

Long lever arm fusions (above L-1) may have a greater fusion rate when APSS is done. Although previous studies have addressed this question, the methods of spinal fixation described were not those currently used. Many factors can influence the success rate, including newer methods of sacral fixation, satisfactory correction of sagittal balance, and the availability of autogenous bone graft, in addition to the general risk factors of pseudarthrosis.

Deficient Posterior Elements

Certain conditions prevent adequate posterior fusions and may be an indication for anterior or APSS. Extensive laminectomy, spina bifida and other congenital abnormalities, or previous infection of a posterior fusion site can decrease the available area for posterior fusion.[5] APSS enhances the fusion mass and can introduce the option for supplemental anterior fixation.

Anterior or Posterior Fusion First?

Anterior Surgery First

Anterior spinal surgery is performed first when a rigid spinal deformity is present. Removal of the intervertebral disk allows mobilization of the deformity when posterior instrumentation is done in the posterior part of surgery. If stiffness in the posterior elements prevents the placement of a rigid structural disk space graft, or if subsequent posterior correction may dislodge the anterior graft, it is preferable to fill the empty disk space with morselized bone graft after decortication of the end plates. Tightly packing bone graft into the disk space of a scoliotic spine may limit the coronal correction during the subsequent posterior surgery.

When restoring lumbar lordosis, it is ideal to open the disk space anteriorly and place a strut graft which will resist axial load. This may be allograft femoral ring with supplemental autogenous graft, metallic cages, or other structural material capable of biologic incorporation. Metallic cages with serrated edges have the additional advantage of resisting anterior dislodgement between the first and second stages.

It may be advantageous for purposes of enhancing the exposure to flex the operating table when the patient is in the lateral decubitus position for the anterior procedure. First stage posterior instrumentation may inhibit this maneuver and thus long posterior instrumentation is best done in the second phase of APSS.

If anterior instrumentation is to be used as part of an APSS, it is usually done in the first stage. Positioning of the patient is easier with a mobile spine.

Posterior Surgery First

Performing the posterior stage first is preferable when immediate stability is necessary and can be provided by posterior instrumentation, such as unusual cases of spinal tumor, fibrous dysplasia, or trauma. When treating nonunion of a short segment lumbar fusion with APSS, I prefer to perform the posterior stage first, so long as no significant deformity exists which would require first stage anterior release and bone graft. When the posterior aspect of the spine is addressed first, ample autogenous bone can be harvested for both the anterior and posterior grafting. The procedure requires less time and the patient is spared the morbidity of an anterior iliac donor site.

Staged Versus Same Anesthetic APSS

The goal of APSS should be to perform the procedure under one anesthetic without exposing the patient to undue risks of excessive blood loss, difficulty in maintaining clotting factors, general medical instability while under prolonged anesthesia, and the mental and psychological fatigue that can affect the surgical team during long and difficult procedures. It is the mark of prudence and not timidity to terminate a difficult APSS if there is impending risk to the patient.

Staged APSS

In many cases it can be determined preoperatively that staged APSS is preferable. If the first stage is predictably long or at significant risk to incur a high blood loss, if intercurrent observation or traction is planned, or if changes in neurologic function between stages is an issue, it is better to plan a staged procedure.

Staged APSS permits preparation for an early in-bed exercise program. Other adjuncts such as sequential compression hose to minimize deep vein thrombosis, mobilization with the assistance of physical therapy, respiratory therapy, and aggressive early nutritional support, should be vigorously pursued.[6] If the patient is unable to take adequate oral nutrition within several days following the first stage surgery, consideration should be given to the placement of a jejunal feeding tube or total parenteral nutrition.

Particularly when a first stage is done in the thoracic region, the substantial stability given to the spine by the intact posterior elements and rib cage allows early ambulation between stages. Vigilance is required to confirm that no neurologic deterioration occurs.

Although there is no absolute time limit, the second stage should be performed at the earliest time permitted by the condition of the patient. Timing depends on the resilience of the patient, return of hematologic and metabolic parameters to acceptable ranges, and the absence of such contraindications as infection or psychosis.

Combined Anterior and Posterior Surgery

When APSS is indicated, it may be expedient to perform both the anterior and posterior stages simultaneously.[7] The prerequisites are the presence of two competent spinal surgeons, each with their own separate support team of instruments and assistants. Both surgeons may be operating at a disadvantage, because most spinal surgeons stand to the patient's back while performing an anterior vertebrectomy or decompression. Thus, this surgeon is in an unfamiliar surgical position if required to stand to the front. The posterior surgeon is also required to perform the planned decompression and/or instrumentation with the patient in the lateral rather than the prone position. Anesthesia support must be aware that the conditions that prompted the choice of this procedure may also motivate the surgeons to work with haste. These factors may predispose to rapid blood loss, and volume replacement must be aggressive. Hypotensive anesthesia techniques are helpful in reducing blood loss.

Although there are no absolute indications for it, a simultaneous procedure can reduce total operating time while allowing controlled mobilization, correction, and stabilization of a spinal deformity.

References

1. Hodgson AR, Stock FE, Fang HSY, et al: Anterior spinal fusion: The operative approach and pathological findings in 412 patients with Pott's disease of the spine. *Br J Surg* 1960;48:172-178.

2. Johnson JR, Holt RT: Combined use of anterior and posterior surgery for adult scoliosis. *Orthop Clin North Am* 1988;19:361-370.

3. Shufflebarger HL, Grimm JO, Bui V, et al: Anterior and posterior spinal fusion: Staged versus same-day surgery. *Spine* 1991;16:930-933.

4. Viviani GR, Raducan V, Bednar DA, et al: Anterior and posterior spinal fusion: Comparison of one-stage and two-stage procedures. *Can J Surg* 1993;36:468-473.

5. Savini R, Cervellati S, Bettini N, et al: Surgical treatment of vertebral deformity due to myelomeningocele. *Ital J Orthop Traumatol* 1991;17:55-63.

6. Mandelbaum BR, Tolo VT, McAfee PC, et al: Nutritional deficiencies after staged anterior and posterior spinal reconstructive surgery. *Clin Orthop* 1988;234:5-11.

7. Spencer DL, DeWald RL: Simultaneous anterior and posterior surgical approach to the thoracic and lumbar spine. *Spine* 1979;4:29-36.

Where to Stop the Fusion Distally in Adult Scoliosis: L4, L5, or the Sacrum?

Keith H. Bridwell, MD

Coronal Principles That Apply for Adolescents and Adults

Whether the patient is an adolescent or an adult, the following principles are important when choosing the distal level. Postoperatively, C7 should bisect the sacrum. Also, the last instrumented vertebra should be centered on the sacrum and centered on the center sacral line. Also, ideally, that last instrumented vertebra should be neutral in rotation and horizontal if it is at L3 or below. The only exception to this is for the surgeon who is dealing with a type II curve pattern and stops at T12 or L1, in which case it is usually necessary to leave some residual tilt in the last instrumented vertebra (Fig. 1, Case 1). For any fusion that is extended down to L3 or lower, the last instrumented vertebra should ideally be horizontal to the sacrum postoperatively (Table 1).

Sagittal Principles That Apply for Adolescents and-Adults

The apex of the lumbar curve in the sagittal plane is usually at L3/L4.[1-3] With surgery, it is important to preserve and, in some cases, even enhance segmental lordosis. The development of some degenerative disk disease is a part of the natural aging process. If a fusion is stopped at L3 or L4 in an adult, it should be anticipated that some degenerative disk disease will probably occur in the unfused segments below as the patient ages. As degenerative

Table 1
Absolute requirements of the last instrumented/fused spinal segment
Horizontal to the sacrum and pelvis if below L2
Bisected by the center sacral line
Bisected by a plumb dropped from C7
Grade I or less rotation

disk disease occurs, the patient will lose distal segmental and total lordosis. To make up for this, adequate segmental lordosis in the upper and middle lumbar spine is necessary. In the sagittal plane, in a long cassette standing lateral radiograph, a plumb dropped from C7 should fall through or behind the lumbosacral disk.[2] The sagittal principles as well as the aforementioned coronal principles are important in determining where to stop distally.

How to Determine if Coronal and Sagittal Correction is Adequate With a One-Stage Posterior Fusion and Posterior Segmental Instrumentation

In the lumbar spine, surgeons usually see two curves. The first curve extends from T12 to L3 or L4, and the second curve swings the other way and extends from L3 or L4 down to the sacrum. Usually the L3/L4 disk is at the junction of these two curves. Therefore, both right and left

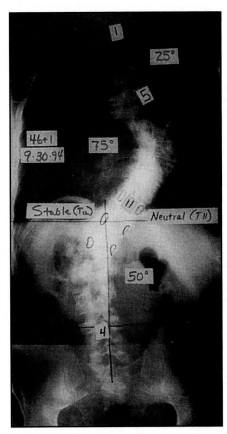

Fig. 1, Case 1 The stable vertebra is the one bisected by the center sacral line. The center sacral line is a line drawn through the center of the sacrum, perpendicular to the level pelvis. In a type II curve pattern, the stable vertebra often is not neutral. Often the neutral vertebra is one or two segments proximal to the stable vertebra. A neutral vertebra demonstrates symmetrical pedicles with reference to the coronal radiograph. This upright coronal radiograph demonstrates the neutral and stable vertebrae.

supine sidebenders are helpful to assess the flexibility of the major lumbar curve above and also the fractional lumbar curve below. If there are no congenital components, usually the fractional curve below in an adolescent or young adult will be totally flexible. But as the person ages, structural changes usually occur in the distal segments of the fractional curve below.

Another very helpful radiograph is what we have coined a "push-prone radiograph." For this film, the patient is placed in a prone position, and an assistant stabilizes the pelvis with both hands. The surgeon applies lateral pressure to the major curve. This gives a radiographic assessment of the flexibility of the major curve and also shows the surgeon the effect of maximal correction of that curve on the fractional curve below. This procedure is better able to predict the effect of correcting one curve on the spine above and below than can be done by simply looking at the sidebending films.

To assess the sagittal flexibility of a curve, we found that a long cassette lateral radiograph taken with the patient supine and with a bump under the apex of the lumbar curve shows the surgeon the sagittal flexibility more effectively than is possible with flexion and extension films. Both this film and the push-prone radiograph on long cassette films show not only flexibility, but also the effect of correction on overall coronal and sagittal balance.

Decision on Distal Fusion Levels in a Young Adult

In a young adult, the fractional curve below is likely to be flexible and is not likely to have much in the way of degenerative changes. The decision must then be made whether to instrument the patient posteriorly or anteriorly.

With anterior instrumentation, it is usually possible to stop the instrumentation at a neutral vertebra rather than a sta-

ble vertebra. This occasionally is the difference between stopping at L4 or L3. Though uncommon, in certain patients it can be the difference between stopping at L5 or L4.

The surgeon should anticipate that any fusion, whether it is done anteriorly or posteriorly, should at least be stopped at a neutral vertebra. If fusion is done posteriorly, instrumentation down to the stable vertebra is usually necessary.

With present-day systems of using either pedicle fixation or multiple hooks, it is possible to instrument posteriorly without taking away the patient's lumbar lordosis. It is necessary to achieve correction either with a rod rotation maneuver or by applying compression forces to the convexity of the curve. Any concave distraction forces should simply be enough to seat the hooks. Generally, the initial force will determine the ultimate sagittal position. For this reason, rod rotation or compression should always be applied to the convex side of every lumbar segment before any distraction is applied to the concave side (Fig. 2, Case 2).

If the primary correction is being achieved with anterior instrumentation, it is extremely important not to take away any segmental lordosis. With the Dwyer system and traditional Zielke systems, even use of the "derotator" tended to take away lumbar lordosis because it shortened the anterior column. It has been our experience that the only way to prevent this is to place structural allograft in the anterior concave disk space. Although Scottish Texas Rite instrumentation reduces the kyphogenic effect of anterior instrumentation, it does not appear to eliminate that problem completely. Placement of structural grafts in the anterior concave disk spaces prior to correction allows lengthening of the anterior column. Rib does not constitute structural graft. Tricortical ilium or something stronger is needed. We have used principally fresh frozen tricortical iliac wedges, and use of this material does seem to pre-

serve and, in some cases, even enhance lumbar lordosis.

If anterior instrumentation is considered to "save a level," then it is necessary preoperatively to demonstrate on a push-prone radiograph that the anticipated last instrumented vertebra can be horizontalized, is centered on the sacrum and center sacral line, and is neutral in rotation at the completion of the instrumentation. Greater correction is possible with anterior instrumentation than with pedicle fixation.

Does a Type II Curve Exist in an Adult With Scoliosis?

King and associates[4] have shown that, in adolescent patients, it is often possible to selectively instrument and fuse the thoracic curve and leave the lumbar curve alone. However, no aspect of adolescent idiopathic scoliosis surgery has met with more debate than the criteria for how and when to fuse the thoracic curve selectively. King and associates[4] have said that this decision should be based principally on the flexibility of the lumbar curve relative to the thoracic curve. Others have suggested that the relative structural nature of the two curves should be assessed on standing radiographs and by physical examination. Suffice it to say that if the thoracic curve has significantly more in the way of structural changes than the lumbar curve, it is at times possible to fix only the thoracic curve, to maintain spinal balance and, in some instances, to achieve some spontaneous correction of the lumbar curve. In the adult population, some of the same flexibility criteria and relative structural characteristic criteria on the standing films can be applied (Fig. 3, Case 3). If the lumbar curve is not symptomatic, and the relative rotation of the lumbar curve and relative deviation of its apex from the midline is small, it may not be necessary to include the lumbar curve. However, if there are multiple rotatory subluxations, and the curve is highly structural in nature and cosmeti-

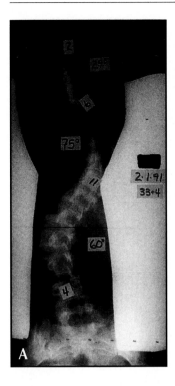
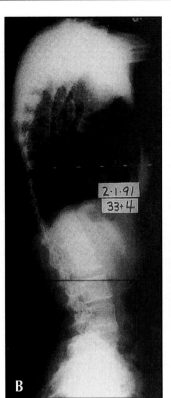
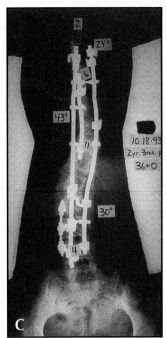
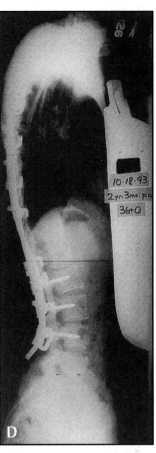

Fig. 2, Case 2 This young adult patient had a double major curve pattern. The lumbar rotation, apical vertebral deviation from the plumb line, and Cobb measurements of the lumbar and thoracic curves, as well as overall flexibility of the two curves, were roughly equal. L4 was a neutral vertebra and stable vertebra. There was no evidence of any rotatory subluxation at L4/L5 or L5/S1. Therefore, the instrumentation was stopped at L4. It was not stopped at L3 because L3 was too close to the apex of that lumbar curve and was not neutrally rotated. In this patient's case, compression forces and rod rotation forces were applied to the convexity of the lumbar curve as the corrective forces, which somewhat enhanced segmental lumbar lordosis. It is hoped that this will reduce the likelihood of breakdown of the L4/L5 and L5/S1 disk spaces as this patient ages. **A** and **B**, Coronal and sagittal upright radiographs preoperatively. **C** and **D**, Same views at ultimate follow-up.

cally deforming, it should be included in the fusion.

Decision Making on Stopping the Distal Fusion Level in the Older Adult

In patients older than 40 years of age, it is quite possible and likely that there are structural changes within the fractional curve.[5-16] Certainly the surgeon should not stop a fusion at a rotatory subluxation. Rotatory subluxations are most likely to occur at L3/L4 or L4/L5. There should be no segmental rotation at the segment below a spinal fusion (Fig. 4, Case 4).

Also, the surgeon should not stop a fusion if the segments below are degenerated and "symptomatic." It is controversial whether or not a fusion can be stopped at L4 or L5 if the segments below have some element of degenerative disk disease. I would define distally degenerated segments as being definitely "symptomatic" if they have either central or lateral recess spinal stenosis, foraminal stenosis, or any evidence of subluxation or instability on flexion-extension films (Table 2).

If the motion segments below show a very small amount of degenerative disk disease with minor loss of disk height,

but appear "black" on magnetic resonance imaging (MRI), it is controversial whether or not those segments should be included. In 1994, Kostuik and Musha reported, at the annual meeting of the Scoliosis Research Society, that they now prefer always to include L5/S1 in a fusion if it is degenerated even if it is not symptomatic. This view is not universally accepted, and more critical analysis is needed in this area.

The test that is reputed to be the most helpful in determining whether or not a degenerated segment below is a significant back pain producer is the provocative diskogram.[11,12] Results of provocative

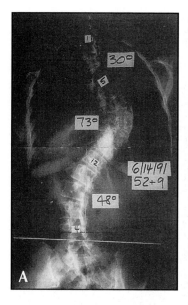
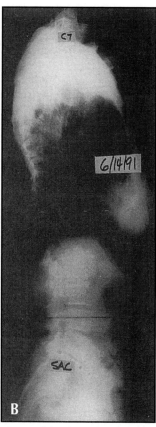
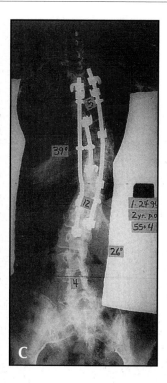
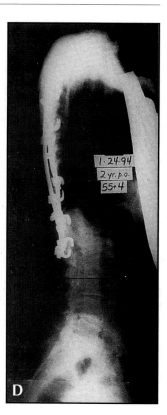

Fig. 3, Case 3 This middle-aged adult had a thoracic and lumbar curve. However, the structural characteristics of the thoracic curve were far more significant than they were for the lumbar curve. Although the patient clearly had some degenerative changes in the lumbar curve, it had been minimally symptomatic. The patient had occasional low back ache, but nothing more. The presenting symptomatology was that of increasing thoracic deformity and increasing thoracic pain. For these reasons, this patient was treated for a type II curve pattern. Selective fusion and instrumentation was performed in the thoracic curve down to only the stable vertebra. A concomitant thoracoplasty was performed as well. Patient satisfaction in this case has been extremely high. **A** and **B,** Coronal and sagittal upright radiographs preoperatively. **C** and **D,** Same views at ultimate follow-up.

diskograms seem to depend to a great extent on the interpretation and technique of the examiner. The true value and limitations of provocative diskograms are still not fully understood.

In 1993, Hu and Bradford, in a poster exhibit at the annual meeting of the Scoliosis Research Society, reported performing an osteotomy above the pedicle of L5 to help horizontalize L4 and reduce the need to instrument down to L5. The opening osteotomy is held open with rib graft, and correction is completed with anterior segmental spinal instrumentation for the segments above. Some cases of excellent patient outcome have been reported, with significant follow-up. To

date, the effect of the osteotomy and correction on the sagittal plane and the long-term follow-up of all patients so treated has not been published or critically analyzed.

If the surgeon is thinking of stopping at L4 based on the principles that are used for an adolescent, he or she should look at the L4/L5 and L5/S1 segments in both the coronal and sagittal planes before deciding that L4 is appropriate. If there is rotatory subluxation at L4/L5, degenerative spondylolisthesis at L4/L5, evidence of spondylolysis at L5/S1, or stenotic problem below, the presence of any of these might influence the surgeon to carry the instrumentation distally.

When Can the Fusion be Stopped at L5 Versus When Does It Need to be Carried to the Sacrum?

If patients have fixed tilt at L4/L5 or stenosis or rotatory subluxations at L4/L5, it is probably mandatory to fuse at least down to L5. At this point, the question arises whether or not the L5/S1 disk can be spared (Table 3).

Situations in which the L5/S1 disk must be included in the fusion include the following: if there is a fixed take-off or fixed tilt at the L5/S1 disk; if there is a bilateral spondylolysis or spondylolisthesis at L5/S1; if there is spinal stenosis at L5/S1 (this is not very common, but it does sometimes occur); if the patient is

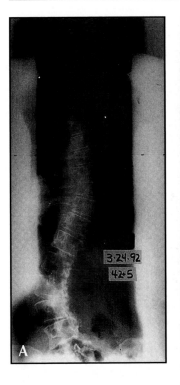
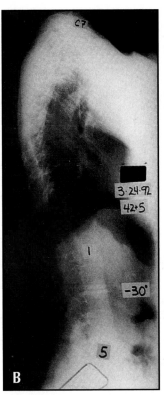
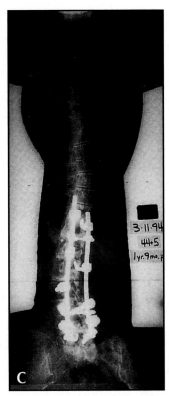
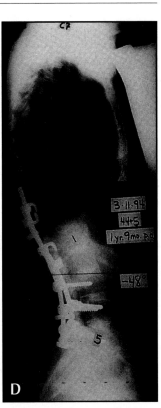

Fig. 4, Case 4 This middle-aged adult presented with increasing lumbar deformity and increasing back pain. If she were treated as an adolescent or a younger adult, her fusion and instrumentation could probably have been stopped at L4. At this point, however, she had structural changes in her L4/L5 disk. She had a rotatory subluxation at that level. At L5/S1, she had preservation of disk height. L5/S1 was well below the intercristal line. She had no posterior column deficiency or stenosis at L5/S1. Her lumbar spine was significantly hypolordotic. For her, the appropriate procedure was to instrument and fuse her lumbar spine down to L5 and to do it in such a way that her lumbar lordosis was increased. This was accomplished by anterior lumbar release and structural grafting followed by posterior instrumentation and fusion in the same anesthesia. At 2-year follow-up, she reports total resolution of her disabling lumbar symptomatology. **A** and **B,** Coronal and sagittal upright radiographs preoperatively. **C** and **D,** Same views at ultimate follow-up.

sagittally out of balance and C7 is in front of the degenerated lumbosacral disk. In any of these situations, it is almost certainly going to be necessary to carry the instrumentation down to the sacrum (Fig. 5, Case 5; and Table 4). To a lesser extent, how deeply seated L5/S1 is below the top of the pelvis and the intercristal line is a factor. Also, if the L5/S1 disk is severely degenerated, then foraminal stenosis may occur at L5/S1, and that may necessitate inclusion of that segment.

Factors Contributing to Breakdown Adjacent to a Previous Spinal Fusion

The following factors seem to be important. The position of the spinal fusion in

Talbe 2
Rules of where not to stop a fusion
Do not stop adjacent to:
A rotatory subluxation
A degenerative spondylolisthesis
An isthmic spondylolisthesis
An area of spinal stenosis
An area of posterior column deficiency

Table 3
When can a fusion be stopped at L5?
"Normal" disk at L5/S1
No posterior column deficiency at L5/S1
No spinal stenosis at L5/S1
L5/S1 under the intercristal line
L5/S1 with large transverse processes

both the coronal and sagittal plane is a factor: (1) whether or not the spine is positioned with physiologic segmental lordosis, and (2) whether or not the top or the bottom of the fusion are perfectly centered on the sacrum in the coronal plane. Also, the length of the spinal fu-

sion is a factor. A longer fusion probably increases stress on the segments below.[17,18] The patient's connective tissues and biology are important also. If the patient is a smoker, is diabetic, or is on prednisone, it is more likely that the spine will break down above or below.

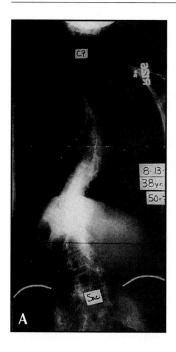
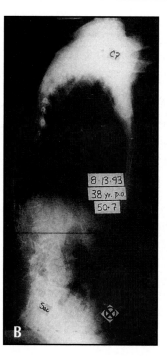
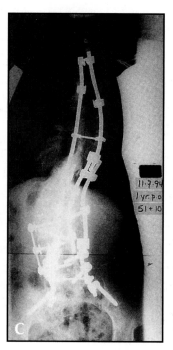
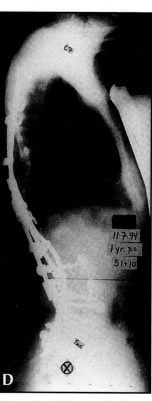

Fig. 5, Case 5 This adult patient had a scoliosis fusion without instrumentation 38 years prior to presentation to the author. Subsequently, she developed degenerative disk disease at L3/L4, L4/L5, and L5/S1. With increasing loss of anterior column height, she was gradually pitched forward more and more. Her sagittal imbalance and flatback syndrome were the presenting symptoms and indications for surgery. Fusion to the sacrum was necessary in order to achieve balance. Anterior column height was restored by placing structural grafts that opened up the 3/4, 4/5, and 5/1 disk spaces. Multiple posterior osteotomies were also required through the posterior fusion. The patient is quite happy with the result at 1-year follow-up. **A** and **B**, Coronal and sagittal radiographs preoperatively. **C** and **D**, Same view at ultimate follow-up. The sagittal plumb line has been shifted from several centimeters in front of L5/S1 to behind L5/S1.

Table 4
When is it not possible to stop at L5 and when is it necessary to fuse to the sacrum?

Severe degenerative disk disease at L5/S1

Central, lateral recess or foraminal stenosis at L5/S1

Deformity at L5/S1
   Fixed tilt
   Listhesis
   In the face of posterior column deficiency at L5/S1

Patient who is sagittally out of balance and has degenerative disk disease at L5/S1

The "normality" of the adjacent segments has been discussed. Although not thoroughly understood, the stiffness of the spinal fusion may be a factor. An anterior and posterior fusion is stiffer than a posterior fusion, and perhaps a posterior fusion with rigid instrumentation is at least initially stiffer than one with more semi-constrained instrumentation.

Summary

Multiple considerations must be weighed and discussed with the patient before deciding on a long fusion down to the middle or distal lumbar spine. The factors outlined above all play a role in the outcome of such surgery.

At the time of this writing, bone screws placed posteriorly into vertebral elements have not been cleared for general use in this specific manner by the Food and Drug Administration (FDA). These are Class III devices. This category includes screws placed transfacetally, within pedicles, or in articular, lateral masses. Some screws for use within the sacrum have been approved as Class II devices.

Some companies have received Class II clearance for use of screws in lumbar pedicles specifically to supplement fusions in the treatment of grade III and IV spondylolisthesis with the proviso that these devices are removed after the arthrodesis has healed. Anterior vertebral body screws (cervical, thoracic, and lumbar) are Class II devices and can be used as labeled in vertebral bodies. Many of the posterior screw-based devices have been shown in laboratory and clinical testing to be useful and can be used in an off-label manner if the physician feels this is appropriate and important for the treatment of the patient. As with all surgeries, informed consent should explain the procedure and why a particular technique has been chosen, as well as its risks and benefits. The question of whether informed consent regarding pedicle screws must include a discussion of the device's FDA clearance status is currently being litigated in several jurisdictions.

References

1. Bernhardt M, Bridwell KH: Segmental analysis of the sagittal plane alignment of the normal thoracic and lumbar spines and thoracolumbar junction. *Spine* 1989;14:717-721.

2. Jackson RP, McManus AC: Radiographic analysis of sagittal plane alignment and balance in standing volunteers and patients with low back pain matched for age, sex, and size: A prospective controlled clinical study. *Spine* 1994;19:1611-1618.

3. Wambolt A, Spencer DL: A segmental analysis of the distribution of lumbar lordosis in the normal spine. *Orthop Trans* 1987;11:92-93.

4. King HA, Moe JH, Bradford DS, et al: The selection of fusion levels in thoracic idiopathic scoliosis. *J Bone Joint Surg* 1983;65A:1302-1313.

5. Benner B, Ehni G: Degenerative lumbar scoliosis. *Spine* 1979;4:548-552.

6. Bradford DS: Adult scoliosis: Current concepts of treatment. *Clin Orthop* 1988;229:70-87.

7. Briard JL, Jegou D, Cauchoix J: Adult lumbar scoliosis. *Spine* 1979;4:526-532.

8. Epstein JA, Epstein BS, Jones MD: Symptomatic lumbar scoliosis with degenerative changes in the elderly. *Spine* 1979;4:542-547.

9. Grubb SA, Lipscomb HJ, Coonrad RW: Degenerative adult onset scoliosis. *Spine* 1988;13:241-245.

10. Jackson RP, Simmons EH, Stripinis D: Incidence and severity of back pain in adult idiopathic scoliosis. *Spine* 1983;8:749-756.

11. Kostuik JP: Decision making in adult scoliosis. *Spine* 1979;4:521-525.

12. Kostuik JP: Adult scoliosis, in Bridwell KH, DeWald RL, Lubicky JP, et al (eds): *The Textbook of Spinal Surgery.* Philadelphia, PA, JB Lippincott, 1991, vol 1, pp, 249-277.

13. Lonstein JE: Adult scoliosis, in Bradford DS, Lonstein JE, Moe JH, et al (eds): *Moe's Textbook of Scoliosis and Other Spinal Deformities,* ed 2. Philadelphia, PA, WB Saunders, 1987, pp 369-390.

14. Robin GC, Span Y, Steinberg R, et al: Scoliosis in the elderly: A follow-up study. *Spine* 1982;7:355-359.

15. Simmons EH, Jackson RP: The management of nerve root entrapment syndromes associated with the collapsing scoliosis of idiopathic lumbar and thoracolumbar curves. *Spine* 1979;4:533-541.

16. Vanderpool DW, James JI, Wynne-Davies R: Scoliosis in the elderly. *J Bone Joint Surg* 1969;51A:446-455.

17. Bartie BJ, Lonstein JE, Winter RB, et al: Long term follow-up of idiopathic scoliosis patients after spinal fusion: An outcome analysis. *Orthop Trans* 1993;17:982.

18. Cochran T, Irstam L, Nachemson A: Long-term anatomic and functional changes in patients with adolescent idiopathic scoliosis treated by Harrington rod fusion. *Spine* 1983;8:576-584.

21

Load Sharing Principles: The Role and Use of Anterior Structural Support in Adult Deformity

Keith H. Bridwell, MD

Introduction

In this manuscript, the clinical significance of load sharing will be discussed. Referable to load sharing, the surgeon must ask himself the following questions: (1) When is anterior and posterior fusion needed rather than just fusion of one column? (2) When instrumenting and correcting a deformity, how can the surgeon maintain correction? (3) What can the surgeon do to prevent instrumentation failure and pull-out in the adult deformity patient? (4) How can the surgeon minimize the pull-out loosening forces on the instrumentation and optimize the environment for incorporation of bone graft, both anteriorly and posteriorly? Ideally, both anterior and posterior bone graft should be loaded in compression.

Importance and Function of the Three Columns of the Spine

The three columns of the spine, as defined by Denis,[1] are the anterior, middle, and posterior columns. The anterior columns include the disks, the anterior vertebral body, and the anterior longitudinal ligament. The middle column includes the posterior vertebral body contiguous to the spinal canal. The posterior columns include the posterior elements and the pedicles.

Of the three columns, the two most important biomechanically, as shown by James and associates,[2] are probably the anterior and posterior columns. In a fracture situation, although the middle column is important for maintenance of neurologic function, the anterior and posterior columns are the principal support structures of the spine.

In the cervical spine, the weightbearing line falls behind the cervical vertebrae and crosses at the cervicothoracic disk. It then falls in front of the thoracic vertebrae, behind the lumbar vertebrae, and just behind or through the lumbosacral disk. As one examines the spine anatomically from cranial to caudal, one will notice that the vertebral bodies gradually become larger. In the lumbar spine, the lumbar disks are increased in height and, in fact, make up the majority of the lordosis in the lumbar spine as shown by Wambolt and Spencer.[3]

The posterior column and musculature of the spine represent the tension side. The anterior column and disks represent the compression/axial loading side. Both columns serve to maintain alignment and resist kyphosis. Haher and associates[4] showed that the normal instantaneous axis of rotation sits just behind the disk. When one column is injured, this axis of rotation shifts to the remaining intact structures. When the surgeon designs a load-sharing construct, the goal is to restore the instantaneous axis of rotation to a position just posterior to the anulus, principally by reconstituting the deficient columns.

Deficiencies of either the anterior or posterior columns will usually lead to increasing kyphosis. Take, for example, acquired spondylolisthesis with bilateral spondylolysis through the pars of L5. The initial defect here is in the posterior column. When this defect first occurs, the anterior column (and anterior disk) is competent. However, with time, the disk inevitably becomes degenerated anteriorly and loses its disk height. This occurs because the disk is overloaded anteriorly. The extent to which a spondylolisthesis either falls into kyphosis or slips forward is a function of the body's reparative processes. These reparative processes include laying down of anterior osteophytes for stabilization and laying down of fiber cartilage to stabilize the spondylolysis bilaterally.

Obvious examples of increasing kyphosis due to anterior column defects include tumors and fractures that destroy vertebral bodies and fall into kyphosis even though the posterior elements, posterior ligaments, and posterior musculature are intact. Likewise, with aging, multiple compression fractures and loss of disk height anteriorly lead to increasing kyphosis and acquired nonsurgical flatback syndromes.

Distribution of Posterior Fixation Points to Achieve Load Distribution

With posterior segmental spinal instrumentation, how many fixation points are needed? With the Harrington distraction rod, there were two fixation points, one on the top and one on the bottom. When

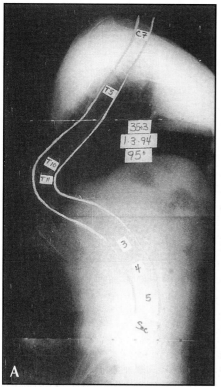 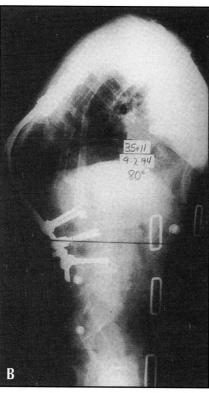

Fig. 1 For this patient, with a very stiff, but painful congenital kyphosis, there was no way to safely normalize the sagittal plane and modest correction had to be accepted. Posterior instrumentation and fusion was performed from a lordotic segment above to a lordotic segment below. Anterior strut grafting was performed along the weightbearing lines from the first kyphotic segment to the last kyphotic segment. Because much of the original deformity had to be accepted, the anterior strut grafts are the most important and critical aspects of the reconstruction. **A,** Preoperative upright sagittal radiograph shows a marked congenital kyphosis. **B,** Same view, showing circumferential reconstruction and placement of several structural grafts anteriorly.

sublaminar wiring and Wisconsin wiring were introduced and employed, the number of fixation points increased.

It is known that the more osteoporotic the patient is, the more desirable it is to have many fixation points. With a long fusion to the sacrum, it probably is desirable to have fixation of L4 and L5 and four screws in the sacropelvic unit. This is preferable to having a fixation point at L3 and then jumping down to the sacrum and pelvis.

For a spondylolisthesis that is being reduced, if structural interbody grafts are used that create a ligamentotaxis effect, placement of two screws above and two screws below is often sufficient if the grafts are positioned perfectly. Alternatively, if anterior interbody grafts are not used, it is mandatory to have four fixation points distally and two fixation points proximally.

There is still considerable discussion regarding the appropriate load-sharing construct for burst fractures.[5,6] Two screws above and two screws below are probably sufficient if a perfectly placed structural graft is used anteriorly. Without a structural graft anteriorly, four screws above and four screws below may be needed to distribute the loads posteriorly. But this construct is probably still not as strong as having a structural anterior column graft.

In general, the more fixation points used posteriorly, the more secure the posterior instrumentation will be. Any cantilever correction must be performed with a minimum of four screws or hooks and two vertebral segments as the base. Precisely how many total fixation points are used will depend on the patient's pathology and bone stock.

Correction of Kyphosis

Kyphosis can be corrected by lengthening the anterior column, by shortening the posterior column, or by a combination of both. Which is needed depends a great deal on the patient's primary pathology (Fig. 1).

If a fracture involves only the anterior and middle columns, and the posterior columns are spared, it may be possible to restore alignment and achieve load sharing with just anterior surgery with anterior structural grafting and instrumentation. However, if a spinal fracture shows loss of anterior and middle column support as well as displacement of the posterior elements with subluxation, it will be necessary to lengthen the anterior column, support the anterior column with the structural graft, and tension the posterior column of the spine with posterior segmental spinal instrumentation (Fig. 2).

Edwards and Osborne[7] and Simmons[8] have noted that with posterior correction of kyphosis by either gradual kyphosis reduction or osteotomy, anterior surgery may not be necessary if the surgeon can shift the weightbearing line so that it is well behind the axis of rotation of the instrumentation and posterior fusion. In other words, by displacing the weightbearing line far enough posteriorly, the anterior column in essence does not have to bear as much axial loading (1) if the surgeon can achieve anatomic correction or over-correction, (2) if the patient's posterior elements are strong enough to hold the instrumentation, and (3) if the patient's biology and connective

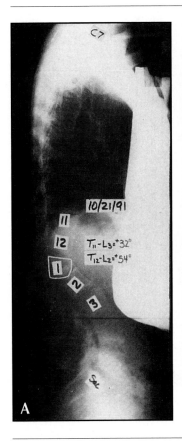
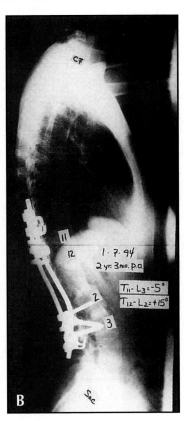

Fig. 2 This patient's initial fracture was not appreciated to include both injury to the anterior column of the spine and the posterior column. Treated conservatively, she fell into an increasing kyphosis. Both anterior and posterior reconstruction was, therefore, necessary. The anterior reconstruction was performed by doing diskectomies and placing structural grafts at each level anteriorly. This afforded the majority of the correction. Posterior instrumentation and fusion was also necessary, to restore the disrupted posterior column. Because of the initial posterior column injury, her instantaneous axis of rotation was shifted anteriorly, thus further loading the already disrupted anterior column. With the anterior and posterior reconstruction, her instantaneous axis of rotation was displaced posteriorly into a more physiologic location. **A,** This upright sagittal radiograph taken 3 years after the initial fracture shows the posttraumatic kyphosis. This deformity evolved slowly. **B,** Same view 2 years after reconstruction.

tissues are conducive to bone formation (Fig. 3).

If anatomic sagittal restoration is not accomplished, greater resistive forces will be applied to the posterior tensioning, significant axial loads will be applied to the anterior column, and the posterior instrumentation will almost certainly fail without anterior column support (Fig. 4).

How to Restore Load Sharing for the Adult Deformity Patient with a Fixed Kyphosis

Osteotomies are often required to restore sagittal profile. If the osteotomies are symmetrically closed so that bone is compressing against bone and the weightbearing line is shifted behind the lumbosacral disk, it may not always be necessary to support the spine anteriorly. However, this assumes stable fixation points on the spine at all levels. It is certainly more difficult to achieve universally stable fixation in the sacrum and

pelvis than it is in the lumbar spine. Factors such as pedicle size, strength of pedicles, and patient osteoporosis also play a role.

For adult degenerative disease, kyphosis almost always plays a role. In adult degenerative disease, shortening the posterior column usually worsens foraminal stenosis. A reasonable alternative is anterior column lengthening, accomplished by resecting the disks anteriorly, opening up the disks anteriorly, and placing structural bone graft (Fig. 5). This lengthening of the anterior column shifts the weight-bearing line posteriorly and more efficiently restores balance between posterior tension and anterior loading while opening up the foramen. These patients often have elements of central or lateral recess spinal stenosis, and these require posterior decompressions that compromise the posterior column. Thus, often anterior and posterior reconstructions are needed to adequately "load share."

Alternatives for Anterior Column Support

Anterior instrumentation cannot, in and of itself, provide anterior column support.[9] Anterior instrumentation is often used to distract/open a disk space. A structural bone graft is then placed into the disk space, which is then compressed down over the bone graft with the instrumentation. The instrumentation, therefore, serves first to achieve the initial correction and is then used to lock the bone graft into place. The structural bone graft serves to resist axial loading and flexion.

Alternatives for anterior column bony support include autograft, fresh frozen allograft, and cages with autograft (Table 1). When allograft is used, fresh frozen bone graft provides better structural support than does freeze dried. Femur, tibia, and full-thickness ilium all seem to have adequate structural support. Ribs do not provide adequate structural support unless they are combined with

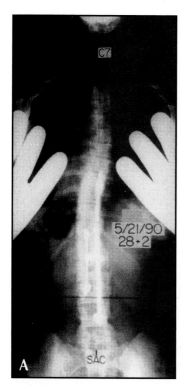 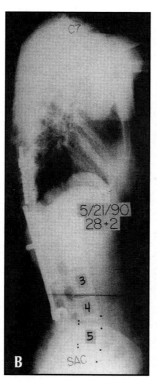 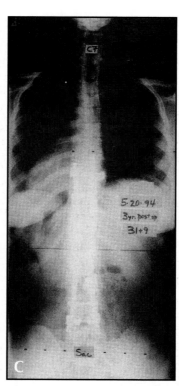 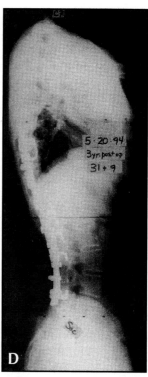

Fig. 3 This patient presented with a segmentally flat lumbar spine in the sagittal plane secondary to Harrington distraction instrumentation. As can be seen in the preoperative radiographs, the L4/L5 disk below must hyperextend to maintain sagittal balance. The diskogram at L4/L5 revealed a normal disk. She was, therefore, treated with multiple posterior osteotomies which restored her sagittal contour throughout the previous fusion as well as the disk below. Because the osteotomies were corrective enough that the weightbearing line was displaced behind the fusion mass and because the patient had multiple fixation points with excellent bone stock, no anterior supportive procedure was necessary. **A** and **B,** Preoperative coronal and sagittal radiographs. **C** and **D,** Same views postoperatively. Note the change in the appearance of the L4/L5 disk space.

Table 1
Structural support for the anterior column

Autograft
   Fibula
   Tricortical ilium
   Vascularized rib with an allograft femoral head

Fresh frozen allograft
   Fresh frozen tricortical ilium
   Fresh frozen full-thickness femur or tibia packed with autogenous morselized bone

Cage or cages packed with autogenous bone

other graft. It is certainly advisable to pack and surround fresh frozen allograft with autogenous bone.

For autograft, suitable grafts include full-thickness ilium, multiple fibular grafts, and a vascularized rib with an allograft. A vascularized rib in and of itself does not provide adequate structural support in the adult patient. Although it may revascularize very quickly, it needs to be supplemented in the initial phases of healing (Table 1).[10]

There is significant morbidity to harvesting anterior full-thickness autograft ilium. The use of fresh frozen allograft bone involves some risk of viral transmission, plus fresh frozen allograft undoubtedly incorporates less rapidly than auto-graft. Very few studies have reported clinical results with fresh frozen allograft and cages with minimum 2-year follow-up.[11] The risk of viral transmission with fresh frozen allograft is remote, but possible.[12] The long-term effect of either carbon fiber or titanium in the front of the spine is not fully known.

Load sharing necessitates a balance between anterior structural bone grafts and posterior segmental instrumentation. Posterior instrumentation should resist posterior tensile forces. Anterior instrumentation and structural bone grafts should resist flexion and axial loading. Several factors are critical to the achievement of effective load sharing. First, it is important to preserve the anterior bony end plates of the vertebral bodies so that cortical bone (of the graft) is on cortical bone (of the vertebral body) rather than

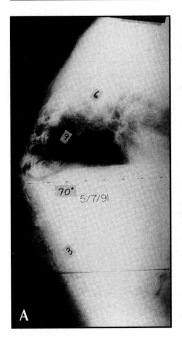
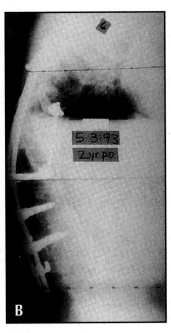

Fig. 4 This patient with ankylosing spondylitis and spondylodiskitis presented with marked kyphosis and myelopathy. He required a posterior extension osteotomy and also a formal anterior decompression. He required posterior instrumentation to compress the extension osteotomy. He required anterior strut grafting both to fill in the hole in the anterior column and also because the extension osteotomy was not corrective enough to displace the weightbearing line behind the osteotomy. **A,** This preoperative upright sagittal radiograph demonstrates the area of spondylodiskitis. **B,** The same view taken after posterior osteotomy and anterior and posterior reconstruction.

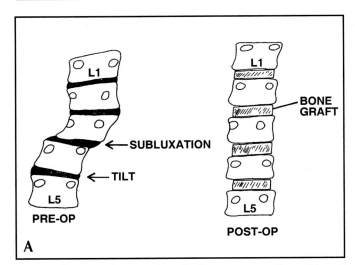
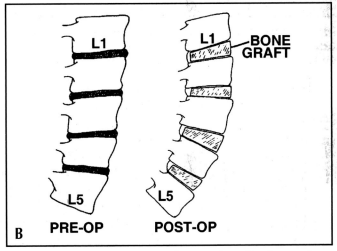

Fig. 5 A, These two drawings show the ligamentotaxis effect achieved by the structural grafting. **B,** These two drawings show the effect on the sagittal plane of placing structural grafts into the anterior disk spaces. The grafting lengthens the anterior column, puts the spine into a position of increased lordosis, and opens up the foramen at each level.

on trabecular bone, which can lead to settling of the graft. It is also important that with any instrumentation placed anteriorly the screws should bite both cortices.[9] Any bone graft should be centered on the vertebral body, placed well over to the other side. Osteoporosis will increase the likelihood of instrumentation failure and increase the likelihood of the axis of rotation being shifted. Both patient biology and osteogenic potential are important factors in achieving load sharing and, ultimately, union.

Conditions Requiring Both Anterior and Posterior Reconstruction to Achieve Load Sharing

These adult conditions consist of those in which there are defects in both the anterior and posterior columns. For burst fractures that require anterior decompression but have intact posterior elements, only anterior reconstruction may be needed. In this situation, following decompression a structural graft anteriorly and anterior segmental spinal instrumentation made up of two screws above, two screws below, two rods, and a crosslink may suffice. On the other hand,

Table 2
Pathologies requiring both anterior and posterior reconstruction

Tumors involving both the anterior and posterior columns

Fractures with collapse of the anterior column and wide displacement of the posterior elements

Post-laminectomy kyphosis

Degenerative scoliosis with sagittal imbalance

if one is dealing with a burst subluxation/dislocation with displaced posterior elements, it is necessary to reconstruct the spine not only anteriorly but also posteriorly, with posterior instrumentation and posterior fusion. Burst fractures with greater initial degrees of kyphosis and comminution are more likely to require anterior structural grafting to reduce the likelihood of failure of posterior fixation systems.[13]

If tumors involve only the posterior elements and the pedicles, only posterior reconstruction may be needed. Alternatively, if the tumor involves only the vertebral body and spares the pedicles and posterior elements, it may be necessary only to reconstruct anteriorly. However, if all three columns of the spine are affected, both anterior and posterior reconstruction will be necessary.

A post-laminectomy kyphosis is a good example of a situation in which both anterior and posterior reconstruction is needed. The posterior column has been rendered deficient by the laminectomy. Anteriorly either wedging of vertebral bodies or failure of the anterior column and anterior disks has resulted in the kyphosis. So in this condition, both anterior and posterior reconstruction is usually necessary.

As mentioned earlier, in severe degenerative scoliosis with sagittal imbalance, it is usually necessary both to structurally graft the spine anteriorly to restore sagittal balance and also to reconstruct the spine posteriorly. The two reasons for the posterior reconstruction are to prevent overload or displacement of the anterior grafts and also to reconstruct the posterior column after the posterior surgery. The posterior surgery usually, to some extent, denervates the posterior spinal muscles, which may further compromise the posterior column. Also, any laminectomy for decompressive purposes further changes the anterior posterior balance (Table 2).

Summary
The goals of load sharing are to restore balance between posterior tension and anterior compression, ideally to maintain the instantaneous axis of rotation just posterior to the anulus and to thereby minimize the forces on the reconstruction. To accomplish this, the surgeon should understand the anatomic column deficiencies of the patient's pathology and the appropriate options for anterior and posterior reconstruction.

References
1. Denis F: The three column spine and its significance in the classification of acute thoracolumbar spinal injuries. *Spine* 1983;8: 817-831.

2. James KS, Wenger KH, Schlegel JD, et al: Biomechanical evaluation of the stability of thoracolumbar burst fractures. *Spine* 1994;19:1731-1740.

3. Wambolt A, Spencer DL: A segmental analysis of the distribution of lumbar lordosis in the normal spine. *Orthop Trans* 1987;11:92-93.

4. Haher TR, O'Brien M, Felmly WT, et al: Instantaneous axis of rotation as a function of the three columns of the spine. *Spine* 1992;17(suppl 6):SI49-SI54.

5. Ebelke DK, Asher MA, Neff JR, et al: Survivorship analysis of VSP spine instrumentation in the treatment of thoracolumbar and lumbar burst fractures. *Spine* 1991;16(suppl 8):S428-S432.

6. McLain RF, Sparling E, Benson DR: Early failure of short-segment pedicle instrumentation for thoracolumbar fractures: A preliminary report. *J Bone Joint Surg* 1993;75A:162-167.

7. Edwards CC, Osborne VA: Abstract: Correction of chronic post-traumatic kyphosis with the kyphoreduction construct and stress-relaxation. Proceedings of the American Academy of Orthopaedic Surgeons 61st Annual Meeting, New Orleans, LA. Rosemont, IL, American Academy of Orthopaedic Surgeons, 1994, p 160.

8. Simmons EH: Relation of vascular complication to the level of lumbar extension osteotomy in ankylosing spondylitis. Proceedings of the American Academy of Orthopaedic Surgeons 61st Annual Meeting, New Orleans, LA. Rosemont, IL, American Academy of Orthopaedic Surgeons, 1994, p 161.

9. Gurr KR, McAfee PC, Shih CM: Biomechanical analysis of anterior and posterior instrumentation systems after corpectomy: A calf-spine model. *J Bone Joint Surg* 1988;70A:1182-1191.

10. McBride GG, Bradford DS: Vertebral body replacement with femoral neck allograft and vascularized rib strut graft: A technique for treating post-traumatic kyphosis with neurologic deficit. *Spine* 1983;8:406-415.

11. Brantigan JW, Steffee AD: A carbon fiber implant to aid interbody lumbar fusion: Two-year clinical results in the first 26 patients. *Spine* 1993;18:2106-2107.

12. Buck BE, Malinin TI, Brown MD: Bone transplantation and human immunodeficiency virus: An estimate of risk of acquired immunodeficiency syndrome (AIDS). *Clin Orthop* 1989;240:129-136.

13. McCormack T, Karaikovic E, Gaines RW: The load sharing classification of spine fractures. *Spine* 1994;19:1741-1744.

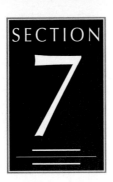

SECTION 7

Cervical Spine Trauma

Cervical Spine Trauma

Cervical spine trauma and acute spinal cord injury are important topics for orthopaedic surgeons and neurosurgeons; a thorough understanding of the evaluation, diagnosis, and the treatment of these patients is critical. Over the past 20 to 30 years, many advances have been made to better understand the acute diagnosis and treatment of these conditions. The two articles in this section, authored by Dr. Alexander Vaccaro and associates and Drs. Andrew Slucky and Frank Eismont, give a broad and sufficiently detailed account of this accumulated knowledge and provide an excellent state-of-the-art review of epidemiology, pathophysiology, and early management of patients with acute spinal cord injury.

Both articles succinctly review proper prehospital and in-hospital emergency care for patients with cervical spine trauma. Proper training of emergency medical technicians and paramedics has standardized prehospital care to include spinal immobilization, patient extrication, and transport to the nearest trauma center. Once a patient arrives at the hospital, the ultimate goal is to provide for a stable, painless spine and an optimal neurologic recovery. For patients with no initial neurologic deficits, the goal is to do no further harm. During early assessment, it is critical to determine whether the patient had a history of transient paralysis after the traumatic event. The neurologic status of some patients may appear normal on arrival at the emergency department, but those who report a brief moment of paralysis immediately after the accident require immediate and careful assessment for a possible unstable cervical spine fracture or dislocation.

Assessment in the emergency department requires a thorough physical examination. After evaluating the trauma ABCs, the first priority in the spine evaluation is to make the appropriate neurologic diagnosis. A carefully documented neurologic examination identifying the sensory and motor levels is critical, especially to note any changes that may occur during the treatment process. The first step is to determine whether the patient has a complete or incomplete spinal cord injury, a root injury, or a normal neurologic status. The more neurologically normal the patient, the more vigilance is needed in protecting the spinal cord from further injury.

The next step is to make the appropriate radiographic diagnosis. In modern emergency departments, radiography and CT of the cervical spine have become routine in all patients believed to have a cervical spine injury, particularly in those with head injuries or loss of consciousness. These patients cannot cooperate with a history and physical examination. In most instances, a lateral view of the cervical spine and a CT scan will confirm one of the following diagnoses: (1) unilateral facet fracture or dislocation, (2) bilateral facet fracture or dislocation, (3) burst fracture, (4) teardrop fracture-dislocation, or (5) other more complex combination injuries. After appropriate neurologic and radiographic diagnoses, a plan for optimal management can be initiated. Although advances in this field have no doubt positively affected the overall outcome of patients with cervical spine trauma, controversy still exists in certain aspects of patient management. I would like to review some of these controversies in the context of my experiences in treating these patients.

The first controversy involves the use of high-dose methylprednisolone in patients with cervical spinal cord injuries. Both articles refer to the original National Acute Spinal Cord Injury Study (NASCIS) by Bracken and associates.[1] This study demonstrated an improvement in the motor scores in patients given high doses of steroids within the first 8 hours of injury. After publication of this report in 1990, most trauma centers routinely began to administer high-dose steroids to any patient with a spinal cord injury; thus, this treatment became the standard of care. More recently, the routine use of methylprednisolone in these patients has come into question. Hurlbert[2] reviewed the available literature and tried to formulate evidence-based recommendations for the use of methylprednisolone in patients with acute spinal cord injuries; he concluded that such a recommendation cannot be made and that prolonged administration of steroids for 48 hours may even be harmful.

The original Bracken study currently appears to be under more scrutiny; criticisms of the methodology and statistical reliability are surfacing that may call into question the study's ultimate conclusions. Most spine surgeons and trauma centers appear to administer steroids because of the medical-legal issues that may surface if they do not. Unfortunately, this is not a scientifically valid rationale for its routine use, especially if there are concerns that steroids may be actually harming patients. On a more pragmatic note, methylprednisolone has been in short supply in this county, which makes further study to determine its true efficacy even more imperative. At my trauma center, as well as others, we are beginning to discontinue the routine use of methylprednisolone for spinal cord injuries.[3]

Another controversy is related to when to order MRI in patients with possible facet injuries. Eismont[4] first reported on a patient who underwent an open reduction of a facet dislocation and woke up a quadriplegic as a result of a herniated disk that presumably compressed the spinal cord during the reduction. Therefore, given the risk for a disk herniation, routine MRI is advocated by some authors for all patients with facet injuries (fractures and dislocations), regardless of neurologic status prior to any reduction. Others advocate early closed reduction of these injuries without MRI. I believe that MRI provides additional information that may be helpful in managing the patient. Therefore, if time permits and the patient can tolerate MRI, I will obtain it. However, I also believe that MRI is not necessary if complete quadriplegia is the diagnosis, particularly if the patient presents within a few hours of the injury.

Emergent reduction of a facet dislocation in an attempt to relieve pressure on the spinal cord may be more important than obtaining an MRI (ie, leaving the spine unreduced for another 1 to 2 hours) for any chance of motor recovery. If MRI is not feasible, closed reduction with tong traction while the patient is awake is a perfectly acceptable and safe procedure with minimal to no chance of neurologic deterioration. However, I also believe that MRI is absolutely indicated in any patient who cannot undergo reduction while awake and therefore must go to the operating room for a closed or open reduction under general anesthesia. Unfortunately, even after all the appropriate precautions are taken, some patients will have neurologic complications that cannot be totally avoided. Therefore, surgeons must be flexible with their protocols, treating each patient individually depending not only on their knowledge and experience but also on their intuition and gestalt.

In summary, orthopaedic spine surgeons face many challenges in diagnosing and treating patients with cervical spine trauma and spinal cord injury. A thorough assessment in the emergency department and a working algorithm used as a guideline for management (not dogmatic protocol) are necessary to optimize patient care and minimize any further injury. Research into the pathophysiology of spinal cord injury may help find new therapeutic modalities to treat such injuries, and it is apparent that more clinical studies are needed to help to clarify some of the existing controversies.

James D. Kang, MD
Associate Professor of Orthopaedic Surgery
University of Pittsburgh School of Medicine
Pittsburgh, Pennsylvania

References
1. Bracken MD, Shepard JM, Collins WF Jr, et al: A randomized, controlled trial of methylprednisolone or naloxone in the treatment of acute spinal-cord injury: Results of the Second National Acute Spinal Cord Injury Study. *N Engl J Med* 1990;322:1405-1411.
2. Hulbert RJ: The role of steroids in acute spinal cord injury. *Spine* 2001;26:S39-S46.
3. Molloy S, Price M, Casey ATH: Questionnaire survey of the view of the delegates at the European Cervical Spine Research Society meeting on the administration of methylprednisolone for acute traumatic spinal cord injury. *Spine* 2001;26:E562-E564.
4. Eismont FJ, Arena MJ, Green BA: Extrusion of an intervertebral disc associated with traumatic subluxation or dislocation of cervical facets: Case report. *J Bone Joint Surg Am* 1991;73:1555-1560.

The Management of Acute Spinal Trauma: Prehospital and In-Hospital Emergency Care

Alexander R. Vaccaro, MD
Howard S. An, MD
Randal R. Betz, MD
Jerome M. Cotler, MD
Richard A. Balderston, MD

Prehospital Care

There are approximately 200,000 people in the United States presently living with some degree of spinal cord injury (SCI) resulting from trauma.[1,2] Of the 7,800 to 11,000 new cases each year, it is estimated that 4% to 14% of such injuries occur in children younger than 15 years of age, with a male-to-female ratio of 2.4:1.[3-6] The causes of spinal cord trauma in the adult are varied and include motor vehicle accidents (40%), falls (21%), acts of violence (15%), sports related injuries (13%), and miscellaneous.[5] Etiologies for pediatric SCI parallel those in adults, with water-related injuries accounting for 13% of the cases and sports-related injuries composing 24% of cases.

In addition to the presence of SCI, 45% to 50% of patients may present with an associated injury, with 15% and 10% of patients having two or three related injuries, respectively.[7] These may include multiple appendicular skeletal fractures, closed head injury and facial fractures, cardiac and pulmonary contusions, thoracic rib fractures, and blunt abdominal injury, including viscus disruption and genitourinary dysfunction. Thoracolumbar and lumbar spine injuries secondary to lap belt injuries in the pediatric patients demand particular attention.

Retroperitoneal injuries have been reported in 30% to 50% of patients presenting with these spine fractures,[8,9] and neurologic deficits occur in 4% to 39%.[10-12] The variance in neurologic deficits in the reported series can be attributed to whether the authors studied patients at a SCI center or patients were seen at random in an emergency room. Of pediatric spinal cord injuries, 25% to 50% may present with concomitant head trauma. Recognition of this head trauma is important because resulting perceptual, speech, and other associated deficits can significantly affect the rehabilitation process.[13,14] An additional complicating factor in the management of SCI patients is the presence of subtle noncontiguous spinal injuries, which may result in great morbidity if overlooked. Thus, individual patient morbidity is often greater than 100%, with each patient having one or more complications during the treatment phase.[15]

Aside from the substantial morbidity complicating SCI, significant patient mortality exists, is most pronounced during the initial hospitalization and treatment period, and is further increased in the elderly patient population.[16] Approximately 10% of patients die during the first year following their injury, with fulminant pneumonia (80%) being the most frequent cause of patient demise, followed by heart disease and septicemia.[5] Studies have shown that 1-year mortality rates for quadriplegic patients may range from 7.5% to 40%.[15] Also, patients who are older than 50 years of age have been found to have an overall mortality rate of 23% at 1 year following their accident.[17]

The successful long-term treatment of the patient with a SCI is contingent on early recognition of the injury, prompt medical resuscitation, mechanical stabilization of the injury, prevention of additional neurologic injury, and avoidance of complications. Therefore, effective care of the traumatized patient begins with a clear and comprehensive prehospital management protocol delivered by a well-organized emergency medical service working in tandem with an in-hospital multidisciplinary trauma team at a qualified receiving health care center.[7,15,18,19] The goal of in-field care is to maximize the potential for neurologic recovery from the scene of the accident to the time of patient arrival at the emergency room.[20] With the birth of qualified regional SCI centers over the last two decades, the ratio of incomplete to complete spinal cord injuries and normalization of life expectancy after the first year of injury has increased, largely as a result of improved sophistication of prehospital care givers and the birth of modern Emergency Medical Services (EMS) and Emergency Medical Technicians (EMT).[21,22]

Emergency Medical Services (EMS)

The principles of in-field resuscitation and stabilization of the patient with a SCI owe their development to the exposure of the deficiencies of prehospital care by a 1966 paper entitled, "Accidental Death and Disability—The Neglected Disease of Modern Society," released by the National Academy of Sciences National Research Council Committee on Shock and The Committee on Trauma.[21] Prior to this report, no organized means of prehospital care for multiple trauma victims existed in the United States. As a result of lack of suspicion of significant spinal injury and improper immobilization prior to transport, Toscano[20] reported a 26% incidence of major neurologic deterioration from the time of the accident prior to arrival to the emergency ward. Factors associated with a delay in diagnosis in the field include an altered state of consciousness, lack of suspicious soft-tissue injuries above the clavicle, and concurrent head trauma.[22] The awareness of the need for more efficient management of multiple trauma set in motion a series of recommendations on the national level, which eventually led to the passage of the National Highway Safety Act of 1966 and the Emergency Medical Services System Act of 1973 and its amendments in 1976. This legislation led to the development of the Division of Emergency Medical Services (DEMS), whose responsibility included the development of Regional Emergency Medical Service delivery systems. This agency was given the responsibility of creating public safety awareness and education programs, raising manpower and training, and developing effective communication systems, patient transfer mechanisms, and disaster planning to better care for medical emergency and multiple trauma patients, SCI, and burn victims, etc. As a result of these founding goals, the function of the emergency medical services regarding the management of patients with spinal cord injuries is to maintain and potentiate vital organ function, prevent further neurologic injury during transport, and provide rapid transportation to a well-qualified hospital center.[21] Today, despite difficulties with funding on the federal level, strong statewide and local programs continue to provide necessary training and in-field support for trauma care patients.

In-Field Personnel

In general, the initial responders to an injury scene are usually the police or fire services. These first responders are individuals who have been trained in general emergency procedures and have the ability to administer basic medical care, open an airway, and apply pressure to external bleeding sites. More highly trained and certified individuals, referred to as Emergency Medical Technicians-Basic (EMT-B), in addition provide basic life support and have been trained in basic extrication techniques, administration of oxygen, and patient immobilization and transport.[21] An EMT-P (paramedic) is a responder who is defined by attainment of certain educational objectives as opposed to the number of hours of training. The duties of these individuals include advanced life support, endotracheal intubation, intravenous line insertion, and administration of intravenous fluids and medications.[21,23]

The in-field responder, usually consisting of EMS personnel, in addition to providing immediate medical attention to the patient, must also make an immediate in-field assessment as to the security of the surrounding environment. After a determination is made as to the safety of the location for both the patient and the care giver, appropriate support personnel are summoned if necessary. Traffic may need to be averted, live electric wires may need to be controlled, and unruly crowds may have to be contained in order to effectively care for the injured. Concomitant with these responsibilities, an initial primary survey of the patient is conducted. This survey includes assessing the patient's airway patency and ventilation, checking for the presence of a pulse, and determining if the patient is conscious. Suspicion of a head or spinal injury may be derived directly, through communication with the patient, or indirectly, through observation of physical deformities or the mechanism of the injury. Definitive evidence of a potential SCI may exist if there is extremity weakness or paralysis, alteration of sensation, soft-tissue lacerations above the clavicle, tenderness on palpation of the spine, and loss of consciousness.

ABCs of EMS Management (Airway, Breathing, and Circulation)

Initially, the highest priority of medical intervention should be to establish a patent and secure airway.[7] Aside from the necessity of respiration, maintaining a patent airway helps prevent secondary injury to the spinal cord as a result of hypoxemia. Any manipulation of the cervical spine must be minimal to prevent injury to the cervical spinal cord in patients with neck trauma. A gentle chin lift or jaw thrust maneuver may prevent detrimental cervical flexion or extension while maintaining an open airway. Appropriate airway control also prevents aspiration of gastric contents, a leading cause of death in patients with SCI. Prior to their arrival at the hospital, frequent suctioning may be necessary in the event of emesis to avoid this complication. For airway control in an awake patient, a standard cutoff oral airway can be used to maintain an open airway and prevent gagging. Airway management in an unconscious patient requires the use of a standard oratracheal or nasopharyngeal airway. Blinded nasotracheal intubation is a useful method of obtaining an airway while preventing hyperextension in a patient with an unstable cervical spine injury. These intubation techniques are equally safe, as long as all intubations are performed with in-line manual cervical immobilization.[7]

After a functioning airway is obtained, ventilation and, most importantly, oxygenation of the patient with a SCI is monitored. All such patients should be given supplemental oxygen (via mask or bag valve) while ventilating. If oxygenation is not monitored, the physiologic effects of SCI, including a loss of sympathetic tone with resultant neurogenic hypotension and decreased respiratory function, may mask the presence of tissue hypoxemia, a major cause of secondary neuronal injury.[22]

Active exsanguination of the patient with a SCI is managed with direct pressure to tamponade bleeding. Penetrating objects should not be removed from the neck or spine in the field to avoid the risk of excessive bleeding, but they should be managed definitively when appropriate operating room facilities and support personnel are available at the hospital.[15] Venous access must be obtained through the placement of two large 14- or 16-gauge peripheral venous catheters. Fluid resuscitation is commenced with strict attention to the patient's vital signs to prevent the signs of hypovolemia or fluid overload.

In the past, Military AntiShock Trousers (MAST), now called Pneumatic AntiShock Garments (PASG), were used frequently to prevent lower extremity pooling of venous blood by constricting the lower extremity vessels and by increasing peripheral vascular resistance. Use of the PASG also allowed for splinting of lower extremity and pelvic fractures and assisted in circulatory support by tamponading interstitial or retroperitoneal hemorrhaging in these fracture situations. Because of the not-so-infrequent reported side effects of these garments, which can include a detrimental increase in intra-abdominal and skeletal compartment pressures as well as increased peripheral ischemia and intracranial pressure as a result of lactic acid buildup, their use has fallen out of favor in many regional trauma centers. In addition, placement of a PASG may aggravate a neurologic injury if there is lower lumbar spinal instability.

Patient Extrication

Motor Vehicle Accident Before a patient can be extricated from an automobile, appropriate spinal immobilization is necessary to prevent neurologic injury during patient movement. Gentle stabilization in an axial direction is applied while a cervical collar is placed. Current recommendations state that the patient's head should be aligned with the axis of the body and in a neutral position for transport; however, this positioning, especially if forced, may result in further spinal cord compression in patients with specific injury patterns such as a cervical dislocation.[23] As a rule, patients should not be forced into a position that results in undue pain or results in a deformity different from their primary posture.[15] Great care must be afforded in the movement of unconscious patients, because 5% to 10% of these patients may have a significant cervical spine injury.[7] It is safest to assume the presence of SCI until proven otherwise.

Patient Immobilization The safest means of patient immobilization is to secure the patient in the supine position on a firm, rigid spine board that extends from the top of the head to the bottom of the buttocks, preferably one that also includes both lower extremities. Various means of patient transfer to a spine board have been investigated, including log-rolling techniques, the four-man lift, or a scoop stretcher, if one is available.[5] A cervical collar should be in place, and it should be one that is light and easily applied.[24] Cervical collars with an opening in the front are preferable for evaluation of tracheal deviation (in the case of tension pneumothorax) or to perform an emergent cricothyroidotomy if necessary.[21] The patient should be secured to the spine board by strapping of the forehead, thorax, and extremities. The chin should not be taped as the sole point for control of the head. In adults, occipital padding may be necessary to place the head in a neutral position as a result of the large trunk-to-head size ratio. In children, however, an occipital recess is usually necessary, to allow the head and neck to be in extension. In children up to 6 years of age, the head is disproportionately large in comparison to the torso, and placing the child flat on a spine board may flex the spine. Placement of a pad behind the child's shoulders and back should allow the cervical spine to be positioned in neutral.[25] Cervical and head side supports attached to the spine board, preferably with Velcro, further stabilize the cervical spine. Unsupported sand bags should not be used, because they can shift during transport and cause a loss in cervical spinal alignment.[21] Cervical traction should not be applied with free weights because they can cause overdistraction during acceleration of the transport vehicle. The principles of spinal immobilization are the same regardless of the setting. In cases of water trauma, patients should be floated flat on their back with the rescuers' hands supporting the victim's head, neck, and spine. The patient is then brought to the edge of the water and slowly floated onto a spine board, which is placed beneath the patient. In a helmeted patient, the patient is securely immobilized on a spine board without removing the helmet in the field, unless the patient's airway is threatened. In the case of a football injury, the shoulder pads should be left in place in order to maintain neutral spinal alignment. The mask or face shell may be removed in the field or in the emergency department, whenever the appropriate tools are present. The helmet shell may then be removed with the help of an assistant to immobilize the neck.

Transportation

If possible, patients should be transported safely to facilities that are equipped to provide a definitive contemporary standard of care.[26] Extra time during transport may be in the patient's best interest, if the patient's vital signs are stable, in order to bring a patient to a registered SCI center. The patient should be transported in the Trendelenburg position (20° to 40°) to maximize cardiovascular function and to avoid gastric aspiration. The feet forward position is the safest, especially in cases of frequent stops, to avoid undue harm to the patient with a cervical spine injury. As stated previously, the goal is to transfer a viable patient from the area of trauma to an emergency room with all systems stabilized in order to enhance the potential for maximal neurologic recovery. The choice of transport vehicle is largely determined by distance, but the patient's vital signs, traffic conditions, and the proximity of a suitable accepting institution must also be considered. In general, for distances less than 50 miles (81 km), an ambulance may be used for transportation; for distances between 51 and 150 miles (81 and 242 km) and during peak traffic for severe injuries, a helicopter; and for distances greater than 150 miles (242 km), a fixed-wing aircraft is useful.[22]

Emergency Room Evaluation

On arrival at the emergency room, a multisystem evaluation is again performed following resurveillance of the basic ABCs of trauma care (Airway, Breathing, and Circulation). A multidisciplinary team approach has been proven to be most effective in the definitive care of the patient with a SCI. Team members include the traumatologist or general surgeon, the orthopaedist, the neurosurgeon, the physiatrist, emergency room personnel, the anesthesiologist, and trained nursing and respiratory personnel. The initial goals are to normalize the patient's vital signs, administer oxygen and appropriate pharmacologic agents, and establish normal spine alignment. The presence of adequate airway patency and ventilation is monitored through arterial blood gases and pulse oximetry. Initially, patients with evidence of a SCI are administered a 40% oxygen humidity mask with a target PaO_2 of 100 torr and a $PaCO_2$ of less than 45 torr.[22] Patients with vital capacities less than 10 mL/kg or $PaO_2/PaCO_2$ ratios < 0.75 should be considered for semiurgent intubation.[7] Following this, appropriate laboratory studies are done, and a large-bore sump nasogastric tube is placed, if not already present, to decompress the stomach as well as to monitor gastric pH and provide a route of administration for antacids. A Foley catheter, again if not already present, is inserted to obtain a sample of urine as well as to monitor urine output and relieve pressure on a hypotense bladder.[26] If the patient presents with an open spinal wound, prophylactic wide-spectrum antibiotics and tetanus prophylaxis should be administered.

The Presence of Hypotension in the Patient With a SCI

During the initial evaluation and monitoring of the patient with a SCI, hypotension caused by either hypovolemia or autonomic dysfunction may be present.[4] It is important to differentiate between these two causes of hypotension, because they are managed differently. Neurogenic shock may be present in injuries above the T6 level, caused by disruption of descending sympathetic pathways with loss of the sympathetic inhibition of the parasympathetic effect of the vagus nerve. This leads to a loss of peripheral sympathetic tone, with increased vessel capacitance, lower extremity venous stasis, and decreased central venous return, resulting in hypotension, often accompanied by hypothermia.[7,22] This is usually accompanied by an increased cardiac output. Patients in neurogenic shock are hypotensive in the presence of bradycardia (pulse rate less than 60), unlike the patient in hypovolemic shock, who presents with a relative tachycardia in the setting of hypotension. In the setting of hemorrhagic shock, the patient's pulse is rapid and irregular; in neurogenic shock, the pulse is usually slow and regular.[22] The presence of hypotension should never be attributed to neurogenic shock in the patient with a spinal injury until occult internal hemorrhage has been ruled out. The treatment of neurogenic shock is similar to the initial resuscitation of hypovolemic shock, except that fluid replacement proceeds in a judicious manner to avoid fluid overload. Initially, these patients are relatively hypovolemic due to loss of peripheral vascular tone, and intravenous fluids resuscitation proceeds expediently. In addition to intravenous fluid replacement, the patient is initially placed in the Trendelenburg position (20° to 40°) to facilitate the central return of venous blood. This is followed, if necessary, by the administration of intravenous atropine (0.4 mg), used for its vagolytic effect, and cardiac pressors (dopamine), to increase peripheral vascular tone and cardiac output. Temporary cardiac pacing is rarely needed,[7] but fluid volume should be followed closely with the placement of a Swan-Ganz catheter.

History and Physical

Following the initial resuscitative phase, a complete history of the mechanism of injury and any prior history of spinal pathology, ie, a known diagnosis of ankylosing spondylitis, kyphoscoliosis, or pre-existing central nervous system dysfunction, is obtained from the patient, family members, or emergency medical personnel.[4,15] The pre-injury neurologic status of the patient is invaluable to determine if any worsening of neurologic function has occurred as the result of the present injury. Also, record any change in the patient's clinical status that has occurred since the initial evaluation. Following the recording of an accurate history, the entire spine should be palpated in search of evidence of injury, including ecchymosis, an abrupt spinal step off, or spine tenderness. If a well-padded rotating bed is available, the patient should be placed on it to decrease the potential for sacral or heel ulcer formation, as well as to avoid further neurologic aggravation from repeated log rolling maneuver during patient care.[26]

The neurologic examination is performed with careful attention to the recording of accurate sensory and motor levels to determine the precise neurologic level of injury. In addition, cranial nerve function must be assessed as well as rectal tone and reflexes. There are 28 dermatomes in the sensory evaluation and 10 myotomes in the motor evaluation.[27] Muscle strength is graded on a 6-point scale: 0 for paralysis, 1 for palpable or visible contractions, 2 for active range of motion with gravity eliminated, 3 for active range of motion against gravity, 4 for active range of motion against moderate resistance, and 5 for active range of motion against full resistance. It should be remembered that children have different motor strengths, and what may be a motor strength of 5 in an adult may not be the same in a child. The sensory examination is determined by evaluation of pin prick and light touch for both sides of the body. There is a 3-point rating scale: 0 for absent, 1 for impaired, and 2 for normal, plus NT for not testable. Together, the numeric results of these tests determine the motor and sensory scores respectively. The presence of motor or pin prick sensation in the S4-S5 distribution carries a favorable prognosis for ambulation, unlike situations in which evidence of sacral sparing is absent after the resolution of spinal shock.

The ASIA (American Spinal Injury Association) impairment scale replaces the modified Frankel classification to which it is similar in many ways. A stands for a complete SCI with no sensory or motor function distal to the level of injury; B represents an incomplete SCI with preservation of sensation, but no motor function distal to the level of injury; C represents an incomplete SCI with motor function present below the level of injury with a motor grade of 3 or less; D represents an incomplete SCI with motor preservation greater than grade 3 below the level of injury, and E represents a normal neurologic examination.[27] In the zone of partial preservation, there are dermatomes or myotomes distal to the level of neurologic injury that remain partially innervated. This information should be recorded in patients with complete cord injuries.

Pathophysiology of SCI

Researchers have attempted to halt or reverse the secondary mechanisms of tissue injury after SCI by influencing the pathophysiologic consequence of tissue hypoxia. The most promising research, in animal models, has shown that only high-dose steroids and gangliosides were of benefit in prospective, randomized, placebo-controlled studies. To understand the potential effectiveness of the various agents being investigated, an overview of the pathophysiology of SCI is necessary.

Beginning with the initial insult, a cascading series of events occur related to both the disruption of blood flow and direct injury to the neuronal membrane. With a decrease in oxygen tension, local tissue metabolism switches from an aerobic to an anaerobic state, with a resultant decrease in local stores of adenosine triphosphate (ATP).[5,22,28] This, along with an increase in tissue lactic acid, and a decrease in intracellular pH, leads to the disruption of Ca^{+2}-dependent K^+ and Na^+ adenosine triphosphatase (ATPase), resulting in an influx of intracellular Ca^{+2} and an efflux of extracellular K^+. Rapid calcium accumulation within the cell causes dysfunction of Ca^{+2}-dependent mitochondrial electron transport, which uncouples oxidative phosphorylation and further depletes ATP stores. Destructive Ca^{+2}-dependent intracellular enzymes are activated, including phospholipases and various neutral proteinases, and this leads to neuronal and neurologic destruction.[5,22,28] In addition, there is a local increase in excitatory amino acid neurotransmitter (glutamate and aspartate), which also contributes to an increase in intracellular Ca^{+2} through specific activated ion channels. The activation of phospholipase A_2 leads, through enzymatic lipid hydrolysis, to the release of various membrane phospholipids, including arachidonic acid and other fatty acids, which are actively metabolized into various eicosanoids, including prostaglandins E_2 and $F_{2\alpha}$, prostacyclins, thromboxanes, leukotrienes, and various free radicals.[3] Specific leukotrienes and prostacyclins, in association with kinins and serotonin, all contribute to an increase in vascular permeability and endothelial wall disruption, leading to edema, polymorphonuclear cell infiltration, vessel thrombosis, and destruction of local neural tissue. The metabolites culminate in cellular destruction, inhibiting neurofilament release and promoting vascular constriction and the release of destructive lysosomes.[5,22,28]

With disruption of Ca^{+2}-dependent mitochondrial electron transport, destructive free radicals are produced, including superoxide anions, hydroxyl radicals, and hydrogen peroxide, which also break down cell membranes.[28] This process of oxidative degradation is referred to as free radical-induced lipid peroxidation and is evidenced by loss of membrane cholesterol with an increase in its auto-oxidation products (ie, 25-hydroxycholesterol) and with a concurrent decrease in tissue vitamin E. Free radicals are also generated from the breakdown of hemorrhagic products through the dislocation or decompartmentalization of intracellular iron complexes from blood components resulting in the release of hemoproteins and ferrous ions. The efflux of K+ itself results in membrane depolarization effectively blocking neurotransmissions.[5,22,28]

On a pathoanatomic level, the initial insult to the spinal cord is followed by the immediate (within minutes to hours) formation of small petechial hemorrhages. Caused by disruption of the microvasculature, these first appear in the central gray matter with eventual centrifugal spread into the surrounding white matter.[5,22] The endothelial lining of the spinal cord microvasculature is disrupted, which allows the deposition of platelets. Eventually, thrombi form and these contribute to further tissue ischemia and loss of vascular autoregulation. The small hemorrhagic foci eventually coalesce into a larger area of central necrosis. Contributing to the destruction of nervous tissue is the extravasation of polymorphonuclear leukocytes into the site of injury and subsequent phagocytosis.[5,22] Within the first few days, vasogenic edema progresses and is identified for up to 2 weeks after the initial insult.[5,22,28]

After 5 to 6 days, hemorrhagic debris is reabsorbed through phagocytosis. Activated glial cells deposit astrophytic fibers, which results in the formation, over the ensuing 3 to 6 months, of scar tissue or extensive gliosis as the result of wallerian degeneration of fiber tracts.[5,22,28]

Drug Therapy

The goal of drug treatment is to minimize the deleterious effects of secondary injury that occur as a result of neuronal hypoxemia and cellular dysfunction. The administration of steroids within 8 hours of SCI is now standard in all trauma centers. The dose of methylprednisolone is 30 mg/kg, given over 15 minutes, followed by a 5.4 mg/kg per hour dosage over 24 hours. The relative contraindications to the use of steroids include any patient with penetrating wounds, pregnancy, patients younger than 13 years of age, and patients with infection or diabetes. Steroid treatment aids neurologic recovery by increasing blood flow to the injured central nervous system, thereby increasing perfusion to the white matter. In addition, steroids reduce edema and inflammation, and they scavenge for oxygen free radicals. Importantly, this drug therapy suppresses the breakdown of cell membranes by inhibiting lipid peroxidation and hydrolysis at the site of injury, thus decreasing the extracellular calcium level. Phase 2 of the National Acute Spinal Cord Injury Study (NASCIS 2) noted the superiority of methylprednisolone over naloxone (an opiate antagonist).[4,22,28-31] In addition, it was noted that if steroids were given within less than 8 hours after SCI, motor scores as well as sensation to pin prick and light touch improved, both in patients with complete and those with incomplete injuries. Very little has been reported on injury modulation in children. Although most treating physicians use methylprednisolone in pediatric SCI, it should be noted that only 15% of the patients in the study by Bracken and associates[29] were aged 13 to 19 years, and the study included no data on patients younger than 13 years. Contrary to these findings, other studies have failed to show an improvement in neurologic function after high dose steroid use.[32]

In addition to steroids, GM-1 gangliosides have also been found useful in the treatment of patients with spinal cord injuries.[33,34] These drugs are complex acidic glycolipids found naturally in cells of the central nervous system. The mechanism of improvement is postulated to be related to an increased axonal survival rate at the site of injury. GM-1 gangliosides are also neurotopic, decrease retrograde neurologic degeneration, and modulate excitatory amino acid endotoxicity and destructive cell membrane enzymatic activity. In addition, these drugs may also reduce the anti-inflammatory effects of high-dose methylprednisolone, effects that can complicate their use when they are given with steroids.[22] Physicians should be aware that separate reports of acute motor neuropathy presenting as Guillain-Barré Syndrome have been noted as soon as 2 weeks after treatment with this drug.[35]

Oxygen free radical scavengers are also being investigated in the treatment of patients with spinal cord injuries. Vitamin E (alpha tocopherol), which functions as an antioxidant and phospholipid membrane stabilizer, and 21 amino steroids, a group of methylprednisolone analogs with antioxidant properties, are examples of extensively studied free radical scavengers. Tirilizad mesylate (U74006F), a 21 amino steroid drug, is currently in a phase-two clinical study, along with extended dose methylprednisolone therapy (48 versus 24 hours), as part of the NASCIS 3 study.

Potassium channel blocking agents, such as 4-aminopyridine (4-AP) are used to overcome the conduction blockades (Na/K ATPase disruption) that occur during the demyelination process in patients with spinal cord injuries.

Naloxone, an opiate receptor antagonist, has been used in the past for the initial treatment of patients with spinal cord injuries. As mentioned previously, no benefit was noted in the NASCIS 2 study. Still, studies indicate that high dosages of naloxone may benefit patients.[32] Naloxone increases spinal cord blood flow by blocking endogenous spinal cord opioid release and the associated systemic hypotension. Thyroid-releasing hormone (TRH), a partial opiate receptor antagonist, may also have the same effects as naloxone, while preserving the analgesic effects of endogenous opioids.[4,5]

Thromboxane inhibitors may increase spinal cord blood flow by reversing or preventing the vasoconstricting effects of thromboxane. The activation of phospholipase as a result of the cascade of SCI releases free fatty acids and arachidonic acid. These substances are metabolized to eicosanoid metabolites such as prostaglandins, thromboxanes, and leukotrienes. Thromboxanes are noted to deleteriously reduce the degree of spinal cord blood flow.

Ca^{+2} channel blockers, considered antihypertensive agents, may be useful in decreasing the post-injury influx of Ca^{+2} that occurs with membrane and enzymatic destabilization. Osmotic diuretics, including mannitol, glycerol, and low-molecular-weight dextran, have also been tried with varying success to decrease post-traumatic spinal cord edema and ischemia. Dimethylsulfoxide (DMSO), also a diuretic agent, contributes to membrane stabilization through free radical scavenging in addition to its anti-inflammatory and vasodilating properties.[4,5]

Medical Therapy

Aside from pharmacologic treatments, other medical modalities are being tested for patient care.[22] Decreasing the spinal cord temperature decreases the metabolic activity and oxygen requirements of the cord, thereby decreasing edema, hemorrhage, and local inflammatory processes. The effects of hypothermia have been reported in animal studies but have not been documented in humans. Direct current fields and functional electrical stimulation may assist in central nervous system fiber tract regeneration. Extracellular matrices are being investigated as a potential spatial framework for axonal migration. Finally, the transplantation of fetal tissues, as witnessed in the canine model, may provide function to compromised spinal cord tissue.

Spinal Imaging

The primary goal in the management of patients with spinal injuries with or without neural deficits is to realign the spinal elements in a position that will relieve abnormal pressure on the neural ele-

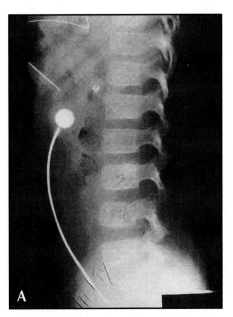
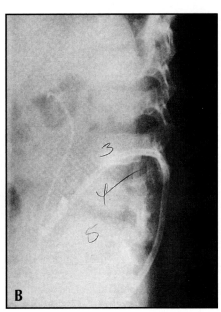

Fig. 1 A, Lateral lumbar radiograph of a 4-year-old who was involved in a motor vehicle accident. She was in a lap belt in the back seat at the time of impact. She was hemodynamically unstable and was rushed to the operating room for repair of retroperitoneal lacerations. The lateral radiograph shows some suggestion of injury at L3-4. **B,** Lateral radiograph of the same patient 24 hours after the first film was taken. Despite careful attempts at positioning this child because of suspected spinal injury, the fracture displaced further. This flexion-distraction injury was then stabilized using posterior interspinous wiring between L3 and L4.

ments. This process begins in the emergency ward with radiographic documentation of the primary and secondary spinal lesions through anteroposterior and lateral plain radiographs of the entire space, including an odontoid view. Patients who are barrel-chested or have a short, wide neck may require arm traction or a swimmer's view to document the cervicothoracic junction. If this area cannot be documented by plain films, a computed tomographic (CT) scan with sagittal reconstruction may be obtained. A coronal CT reconstruction of the odontoid is useful in patients who are intubated and cannot provide an open mouth view of this region. Tomography may be extremely useful in documenting a transverse fracture of the odontoid or subtle lateral mass fractures. Such fractures may be missed on computed tomography, either because of the slice thickness of image or because the imaging is outside the plane of fracture.

In the pediatric patient with a known lap belt injury, the spine must be carefully evaluated radiographically, preferably before the patient is taken to the operating room. The flexion-distraction spine fracture secondary to a lap belt injury must be diagnosed on a plain radiograph. This fracture is extremely difficult to diagnose on CT scan, because the plane of the distraction of the spine injury is the same as the axial CT cut.[36] If the spine cannot be evaluated radiographically because the patient is unstable hemodynamically, it should be assumed that a fracture is present until it is determined that it is not. Cases have been reported in which children who were previously neurologically intact have awakened paralyzed after an abdominal procedure. In such cases, the paralysis probably occurred during manipulation on the operating room table (Fig. 1). Oblique radiographs are helpful to confirm or rule out a facet or uncinate process fracture. In the neurologically in-

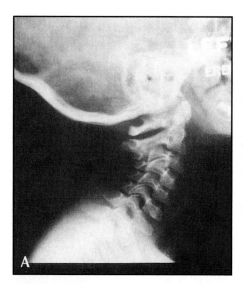

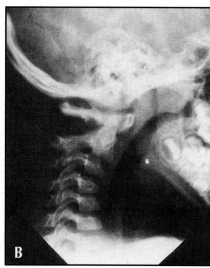

Fig. 2 A, Lateral extension radiograph of the cervical spine. **B,** Lateral flexion radiograph shows pseudosubluxation of the anterior vertebral body of C2-C3. The posterior intralaminar line (Line of Swichuk) is intact.

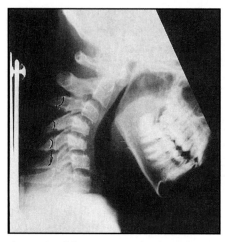

Fig. 3 Lateral flexion cervical radiograph shows subluxation after C3-C4. Posterior interlaminar line is disrupted to confirm that this is true instability.

tact but symptomatic patient (one with neck pain), flexion and extension lateral plain radiographs are deferred until cervical paraspinal muscle spasm subsides in order not to mask subtle instability patterns obscured by muscular guarding.

Careful scrutiny of the plain radiographs with a knowledge of normal radiologic skeletal relationships allows the treating physician to infer the primary and secondary force vectors of injury and to determine which anatomic structures are disrupted. A flexion force resulting in spinal injury will manifest as widening of the interspinous, interlaminar, and facet joint spaces with or without evidence of vertebral body subluxation or dislocation. The vertebral body may show evidence of asymmetric loss of height. On a lateral radiograph, compression is greater anteriorly than posteriorly, with associated loss of subadjacent disk space height.

An extension injury may reveal widening of the disk space anteriorly with or without a bony avulsion fracture. There may be evidence of retrolisthesis of the proximal vertebral body on the subadjacent vertebral body with bony failure of the posterior elements, including the pars interarticularis, lamina, or spinous process. A rotational injury will manifest as malalignment of the spinal column on an anteroposterior or lateral view. Above the level of injury, the spine appears to be out of plane from the spinal elements below the level of injury. Associated fractures or soft-tissue disruption may be present with this injury mechanism. A shear force is manifested as a displacement of the spinal elements at the level of injury in the direction of force application (horizontal with or without rotation), with complete disruption of the bony and soft-tissue elements at the level of injury.

Abnormal soft-tissue relationships, especially swelling in the paravertebral region, must be scrutinized, as they may be the only indication of a subtle vertebral body injury. During the radiographic assessment of the child, it is necessary to keep normal radiographic variants in mind. Pseudosubluxation of C2 on C3 is troublesome when seen on initial evaluation in the emergency room, especially in a child who may have sustained neck trauma. If the posterior intralaminar line is not displaced, the pseudosubluxation seen is a normal variant[37] (Fig. 2). If the line is disrupted, it is pathologic (Fig. 3). Radiographs of the cranium may be necessary when head trauma is present in order to avoid missing a skull defect at the site of anticipated skeletal tong placement.

If a spinal lesion is identified, the treating physician must decide whether to pursue more advanced imaging studies, such as MRI, to exclude soft-tissue encroachment on the neural elements or to proceed immediately with attempted spinal realignment through closed traction techniques in the emergency ward. Eismont and associates[38] recommend using MRI before attempting closed reduction, because a high incidence of disk herniation is associated with cervical dislocations, and therefore there is a potential for neurologic worsening as a result of further spinal cord compression with cervical manipulation. A review of the case reports in which neurologic injury was associated with a closed reduction reveals that the reductions were performed under general anesthesia. On the other hand, if the reduction is performed in awake and alert patients, closed reduction is highly successful without reported neurologic complications.[39,40] Therefore,

MRI is not mandatory prior to attempted closed reduction in appropriately selected patients. MRI is recommended in obtunded patients, those cases in which neurologic function deteriorates temporarily while adding weights during attempted closed reduction, and in any patient requiring open reduction. In all patients, MRI should be obtained after closed reduction is accomplished to rule out spinal cord compression by a herniated disk. If a herniated disk is found, anterior decompression should precede any posterior instrumentation or any attempt at reduction under general anesthesia.

Once patients are stabilized in the emergency ward, advanced spinal imaging such as MRI or CT scanning may be obtained if necessary. Flanders and associates[41] have documented, through MRI, that disk herniations of varying degrees occur in cervical dislocations and fracture subluxations 30% to 50% of the time. An interesting benefit of noninvasive MRI technology is the ability to evaluate the integrity of the extracranial circulation with MRI angiography. We prospectively evaluated 60 patients with cervical spine injuries at Thomas Jefferson University and identified 12 patients (20%) with vertebral artery disruptions. The clinical significance of these injuries is unclear, because only three of the patients manifested symptoms of vertebral artery insufficiency.

MRI following pediatric SCI can show problems not visible on plain radiographs. MRI also can be beneficial in delineating spinal column injury in difficult-to-see areas such as C7-T1 (Fig. 4).[42] SCIWORA (SCI without radiographic abnormality) has been reported in 10% to 20% of children with SCI.[43-46] In very young children (3 to 4 years of age), the association of SCIWORA with a Chiari malformation has been reported.[47] It is important to recognize the Chiari malformation because decompression of C1 and the foramen magnum has been reported to help with some recovery of

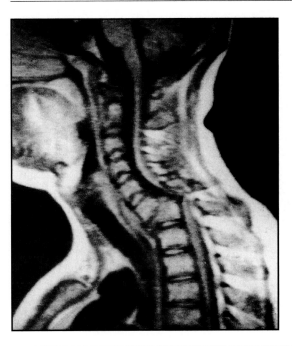

Fig. 4 Sagittal cervical magnetic resonance image of a football player with a T7 complete spinal cord injury. Radiographs were indeterminate in defining the spinal column injury.

function, especially when the lesion is incomplete. Growth plate injuries may be seen on MRI that may not be visible on plain radiographs, and any external dural compression caused by the fragments may be relieved by removing them.[48-50]

Technique of Closed Cervical Reduction for Cervical Facet Dislocations

The goals of closed cervical reduction are to restore anatomic alignment of the spine, thereby restoring the space for the spinal cord. In order to maximize neurologic recovery, closed reduction is performed as quickly and safely as possible, usually within 2 to 3 hours after the patient is brought to the emergency room.

Following the general trauma evaluation, the patient is placed in the supine position on a Stryker frame (Stryker Corp, Kalamazoo, MI). Gardner-Wells tongs (Zimmer, Inc, Warsaw, IN) are usually applied without removing the patient's hair. The areas are thoroughly prepped, and tongs are inserted using local anesthesia. For straight traction, pins are inserted 1 cm superior to the middle of the pinna of the ear. The pins

should be tightened until the pressure indicator protrudes 1 mm. For a flexion moment, pins may be inserted slightly posterior to the pinna. A further flexion moment may be added by removing the bed springs caudal to the injury. If an extension moment is desired, the pins may be inserted slightly anterior to the pinna. A small pad may be placed under the upper back between the scapulae if more extension of the neck is needed. The mean pull-out strength of stainless steel Gardner-Wells tongs is up to 300 lb, whereas MRI-compatible titanium tongs fail at an average of 75 lb.[51] For this reason, stainless steel tongs are recommended for closed reduction, particularly if high weight reduction is anticipated.

The initial amount of traction applied should be 10 lb, to rule out upper cervical spine injuries. Weight is added sequentially, in 10 lb increments every 10 or 15 minutes, until reduction is obtained. Immediately after each application of weight, a neurologic examination is performed and a lateral radiograph is obtained. As weight exceeds 50 lb, the Stryker bed should be placed in a reverse Trendelenburg position to provide some

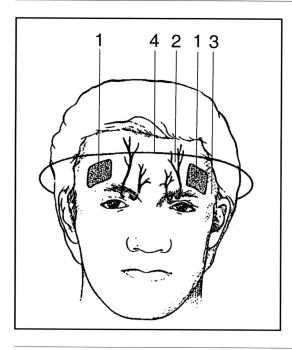

Fig. 5 (1) Safety zones for the anterior pin sites. **(2)** Medially, over the medial one third of the orbit are the supraorbital and supratrochlear nerves and artery. **(3)** The temporal fossa has very thin bone, which should be avoided. **(4)** The pins are inserted below the equator line or the largest circumference of the skull. (Reproduced with permission from Mubarak SJ, Camp JF, Vuletich W, et al: Halo application in the infant. *J Pediatr Orthop* 1989;9:612-614.)

Table 1
Ten steps of halo vest application in the adult patient

1. Have patient lie supine over the edge of the table or bed.

2. Determine the correct ring and vest size. The ring is placed about 1 cm above the ears, and the anterior ring is slightly more cephalad than the posterior ring so that the head is slightly extended. The ring of the halo should be inferior to the equator or widest diameter of the skull.

3. Identify the pin site locations by holding the ring in place. A 3 cm by 3 cm hair trim, shave, and prep is carried out just superior and posterior to the ear. The halo ring is positioned, using temporary positioning posts.

4. Prepare pin sites with povidone-iodine solution and 1% lidocaine. Approximately 5 mL is injected down to and including the periosteum of the skull.

5. Insert the pins and tighten to 8 in/lb at 2 in/lb increments.

6. Apply the posterior vest first by log rolling or raising the patient's trunk to 30°.

7. Apply the anterior vest and connect it to the posterior vest.

8. Apply four upright posts and tighten linkages.

9. Obtain cervical spine radiographs to check reduction and alignment.

10. Retighten the pins to 8 in/lb and recheck all nuts and screws 24 hours later.

countertraction. Up to 140 lb of traction can be used to reduce dislocations in awake and cooperative patients.[39] Once the facets have been unlocked, reduction usually occurs spontaneously. When the tips of the facets are perched, a gentle manual reduction maneuver may help reduction. Once reduction is confirmed with a lateral radiograph, 10 to 15 lb of traction is retained to maintain reduction.

In 200 consecutive patients, this technique of closed reduction was successful in approximately 90% of cases with no permanent worsening or progressive neurologic deficit.[52] Even if complete reduction is not achieved, at least the canal's volume has been increased and a significant degree of cord decompression obtained. After the closed reduction, the patient may undergo surgery while still in

traction or a halo vest may be applied.

Cervical traction in children younger than 12 years of age is associated with greater risk than in adults, and primary halo traction may be preferred. Martinez-Lage and associates[53] reported dural leaks with Crutchfield tongs in patients younger than 12 years.

Halo Vest Application
The advantages of preoperative halo vest immobilization include increased ease and safety of patient transfer and transport, improved pulmonary care, and facilitation of MRI. At surgery, either the anterior or posterior bars of the halo vest may be taped to the Stryker frame and the opposite vest and bars removed for either an anterior or posterior cervical approach.

Additionally, the halo vest may be used for nonoperative management in patients with C1 fractures (Jefferson's fracture), C2 hangman's fractures, odontoid fractures, stable compression fractures, axial loading burst fractures, and flexion-compression fractures with minimal ligamentous disruption in the absence of a neurologic deficit. The halo vest is frequently used for adjunctive support following surgical stabilization with nonrigid internal fixation as in long segment anterior cervical corpectomies and plating or posterior wiring procedures for the upper and lower cervical spine.

There are many varieties of Halo rings and vests available on the market (Table 1). A posteriorly opened ring gives surgical access to the occiput and upper cervical spine and is easy to apply with the patient in the supine position. Lightweight and MRI-compatible rings are preferred. Appropriate pin site placement is crucial. Anterior pins are placed anterolaterally approximately 1 cm above the orbital rim, below the equator of the skull and cephalad to the lateral two thirds of the orbit (Fig. 5). Posterior pins should be directly opposite the anterior pins. Anterior pins should be tightened

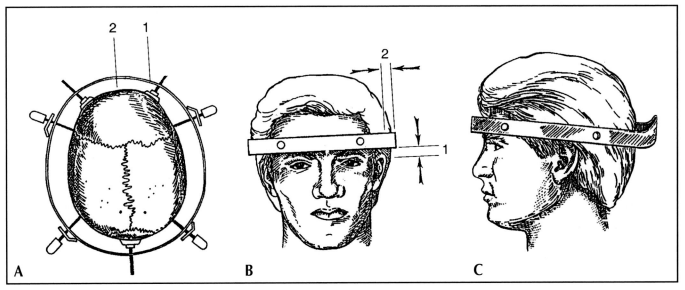

Fig. 6 Proper positioning of the halo ring. **A, (1)** Top view showing the ring with 1 cm clearance around the circumference of the skull. **(2)** Temporary positioning posts. **B, (1)** Front view showing the ring about 1 cm above the ear and eyebrows and **(2)** 1 cm clearance from the skull. **C,** The ring is placed about 1 cm above the ears, and the anterior ring is slightly more cephalad than the posterior ring so that the head is slightly extended. The ring of the halo should be inferior to the equator or widest diameter of the skull.

with the patient's eyes closed. Structures that are at risk anteriorly during pin placement include the frontal sinus, which usually is located centrally cephalad to the bridge of the nose but which can extend to a variable extent above the medial aspect of the orbit.[54] Medially, over the medial one third of the orbit are the supraorbital and supratrochlear nerves and artery. Laterally, cephalad to the orbital ridge and eyebrow over the lateral one half of the orbit, there are no significant structures and, therefore, this is the optimum location for pin placement. The temporal fossa has very thin bone that may fracture or be penetrated by a pin that is too tightly torqued. Additionally, muscles of mastication are located in the temporal fossa. Posterior to the temporal fossa there are no significant anatomic structures of risk and this area is an acceptable alternative pin placement site (Fig. 6). The torque of insertion should be 8 in/lb, applied at increments of 2 in/lb with opposite pins being tightened alternatively.[54] Pins should be retightened once to 8 in/lb at 24 hours

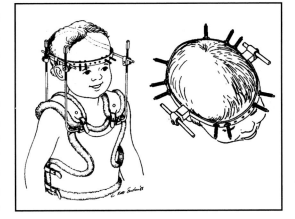

Fig. 7 Schematic of halo placement in an infant. Note the increased number of pins from 4 to 8 or 10. Use 2 lb/in of torque instead of 8. (Reproduced with permission from Mubarak SJ, Camp JE, Vuletich W, et al: Halo application in the infant. *J Pediatr Orthop* 1989;9:612-614.)

later. Following halo ring application, a well-fitting vest is applied. The posterior vest is applied first by log rolling or raising the patient's trunk to 30°. The connection mechanism between the halo ring and upright posts may allow for additional flexion-extension, anterior-posterior translation, or compression-traction manipulation. Halo fixators can safely be used in children,[55] but the number of pins must be increased to 8 or 10 and the torques reduced to 2 lb instead of 8. If standard halo rings are used, addi-

tional holes must be drilled in them (Fig. 7).[56,57] For children younger than 6 years of age, CT scans of the head are recommended to help determine the best pin sites.[58,59] Should the halo become loose, or if for some reason it cannot be applied, a Minerva type of cervicothoraco-lumbosacral orthosis (CTLSO) may be an option.

In conclusion, successful management of the patient with a SCI requires a multidisciplinary team approach beginning with an organized emergency medical service and effective utilization of regional centers that specialize in the care of these devastating injuries. As further research defines the precise pathophysiology of acute SCI as well as reinjury from the secondary byproducts of tissue dysfunction, more selective pharmacologic and physical modulations may be chosen to improve the overall neurologic prognosis. It is imperative that patients with spinal injury be immobilized and stabilized as quickly and safely as possible in order to maximize their neurologic function and rehabilitation.

References

1. DeVivo MJ, Fine PR, Maetz HM, et al: Prevalence of SCI: A reestimation employing life table techniques. *Arch Neurol* 1980;37:707-708.

2. Harvey C, Rothschild BB, Asmann AJ, et al: New estimates of traumatic SCI prevalence: A survey-based approach. *Paraplegia* 1990;28:537-544.

3. Burke DC: Injuries of the spinal cord in children, in Vinken PJ, Bruyn GW, Braakman R, et al (eds): *Handbook of Clinical Neurology: Injuries of the Spine and Spinal Cord. Part 1*. Amsterdam, The Netherlands, North Holland Publishing, 1976, vol 25, pp 175-195.

4. Maroon JC, Abla AA: Classification of acute spinal cord injury, neurological evaluation, and neurosurgical considerations. *Crit Care Clin* 1987;3:655-677.

5. Sonntag VK, Douglas RA: Management of spinal cord trauma. *Neurosurg Clin North Am* 1990;1:729-750.

6. Kewalramani LS, Taylor RG: Multiple noncontiguous injuries to the spine. *Acta Orthop Scand* 1976;47:52-58.

7. Cohen M: Initial resuscitation of the patient with spinal cord injury. *Trauma Quarterly* 1993;9:38-43.

8. Glassman SD, Johnson JR, Holt RT: Seatbelt injuries in children. *J Trauma* 1992;33:882-886.

9. Rumball K, Jarvis J: Seat-belt injuries of the spine in young children. *J Bone Joint Surg* 1992;74B:571-574.

10. Gumley G, Taylor TK, Ryan MD: Distraction fractures of the lumbar spine. *J Bone Joint Surg* 1982;64B:520-525.

11. Rizzolo SJ, Piazza MR, Cotler JM, et al: Intervertebral disc injury complicating cervical spine trauma. *Spine* 1991;16(suppl 6):S187-S189.

12. Womack MS, Kehl DK, Baggett A, et al: Pediatric spine injuries associated with lap seat belts. Proceedings of the American Academy of Orthopaedic Surgeons 60th Annual Meeting, San Francisco, CA. Rosemont, IL, American Academy of Orthopaedic Surgeons, 1993, p 140.

13. Desmond, J: Paraplegia: Problems confronting the anaesthesiologist. *Can Anaesth Soc J* 1970;17:435-451.

14. Nand S, Goldschmidt JW: Abstract: Hypercalcemia and hyperuricemia in young patients with spinal cord injury. *Arch Phys Med Rehabil* 1976;57:553.

15. Green BA, Eismont FJ, O'Heir JT: Spinal cord injury: A systems approach. Prevention, emergency medical services, and emergency room management. *Crit Care Clin* 1987;3:471-493.

16. Spivak JM, Weiss MA, Cotler JM, et al: Cervical spine injuries in patients 65 and older. *Spine* 1994;19:2302-2306.

17. Alander DH, Andreychik DA, Stauffer ES: Early outcome in cervical spinal cord injured patients older than 50 years of age. *Spine* 1994;19:2299-2301.

18. Green BA, Eismont EJ, Klose KJ: Management of cervical cord lesions including advances in rehabilitative engineering, in Camins MB, O'Leary PF (eds): *Disorders of the Cervical Spine*. Baltimore, MD, Williams & Wilkins, 1992, pp 351-367.

19. Green BA, Mose KJ, Eismont FJ, et al: Immediate management of the spinal cord injured patient, in Lee BY, Ostrander LE, Cochran GVB, et al (eds): *The Spinal Cord Injured Patient: Comprehensive Management*. Philadelphia, PA, WB Saunders, 1991, pp 24-33.

20. Toscano J: Prevention of neurological deterioration before admission to a spinal cord injury unit. *Paralegia* 1988;26:143-150.

21. Ramzy AI, Parry JM, Greenberg J: Head and spinal injury: Prehospital care, in Greenberg J (ed): *Handbook of Head and Spine Trauma*. New York, NY, Marcel Dekker, 1993, pp 29-44.

22. Slucky AV, Eismont FJ: Treatment of acute injury of the cervical spine. *J Bone Joint Surg* 1994;76A:1882-1896.

23. Crosby LA, Lewallen DG (eds): *Emergency Care and Transportation of the Sick and Injured*, ed 6. Rosemont, IL, American Academy of Orthopaedic Surgeons, 1995.

24. Chandler DR, Nemejc C, Adkins RH, et al: Emergency cervical-spine immobilization, *Ann Emerg Med*. 1992;21:1185-1188.

25. Fielding JW: Fractures of the spine: Part I. Injuries of the cervical spine, in Rockwood CA Jr, Wilkins KE, King RE (eds): *Fractures in Children*. Philadelphia, PA, JB Lippincott, 1984, pp 683-705.

26. Pasarin GA, Green BA: Emergency room assessment and stabilization of spinal injury, in Greenberg J (ed): *Handbook of Head and Spine Trauma*. New York, NY, Marcel Dekker, 1993, pp 413-425.

27. American Spinal Injury Association International Medical Society of Paraplegia: *International Standards for Neurological and Functional Classification of Spinal Cord Injury*. Chicago, IL, American Spinal Injury Association, 1992.

28. Anderson DK, Hall ED: Pathophysiology of spinal cord trauma. *Ann Emerg Med* 1993;22:987-992.

29. Bracken MB, Shepard MJ, Collins WF, et al: A randomized controlled trial of methylprednisolone or naloxone in the treatment of acute spinal-cord injury: Results of the Second National Acute Spinal Cord Injury Study. *N Engl J Med* 1990;322:1405-1411.

30. Bracken MB, Shepard MJ, Collins WF Jr, et al: Methylprednisolone or naloxone treatment after acute spinal cord injury: 1-year follow-up data. Results of the Second National Acute Spinal Cord Injury Study. *J Neurosurg* 1992;76:23-31.

31. Bracken MB: Pharmacological treatment of acute spinal cord injury: Current status and future projects. *J Emerg Med* 1993;11(suppl 1):43-48.

32. Segal JL: Clinical pharmacology of spinal cord injury, in Young RR, Woolsey RM (eds): *Diagnosis and Management of Disorders of the Spinal Cord*. Philadelphia, PA, WB Saunders, 1995, pp 414-433.

33. Geisler FH, Dorsey FC, Coleman WP: GM-1 ganglioside in human spinal cord injury. *J Neurotrauma* 1992;9(suppl 2): S517-S530.

34. Geisler FH, Dorsey FC, Coleman WP: Past and current clinical studies with GM-1 ganglioside in acute spinal cord injury. *Ann Emerg Med* 1993;22:1041-1047.

35. Nobile-Orazio E, Carpo M, Scarlato G: Gangliosides: Their role in clinical neurology. *Drugs* 1994;47:576-585.

36. Taylor GA, Eggli KD: Lap-belt injuries of the lumbar spine in children: A pitfall in CT diagnosis. *Am J Roentgenol* 1988;150:1355-1358.

37. Swischuk LE: Anterior displacement of C2 in children: Physiologic or pathologic? A helpful differentiating line. *Radiology* 1977;122:759-763.

38. Eismont FJ, Arena MJ, Green BA: Extrusion of an intervertebral disc associated with traumatic subluxation or dislocation of cervical facets: Case report. *J Bone Joint Surg* 1991;73A:1555-1560.

39. Cotler JM, Herbison GJ, Nasuti JF, et al: Closed reduction of traumatic cervical spine dislocation using traction weights up to 140 pounds. *Spine* 1993;18:386-390.

40. Star AM, Jones AA, Cotler JM, et al: Immediate closed reduction of cervical spine dislocations using traction. *Spine* 1990;15:1068-1072.

41. Flanders AE, Tartaglino LM, Friedman DP, et al: Magnetic resonant imaging in acute spinal injury. *Semin Roentgenol* 1992;27:271-298.

42. Betz RR, Gelman AJ, DeFilipp GJ, et al: Magnetic resonance imaging (MRI) in the evaluation of spinal cord injured children and adolescents. *Paraplegia* 1987;25:92-99.

43. Anderson JM, Schutt AH: Spinal injury in children: A review of 156 cases seen from 1950 through 1978. *Mayo Clin Proc* 1980;55:499-504.

44. Hadley MN, Zabramski JM, Browner CM, et al: Pediatric spinal trauma: Review of 122 cases of spinal cord and vertebral column injuries. *J Neurosurg* 1988;68:18-24.

45. Pang D, Wilberger JE Jr: Spinal cord injury without radiographic abnormalities in children. *J Neurosurg* 1982;57:114-129.

46. Yngve DA, Harris WP, Herndon WA, et al: Spinal cord injury without osseous spine fracture. *J Pediatr Orthop* 1988;8:153-159.

47. Bondurant CP, Oro JJ: Spinal cord injury without radiographic abnormality and Chiari malformation. *J Neurosurg* 1993;79:833-838.

48. Keller RH: Traumatic displacement of the cartilagenous vertebral rim: A sign of intervertebral disc prolapse. *Radiology* 1974;110:21-24.

49. Lawson JP, Ogden JA, Bucholz RW, et al: Physeal injuries of the cervical spine. *J Pediatr Orthop* 1987;7:428-435.

50. Ogden JA (ed): Spine, in *Skeletal Injury in the Child*. Philadelphia, PA, Lea & Febiger, 1982, pp 385-422.

51. Blumberg KD, Catalano JB, Cotler JM, et al: The pull-out strength of titanium alloy MRI-compatible and stainless steel MRI-incompatible Gardner-Wells tongs. *Spine* 1993;18:1895-1896.

52. Rizzolo SJ, Vaccaro AR, Cotler JM: Cervical spine trauma. *Spine* 1994;19:2288-2298.

53. Martinez-Lage JF, Perez-Espejo MA, Masegosa J, et al: Bilateral brain abscesses complicating the use of Crutchfield tongs. *Childs Nerv Syst* 1986;2:208-210.

54. Botte MJ, Garfin SR, Byrne TP, et al: The halo skeletal fixator: Principles of application and maintenance. *Clin Orthop* 1989;239:12-18.

55. Garfin SR, Botte MJ, Waters RL, et al: Complications in the use of the halo fixation device. *J Bone Joint Surg* 1986;68A:320-325.

56. Botte MJ, Byrne TP, Garfin SR: Application of the halo device for immobilization of the cervical spine utilizing an increased torque pressure. *J Bone Joint Surg* 1987;69A:750-752.

57. Mubarak SJ, Camp JF, Vuletich W, et al: Halo application in the infant. *J Pediatr Orthop* 1989;9:612-614.

58. Garfin SR, Roux R, Botte MJ, et al: Skull osteology as it affects halo pin placement in children. *J Pediatr Orthop* 1986;6:434-436.

59. Letts M, Kaylor D, Gouw G: A biomechanical analysis of halo fixation in children. *J Bone Joint Surg* 1988,70B:277-279.

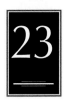

Treatment of Acute Injury of the Cervical Spine

Andrew V. Slucky, MD
Frank J. Eismont, MD

Acute injury of the cervical spine presents the treating physician with numerous diagnostic and management issues. Successful long-term treatment is contingent on early recognition of the injury, prompt resuscitation of the patient, stabilization of the injury, prevention of additional neurologic injury, and avoidance of complications.

The improvement of emergency medical procedures, including the education of pre-hospital personnel with an emphasis on the recognition and stabilization of spinal injury at the trauma scene, combined with the development of centers for the treatment of acute spinal-cord injuries, has proved to be of benefit in the management of patients who have such an injury.[1-5] Tator and associates[5,6] compared a regional group of 351 patients managed before and 201 patients managed after the establishment of a unit for the treatment of acute spinal-cord injuries. After the establishment of the unit, the proportion of complete spinal-cord injuries decreased from 65% to 46%, and overall mortality decreased from 20% to 9%. Similar results were reported by Meyer and Carle,[3] with the proportion of neurologically complete injuries decreasing from 50% to 39% after the development of the Midwest Regional Spinal Cord Injury Care System.[3,7]

The expense to society of spinal-cord injuries is overwhelming, with average hospitalization costs, in 1987 dollars, of $50,000 to $90,000 for patients who had

low-level paraplegia and $170,000 to $250,000 for those who had high-level quadriplegia and were respirator-dependent.[1,8] The individual tragedy and the cost of lost productivity are immeasurable and underline the need for a systematic approach to the treatment of acute injuries of the cervical spine.

Epidemiology

The National Head and Spinal Cord Injury Statistical Center estimated that 14,000 spinal-cord injuries occur each year, with 10,000 individuals surviving the initial accident.[9-11] The reported annual incidence has varied, with most studies demonstrating a rate of 3.2 to 5.3 new spinal-cord injuries per 100,000 persons at risk in the United States.[11,12] The peak months of occurrence of the injury are the late spring and summer months.[13,14]

The injury has a bimodal distribution in terms of the age of occurrence, with

the highest prevalence in people who are between 15 and 24 years of age and a second, smaller peak in people who are older than 55.[14] Spinal-cord injury is more frequent in boys and men than in girls and women, with several studies demonstrating variable male-to-female ratios ranging from 0.8:1 to 3.5:1, and there is a slightly higher prevalence in black people than in white people, a finding that is consistent with the higher accidental death rate observed among black people.[12,14]

The causes of spinal-cord injury vary regionally; however, with few exceptions, most spinal-cord injuries result from motor-vehicle accidents (42% to 56%), falls from a height (19% to 30%), gunshots (12% to 21%), and sports-related activities (6% to 7%) (primarily diving) (Table 1).[11,13,15] The mechanism of injury varies with age; motor-vehicle and water sports-related accidents account for most of the injuries in individuals who are

Table 1				
Causes of Spinal Cord Injury in Other Studies*				
Cause of Injury	**Kraus et al[11] (1975)**	**Fine et al[13] (1979)**	**Fife and Kraus[15]† (1986)**	**Total**
Motor-vehicle accident	338 (56)	152 (42)	259 (47) [169]	749 (50)
Fall	116 (19)	106 (30)	120 (22) [64]	342 (23)
Gunshot wound	74 (12)	76 (21)	73 (13) [27]	223 (15)
Recreational accident	43 (7)	25 (7)	33 (6) [32]	101 (7)
Other	33 (5)	—	65 (12) [39]	98 (6)
Total	604 (100)	359 (100)	550 (100) [331]	1513 (100)

*The numbers in each column indicate the number of injuries in each study, with the percentage given in parentheses.
†The numbers in brackets indicate the number of patients who had an injury of the cervical spine.

younger than 30, while falls and gunshots are more common causes in individuals who are older than 35.[9] In recent years, gunshot wounds have accounted for an increasing number of spinal-cord injuries in younger patients.[16]

The anatomic location of the spinal-cord injury bears a distinct relationship to the cause and mechanism of the injury. Fife and Kraus[15] reviewed the cause and anatomic location of 550 fatal and non-fatal spinal-cord injuries; 331 (60%) of these injuries involved the cervical spine (Table 1). Of 259 injuries sustained in a motor-vehicle accident, 169 (65%) involved the cervical spine; of 120 injuries sustained in a fall from a height, 64 (53%) were cervical injuries; and of 73 gunshot wounds, only 27 (37%) were cervical injuries. Although diving accidents accounted for less than 10% of the spinal-cord injuries, those injuries had the highest rate of involvement of the cervical spine (32 [97%] of 33 injuries). Within the cervical region, the greatest frequency of injury is at the level of the first cervical vertebra, followed by the fifth, sixth, and seventh cervical vertebrae.[15] Injuries from a motor-vehicle accident are most frequent at the levels of the first, fifth, sixth, and seventh cervical vertebrae, while injuries resulting from a fall or a diving accident predominantly involve the caudad cervical regions (the fifth, sixth, and seventh cervical vertebrae). Gunshot injuries have a random distribution. Given these findings, the mechanism of injury and the age of the patient should alert the physician to the probable level of the injury.

Pathophysiology
Injury Mechanism
The spinal cord is particularly prone to injury in the cervical region because of the coupling of a large mass, the head, to a lever arm of great flexibility, the cervical spine. The spinal cord is injured when the ligaments, muscles, and osseous structures between the skin and the spinal cord fail to dissipate the energy of impact.[17,18] The spinal cord can be injured directly, by means of excessive flexion, extension, rotation, or axial loading, or indirectly, by the impact of a displaced disk or bone fragments, or both. Fracture-dislocation is the most common cause of cervical spinal-cord injury;[19] however, the spinal cord also can be injured without radiographic evidence of injury to the vertebral column. This latter condition is called spinal-cord injury without radiographic abnormality, and it typically occurs in very young patients or in older individuals who have cervical spondylosis.[4]

The biomechanics of injury of the cervical spine have been studied extensively. Allen and associates[20] classified closed, indirect fracture-dislocations of the cervical spine into six groups that were based on the mechanism of injury: compressive flexion, distractive flexion, vertical compression, compressive extension, distractive extension, and lateral flexion. Each of these groups then was subdivided according to the severity of the injury on the basis of radiographic findings. White and associates[21] further defined cervical instability on the basis of disrupted anatomy, radiographic signs of malalignment (sagittal-plane translation, rotation, or distraction), clinical signs (spinal-cord or nerve-root damage), or the anticipation of dangerous loading after the injury (for example, in an interior lineman on a professional football team). Typically, unstable fracture patterns include bilateral facet dislocations, fracture-dislocations, or cervical vertebral fractures with more than 11.5° of angular rotation compared with adjacent levels, or 3.5 mm of sagittal translation, and clinical signs of injury of the medulla or of at least one nerve root.

The risk of spinal-cord injury with damage to cervical vertebrae is greater in individuals who have narrow spinal-canal diameters.[22,23] Patients who have a narrow midsagittal spinal-canal diameter have an increased chance of sustaining a severe neurologic injury in association with a given spinal fracture or dislocation, or both, compared with patients who have a larger midsagittal canal diameter.[22] Patients at risk include those who have cervical stenosis radiographically and who had an episode of neurapraxia in association with an event of axial compression of the cervical spine (for example, during a competitive dive from a 10-m height).[23] According to Torg and associates,[23] a patient has cervical stenosis when the ratio of the diameter of the cervical canal to the width of the cervical body is less than 0.8 as seen on the lateral radiograph.

Spinal-Cord Injury
Transmission of the energy of impact to the cervical spinal cord results in microhemorrhage in the central gray matter and loss of neuroconduction in the adjacent white matter. Following this primary injury event, there is a deleterious secondary-injury pattern that is characterized by a biochemical cascade that destabilizes the neurologic membrane of the axon, with a resultant progressive and heretofore irreversible pattern of spinal-cord cystic degeneration and neurolysis.[18,24-26]

There are two theories on how this spinal-cord lesion progresses. *A vascular theory* suggests that reduced or interrupted blood flow secondary to microvascular endothelial damage and thrombus formation results in ischemia in the central gray matter. The ischemia in the gray matter and an associated loss of vascular autoregulation contribute to ischemic changes in the adjacent white matter.[25,27-30] *A neuronal theory* postulates a traumatic distortion of the neurologic membrane of the axon at the instant of injury, with resultant paraplegia and the initiation of a secondary injury cascade.[31] This theory is supported by studies of focal blood flow in experimental animals that had functional paraplegia, which have shown increased post-injury blood flow to the lateral axon tracts of the white matter.[31,32]

Despite the uncertainty regarding the exact etiology, it is clear that the primary injury produces a complex cascade of metabolic abnormalities, which results in secondary injury to the neurologic tissues within minutes to hours after the initial insult (Fig. 1).[18,24-26] Within an ischemic environment, adenosine triphosphate stores are depleted, leading to an inactivation of calcium-dependent adenosine triphosphatase. This factor, as well as the fact that the neuronal membrane is depolarized by potassium and sodium fluxes following similar inactivation of the membrane-bound sodium and potassium adenosine triphosphatase pump, leads to an uncontrolled influx of calcium ions, with resultant uncoupling of mitochondrial oxidative phosphorylation, further loss of adenosine triphosphate production, and exacerbation of ischemia caused by local vasospasm.[18,26,33]

In addition, the uncontrolled influx of calcium ions promotes the activation of calcium-dependent phospholipase A$_2$, with resultant liberation of membrane phospholipid arachidonic acid, generation of free radicals, and peroxidation of membrane lipids, leading to membrane degradation.[26] Additional generation of free radicals occurs from hemorrhagic products, which release ferrous ions and hemoproteins into the cellular environment.

The primary cord injury leads to altered autonomic tone, loss of autoregulation, depressed cardiovascular function, and hypotension, thus promoting ischemia in the area of the injury.[18,26,30] Additionally, the inflammatory response to the injury, modulated by the migration of polymorphonuclear leukocytes and coupled with the generation of free radicals, contributes to further neuronal necrosis and edema.[25,34] After a spinal-cord injury has occurred, the current pharmacologic treatment is concerned with minimizing the deleterious effects of this secondary injury biochemical cascade.

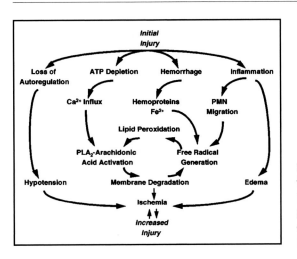

Fig. 1 Biochemical cascade effect following primary spinal-cord injury. ATP = adenosine triphosphate, PMN = polymorphonuclear leukocytes, and PLA$_2$ = phospholipase A$_2$.

Neurologic Classification

Spinal cord lesions are classified as complete or incomplete. A patient who has a complete cord injury has no sensory or motor function caudad to the level of the injury. If the lesion is complete and remains so for 48 hours, no return of sensation or motor function will occur.[35] In a review of the cases of 359 patients who had been managed consecutively at an acute spinal-cord-injury unit, Fine and associates[13] reported a neurologically complete lesion in 77 (46%) of 169 patients who had a cervical injury.

Anterior Cord Syndrome This is the loss of neurologic function in the anterior two thirds of the spinal cord. Affected regions include the spinothalamic (pain and temperature) and corticospinal (motor function) tracts. Patients have complete loss of sharp pain and temperature sensation and of motor function, but they retain proprioception and the ability to sense vibration and deep pressure.[35,36] This syndrome usually is associated with a flexion injury, a fracture-dislocation, or a burst fracture. The prognosis is poor, with a chance of recovery of one nerve-root level of motor function and a minimum chance of a return of functional walking.[35,37,38] Preservation of the spinothalamic tract (retained pinprick sensation) conveys a better prognosis.[39]

Central Cord Syndrome This syndrome typically results from a hyperextension injury with pinching of the spinal cord between the ligamentum flavum and the intervertebral disk and posterior vertebral body bone spurs. Central cord injury and hemorrhage occur with compression of adjacent white-matter tracts. The syndrome is characterized by a mixed upper and lower-motor-neuron lesion, with flaccid paralysis of the upper extremities (indicative of involvement of the lower motor neurons) and spastic paralysis of the lower extremities (indicative of involvement of the upper motor neurons).[39] The more peripheral positioning of the lower extremity axons within the spinal cord tracts accounts for the injury pattern. The prognosis for recovery is fair; in one series, 23 (59%) of 39 patients achieved functional walking.[35]

Brown-Séquard Syndrome This syndrome results from hemitransection of the spinal cord with unilateral damage to the spinothalamic and corticospinal tracts and resultant loss of ipsilateral motor and dorsal column function and of contralateral pain and temperature sensation. Common injury mechanisms include penetrating trauma or unilateral facet fracture or dislocation. Little and Halar,[40] in a review of the literature, noted a substantial recovery of voluntary

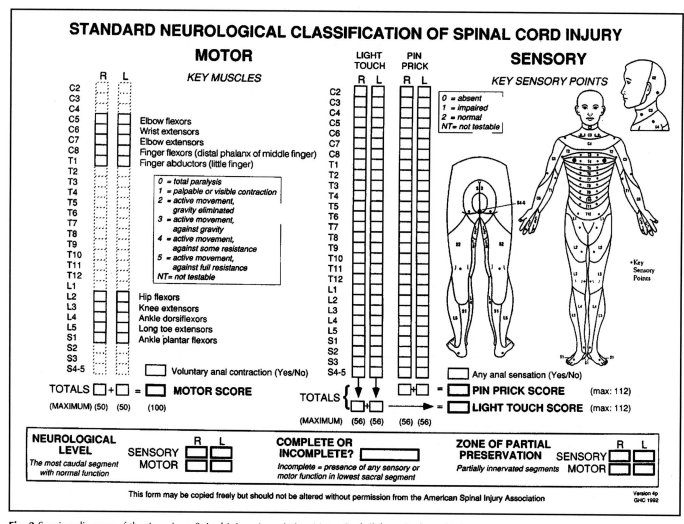

Fig. 2 Scoring diagram of the American Spinal Injury Association Motor Scale[42] for spinal-cord injury.

strength of the lower extremities and functional walking in 55 (93%) of 59 patients within a period of 6 months after the injury.

Posterior Cord Syndrome This rare syndrome is characterized by the loss of dorsal column function (deep pressure and proprioception). The prognosis is good, as motor function is preserved; however, walking is extremely difficult or impossible because of persistent impairment of proprioception.[35,39]

Cervical Root Syndrome This is an isolated deficit in a specific nerve root. It commonly is associated with acute disk protrusion or facet dislocation, often with associated vertebral-body rotation.[39]

The extent of a spinal-cord injury is classified according to functional criteria. The level of the injury is defined as the most caudad nerve root that innervates muscles that demonstrate at least antigravity strength, provided that the next cephalad level is normal. The classification system of Frankel and associates[41] subdivides injuries according to sensory loss and the amount of preserved motor function. The American Spinal Injury Association Motor Scale is based on a numeric strength score for specific bilateral motor groups of both the upper and the lower extremities and is the classification system most often recommended for current studies (Fig. 2).[42]

Immediate Patient Care
Accident Scene Management

The first step in the management of a patient who has an injury of the cervical spine is the recognition or suspicion of cervical injury. In a review of the cases of 300 patients who had been hospitalized because of an injury of the cervical spine, Bohlman[43] reported a delayed or missed diagnosis in 100 patients (33%). In another multiregional study, 33% of 371 patients who had an injury of the cervical spine were transferred from the field to the hospital with only a soft collar or no cervical immobilization.[44] Factors leading to delayed diagnosis have included concurrent head injury, an altered state of consciousness, and poor radiographic visualization in the hospital setting.[45] In many patients, multiple injuries may mask the spinal-cord injury; conversely, spinal-cord injury can mask other injuries, such as visceral rupture or long-bone fracture.[2,46]

Evaluation of the patient begins with general observation. Abrasions, lacerations, or deformities of the upper part of the thorax, neck, or head suggest that substantial force vectors were applied to the cervical region. Pain or tenderness should be evaluated only by palpation—not by movement—of the neck or spine.[2] An abbreviated neurologic examination should be specific for motor signs (weakness or paralysis of the extremities or trunk muscles), sensory signs (absence or alteration of sensation of the trunk or extremities), and incontinence (loss of control of the bladder or bowel, or both).[2] Patients who are unconscious or inebriated should be considered to have a spinal cord or spinal column injury until it has been proved otherwise.[2,45] Bohlman[43] noted that 14 of 100 patients who had a misdiagnosed cervical injury had been intoxicated due to alcohol or drugs. Other investigators have noted similar alcohol or drug involvement.[6,44,47]

With recognition of the potential for an injury of the cervical spine, primary treatment should then focus on the ABCs of resuscitation: airway, breathing, and circulation.

Airway and Breathing

An unobstructed airway is necessary in all patients. Aspiration of gastric contents and shock are the two most common causes of prehospital death in patients who have a spinal-cord injury.[48] In a patient who is awake, a standard cut-off oral airway or tongue-blade wrapped in tape will suffice. In a patient who is unconscious, a full standard oral airway or esophageal obturator should be inserted. In the event of emesis in the acute setting, the oral cavity should be suctioned

until clear. The neck should never be moved out of position in order to establish an airway in any patient suspected of having a spinal injury.

If insertion of a device into the airway does not improve ventilation as determined by lung auscultation, the patient should be intubated. Use of an esophageal obturator (that is, pharyngeal intubation) or blind nasotracheal intubation is preferable at the accident scene because of the comparative ease of placement without the need to hyperextend the head or neck.[2,9] In the event of insufficient ventilation or respiratory excursion, artificial assistance should be initiated immediately. Paralysis of intercostal muscles or diaphragm muscles, or both; atelectasis; aspiration; and chest trauma all act to compromise ventilation.

Patients who have a spinal-cord injury should receive supplemental oxygen at all times during the acute-care and transportation sequence. The physiologic effects of cervical spinal-cord injury, including the loss of sympathetic tone, bradycardia, hypotension, and decreased respiratory excursion, all act to compromise oxygenation despite the appearance of adequate breathing. Uncorrected hypoxia further compounds the localized ischemia at the level of the cord injury.[49,50] In the acutely injured patient, the goal should be to maintain a minimum PaO_2 of at least 100 torr (13.3 kPa) and a $PaCO_2$ of less than 45 torr (6.0 kPa).[2,51]

Circulation and Shock

Active bleeding should be controlled with direct pressure. Objects that have penetrated the head or neck should not be removed until the patient is in a more controlled, hospital setting. If necessary, a penetrating object may be shortened at the point of entry, with great care taken not to manipulate the object or the head or neck.

The maintenance of adequate circulation and cardiac function is essential and minimizes secondary spinal-cord in-

jury.[49,50,52] In specific instances of asystole or arrhythmia, manual cardiopulmonary resuscitation and defibrillation is necessary to maintain adequate cardiac and neurologic perfusion.[2] Care must be taken to avoid manipulation of the neck during ventilation attempts.[53]

Depending on the associated injuries, patients who have a spinal-cord injury may be in neurogenic shock or hemorrhagic shock, or both. Both types of shock are characterized by hypotension and decreased body temperature. The keys to differentiation of the two types are the rate and character of the pulse. Bradycardia (a pulse of less than 60 beats per minute) and a regular pulse are characteristic of neurogenic shock, while tachycardia (a pulse of more than 100 beats per minute) and an irregular pulse are indicative of hemorrhagic shock.[2]

Neurogenic shock associated with a cervical spinal-cord injury is due to the loss of peripheral sympathetic vascular tone, with resultant pooling of blood in the extremities and inadequate central venous return. Bradycardia results from a loss of sympathetic stimulation, which allows the parasympathetic effects of the vagus nerve to predominate. Patients in neurogenic shock typically have a systolic blood pressure of 70 mm Hg (9.3 kPa) or less and a pulse of less than 60 beats per minute.

Resuscitation from neurogenic shock begins with the placement of the patient in the Trendelenburg position, which immediately reduces pooling of peripheral blood and increases central venous return. Such positioning also reduces the chance of aspiration of gastric contents with emesis. A pneumatic counterpressure suit also can be used to complement central venous return, provided that the application of the suit does not compromise the positioning of the spine.[51,54] Intravenous administration of atropine (0.4 mg) helps to block the dominant vagal effects causing the bradycardia. The overriding consideration must be to maintain perfusion to the vital organs, including the spinal cord, during the early minutes or hours after the injury.[2] Fluid resuscitation must proceed with caution, because blood volume is sufficient in patients in neurogenic shock, which is instead a problem with blood distribution. The administration of a large volume of intravenous fluid in an attempt to increase central venous return may cause congestive heart failure.

Immobilization and Extrication
After medical stabilization, acute-care efforts should be directed toward immobilization of the injured spine, preferably before the removal of the patient from the injury scene (for example, from the water after a diving injury). Regardless of the posture in which the patient was found after the accident, the patient should be placed in a neutral supine position and a splint should be applied from the top of the head to the bottom of the buttocks.[2] When the patient is being moved, the head must be held in neutral position with respect to the long axis of the body, and great care must be taken to avoid flexion, extension, or rotation of the neck. Very gentle traction can be applied, with the hands of the rescue worker locked under the jaw and neck of the patient to help move the head into the neutral body plane. Once the neck is in neutral position, a cervical collar can be placed for additional support. Recently developed two-piece cervical collars allow placement without undue motion of the neck. Traction with weights should not be used in the field because of the risk of overdistraction of certain cervical injuries. Once in neutral position, the patient is ready for transfer to a rigid splint (backboard). Previously advocated transfer maneuvers, including the log-roll or four-man lift, are discouraged. Recent cadaveric and human studies have demonstrated that such transfers do not offer any marked degree of stability.[55] Currently, it is recommended that a scoop-style stretcher be used to lift and transfer the patient to a backboard, with both elements then being secured for complete support. The head and neck then are stabilized with sandbags. The thorax and extremities are secured with straps, with care being taken not to compromise respiratory excursion. When a patient who has an injury of the spinal cord is to be moved, the most important factors are the evaluation at the accident scene and the development of an organized extrication plan.[2]

Transportation
As with all critical-care transport, emphasis should be placed on life support and on the stability of the patient as opposed to unwarranted rapid transport. Patients should be transported in the Trendelenburg position to maximize cardiovascular function and to avoid aspiration of gastric contents with emesis.[48] In the ambulance, the patient should be positioned with the feet facing forward so as to avoid inadvertent cervical injury from the forward momentum of a sudden stop.

Selection of the transport vehicle depends on a combination of factors: patient stability, equipment availability, and the logistics of time, distance, weather, and local conditions. Recommended guidelines are as follows: use of an ambulance for distances of less than 50 miles (81 km), although a helicopter may be used at peak traffic periods or when associated injuries require more rapid transport; use of a helicopter for distances of between 50 and 150 miles (81 and 242 km); and use of a fixed-wing aircraft for distances of more than 150 miles (242 km).[39] Before prolonged transport, the placement of intravenous lines, a nasogastric tube, and a Foley catheter is recommended.[2,39]

The selection of hospital destination is contingent on patient stability. For patients who have concurrent destabilizing injuries, transport to the nearest emergency facility is necessary for resuscitation, stabilization, and immobilization. Secondary transport to an appropriate facility then should be initiated as soon as possible. It is recommended that patients in whom the spinal-cord injury is physiologically stable be transferred directly to a level-I trauma center or a similar tertiary-care facility within a reasonable transport distance (that is, one that is less than 1 hour away).[7,18]

Hospital Management
Resuscitation
On arrival at the appropriate emergency facility, the respiratory and circulatory status of the patient must be reevaluated. For patients who have concurrent injuries of the cervical spine and spinal cord, peripheral or central venous access should be obtained. The levels of blood gases and electrolytes and the hematocrit should be evaluated and corrected as necessary. A nasogastric tube and a Foley catheter should be inserted. Appropriate respiratory and cardiovascular support should be initiated to maintain adequate systemic and spinal-cord perfusion.

Assessment and Physical Examination
After resuscitation and stabilization, a thorough assessment and complete physical examination of the patient should be carried out. Particular attention should be directed toward the accident history, the mechanism of injury, and any change in the condition of the patient during transport. The detailed neurologic examination must include an assessment of cranial nerve function, sensory and motor function, and rectal tone, as well as testing of reflexes, including the bulbocavernosus reflex.

Spinal shock represents a condition of altered spinal-cord conduction with transient loss of all motor, sensory, and reflex function caudad to the level of the injury; it can persist for 48 hours and occasionally longer. The definitive neurologic status cannot be assessed until the cessation of spinal shock. The return of a bulbocavernosus or anal wink reflex signals the end of spinal shock and allows an accurate classification of the neurologic injury.

An accurate physical examination cannot be performed for an unconscious patient. In this situation, suspicion of an injury of the cervical spine must be confirmed by radiographic evaluation.

Radiographic Examination

The evaluation of a patient who has had cervical trauma should follow an orderly progression of diagnostic steps (Fig. 3). Radiographic examination of the cervical spine is indicated for all alert, sober patients who have neck pain or tenderness; for patients who have a neurologic deficit, polytrauma, or craniofacial injuries; and for all inebriated or unconscious patients who have sustained trauma.[56-58] The standard radiographic study is the five-view series, in which lateral, anteroposterior, odontoid, and right and left oblique radiographs are made. The lateral radiograph should be made first, as an initial assessment. A standard target-to-film distance of 72" (183 cm) eliminates magnification distortion. Every attempt must be made to visualize the entire lateral part of the cervical spine to the cervicothoracic junction. A substantial number of patients who have an injury of the cervical spine demonstrate additional fractures at other levels of the cervical spine.[59] When the cervicothoracic junction cannot be seen on the routine lateral radiograph, a so-called swimmer's (Twinning) radiograph will allow evaluation of the cervicothoracic junction.[60] Additional radiographs of the thoracic spine, the lumbar spine, and extremities in which an injury is suspected should be made for all patients who have multiple injuries, who are unconscious, or who have neurologic compromise. In one review, 39 (10%) of 372 consecutive patients had noncontiguous vertebral injuries, typically at the cervicothoracic or thoracolumbar juncture.[61] Patients who

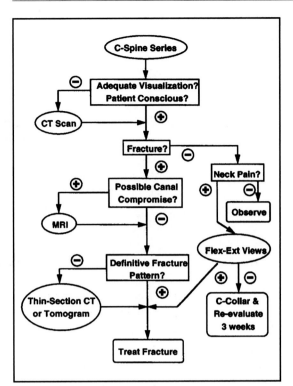

Fig. 3 Diagram of diagnostic steps to be taken in the evaluation of cervical trauma. C = cervical, CT = computed tomography, and MRI = magnetic resonance imaging.

have a spinal-cord injury often have concurrent osseous injury.[9,51,62] Soderstrom and Brumback[51] reported the additional diagnosis of a thoracic, pelvic, or long-bone fracture in 87 (21%) of 408 patients who had cervical spine trauma.

Computed Tomography

If available, a computed tomographic scan is warranted for an unconscious patient and for a patient who has suspicious or inadequate cervical radiographic findings. The standard tomographic evaluation includes 5-mm sections in a spiral format. Suspect areas on standard radiographs should be evaluated with a high-resolution, thin-section (2 to 3mm), nonspiral format to minimize the image-averaging artefact. Thin-section acquisition also allows for sagittal reconstruction in select patients.[18,58]

Magnetic Resonance Imaging

In recent years, because of improved technique and availability, magnetic resonance imaging (MRI) has played an ex-

panding role in the assessment of acute injuries of the cervical spine. The advantages of MRI include excellent visualization of spinal soft-tissue structures and clear definition of canal compromise, when it exists, as well as demonstration of areas of hemorrhage and extraspinal soft-tissue edema.[58,63,64] In addition, studies have shown a direct relationship of the pathological characteristics of spinal-cord injury with image changes seen on MRI.[64,65]

The disadvantages of MRI include its limited availability, high expense, poor resolution due to motion of the patient (typically due to coughing by a patient who has respiratory compromise), and the requirement of compatible (nonferrous) equipment (such as graphite Gardner-Wells tongs) and shielded cardiac-monitoring devices.

MRI is indicated for patients who have a complete or incomplete neurologic deficit, for assessment of the degree of spinal-cord compression; for patients whose neurologic status has deteriorated;

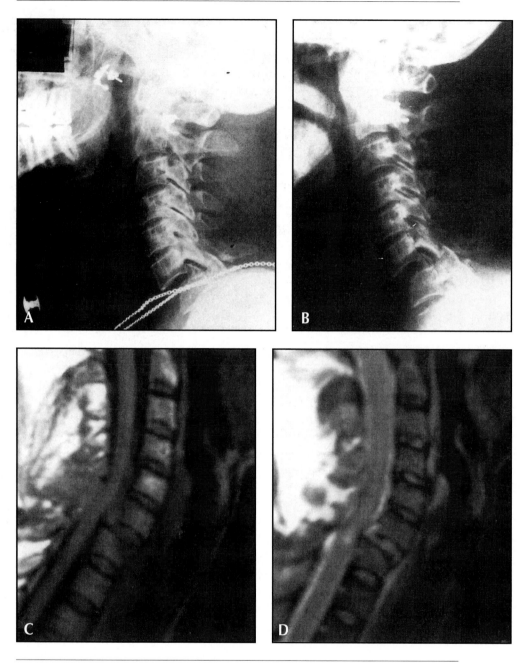

Fig. 4 A 65-year-old woman fell and struck her head after a syncopal episode. The patient was seen in the emergency room because of bilateral weakness and paresthesias of the upper extremity. Physical examination showed weakness (grade 3 of 5) of the triceps, wrist flexors, finger extensors and flexors, and intrinsic muscles of both hands. The strength of the other muscles in the arms and lower extremities was normal. The lower extremities were hyperreflexic. **A,** Lateral cervical radiograph demonstrating a unilateral dislocation of the sixth and seventh facets. **B,** Lateral radiograph made with the patient in traction. T1-weighted **(C)** and T2-weighted **(D)** mid-sagittal MRI demonstrating herniated disk material behind the body of the sixth cervical vertebra.

and for patients in whom there is a suspicion of disk retropulsion with canal compromise or possible posterior ligamentous injury (Fig. 4).[66] Several studies have demonstrated the herniation of intervertebral disks in association with fracture or dislocation, or both, and subsequent catastrophic compression of the spinal cord during reduction and realignment.[67,68] This problem is associated with such injuries as facet dislocations (unilateral or bilateral) and flexion-compression patterns. MRI is contraindicated for patients who have a pacemaker, aneurysm clips, metallic fragments in the eye or spinal cord, or severe claustrophobia.[66]

Tomograms

Tomograms can be used to evaluate patients who have a slightly displaced horizontal fracture of the odontoid process, to assess the extent of a facet or a lateral mass injury, or as a complement to thin-section computed tomographic sagittal reconstructions.

Flexion-Extension Radiographs

Flexion-extension radiographs are useful in the evaluation of patients who have neck pain despite normal neurologic and plain radiographic findings. Flexion-extension radiographs for these patients should be made under the supervision of a physician, with the patient moving the head and neck through a pain-free range of motion. No attempt at forced motion should be made. If these radiographs are normal, it is recommended that the patient be managed with a cervical collar and reevaluated with flexion-extension radiographs after three weeks; Herkowitz and Rothman[69] reported on several patients who had a late onset of cervical instability despite initially normal radiographic findings.

Immobilization and Realignment

In patients who have instability of the cervical spine, initial immobilization is achieved with skeletal traction. Gardner-Wells tongs that are compatible with MRI are applied 1 cm above the tips of the ears and in line with the external auditory meatus. Shaving of the skin is not necessary. After placement of the tongs, the patient is transferred to a rotating bed (Rotorest; Kinetic Concepts, San Antonio, Texas) by means of the transport backboard. Ten pounds (4.5 kg) of weight then is gently applied to the tongs, with close attention being paid to the maintenance of neutral alignment of the head and neck. The patient must be monitored closely for any change in neurologic condition. Post-traction alignment must be confirmed immediately by a lateral radiograph. Overdistraction should be avoided.

Closed reduction should be attempted for all patients who have an injury of the cervical spine associated with malalignment.[41,66] Before reduction, the injury mechanism must be assessed. Certain injury patterns, particularly facet dislocations, frequently are accompanied by marked disk herniation into the anterior part of the spinal canal. In patients who have such an injury, catastrophic compression of the spinal cord can result from an uncontrolled facet reduction. Eismont and associates[67] reported intervertebral disk herniation with marked protrusion of disk material into the spinal

canal in six (9%) of 68 patients who had subluxation or dislocation of a cervical facet. MRI is recommended for such patients before reduction or surgical intervention is attempted.

Reduction must be done under the supervision of a physician, with close monitoring of the neurologic and radiographic status of the patient, preferably when the patient is awake and alert. Skeletal traction, patient positioning, and postural bumps assist in reduction. Traction weight is added incrementally, with radiographs being made after each addition. As a general rule, 10 lb (4.5 kg) is added for the occiput, and an additional 5 lb (2.3 kg) for each vertebra to the level of the injury (for example, a fracture at the level of the fifth cervical vertebra would require 35 lb [15.8 kg] of traction). The maximum amount of traction weight that can be applied safely is unknown.[66] Generally, as much as 20 lb (9.1 kg) can be applied in the upper cervical region (first and second cervical vertebrae) and as much as 50 lb (22.5 kg) can be applied in the lower cervical region (third through seventh cervical vertebrae) with close supervision;[70] however, some authors have recommended that a much greater force be used.[71] Attempts at closed reduction should be discontinued when reduction is achieved, when more than 1 cm of distraction occurs at the site of the injury or at any other level, when the neurologic status of the patient deteriorates, or when it is evident that reduction cannot be achieved safely with this method.[66] Once reduction has been achieved, the traction weight can be reduced to 20 lb (9.1 kg) or less to maintain alignment.[66]

Pharmacologic Treatment

Recently, clinical studies have demonstrated the potential benefits of pharmacologic treatment as an adjunct to the principles of stabilization and reduction of a spinal injury. The treatment is directed toward interruption of the path-

way of the secondary injury mechanism associated with spinal-cord damage.

Methylprednisolone

Numerous animal studies and a multicenter clinical trial of 487 patients have demonstrated the benefit of high-dose methylprednisolone in the treatment of acute spinal-cord injury.[72-75] Its mechanisms of action are believed to be the reduction of edema, an anti-inflammatory effect, and the protection of neuronal membranes by the scavenging of oxygen free radicals.[76] Bracken and associates,[74] in the multicenter National Acute Spinal Cord Injury Study (Phase 2), at the time of follow-up 6 months after the treatment, reported improvement in the motor scores of 47 patients who had an incomplete motor lesion and who had been managed within 8 hours after the injury with high-dose methylprednisolone compared with those of similar patients who had been managed with naloxone (37 patients) or a placebo (46 patients). No significant difference was noted between treatment groups, consisting of 337 patients, managed 8 hours after the injury. Complications after treatment with steroids included an increased, although not significantly so, prevalence of wound infection (8%, 3%, and 4% for patients given methylprednisolone, naloxone, and placebo, respectively [$p = 0.21$]) and gastrointestinal hemorrhage (5%, 2%, and 3% for patients given methylprednisolone, naloxone, and placebo, respectively [$p = 0.44$]). Criticisms of the study have included the lack of control for subsequent surgical intervention in the long-term follow-up period, stratification of the patient population, use of summed motor scores, and absence of functional assessment with respect to improvement in motor scores.[77] In a subsequent review of the data after a 1-year follow-up interval, Young and Bracken[78] addressed several of the shortcomings of the design. At 1 year, the number of surgical approaches and overall patient mortality did not significantly differ among the three treatment groups. At 6 weeks after the injury, the odds ratio for patients who had been managed with methylprednisolone to improve from one motor category to a better one was 2.04 (95% confidence interval, 0.81 to 5.21).[74] At 1 year after the injury, the probability of improved motor function was greater in patients who had been managed with methylprednisolone (odds ratio, 1.29; 95% confidence interval, 0.64 to 3.03) than in patients who had received a placebo.[78] Separate analysis of the lumbosacral segments revealed significantly improved motor scores (11.8%; 95% confidence interval, 2.9% to 25.5%) for the patients who had received methylprednisolone within 8 hours compared with those of the patients who had received a placebo. These results suggest that the beneficial effects of methylprednisolone were not limited to segments close to the site of the injury.

Despite uncertainty regarding the ultimate role of high-dose methylprednisolone in the treatment of cervical spine injuries, the current recommendation is intravenous administration of a bolus of 30 mg/kg of body weight over 15 minutes, followed by an infusion of 5.4 mg/kg of body weight per hour for 23 hours for all patients who are managed within 8 hours after blunt trauma involving the spinal cord.

GM-1 Ganglioside

Gangliosides are complex acidic glycolipids that are present in high concentration in the cells of the central nervous system; they form a major component of the cell membrane, predominantly in the outer leaflet of the lipid bilayer of the membrane.[79,80] In a small prospective, randomized, placebo-controlled clinical trial, the administration of GM-1 ganglioside was shown to markedly enhance neurologic motor function at a 1 year follow-up.[79] Thirty-four patients were given either 100 mg of GM-1 ganglioside or a placebo intravenously each day for 18 to 32 days, with the first dose being taken within 72 hours after the injury. All patients also received a bolus of 250 mg of methylprednisolone followed by intravenous administration of 125 mg of methylprednisolone every 6 hours for 72 hours. The improvement was attributed to the return of useful motor strength to initially paralyzed muscles rather than to the strengthening of paretic muscles. This finding was derived from studies of experimental injuries in which an increase in axonal survival, from less than 3% to more than 6%, at the site of the injury allowed neurologic function to return caudad to the site of the injury (that is, paralyzed muscles regained normal movement).[81] It has been postulated that the mechanism of GM-1 ganglioside is the facilitation of neurite growth, the attenuation of retrograde neurologic degeneration, the modulation of glutamate-mediated endotoxicity and protein-kinase activity, or a combination of these actions.[79,80,82] Studies of larger patient populations are planned.[79]

A controversial issue is the concurrent use of GM-1 ganglioside and high-dose methylprednisolone in the acute setting. Recent studies have demonstrated that GM-1 ganglioside induces a blockade of the lipocortin-mediated anti-inflammatory effects of high-dose methylprednisolone.[82] Additional investigations, of the use of interval dosing to maximize the acute injury protective effects of high-dose methylprednisolone and the potential neuronal recovery effects of GM-1 ganglioside, are warranted.

21-Aminosteroids (Tirilizad Mesylate-U74006F)

Clinical trials of 21-aminosteroid compounds are currently in progress. This is a group of methylprednisolone analogs without the 11-beta-hydroxyl function that is known to be essential for glucocorticoid-receptor binding.[83] The presumed mechanism of action is through an anti-oxidant protective effect. These drugs lack the drawbacks of the glucocorticoid-modulated systemic effects.[84] Many studies of animals that had an acute spinal-cord injury have shown a substantial neuroprotective effect, with a greater anti-oxidant efficacy than is achieved with high-dose methylprednisolone.[83,85-87]

Naloxone and Thyrotropin-Releasing Hormone

Both naloxone and thyrotropin-releasing hormone are opiate-receptor antagonists. The theoretic benefit of the compounds is the blockade of the release of endogenous spinal-cord opioids with a reversal of injury-induced systemic hypotension and its coupled decrease in spinal-cord blood flow. Despite controversial success in animal studies, the inclusion of naloxone in the National Acute Spinal Cord Injury Study (Phase 2), demonstrated no apparent clinical benefit.[72-74,78] Recent work with other opiate receptors has suggested that kappa receptor-mediated mechanisms may be protective of spinal cord blood flow after an acute spinal-cord injury.[88,89]

Thyrotropin-releasing hormone is a pituitary tripeptide that has many physiologic effects, including the ability to act in vivo as a partial physiologic opiate antagonist. Thyrotropin-releasing hormone differs pharmacologically from naloxone in that it does not act as an opiate receptor and it reverses opioid autonomic and behavioral effects while maintaining opioid analgesic effects.[90] In several animal models, thyrotropin-releasing hormone and associated analogs have been shown to improve neurologic recovery from experimental spinal-cord injury, suggesting that it has therapeutic clinical potential.[91,92]

Other Pharmacologic Agents

Vitamin E Preinjury treatment with vitamin E (alpha tocopherol) has been shown to reduce morbidity after a spinal-cord injury in experimental models.[93] The presumed mechanism of action is through an antioxidation effect and phospholipid membrane stabilization. Clinical shortcomings include the need for preinjury treatment, thus limiting the benefit in the treatment of acute injuries.

Calcium-Channel Blockers The benefit of calcium-channel agents with regard to posttraumatic spinal-cord ischemia is controversial. The presumed mechanism of action is through stabilization of postinjury calcium influx, minimizing the deleterious calcium-modulated elements of the secondary injury cascade. Numerous calcium-channel blockers (nifedipine, nimodopine, and flunarizine) have decreased posttraumatic spinal-cord ischemia in some models[94,95] and not in others.[96,97]

Osmotic Diuretics Despite experimental success with these edema-reducing agents, including mannitol, glycerol, and low-molecular-weight dextran, there has been no compelling evidence of clinical effectiveness with regard to posttraumatic spinal-cord ischemia.[25,26]

Physical Approaches
Hypothermia
Cooling of traumatized spinal-cord segments has been shown to be of some benefit.[26,98,99] A combined review of 11 clinical trials demonstrated that 28 (45%) of 62 patients who had an injury of the spinal cord with no motor or sensory sparing had neurologic improvement and ten (16%) regained the ability to walk.[98] These results can be compared with the historically poor results of conventional treatment, in which only 2% to 10% of patients who had a complete injury on presentation exhibited substantial distal motor function after the period of spinal shock.[35,37,100] However, the clinical results of cord-cooling have been clouded by the concurrent use of steroids in many of the studies. The theoretic mechanism of action of cord-cooling is a local decrease of spinal cord metabolism and oxygen consumption, with a resultant reduction of edema and the blockade of the secondary

injury biochemical cascade. Mathematic modeling studies have suggested that additional benefit is derived from cerebrospinal fluid convection within injured spinal levels.[101]

Controversy exists with regard to the degree and duration of cooling that is required for benefit. Recent experimental studies have demonstrated moderate temperature decreases of 1° to 3° C to be of value.[99]

Cooling has serious disadvantages: the need for acute surgical intervention in a traumatized patient, the need for a wide multilevel laminectomy and prolonged surgical exposure, and the technical difficulties inherent in the currently available cooling devices.[25,98,99] At this time, the clinical role of cord-cooling is experimental.

Indications for Acute Surgical Treatment
The value of late surgical decompression of cervical spine nerves has been well documented in the literature.[70,102] The role of acute surgical decompression (within 48 hours after the injury) is more controversial and less clear. The theoretic benefits include removal of mechanical compression, correction of malalignment, and improved neurologic circulation. Opponents think that the maximum damage to the cervical spinal cord occurs at the time of the injury and with the secondary injury biochemical cascade, and that no substantial benefit can be achieved by acute surgical intervention.[103,104]

In a recent multicenter study, neurologic deterioration was noted in four of 26 patients who had had surgery within 5 days after a spinal-cord injury, but in none of the 108 patients who had had an operation after the fifth day.[105] In 44 patients who had been managed consecutively because of a cervical injury, Wagner and Chehrazi[106] noted no difference in long-term neurologic recovery whether decompression had been early (within 8 hours after the injury) or late (9 to 48 hours after the injury).

Current recommendations for the treatment of acute injuries of the cervical spinal cord stress patient resuscitation, immobilization, and skeletal traction for fracture reduction and alignment. In our experience, approximately 40% of these injuries have been most appropriately treated nonsurgically. Surgical treatment plays a role in decompression and stabilization in the elective setting, after patient stabilization. Most surgeons would agree that an absolute indication for emergent surgical intervention is progressive neurologic deterioration in the presence of irreducible canal compromise.[107] Other relative indications for an operation include a stable neurologic deficit with irreducible canal compromise, an incomplete lesion with initial improvement and a subsequent early plateau, and grossly unstable osseous or ligamentous injury patterns. A contraindication to surgical treatment is deteriorating neurologic status without evidence of canal compromise; this condition suggests irreversible ascending necrosis of the cord.[43]

Future Directions
Future research trends in the treatment of spinal-cord injury include efforts at blocking the secondary injury biochemical cascade, direct manipulation of central nervous-system regeneration and plasticity, and enhancement of neuronal function after the injury. Numerous efforts are underway with regard to axonal regeneration[61,108] and neurologic tissue transplantation.[108-112] For example, the ability of 4-aminopyridine to enhance conduction in demyelinated nerve fibers in patients who have chronic spinal-cord injury recently has been documented.[113-115]

Despite encouraging research and improvements in treatment, successful treatment of cervical spinal-cord injuries rests with prevention. Public awareness campaigns, injury-prevention programs, promotion of automotive safety devices, and civil legislation with regard to seatbelt laws, alcohol abuse, and gun-control enforcement are the most effective ways to reduce the costs, to the individual and society, of this devastating injury.

References

1. De Vivo MJ, Kartus PL, Stover SL, et al: Benefits of early admission to an organised spinal cord injury care system. *Paraplegia* 1990;28:545-555.

2. Green BA, Eismont FJ, O'Heir JT: Pre-hospital management of spinal cord injuries. *Paraplegia* 1987;25:229-238.

3. Meyer PR, Carle TV: Midwestern Regional Spinal Cord Injury Care System. Northwestern University and Rehabilitation Institute of Chicago Progress Report No. 9. Chicago, Northwestern University, 1980.

4. Tator CH: Spine-spinal cord relationships in spinal cord trauma. *Clin Neurosurg* 1983;30: 479-494.

5. Tator CH, Duncan EG, Edmonds VE, et al: Abstract: Demographic analysis of 552 patients with acute spinal cord injury in Ontario, Canada, from 1948 to 1981. *Paraplegia* 1988;26:112-113.

6. Tator CH, Duncan EG, Edmonds VE, et al: Changes in epidemiology of acute spinal cord injury from 1947 to 1981. *Surg Neurol* 1993;40:207-215.

7. Gunby I: New focus on spinal cord injury. *JAMA* 1981;245:1201-1206.

8. Whiteneck GG, Menter RR, Charlifue SW, et al: Abstract: Initial and long-term costs of spinal cord injury. *Paraplegia* 1988;26:135.

9. Garfin SR, Shackford SR, Marshall LF, et al: Care of the multiply injured patient with cervical spine injury. *Clin Orthop* 1989;239:19-29.

10. Kalsbeek WD, McLaurin RL, Harris BS III, et al: The national head and spinal cord injury survey: Major findings. *J Neurosurg* 1980;53(suppl):S19-S31.

11. Kraus JF, Franti CE, Riggins RS, et al: Incidence of traumatic spinal cord lesions. *J Chronic Dis* 1975;28:471-492.

12. Stover SL, Fine PR: The epidemiology and economics of spinal cord injury. *Paraplegia* 1987;25:225-228.

13. Fine PR, Kuhlemeier KV, DeVivo MJ, et al: Spinal cord injury: An epidemiologic perspective. *Paraplegia* 1979;17:237-250.

14. Kraus JF: A comparison of recent studies on the extent of the head and spinal cord injury problem in the United States. *J Neurosurg* 1980;53(suppl):S35-S43.

15. Fife D, Kraus J: Anatomic location of spinal cord injury: Relationship to the cause of injury. *Spine* 1986;11:2-5.

16. Capen DA, Nelson RW, Nagelberg S, et al: Etiology of spinal cord injuries: Significant changes over ten years. *Orthop Trans* 1994;17:1035.

17. Bunegin L, Hung TK, Chang GL: Biomechanics of spinal cord injury. *Crit Care Clin* 1987;3:453-470.

18. Sonntag VK, Douglas RA: Management of cervical spinal cord trauma. *J Neurotrauma* 1992;9(suppl 1):S385-S396.

19. Riggins RS, Kraus JF: The risk of neurologic damage with fractures of the vertebrae. *J Trauma* 1977;17:126-133.

20. Allen BL Jr, Ferguson RL, Lehmann TR, et al: A mechanistic classification of closed, indirect fractures and dislocations of the lower cervical spine. *Spine* 1982;7:1-27.

21. White AA, Southwick WO, Panjabi MM: Clinical instability in the lower cervical spine: A review of past arid current concepts. *Spine* 1976;1:15-27.

22. Eismont FJ, Clifford S, Goldberg M, et al: Cervical sagittal spinal canal size in spine injury. *Spine* 1984;9:663-666.

23. Torg, JS, Pavlov H, Genuario SE, et al: Neurapraxia of the cervical spinal cord with transient quadriplegia. *J Bone Joint Surg* 1986; 68A:1354-1370.

24. Bauer RD, Errico TJ, Waugh TR, et al: Evaluation and diagnosis of cervical spine injuries: A review of the literature. *Cent Nerv Sys Trauma* 1987;4:71-93.

25. de la Torre JC: Spinal cord injury: Review of basic and applied research. *Spine* 1981;6: 315-335.

26. Janssen L, Hansebout RR: Pathogenesis of spinal cord injury and newer treatments: A review. *Spine* 1989;14:23-32.

27. Collins WF, Piepmeier J, Ogle E: The spinal cord injury problem: A review. *Cent Nerv Syst Trauma* 1986;3:317-331.

28. Nelson E, Gertz SD, Rennels ML, et al: Spinal cord injury: The role of vascular damage in the pathogenesis of central hemorrhagic necrosis. *Arch Neurol* 1977;34:332-333.

29. Senter HJ, Venes JL: Loss of autoregulation arid posttraumatic ischemia following experimental spinal cord trauma. *J Neurosurg* 1979;50:198-206.

30. Tator CH: Hemodynamic issues and vascular factors in acute experimental spinal cord injury. *J Neurotrauma* 1992;9:139-141.

31. Kobrine AI, Doyle TF, Martins AN: Local spinal cord blood flow in experimental traumatic myelopathy. *J Neurosurg* 1975;42:144-149.

32. Locke GE, Yashon D, Feldman RA, et al: Ischemia in primate spinal cord injury. *J Neurosurg* 1971;34:614-617.

33. Clendenon NR, Allen N, Gordon WA, et al: Inhibition of Na+-K+-activated ATPase activity following experimental spinal cord trauma. *J Neurosurg* 1978;49:563-568.

34. Anderson DK: Chemical and cellular mediators in spinal cord injury. *J Neurotrauma* 1992;9: 143-146.

35. Bosch A, Stauffer ES, Nickel VL: Incomplete traumatic quadriplegia: A ten-year review. *JAMA* 1971;216:473-478.

36. Anderson PA: Spinal cord injuries, in Hansen ST Jr, Swiontkowski MF (eds): *Orthopaedic Trauma Protocols.* New York, NY, Raven Press, 1993, pp 193-198.

37. Ducker TB, Russo GL, Bellegarrique R, et al: Complete sensorimotor paralysis after cord injury: Mortality, recovery, and therapeutic implications. *J Trauma* 1979; 19:837-840.

38. Stauffer ES: Neurologic recovery following injuries to the cervical spinal cord and nerve roots. *Spine* 1984;9:532-534.

39. Meyer PR Jr, Rosen JS, Hamilton BB, et al: Fracture-dislocation of the cervical spine: Transportation, assessment, and immediate management, in Evans EB (ed): *American Academy of Orthopaedic Surgeons Instructional Course Lectures XXV.* St. Louis, MO, CV Mosby, 1976, pp 171-183.

40. Little JW, Halar E: Temporal course of motor recovery after Brown-Séquard spinal cord injuries. *Paraplegia* 1985;23:39-46.

41. Frankel HL, Hancock DO, Hyslop G, et al: The value of postural reduction in the initial management of closed injuries of the spine with paraplegia and tetraplegia: Part I. *Paraplegia* 1969; 7:179-192.

42. Lucas JT, Ducker TB: Motor classification of spinal cord injuries with mobility, morbidity, and recovery indices. *Am Surg* 1979; 45: 151-158.

43. Bohlman HH: Acute fractures and dislocations of the cervical spine: An analysis of three hundred hospitalized patients and a review of the literature. *J Bone Joint Surg* 1979;61A: 1119-1142.

44. Garfin SR, Marshall LF, Eisenberg HM, et al: Abstract: Spinal cord injury in three regions in the United States. *Paraplegia* 1988;26:113.

45. Bohlman HH: The neck, in D'Ambrosia RD (ed): *Musculoskeletal Disorders, Regional Examination and Differential Diagnosis,* ed 2. Philadelphia, PA, JB Lippincott, 1986, pp 219-286.

46. Soderstrom CA, McArdle DQ, Ducker TB, et al: The diagnosis of intra-abdominal injury in patients with cervical cord trauma. *J Trauma* 1983;23:1061-1065.

47. Ersmark H, Dalen N, Kalen R: Cervical spine injuries: A follow-up of 332 patients. *Paraplegia* 1990;28:25-40.

48. Green BA, Callahan RA, Klose KJ, et al: Acute spinal cord injury: Current concepts. *Clin Orthop* 1981;154:125-135.

49. Ducker TB, Salcman M, Perot PL Jr, et al: Experimental spinal cord trauma: I. Correlations of blood flow, tissue oxygen and neurologic status in the dog. *Surg Neurol* 1978;10:60-63.

50. Ducker TB, Salcman M, Lucas JT, et al: Experimental spinal cord trauma: II. Blood flow, tissue oxygen, evoked potentials in both paretic and plegic monkeys. *Surg Neurol* 1978;10:64-70.

51. Soderstrom CA, Brumback RJ: Early care of the patient with cervical spine injury. *Orthop Clin North Am* 1986;17:3-13.

52. Rawe SE, Lee WA, Perot PL Jr: The histopathology of experimental spinal cord trauma: The effect of systemic blood pressure. *J Neurosurg* 1978;48:1002-1007.

53. Mesard L, Carmody A, Mannarino E, et al: Survival after spinal cord trauma: A life table analysis. *Arch Neurol* 1978;35:78-83.

54. Rockwell DD, Butler AB, Keats TE, et al: An improved design of the pneumatic counter-pressure trousers. *Am J Surg* 1982;143:377-379.

55. McGuire RA, Neville S, Green BA, et al: Spinal instability and the log-rolling maneuver. *J Trauma* 1987;27:525-531.

56. Clark CR, Igram CM, el-Khoury GY, et al: Radiographic evaluation of cervical spine injuries. *Spine* 1988;13:742-747.

57. Harris JH Jr: Radiographic evaluation of spinal trauma. *Orthop Clin North Am* 1986;17:75-86.

58. Kaye JJ, Nance EP Jr: Cervical spine trauma. *Orthop Clin North Am* 1990;21:449-462.

59. Vaccaro AR, An HS, Lin SS, et al: Non-contiguous injuries of the spine. *J Spinal Disord* 1992;5:320-329.

60. Ballinger PW (ed): *Merrill's Atlas of Radiographic Positions and Radiologic Procedures,* ed 7. St. Louis, MO, Mosby-Year Book, 1991, vol 1, pp 318-319.

61. Schwab ME: Regeneration of lesioned CNS axons by neutralization of neurite growth inhibitors: A short review. *J Neurotrauma* 1992;9(suppl 1):S219-S221.

62. Meinecke FW: Frequency and distribution of associated injuries in traumatic paraplegia and tetraplegia. *Paraplegia* 1968;5:196-209.

63. Beers GJ, Raque GH, Wagner GG, et al: MR imaging in acute cervical spine trauma. *J Comput Assist Tomog* 1988;12:755-761.

64. Goldberg AL, Rothfus WE, Deeb ZL, et al: The impact of magnetic resonance on the diagnostic evaluation of acute cervicothoracic spinal trauma. *Skeletal Radiol* 1988;17:89-95.

65. Weirich SD, Cotler HB, Narayana PA, et al: Histopathologic correlation of magnetic resonance imaging signal patterns in a spinal cord injury model. *Spine* 1990;15:630-638.

66. Rizzolo SJ, Cotler JM: Unstable cervical spine injuries: Specific treatment approaches. *J Am Acad Orthop Surg* 1993;1:57-66.

67. Eismont FJ, Arena MJ, Green BA: Extrusion of an intervertebral disc associated with traumatic subluxation or dislocation of cervical facets: Case report. *J Bone Joint Surg* 1991;73A:1555-1560.

68. Pratt ES, Green DA, Spengler DM: Herniated intervertebral discs associated with unstable spinal injuries. 1990;15:662-666.

69. Herkowitz HN, Rothman RH: Subacute instability of the cervical spine. *Spine* 1984;9:348-357.

70. Bohlman HH, Anderson PA: Anterior decompression and arthrodesis of the cervical spine: Long-term motor improvement: Part I. Improvement in incomplete traumatic quadriparesis. *J Bone Joint Surg* 1992;74A:671-682.

71. Cotler JM, Herbison GJ, Nasuti JF, et al: Closed reduction of traumatic cervical spine dislocation using traction weights up to 140 pounds. *Spine* 1993;18:386-390.

72. Bracken MB, Holford TR: Effects of timing of methylprednisolone or naloxone administration on recovery of segmental and long-tract neurological function in NASCIS 2. *J Neurosurg* 1993;79:500-507.

73. Bracken MB, Shepard MJ, Collins WF, et al: Methylprednisolone or naloxone treatment after acute spinal cord injury: 1-year follow-up data. Results of the Second National Acute Spinal Cord Injury Study. *J Neurosurg* 1992;76:23-31.

74. Bracken MB, Shepard MJ, Collins WF Jr, et al: A randomized, controlled trial of methylprednisolone or naloxone in the treatment of acute spinal-cord injury: Results of the Second National Acute Spinal Cord Injury Study. *N Engl J Med* 1990;322:1405-1411.

75. Xu J, Qu ZX, Hogan EL, et al: Protective effect of methylprednisolone on vascular injury in rat spinal cord injury. *J Neurotrauma* 1992;9:245-253.

76. Hall ED, Braughler JM, McCall JM: Antioxidant effects in brain and spinal cord injury. *J Neurotrauma* 1992;9(suppl 1):S165-S172.

77. Bohlman HH, Ducker TB: Spine and spinal cord injuries, in Rothman RH, Simeone FA (eds): *The Spine,* ed 3. Philadelphia, PA, WB Saunders, 1992, pp 973-1103.

78. Young W, Bracken MB: The Second National Acute Spinal Cord Injury Study. *J Neurotrauma* 1992;9 (suppl 1):S397-S405.

79. Geisler FH, Dorsey FC, Coleman WP: Recovery of motor function after spinal-cord injury: A randomized, placebo-controlled trial with GM-1 ganglioside. *N Engl J Med* 1991;324:1829-1838.

80. Geisler FH, Dorsey FC, Coleman WP: GM-1 ganglioside in human spinal cord injury. *J Neurotrauma* 1992;9 (suppl 1):S407-S416.

81. Young W: Recovery mechanisms in spinal cord injury: Implications for regenerative therapy, in Seil FJ (ed): *Neural Regeneration and Transplantation, Frontiers of Clinical Neurosciences.* New York, NY, Alan R. Liss, 1989, vol 6, pp 157-169.

82. Constantini S, Young W: The effects of methylprednisolone and the ganglioside GM1 on acute spinal cord injury in rats. *J Neurosurg* 1994;80:97-111.

83. Hall ED, Yonkers PA, Andrus PK, et al: Biochemistry and pharmacology of lipid antioxidants in acute brain and spinal cord injury. *J Neurotrauma* 1992;9(suppl 2):S425-S442.

84. Hall ED: Effects of the 21-aminosteroid U74006F on posttraumatic spinal cord ischemia in cats. *J Neurosurg* 1988;68:462-465.

85. Anderson DK, Hall ED, Braughler JM, et al: Effect of delayed administration of U74006F (tirilazad mesylate) on recovery of locomotor function after experimental spinal cord injury. *J Neurotrauma* 1991;8:187-192.

86. Francel PC, Long BA, Malik M, et al: Limiting ischemic spinal cord injury using a free radical scavenger 21-aminosteroid and/or cerebrospinal fluid drainage. *J Neurosurg* 1993;79:742-751.

87. Hall ED, Braughler JM, McCall JM: New pharmacological treatment of acute spinal cord trauma. *J Neurotrauma* 1988;5:81-89.

88. Faden AI: Opioid and nonopioid mechanisms may contribute to dynorphin's pathophysiological actions in spinal cord injury. *Ann Neurol* 1990;27:67-74.

89. Hall ED, Wolf DL, Althaus JS, et al: Beneficial effects of the kappa opioid receptor agonist U-50488H in experimental acute brain and spinal cord injury. *Brain Res* 1987;435:174-180.

90. Faden AI, Jacobs TP, Holaday JW: Thyrotropin-releasing hormone improves neurologic recovery after spinal trauma in cats. *N Engl J Med* 1981;305:1063-1067.

91. Faden AI: TRH analog YM-14673 improves outcome following traumatic brain and spinal cord injury in rats: Dose-response studies. *Brain Res* 1989;486:228-235.

92. Faden AI, Jacobs TP, Smith MT: Thyrotropin-releasing hormone in experimental spinal injury: Dose response and late treatment. *Neurology* 1984;34:1280-1284.

93. Anderson DK, Waters TR, Means ED: Pretreatment with alpha tocopherol enhances neurologic recovery after experimental spinal cord compression injury. *J Neurotrauma* 1988;5:61-67.

94. De Ley G, Leybaert L: Effect of flunarizine and methylprednisolone on functional recovery after experimental spinal injury. *J Neurotrauma* 1993;10:25-35.

95. Pointillart V, Gense D, Gross C, et al: Effects of nimodipine on posttraumatic spinal cord ischemia in baboons. *J Neurotrauma* 1993;10:201-213.

96. Faden AI, Jacobs TP, Smith MT: Evaluation of the calcium channel antagonist nimodipine in experimental spinal cord ischemia. *J Neurosurg* 1984;60:796-799.

97. Shi RY, Lucas JH, Wolf A, et al: Calcium antagonists fail to protect mammalian spinal neurons after physical injury. *J Neurotrauma* 1989;6:261-278.

98. Hansebout RR, Tanner JA, Romero-Sierra C: Current status of spinal cord cooling in the treatment of acute spinal cord injury. *Spine* 1984;9:508-511.

99. Martinez-Arizala A, Green BA: Hypothermia in spinal cord injury. *J Neurotrauma* 1992;9(suppl 2):S497-S505.

100. Hansebout RR: A comprehensive review of methods of improving cord recovery after acute spinal cord injury, in Tator CH (ed): *Seminars in Neurological Surgery: Early Management of Acute Spinal Cord Injury.* New York, NY, Raven Press, 1982, pp 181-196.

101. Goetz T, Romero-Sierra C, Ethier R, et al: Modeling of therapeutic dialysis of cerebrospinal fluid by epidural cooling in spinal cord injuries. *J Neurotrauma* 1988;5:139-150.

102. Anderson PA, Bohlman HH: Anterior decompression and arthrodesis of the cervical spine: Long-term motor improvement: Part II. Improvement in complete traumatic quadriplegia. *J Bone Joint Surg* 1992;74A:683-692.

103. Guttmann L (ed): *Spinal Cord Injuries: Comprehensive Management and Research.* Oxford, Blackwell Scientific, 1973, pp 122-157.

104. Ikata T, Iwasa K, Morimoto K, et al: Clinical considerations and biochemical basis of prognosis of cervical spinal cord injury. *Spine* 1989;14:1096-1101.

105. Marshall LF, Knowlton S, Garfin SR, et al: Deterioration following spinal cord injury: A multicenter study. *J Neurosurg* 1987;66:400-404.

106. Wagner FC Jr, Chehrazi B: Early decompression and neurological outcome in acute cervical spinal cord injuries. *J Neurosurg* 1982;56:699-705.

107. Ducker TB, Bellegarrigue R, Salcman M, et al: Timing of operative care in cervical spinal cord injury. *Spine* 1984;9:525-531.

108. Bunge RP, Bunge MB: Prospects for treatment of chronic human neural injury. *J Neurotrauma* 1993;10(suppl):S123.

109. Anderson DK, Reier PJ: Transplantation and spinal cord repair in higher vertebrates. *J Neurotrauma* 1993;10(suppl):S117.

110. Kuhlengel KR, Bunge MB, Bunge RP: Implantation of cultured sensory neurons and Schwann cells into lesioned neonatal rat spinal cord: I. Methods for preparing implants from dissociated cells. *J Compar Neurol* 1990;293:63-73.

111. Kuhlengel KR, Bunge MB, Bunge RP, et al: Implantation of Cultured sensory neurons and Schwann cells into lesioned neonatal rat spinal cord: II. Implant characteristics and examination of corticospinal tract growth. *J Compar Neurol* 1990;293:74-91.

112. Reier PJ, Anderson DK, Thompson FJ, et al: Neural tissue transplantation and CNS trauma: Anatomical and functional repair of the injured spinal cord. *J Neurotrauma* 1992;9(suppl 1):S223-S248.

113. Blight AR, Toombs JP, Bauer MS, et al: The effects of 4-aminopyridine on neurological deficits in chronic cases of traumatic spinal cord injury in dogs: A phase I clinical trial. *J Neurotrauma* 1991;8:103-119.

114. Hansebout RR, Blight AR, Fawcett S, et al: 4-aminopyridine in chronic spinal cord injury: A controlled, double-blind, crossover study in eight patients. *J Neurotrauma* 1993;10:1-18.

115. Waxman SG: Aminopyridines and the treatment of spinal cord injury. *J Neurotrauma* 1993;10:19-24.

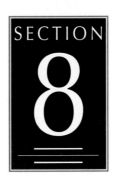

SECTION 8

Thoracolumbar Spine Trauma

Thoracolumbar Spine Trauma

Thoracolumbar spine trauma is an important topic for orthopaedic surgeons, neurosurgeons, physical medicine and rehabilitation physicians, emergency physicians, and any other personnel who are involved in the care of these patients. Dr. Jerome Cotler, who was one of my most revered mentors at Thomas Jefferson Medical Center, introduces this section with an article on the incidence of these injuries, anatomic differences among the thoracic, thoracolumbar, and lower lumbar regions, neurologic assessment and preservation, and the need to adhere to careful and logical thought processes to manage these conditions either surgically or nonsurgically. Dr. Cotler has taught me much, as he did to so many other residents and spine fellows over 30 years, and his teachings on these fundamentals will remain classics for many years.

Dr. Adam Flanders presents an overview of imaging for thoracolumbar trauma using plain radiographs, CT, and MRI. The multi-planar reconstructions obtained with spiral CT are also extremely helpful in the management of trauma patients. Plain radiographs and CT should be the first imaging studies obtained in the evaluation of acutely injured patients. MRI is reserved for patients with acute spinal cord injuries whose neurologic deficits are not explained by radiographs or CT findings. MRI is helpful in evaluating the degree of canal compromise or cord compression in the presence of displaced fractures and before surgical stabilization to exclude the presence of a disk herniation, epidural hematoma, and/or ligamentous injuries. MRI can also be used as a prognostic tool, as patients with spinal cord hemorrhage do not fair as well as those who do not exhibit cord hemorrhage.

Dr. Glenn Rechtine presents a discussion of nonsurgical treatment options for thoracic and lumbar fractures; nonsurgical treatment is still a viable and effective option in the 21st century. Initial nonsurgical management can be considered for the following: (1) stable fractures such as compression fractures, bony distractive-flexion injuries, or stable burst fractures without significant kyphosis or canal compromise; (2) fractures that are not associated with neurologic deficit; or (3) multiple-level noncontiguous fractures that would be very difficult to treat surgically.

Controversy continues on the treatment of unstable burst fractures and thoracic fractures with complete spinal cord injury, but many orthopaedic spine surgeons believe that these problems require prompt treatment by adequate decompression and stabilization to maximize neurologic recovery and facilitate rehabilitation, as long as the rate of surgical complications is minimized and does not exceed that of nonsurgical treatment. As Dr. Rechtine points out, nonsurgical treatment does not equal benign neglect. It requires careful monitoring with specific protocols such as turning frames, thoracolumbar casting or orthosis, and frequent follow-up examinations.

Dr. Daniel Capen's principles on classification of thoracolumbar fractures and posterior instrumentation still apply today. Among the many classifications mentioned, Ferguson and Allen have enhanced our understanding of the mechanism of injury that is helpful in developing appropriate treatment plans. The McAfee's classification is noteworthy in that it separates the Denis' burst fractures into stable and unstable fractures, which again is important in choosing a treatment strategy[1]. McCormack and associates[2] further divided the burst fractured body into comminution, apposition, and kyphosis components that may be important in the load-sharing capacity of the anterior column. At a minimum, surgeons should be familiar with the Frankel grades and the American Spine Injury Association (ASIA) scoring system to assess each patient neurologically.

Dr. Capen's discussion of surgical treatment includes indications and techniques of posterior approaches, and Dr. Alexander Vaccaro describes a combined anterior and posterior approach for thoracolumbar fractures. What is missing from their articles is a discussion of the anterior approach alone, which may be done in some cases. In the last two decades, important developments and advances have improved the surgical management of spinal injuries. In choosing a particular approach, numerous factors should be considered, including the mechanism of injury, the neurologic status of the patient, the level of injury, the stability of the fractures, and the overall status of the patient. As Dr. Capen pointed out, distractive-flexion injuries should be approached posteriorly. If surgery has been chosen, most unstable burst fractures without significant canal compromise or neurologic deficits can be approached posteriorly by applying fusion with rigid instrumentation.

What has changed over the last 10 to 15 years is the choices for instrumentation, such as more rigid pedicle screw constructs. A stable construct can be obtained by two above and one below the fracture, whereas three above and two below fusion is generally recommended for hook-rod systems. Pedicle screw constructs spanning one above and one below the vertebrae are prone to failure, especially at the thoracolumbar junction. It should be remembered that the posterior constructs for burst fractures are load-bearing constructs as opposed to load-sharing constructs; therefore, the spinal instrumentation should be as rigid as possible with copious bone grafts posterolaterally, spanning the entire instrumented motion segments. These patients should be braced postoperatively to protect the surgical construct.

Thoracolumbar injuries that are associated with large retropulsed bone fragment and neurologic deficits are best approached anteriorly, as suggested by Dr. Vaccaro. Because decompression of the spinal canal is the most important part of surgery in these cases, an anterior extensile approach would be advantageous over posterolateral or transpedicular decompression procedures. With modern-strut grafting techniques and with the availability of compression plate or rod systems, these injuries may be treated by an anterior approach alone, as reported by Kaneda and associates.[3] Again, use of a postoperative orthosis for 3 months is recommended for these patients. The anterior construct may not be stable in certain circumstances, particularly in the osteoporotic spine. In these cases, posterior stabilization should be added. As pointed out by both Drs. Capen and Vaccaro, fracture-dislocations should be approached posteriorly first, followed by an anterior load-sharing construct if necessary. Some surgeons advocate treating all burst fractures with the combined anterior and posterior approach, which provides a biomechanically superior construct, but it may be an "overkill" approach that may increase patient morbidity.

In summary, these articles on the diagnosis and management of thoracolumbar fractures are concise and informative, and most of the principles will remain as classics for many years. Spinal instrumentation is evolving, however, with ongoing advances and innovations in spinal surgery, and the understanding of the underlying spinal instability and biomechanical principles of various constructs has become more important. The orthopaedic spine surgeon should treat each patient based on the type and mechanism of fracture and neurologic status, and with the basic foundation of knowledge in biomechanics, spinal instrumentation, and evidence-based literature.

Howard S. An, MD
The Morton International Professor of Orthopaedic Surgery
Director, Division of Spine Surgery and Spine Fellowship Program
Rush-Presbyterian-St. Luke's Medical Center
Chicago, Illinois

References
1. McAfee PC, Yuan HA, Frederickson BE, Lubicky JP: The value of computed tomography in thoracolumbar fractures: An analysis of one hundred consecutive cases and a new classification. *J Bone Joint Surg Am* 1983;65:461-473.
2. McCormack T, Karaikovic E, Gaines RW: The load sharing classification of spine fractures. *Spine* 1994;19:1741-1744.
3. Kaneda K, Taneichi H, Abumi K, Hashimoto T, Satoh S, Fujiya M: Anterior decompression and stabilization with the Kaneda device for thoracolumbar burst fractures associated with neurological deficits. *J Bone Joint Surg Am* 1997;79:69-83.

Introduction to Thoracolumbar Fractures

Jerome M. Cotler, MD

Injuries to the thoracolumbar spine are frequently encountered by orthopaedic surgeons. The incidence of such injuries that are associated with some type of neurologic deficit is approximately 1 per 20,000 per year. As with most injuries of the spine, the majority of thoracolumbar injuries occur in males, generally males between the ages of 15 and 29 years. In a multicenter review of more than 1,000 patients by the Scoliosis Research Society, 16% of injuries occurred between T1 and T10, 52% between T11 and L1, and 32% between L1 and L5.[1] The T2 to T10 area has the smallest ratio of canal size to cord diameter in the spine, which is why this area has the least tolerance to injury and a higher risk of loss of neural function. In addition, the cord area between T2 and T10 is a circulatory watershed area. The artery of Adamkiewicz provides the spinal blood supply at approximately T9 and below, and the blood supply for the area above comes from the upper thoracic area. Injuries in this area with severe thoracic fractures usually have a 6 to 1 ratio of complete to incomplete neural deficits.

The T11 to L1 area is the junction between the thoracic spine and the lumbar spine. The relative immobility of the thoracic spine and the mobility of the lumbar spine make this transition area much more vulnerable to injury, which accounts for the fact that 52% of injuries occur here. The neural elements in this area, particularly at the junction, are a commingling of cord, conus, and cauda equina, and for this reason, it is difficult to ascertain which of these elements is injured and what the ultimate outcome is likely to be. Injury to the cauda equina carries a far better prognosis, because it is a peripheral nerve and has regenerative powers not normally seen in the cord or conus. Although the lumbar spine has more sagittally oriented facets, making it more mobile in the flexion/extension mode, it nonetheless has a far better prognosis because of its increased ratio of canal area to neural tissue. Also, most of the neural tissue here is peripheral nerve tissue and is less susceptible to permanent neural damage.

Treating physicians must not lose sight of the responsibility imparted to them when seeing patients with thoracolumbar injuries. The determination must be made rapidly whether the patient is neurally intact or has an incomplete or a complete neural deficit. These baseline assessments of neural function are important, and so are early baseline assessments of the presence of bony lesions. In addition, the earliest medical status must be ascertained and recorded, and care taken not to allow any further harm or loss of function to come to the patient if at all possible. Thus, the physician must protect the neural elements and accomplish the earliest possible decompression either surgically or through closed reduction and stabilization, with the hope of obtaining some return of neural function. The physician must also determine if the patient's injury is solely in the spine or if other systems must be considered. Depending on the type of fracture, associated injuries occur in up to 50% of patients.[2-6] Half of the associated injuries result from a distraction force and involve an intra-abdominal injury, such as a rupture of a visceral organ.[7] Pulmonary injuries also occur in approximately 20% of these patients, while intra-abdominal bleeding secondary to liver and splenic injury occurs in about 10%.[8] In addition, contiguous and noncontiguous spine injuries are present in between 6% and 15%. Because the mortality rate in the first year for thoracic level paraplegia is approximately 7%,[9] the primary goal is to protect the neural elements and to maximize neural return by whatever means possible, using the pharmacologic agents available today. It also is necessary to attempt to reduce the bony deformity, whether it is a fracture-subluxation or a dislocation. Frequently, this can be done by using a traction apparatus, thus avoiding early surgery, while the patient is being stabilized and evaluated. The ultimate goal is that stabilization of the fracture will enable the patient to once again have a pain-free, stable spine and to return to the work force as a productive member of society.

Injuries at the thoracolumbar area can also lead to slow progressive deformity and vertebral body collapse (HS An, MD, personal communication). Some underlying processes that may be involved include tumors, metabolic bone disease, osteomyelitis, or osteoporosis. Of course, these latter patient groups are usually the elderly and, unfortunately, elderly females, because of their propensity to osteoporosis. Some of the issues to be addressed in subsequent chapters

include thorny ones that truly require clarification, such as those in the surgical area. What are the indications for surgery, when should these types of procedures be carried out, and which is the best approach for decompression or fusion? It is also necessary to decide whether the approach should be posterior, anterior, or combined.

References

1. Gertzbein SD: Scoliosis Research Society: Multicenter spine fracture study. *Spine* 1992; 17:528–540.

2. Cotler JM, Vernace JV, Michalski JA: The use of Harrington rods in thoracolumbar fractures. *Orthop Clin North Am* 1986;17:87–103.

3. Gertzbein SD, Court-Brown CM: Flexion-distraction injuries of the lumbar spine: Mechanism of injury and classification. *Clin Orthop* 1988;227:52–60.

4. Gumley G, Taylor TK, Ryan MD: Distraction fractures of the lumbar spine. *J Bone Joint Surg* 1982;64B:520–525.

5. Saboe LA, Reid DC, Davis LA, Warren SA, Grace MG: Spine trauma and associated injuries. *J Trauma* 1991;31:43–48.

6. Weinstein JN, Collalto P, Lehmann R: Thoracolumbar "burst" fractures treated conservatively: A long-term follow-up. *Spine* 1988;13:33–38.

7. Levine AM, Bosse M, Edwards CC: Bilateral facet dislocations in the thoracolumbar spine. *Spine* 1988;13:630–640.

8. Ducker TB, Russo GL, Bellegarrique R, Lucas JT: Complete sensorimotor paralysis after cord injury: Mortality, recovery, and therapeutic implications. *J Trauma* 1979;19:837–840.

9. Shikata J, Yamamuro T, Iida H, Shimizu K, Yoshikawa J: Surgical treatment for paraplegia resulting from vertebral fractures in senile osteoporosis. *Spine* 1990;15:485–489.

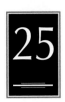

Thoracolumbar Trauma Imaging Overview

Adam E. Flanders, MD

Some of the most essential tools in the evaluation of thoracolumbar trauma are the various types of diagnostic imaging. Today, imaging of the spine and spinal axis can be performed using numerous techniques. These include plain radiographs, multiplanar tomography, myelography, computed tomography (CT) and magnetic resonance imaging (MRI). The use of these techniques is guided by the clinical assessment of the individual patient and by diagnostic algorithms.

In general, isolated thoracic spine fractures are less common than isolated cervical or lumbar fractures. The structural stability of the thoracic cage offers to the thoracic spine some protection against injury.[1] Higher forces are required to induce an injury. As a result, one half of all thoracic injuries produce a neurologic deficit.[2,3] This is attributed to the relatively smaller spinal cord diameter to spinal canal diameter ratio and the higher energies expended during injury.[2,3] Because there is relative resistance to rotation, most thoracic injuries occur in flexion and axial loading; therefore, fracture dislocations are more common than compression/burst fractures.[2]

Nondisplaced fractures of the thoracic spine may be difficult to identify on plain radiographs. Regardless, plain radiography remains the initial imaging study of choice for evaluation of thoracolumbar trauma. Standard anterior-posterior (AP) and lateral radiographs are necessary for initial evaluation because more than half of fractures are undetectable on the AP view alone.[4,5]

Lumbar level fractures are more common than thoracic injuries because of the increased mobility of the lumbar spine. The thoracolumbar junction is especially prone to injury. Anatomic differences that predispose the lumbar spine to fracture compared to the thoracic spine include the absence of ribs, the different orientation of the facet joints, and the transition from a kyphotic to a lordotic curvature.[6-8] Most lumbar fractures are classified using a variation of the Denis or McAfee schema.[9-11] The mechanisms of injury are based on the 2- and 3-column models of spinal injury proposed by Holdsworth and Denis respectively. The major difference between the 2 classification systems is the distinction between stable and unstable burst fractures in the McAfee system. The fracture subtypes include the simple compression fracture, the burst fracture, the seat belt type injury (including Chance fractures), the flexion-distraction injury, and the translational injury.[9-12]

Standard chest films are inadequate for evaluation of the spine; the radiographs must be exposed properly to optimize visualization of the spine. In the setting of acute trauma, it may be technically difficult to obtain diagnostic quality radiographs. On lateral radiographs, the upper thoracic spine is often obscured by the shoulders, and patient motion and respiration can blur bony details. A swimmer's view can prove helpful in improving the visibility of the cervicothoracic junction. In addition, cross table lateral films that are deliberately blurred by breathing artifact can improve the visibility of the spine. CT is usually reserved for imaging areas of the spine that are inadequately demonstrated on conventional radiographs. Indirect signs of thoracic fracture include a paraspinal mass, mediastinal widening, fracture of the sternum, fractures of the posterolateral or posteromedial ribs, identification of 2 spinous processes at 1 level on a frontal radiograph, and a hemothorax on a chest radiograph.[5,6]

The radiographic and clinical findings of thoracic spine fracture and traumatic aortic dissection have many similarities. Widening of the mediastinum, pleural effusions, paravertebral hematomas, and neurologic symptoms can be identified with both entities. Important distinguishing features of aortic injury on radiographs include depression of the main stem bronchus, displacement of a nasogastric tube to the right, and indistinct margins of the aortic knob.[7] Dynamic contrast CT or conventional aortography may be necessary for confirmation.

Although conventional tomography has been largely supplanted by CT in the evaluation of the spine, it is still used at many centers to delineate complex fractures. It is technically more difficult to perform than CT and requires more patient cooperation. The best application of conventional tomography is in the postoperative spine with instrumentation, because the artifacts produced by hardware degrade CT or MRI images.

CT yields significantly more diagnostic information regarding the extent of bony injury than plain radiographs. It remains the study of choice for depicting the extent of injury, as modern CT equipment with bone reconstruction algorithms provides the highest sensitivity for detecting subtle cortical abnormalities. CT has the additional advantage of computer reformatting 2-dimensional or cross-sectional information into other 2-dimensional (sagittal or coronal) or 3-dimensional views in an infinite number of potential orientations. The biggest disadvantage of CT is its limited capability for depicting soft-tissue injuries (disk herniation, epidural hematoma, ligamentous disruption, or spinal cord injury). Modern CT scanners can acquire all of the image dataset in one helical acquisition. This technique allows rapid acquisition of the clinical data with a minimum of patient cooperation. The data can then be post-processed into additional projections off-line. The quality of reconstructed images is indirectly proportional to the in-plane resolution or slice thickness.

MRI has emerged as the definitive diagnostic modality in the evaluation of spinal and spinal cord injury. The primary reason is MRI's unequaled capacity to demonstrate the soft-tissue component of spinal injury.

Formerly, soft-tissue injuries such as ligament and disk damage were inferred by the extent and type of osseous injury.[13,14] Moreover, MRI has completely supplanted myelography in the evaluation of spinal cord injury. The majority of spinal injured patients can be safely imaged with MRI during the acute period, prior to or following closed reduction of the injury. MRI-compatible monitoring and life-support equipment is also available for medically unstable patients. Absolute contraindications to MR imaging include certain biomedical implants, such as cardiac pacemakers and aneurysm clips.

While it is acknowledged that MRI is less sensitive to fractures than CT, compressive injuries to the vertebral body usually induce changes in the marrow elements, which are readily detectable with MRI. Fractures of the posterior elements, as well as nondisplaced fractures of the anterior and middle columns, are difficult to resolve on MRI. Despite these shortcomings, MRI is capable of revealing the majority of clinically significant fractures and can be used to tailor detailed imaging with CT at specific levels in question.[15] MRI also reliably demonstrates vertebral alignment and integrity.

MRI is particularly well suited for demonstrating the spectrum of soft-tissue injuries associated with spinal and spinal cord injury. The fracture classification schemes commonly in use today are based on the appearance of an injury on plain radiographs. These classification systems are useful because they attempt to predict the degree of instability and associated ligamentous damage based on the appearance on standard radiographs. The primary benefit that MRI offers over standard radiographs is direct visualization of the injured ligamentous complexes.[16]

Using MRI, spinal injury can be subdivided into 5 general injury categories: (1) vertebral fractures, subluxations, and compressive injury, (2) disk injury and herniation, (3) ligamentous disruption, (4) epidural and paravertebral hematoma, and (5) spinal cord edema and hemorrhage.

It is difficult to produce an imaging algorithm or protocol that effectively manages appropriate use of diagnostic imaging in thoracolumbar trauma. Standard, high-quality radiographs of the thoracolumbar spine should be obtained initially in any patient with a clinical examination or historical information suggestive of thoracolumbar injury. CT should be obtained through any areas of fracture and of areas that have been incompletely evaluated on the radiographs. MRI should be obtained on any patient with a neurologic deficit, regardless of the existence of a concomitant bony injury. If there is compelling evidence for a traumatic aortic injury (eg, paraspinal mass, indistinct aortic knob on chest radiograph, high speed deceleration mechanism, etc), emergent arteriography may be necessary.

References

1. Andriacchi T, Schultz A, Belytschko T, Galante J: A model for studies of mechanical interactions between the human spine and rib cage. *J Biomech* 1974;7:497–507.

2. Hanley EN Jr, Eskay ML: Thoracic spine fractures. *Orthopedics* 1989;12:689–696.

3. Meyer S: Thoracic spine trauma. *Semin Roentgenol* 1992;27:254–261.

4. Dennis LN, Rogers LF: Superior mediastinal widening from spine fractures mimicking aortic rupture on chest radiographs *Am J Roentgenol* 1989;152:27–30.

5. el-Khoury GY, Moore TE, Kathol MH: Radiology of the thoracic spine. *Clin Neurosurg* 1992; 38:261–295.

6. el-Khoury GY, Whitten CG: Trauma to the upper thoracic spine: Anatomy, biomechanics, and unique imaging features. *Am J Roentgenol* 1993;160:95–102.

7. Kram HB, Appel PL, Wohlmuth DA, Shoemaker WC: Diagnosis of traumatic thoracic aortic rupture: A 10-year retrospective analysis. *Ann Thorac Surg* 1989;47:282–286.

8. Kaye JJ, Nance EP Jr: Thoracic and lumbar spine trauma. *Radiol Clin North Am* 1990; 28:361–377.

9. Denis F: Spinal instability as defined by the three-column spine concept in acute spinal trauma. *Clin Orthop* 1984;189:65–76.

10. Denis F: The three column spine and its significance in the classification of acute thoracolumbar spinal injuries. *Spine* 1983;8:817–831.

11. McAfee PC, Yuan HA, Fredrickson BE, Lubicky JP: The value of computed tomography in thoracolumbar fractures: An analysis of one hundred consecutive cases and a new classification. *J Bone Joint Surg* 1983;65A:461–473.

12. Holdsworth FW: Fractures, dislocations, and fracture-dislocations of the spine. *J Bone Joint Surg* 1963;45B:6–20.

13. Schaefer DM, Flanders AE, Osterholm JL, Northrup BE: Prognostic significance of magnetic resonance imaging in the acute phase of cervical spine injury. *J Neurosurg* 1992;76: 218–223.

14. Flanders AE, Spettell CM, Tartaglino LM, Friedman DP, Herbison GJ: Forecasting motor recovery after cervical spinal cord injury: Value of MR imaging. *Radiology* 1996;201:649–655.

15. Silberstein M, Tress BM, Hennessy O: Prediction of neurologic outcome in acute spinal cord injury: The role of CT and MR. *Am J Neuroradiol* 1992;13:1597–1608.

16. Yamashita Y, Takahashi M, Matsuno Y, et al: Chronic injuries of the spinal cord: Assessment with MR imaging. *Radiology* 1990;175:849–854.

Nonsurgical Treatment of Thoracic and Lumbar Fractures

Glenn R. Rechtine, MD

Introduction

The treatment of thoracic and lumbar fractures remains as controversial as it has been over the past 50 years. Surgical and nonsurgical treatment have had their advocates with successful series in both.[1-9] There are advantages and disadvantages with each. The assumption has been that nonsurgical treatment is plagued with problems, such as pneumonia, pulmonary problems, venostasis, pulmonary emboli, late deformity, late neurologic compromise, and other complications, related to the prolonged immobilization. Over the past 25 years, with the development of more sophisticated spinal instrumentation, surgical techniques have become much more prevalent. The hypothesis is that anatomic restoration of spinal alignment and spinal canal reconstruction would result in a better functional outcome for the patient. The actual results from these techniques have not been nearly as conclusive as the initial hypothesis.

The initial treatment of any spinal injury is adequate immobilization. Once a spinal injury is suspected the patient should be immobilized. In the field, this should be done initially with extraction equipment and a spine board. On the patient's arrival at the treatment facility, the patient's hemodynamic stability and other injuries need to be evaluated and addressed. There is a high incidence of multiple

level injuries; the identification of one is the key to look for others. In a study by Henderson and associates[10] of 508 patients with spinal injuries, 15% of patients had multiple noncontiguous spinal injuries. Once the spinal injury has been identified on plain radiograph, it is prudent to follow this up with a computed tomography (CT) scan to also determine the extent of the spinal injury. A plain radiograph is not necessarily accurate in determining whether the fracture involves the middle column or creates an instability.[11] Some injuries are much more common and certain spinal injuries carry a high incidence of associated injuries. Chance-type fractures have a high association with intra-abdominal injuries. Low lumbar burst fractures are associated with high-energy injuries and are usually associated with multiple trauma as well. There is also a high association between spinal injuries and sacral and pelvic fractures. Twenty-six percent of sacral fractures will have an associated spinal fracture and almost 8% of pelvic fractures will have an associated spinal fracture.[12] When a sacral or pelvic fracture is identified, attention should be directed toward the spine, to look for an injury there as well.

The complicated biomechanics and pathophysiology of spine trauma and spinal cord injury contribute to the difficulty in being able to draw conclusions as to the most effective

treatment for these injuries. Panjabi and associates[13] pointed out in an in vitro study that the injury itself is a dynamic situation. The maximum canal compromise was 85% greater than the residual at the time the patient would have arrived for treatment at the hospital.[13] This information helps to explain papers that have reported no association between spinal canal narrowing and neurologic deficits or decompressions with neurologic recovery.[14,15] At the time of the injury, the spinal canal is markedly compromised and may already be relatively decompressed. The spinal cord injury occurred at the time of the impact.

One argument for surgical treatment is that the spinal canal must be decompressed in patients with marked canal compromise even if they are neurologically intact. The concern is that these patients will develop spinal stenosis symptoms in the future; however, they do not do so in reality. There are only rare reports of spinal stenosis symptoms developing in the future, probably because spinal canal compromise remodels spontaneously over time through an expression of Wolfe's Law.[8,16,17]

Methods of Treatment
Bracing

Bracing is one of the oldest treatment methods available. Biomechanical in vitro testing shows that an orthosis will accommodate for approximately 50% loss of stiffness at 1 level and 25% at 2 levels.[7] Cantor and associates[1] reported excellent results in a series of 33 patients who had no ligamentous injury and no neurologic deficit and were treated with bracing. Most patients were discharged within a week to 10 days after their injury.[1]

Nonsurgical Treatment of Patients Without Neurologic Deficit

There are several series in which bed rest and nonsurgical treatment were used for patients with spinal injuries. Weinstein and associates[9] presented a series of 42 patients with no neurologic deficits; at a 20-year follow-up, 2 of these patients had subsequent late surgery. In a series of 34 patients with spinal cord injuries treated nonsurgically, Davies and associates[2] reported complications of 2 pulmonary emboli and no deaths. There was no discussion as to deep venous thrombosis prophylaxis. In another report, Chan and associates[18] showed excellent results in patients treated with a combination of casts and bed rest.

Bone Remodeling

In a series of 41 neurologically intact patients, two thirds of the retropulsed bone resorbed at long-term follow-up. These data again are a reflection of bone stress and stress shielding; once the bone is no longer loaded it is resorbed.[6]

Nonsurgical Treatment of Patients With Neurologic Defects

Sandor and Barabas[8] showed that a patient with as much as 93% canal compromise resorbed the spinal canal over time with nonsurgical treatment. In a series of 63 patients with neurologic deficits, Dendrinos and associates[3] showed that there was no correlation of the neurologic deficit with canal compromise or resolution of

the deficit with decompression. In Kinoshita and associates'[5] study of 23 patients, 13 of whom had neurologic deficits, there was only 1 late surgery for progressive kyphosis. In my series of 32 patients, 12 had neurologic deficits: 3 complete and 9 incomplete. The incomplete neurologic deficits all improved at least 1 Frankel grade. The complications were 1 heel ulcer and 1 deep venous thrombosis. These did not prolong the hospitalization.

In determining which patients are candidates for nonsurgical treatment, an accurate assessment of the injury is critical. Ligamentous injuries are not candidates for nonsurgical treatment because there is a low likelihood that the ligamentous injury will heal over time. The greater the bony injury, the more likely the patient will do well with nonsurgical treatment. Multiple level injuries, particularly noncontiguous injuries, are a very good indication for nonsurgical treatment. Surgical stabilization would require immobilization of large portions of the patient's spinal column. This is particularly important when dealing with lumbar fractures where residual motion is more important.

Types of Injuries

Spinal injuries can be divided into 3 different groups because they have different characteristics both biomechanically and neurologically. Upper thoracic fractures occurring from T1 to T9-10 have the stability of the ribs, and the blood supply to the spinal cord is poor. These 2 factors combined mean that the patient is usually neurologically intact or has sustained complete neurologic injury because the stability has been overcome and the thoracic spinal cord has not withstood the high-energy injury that took place. Patients who are intact or have complete injuries are excellent candidates for nonsurgical treatment.

The thoracolumbar junction (T10 to L2) is the most common level for trauma. This is a reflection biomechanically of the junction between the stiff thoracic spine and the mobile lumbar spine. This area has the potential for any combination of neurologic injury. The neurologic injury is a combined upper motor neuron lesion and lower motor neuron lesion with injury to the conus and the cauda equina. These patients may be candidates for nonsurgical treatment because stabilization at this area, involving short-segment fixation, has a significant failure rate as a result of the high stresses involved, and using longer segment fixation will reduce significant amounts of lumbar motion.

Low lumbar fractures from L3 to L5 tend to be different both biomechanically and physiologically. These tend to be high-energy injuries, and the neurologic injury is a cauda equina injury or a lower motor neuron injury. Mick and associates[19] point out that patients with neurologic deficits and L5 fractures have more predictable results with surgery, but this is such a small series this conclusion may not be valid.

Ligamentous lumbosacral dislocations are relatively uncommon. There is a case report of 1 being reduced and treated nonsurgically, but the consensus is that this injury is best reduced open and stabilized surgically.[20] The comminuted bony injury can be treated nonsurgically.

Plan of Treatment

The protocol for nonsurgical treatment that I have used over the past 10 years includes the use of a kinetic bed with the patient rotating 40° each direction continuously. The patient must be rotating at least 6 of every 8 hours. Deep venous thrombosis prophylaxis is carried out with compression stockings and sequential compression devices. The patient is started on an active exercise program using rubber bands and weights as soon as the medical condition will allow. If the patient had other fractures and other injuries, he or she may be placed on a continuous passive motion device while on the kinetic bed. Each hatch on the kinetic bed is opened each nursing shift and the skin is inspected and massaged.

Using this protocol, the experience in Tampa now extends over 10 years. One hundred fifty patients have been treated with long-term bed rest on the kinetic bed. I also have reviewed 120 patients who were treated surgically within the same time period. The groups are comparable in age, with the average age of 32 to 33 years. There is a 70% male population, as is common with trauma. The fracture patterns are similar with slightly more burst fractures in the surgical group. There were 21% multiple-level spinal injuries with 9% noncontiguous spinal injuries. There were more complete spinal cord injuries in the nonsurgical group and more incomplete injuries in the surgically treated group. The multiple system trauma was comparable. Complications totaled 32% in the surgical group and 22% in the nonsurgical group. The difference was the 9% infection rate. Mortality was 3.3% in the surgical group and 2% in the nonsurgical group. One of the 2 fatalities in the nonsurgical group was a patient who was actually scheduled for surgery on several occasions but never stabilized medically from the time of his initial hospitalization to be a candidate for surgical treatment. The other fatality was due to a pulmonary embolus in a paraplegic patient that occurred 2 ½ weeks into his hospitalization. It is also of note that the patient had a negative color Doppler within 48 hours

prior to his fatal pulmonary embolus. Decubiti are associated with prolonged immobilization on a back board. The length of stay was longer in the nonsurgical group (41 versus 25 days) as would be expected, but in a previous study we were able to demonstrate that the overall cost was not significantly different. Without costs for surgeries and anesthesiologists, complications, and rehospitalization, the cost difference in billings is $13,000.

The key to nonsurgical treatment is an aggressive treatment plan. This is not as simple as placing the patient in a bed and ignoring him or her for 6 weeks. Some sort of kinetic bed must be used for effective immobilization. The nursing staff must be familiar with the bed and familiar with the treatment plan in order to be able to maximize the patient's eventual outcome. The patient should be exercising as early as the first injury day if possible. I am trying to avoid not only the complications of venostasis and pulmonary emboli, but also to eliminate the decreased muscle tone and muscle loss from prolonged immobilization. The patient should also have deep venous thrombosis prophylaxis with sequential compression devices and thromboembolic disease stockings, and each individual institution can decide about future prophylaxis with anticoagulation. In the initial postinjury period, anticoagulation is contraindicated for fear of creating an epidural hemaotoma.

Conclusion

The main indication for surgical treatment in a patient with a thoracic or lumbar spine injury would be to mobilize the patient sooner. This mobilization saves the patient approximately 2 weeks in acute hospitalization. The patient with a spinal cord injury will start rehabilitation

sooner. The price paid is increased mortality and morbidity, the most significant of which is an infection rate that in various series can vary anywhere from 7% to 15%. In my particular setting this rate has been approximately 9%. In my experience, which is also consistent with that of the literature, several myths associated with thoracic and lumbar trauma have evolved over time.

Myth Number 1
Any patient with a neurologic deficit requires surgical treatment. As I have already pointed out, complete injuries may be mobilized sooner but with the cost of higher complications and infection. Incomplete neurologic injuries tend to improve even with nonsurgical treatment, and if they do not improve with nonsurgical treatment, surgical treatment can be carried out at a later date with the ability to obtain similar end results.

Myth Number 2
Greater than a 50% compression of the vertebral height requires surgical restoration. To my knowledge, there has never been a study to substantiate this. Patients with multiple-level compression fractures, as long as they have been adequately immobilized and treated nonsurgically, do as well or better than those surgically treated.

Myth Number 3
Forty percent canal compromise requires surgery. This again cannot be justified in and of itself. Spinal canal compromise will resolve spontaneously over time and if the patient is asymptomatic, it is very difficult to improve that situation.

Myth Number 4
Multiple spinal fractures require surgery. Just the opposite is true. The

more injuries there are, the most likely the patient should be treated nonsurgically and that the surgical stabilization would take away too much spinal motion because of the long levels of fusion required.

Myth Number 5

Nonsurgical treatment should not be used because of the increased incidence of deep venous thrombosis and pulmonary emboli. In actuality, as long as the nonsurgical treatment is done aggressively with prophylaxis, I found either the same or lower incidence in the group treated nonsurgically as in the group treated surgically.

Myth Number 6

Nonsurgical treatment should not be used because of the higher complication rates. In actuality, I have found that the complication rates and particularly significant morbidity and mortality are much lower with nonsurgical treatment.

Myth Number 7

There was less pain long term if the spine was surgically stabilized. We found this to be just the opposite. In fact, there was more pain in the groups that had fusions. There were also more patients who required late surgery in the group initially treated with surgery than in the group initially treated nonsurgically. Most of the instrumentation was removed either by protocol or rod-long and fuse short techniques.

Myth Number 8

There is better neurologic recovery with surgery. This was not substantiated in our series or in other series.[4]

Myth Number 9

Canal compromise correlates with neurologic deficits. Again, this is not

true as evidenced by several studies already discussed.

Myth Number 10

Neurologic recovery correlates with spinal canal decompression. This again has been shown in several studies not to be the case. As was pointed out, it is probably biomechanically related to the fact that a great deal of the neurologic picture is determined at the time of the injury, both by the maximum canal compromise that takes place at the time of impact and by the speed of loading and the energy applied. Patients with incomplete injuries that have been stabilized can be decompressed electively.

Summary

The treatment of thoracolumbar trauma remains controversial. As more and more data are collected, there appears to be information that substantiates both surgical and nonsurgical treatment. Orthopaedic surgeons must all be cognizant of the fact that we draw our conclusions from data and not subjective prejudicial opinions. Nonsurgical treatment is still a viable and effective treatment for thoracic and lumbar fractures and should be part of the armamentarium available to all practitioners involved in the treatment of these patients.

References

1. Cantor JB, Lebwohl NH, Garvey T, Eismont FJ: Nonoperative management of stable thoracolumbar burst fractures with early ambulation and bracing. Spine 1993;18:971–976.

2. Davies WE, Morris JH, Hill V: An analysis of conservative (non-surgical) management of thoracolumbar fractures and fracture-dislocations with neural damage. J Bone Joint Surg 1980;62A:1324–1328.

3. Dendrinos GK, Halikias JG, Krallis PN, Asimakopoulos A: Factors influencing neurological recovery in burst thoracolumbar fractures. Acta Orthop Belg 1995;61:226–234.

4. Hartman MB, Chrin AM, Rechtine GR: Nonoperative treatment of thoracolumbar fractures. Paraplegia 1995;33:73–76.

5. Kinoshita H, Nagata Y, Ueda H, Kishi K: Conservative treatment of burst fractures of the thoracolumbar and lumbar spine. Paraplegia 1993;31:58–67.

6. Mumford J, Weinstein JN, Spratt KF, Goel VK: Thoracolumbar burst fractures: The clinical efficacy and outcome of nonoperative management. Spine 1993;18:955–970.

7. Patwardhan AG, Li SP, Gavin T, Lorenz M, Meade KP, Zindrick M: Orthotic stabilization of thoracolumbar injuries: A biomechanical analysis of the Jewett hyperextension orthosis. Spine 1990;15:654–661.

8. Sandor L, Barabas D: Spontaneous "regeneration" of the spinal canal in traumatic bone fragments after fractures of the thoraco-lumbar transition and the lumbar spine. Unfallchirurg 1994;97:89–91.

9. Weinstein JN, Collalto P, Lehmann TR: Thoracolumbar "burst" fractures treated conservatively: A long-term follow-up. Spine 1988;13:33–38.

10. Henderson RL, Reid DC, Saboe LA: Multiple noncontiguous spine fractures. Spine 1991;16:128–131.

11. Ballock RT, Mackersie R, Abitbol JJ, Cervilla V, Resnick D, Garfin SR: Can burst fractures be predicted from plain radiographs? J Bone Joint Surg 1992;74B:147–150.

12. Albert TJ, Levine MJ, An HS, Cotler JM, Balderston RA: Concomitant noncontiguous thoracolumbar and sacral fractures. Spine 1993;18:1285–1291.

13. Panjabi MM, Kifune M, Wen L, et al: Dynamic canal encroachment during thoracolumbar burst fractures. J Spinal Disord 1995;8:39–48.

14. Lemons VR, Wagner FC Jr, Montesano PX: Management of thoracolumbar fractures with accompanying neurological injury. Neurosurgery 1992;30:667–671.

15. Shuman WP, Rogers JV, Sickler ME, et al: Thoracolumbar burst fractures: CT dimensions of the spinal canal relative to postsurgical improvement. Am J Neuroradiol 1985;6:337–341.

16. Chakera TM, Bedbrook G, Bradley CM: Spontaneous resolution of spinal canal deformity after burst-dispersion fracture. Am J Neuroradiol 1988;9:779–785.

17. Yazici M, Atilla B, Tepe S, Calisir A: Spinal canal remodeling in burst fractures of the thoracolumbar spine: A computerized tomographic comparison between operative and nonoperative treatment. J Spinal Disord 1996;9:409–413.

18. Chan DP, Seng NK, Kaan KT: Nonoperative treatment in burst fractures of the lumbar spine (L2–L5) without neurologic deficits. Spine 1993;18:320–325.

19. Mick CA, Carl A, Sachs B, Hresko MT, Pfeifer BA: Burst fractures of the fifth lumbar vertebra. Spine 1993;18:1878–1884.

20. Boyd MC, Yu WY: Closed reduction of lumbosacral fracture dislocations. Surg Neurol 1985;23:295–298.

Classification of Thoracolumbar Fractures and Posterior Instrumentation for Treatment of Thoracolumbar Fractures

Daniel A. Capen, MD

Neurologic and Structural Classifications

In treating an injury to the thoracolumbar spine, several factors must be considered before treatment can be implemented. Outcome is governed as much by the decision-making process as by surgical or non-surgical care. Several classification systems are available that provide the practitioner with the information needed to plan successful treatment of the injury. Any classification system must provide a guide for the clinician to permit an understanding of the injury and to allow correct treatment choice.

Injuries to the thoracolumbar spine can result from many types of trauma. Anatomic proximity to abdominal structures and intrathoracic structures often creates life-threatening injury that requires emergent attention. Head injury can also accompany spine injury, especially when high-energy trauma has occurred, such as vehicular injury or fall from heights. Once multisystem assessment is complete and life-threatening problems are cleared, the spinal surgeon can safely treat the patient's spinal injury.

The planning of treatment begins, however, with initial patient contact. A checklist can be used to glean important bits of information that

will lead to appropriate treatment planning. (1) Is the injury high energy or low energy? Low-velocity gunshot wounds rarely destabilize the spine, and injuries that result from insignificant traumas, especially in older patients, must lead the practitioner to seek metabolic, metastatic, or infectious causes of the fracture. (2) Is the spinal column acutely unstable? High-energy trauma often creates an acutely unstable spine that requires emergent spine precautions. Care of life-threatening injury may delay spine surgery but must not delay spine supervision and appropriate precautions to prevent neurologic injury. If the spine is unstable acutely, does the patient need stabilization or orthotic treatment? (3) Is the neural column safe, threatened, or damaged? Imaging information may be important, but the neurologic examination is critical for appropriate decision making. Serial neurologic evaluation and appropriate grading will produce a treatment plan for successful outcome. (4) Is surgery required urgently? If canal compromise and neural deficit are documented and deterioration occurs, emergent surgery can help. If instability threatens further neurologic injury, emergent surgery can help. (5) Is surgery required for stability, neural recovery, or both?

These decisions require an understanding of the complete clinical picture. Radiographs taken of the spine at initial evaluation can often be used to diagnose spinal column injury. Computed tomography (CT) and magnetic resonance imaging (MRI) in the thoracolumbar region further clarify the picture of the spinal canal and can reveal posterior column injury, but most information regarding acute and chronic instability is present on plain radiographs. An understanding of Denis's classification of the 3-column spine will permit treatment planning for stabilization.[1] In addition to restoring spinal alignment, protecting neural elements, and preventing further injury, it is also important to avoid unneeded surgery. Even if well-performed, surgery for the wrong reason or without regard for the area of instability is subject to risk and may require revision. If appropriately applied, the Denis classification will assist the practitioner in planning the required procedure.

A mechanistic approach to thoracolumbar injury is well described by Ferguson and Allen.[2] This approach enhances the understanding of the forces applied to the spinal column at injury and helps the clinician to direct the treatment to the unstable

Table 1
Recommended treatment for various types of injury

Injury	Stability	Treatment
Vertical compression fracture	Stable	Orthosis
Missile injury	Stable	Orthosis
Distraction extension	Acutely	Surgical stabilization
Distraction flexion	Unstable	Rod-hook Screw-hooks
Translational injuries	Unstable	Reduction Rod-hooks Screw-hooks

area. From experience with the Allen classification of cervical trauma,[3] there is also some predictive information to allow nonsurgical treatment for fractures that are stable long-term. Flexion, distraction, compression, and rotational forces all produce radiographic pictures that are described in this classification.

The McAfee classification,[4] which describes 6 injury types that require CT for evaluation, also provides information regarding the forces applied at injury. This system also helps the clinician direct treatment to the area of spinal column failure. Wedge-compression, stable burst, unstable burst, Chance, flexion-distraction, and translational injuries are described, and pathology to the anterior, middle, and posterior columns associated with these injuries is described. I rely on the Allen classification because it is truly a total spine classification. However, the crucial factor is to use and become familiar with a system that will assist in understanding the pathoanatomy and enable the surgeon to plan appropriate treatment. Table 1 reflects injury type and recommended treatment.

The next factor for consideration in thoracolumbar trauma is the patient's neurologic status. Without this information, the clinician cannot plan appropriate care. Frankel grading, the standard system for many

decades,[5] is generally too generic. At present, the American Spinal Injury Association (ASIA) Scoring System[6] is widely used as the standard for determining status. Waters and associates[7–9] at Rancho Los Amigos, have followed large numbers of neurologic injuries by ASIA scores to determine anticipated outcomes. The surgeon is encouraged to use this information before completing the treatment plan.

The International Standards for Neurological and Functional Classification of Spinal Cord Injury[6] defines tetraplegia as loss or impairment of motor and/or sensory function in the cervical cord. Paraplegia is loss of motor and/or sensory function in the thoracic, lumbar, or sacral cord, including caudal and conus injuries. The neurologic level is the most caudal level of bilaterally normal motor and sensory function. Incomplete injury is defined by partial motor and/or sensory function below the neurologic level. Complete injury is defined as absence of sensory and motor function in the lowest sacral segment.

The ASIA scoring system for sensory function rates dermatomes as absent = 0, impaired = 1, and normal = 2. Motor scoring is done by testing 5 muscles in the upper and 5 in the lower extremities. All tests are scored 0 to 5, and all testing is done supine. Deltoid or biceps, wrist extensors, triceps, flexor profundus,

and hand intrinsics are tested for upper extremity scores. Iliopsoas, quadriceps, ankle dorsiflexors, extensor hallucis longus, and the gastrocnemius-soleus complex are scored in the lower extremities, to make a possible total of 100 points. Repeat examinations permit accurate tracking of improvement or deterioration, and pre- and postsurgical scoring is objectified.

Timing of Surgery

Complete injury is defined as the absence of motor and sensory function below the level of injury following emergence from spinal shock. Return of spinal bulbocavernosus reflex heralds emergence from spinal shock. After documentation of this, the likelihood of further neural recovery of significance is extremely small.[6] There is no current scientific justification for emergent surgery for decompression for the purpose of cord recovery in these patients. Focus must be turned to surgical or nonsurgical stabilization for enhancement of rehabilitation.[10] Needless surgery and postsurgical complications can be avoided if this is borne in mind. Some authors cite the zone of partial preservation as the target for decompression of complete injury. Some support for this viewpoint has been presented at the North American Spine Society 10th Annual Meeting by Rabinowitz (personal communication, 1995) in an animal study in which methylprednisolone was combined with decompression to produce better neural recovery, but the surgery must have reasonable likelihood of improving functional outcome.

The other group of patients with thoracolumbar trauma for whom treatment is clearly defined is the group with a perfect ASIA score, that is, normal neurologic function. This group includes patients with stable compression and burst type injuries and a few with unstable or potentially unstable injuries. It is generally agreed that, in these cases, improvement on normal neural function is impossible, while iatrogenic injury is possible.

Regardless of imaging studies, there is no justification for prophylactic decompression. In a tertiary center, such as Rancho Los Amigos Medical Center, however, it has been my experience that not all clinicians follow that caveat. The group of patients with incomplete cord injury syndromes presents the area of greatest variation in opinion and approach as to the timing and extent of surgery. The cord syndromes most frequently encountered are central, anterior, Brown-Sequard, conus, and cauda equina. Ditunno, in the ASIA standards, eloquently describes all these lesions.[6] Waters and associates[11] also describe anticipated outcomes in nonsurgical treatment for all these injuries. Before emergency intervention, the clinical status must be identified. Literature regarding cord recovery in animals by Bohlman and associates[12] and Delamarter and associates[13] has been cited most often to support emergency decompression.

The clear information is that within 6 hours after injury, the removal of compressing bone, disk, and deformity has some benefit. After 6 hours, no scientific evidence supports time as a factor in performance of decompression. I wish to stress that the time is 6 hours from time of injury, which reduces the number of patients eligible. Consideration of this factor should reduce needless high-risk surgery at midnight hours by ill-prepared surgical teams. Documented loss of neurologic function remains the 1 true indication for emergency surgery. Increased deformity, accumulation of hematoma, and cord edema remain the most frequent causes. After adequate study, efforts should focus on both decompression and stabilization to minimize revision surgery. Laminectomy alone is to be avoided, because it serves only to further destabilize the thoracolumbar spine and often fails to adequately decompress anterior bone and disk.

In addition to maximum attention to skeletal and neurologic classification, and optimal performance of surgery, 2 other factors must be stressed. First, in most high-energy thoracolumbar patients, early surgery is likely to be adversely impacted by increased blood loss, pulmonary complications, and the sequelae of multisystem injury. Second is the incidence of neurologic complication as a result of early intervention. Marshall and associates[14] described a 2.9% complication rate in 134 cases of surgery within 48 hours. Compromised hemodynamics will compromise cord environment and injury edema also adversely affects canal manipulation.

Spine traumas that produce ligamentous and bony instability, such as Chance-type fractures, distractive flexion injuries, and translational injuries, are the most unstable of injuries to the thoracolumbar region. The preferred treatment is to stabilize the spine initially with a combination of rods, with distraction-compression type hooks above the injury and, in the very lower thoracic and lumbar spine, to use intrapedicular bone screws. Cross-links are used. In many of these fractures, especially in the L1-2 area, a posterolateral decompression can be done as well. If it is also necessary to perform anterior decompression, this can be done once the spine is reduced and stabilized. Posterior instrumentation does permit contouring of rods to preserve lumbar lordosis and thoracic kypho-sis. Sagittal spinal balance is important for ambulation and wheelchair sitting. Unless secure fixation can be obtained with short segment fixation, at least 2 levels above and 2 levels below the injury must be incorporated. Newer FDA-approved combination rods, with pedicular hooks, transverse process hooks, and laminar hooks, provide sufficient stabilization to prevent later deformity.

As with all injuries, overdistraction or excessive compression across the traumatized area can result in neurologic worsening, because of the risk of retropulsion of bone and disk into the canal. This risk must be evaluated at the time of surgery to avoid iatrogenic neurologic injury. Understanding the mechanism of trauma and the classification of injury, together with intraoperative evaluation by radiographs, are the best methods for assurance of avoiding this complication.

In preoperative planning, if any of the posterior rod, hook, and screw combinations are going to be used, it is essential to ascertain the continuity of the planned bony structures for fixation. Ruling out occult lamina fracture, transverse process fracture, and pedicular fracture is essential. Noncontiguous spinal injury can occur, and appropriate imaging, whenever practical, can help to avoid the necessity for intraoperative change in plan.[15,16]

I prefer spinal-cord monitoring during the performance of decompression and fixation posteriorly for thoracolumbar fractures in any patient other than those with a complete neurologic injury. Even with anterior cord syndrome, monitoring impulses should be kept stable, and any manipulation of the spine must be documented. These precautions will help avoid iatrogenic neurologic worsening.

Table 2
Recommended methods for dealing with various thoracolumbar fractures

Spine Structure	Neurologic	Treatment
Stable	Normal	Nonsurgical
Stable	Complete	Nonsurgical
Stable	Incomplete	Decompression and stabilization
		Anterior or posterolateral
Unstable	Complete	Posterior stabilization
Unstable	Incomplete	Decompression and arthrodesis
		Anterior with plates
		Posterior or 360°

Posterior Instrumentation for Treatment of Thoracolumbar Fractures
Indications

The clinician must use the information contained in the classification of thoracolumbar injuries together with information regarding the patient's neurologic status in planning surgery. If the skeletal injury, the neurologic status, and the patient's multisystem health permits surgery, selection of a device for surgical fixation is the next important choice the surgeon must make.

Since the introduction of Harrington rod fixation,[17–23] there has been progressive development of instrumentation for spinal fracture fixation. Recognizing that each era had surgeons who were convinced that the "current technique" was optimal, we now have at our disposal fixation rod, hook, and cross-link systems that have been biomechanically tested. These devices are documented to provide secure fixation. The health-care industry has seen a remarkable proliferation of manufacturers of equipment, and, as a result, the surgeon can now select from multiple products.

The goals of posterior surgical treatment remain threefold. Realignment of the spine, restoration of canal anatomy, and protection against late deformity and instability are the 3 purposes for surgical intervention. The instrumentation available for treatment of thoracolumbar spine fractures permits the surgeon to create a construct that spans the area of instability and is fixed to the areas above and below the instability.

While Luque rod and wire stabilization has been shown to stabilize most fractures, the undesirable aspect of placing wires in the spinal canal adjacent to neural elements was a major drawback. Also, no distraction was possible. Current constructs, such as the Sofamor-Danek Horizon system and Acromed systems, have screw fixation systems for the pedicles below the thoracolumbar injury, and these screws are connected by a rod system to sublaminar claw and pedicular hook devices placed above the area of injury to actually grasp the spinal posterior elements. Some transverse process hooks are also available to maximize fixation above the thoracolumbar injury and to minimize the need for intracanal instrumentation. All constructs currently available emphasize the option for rods that are contoured to the spine to maintain normal or near normal sagittal balance. Numerous studies have stressed the importance of avoiding fixation in excessive kyphosis or lordosis.

The surgeon is encouraged to become familiar with a particular system and to practice working with that one instrument system until the entire operating team is aware of all the nuances of the particular device. These devices allow fixation of the minimal number of segments with maximum strength. I prefer the Horizon system by Sofamor-Danek, but this by no means indicates that other systems will not work as well. It merely reflects my familiarity with that particular device.

The success of posterior surgical treatment of thoracolumbar injuries depends on surgical judgment and appropriate indications, health of the patient at the time of the surgery, and appropriate uncomplicated application of the device at the time of the spinal surgery. Extensive operating time, staff unfamiliar with the device, and incomplete equipment can lead to substantial complications. The timing of surgery can also create hazards for the patient and intolerance of the surgical procedure. Successful outcome requires understanding and applying information from fracture classification and neurologic classification to provide appropriate treatment. Table 2 indicates the methods I prefer to use in dealing with various thoracolumbar fractures. This suggested guideline incorporates skeletal injury, neurologic status, and selected techniques for surgical intervention.

As shown in Table 2, there are several situations in which surgical intervention is not recommended. There remain indications for anterior surgery that are addressed in the anterior approaches to the thoracolumbar spine. The posterior surgical indications remain foremost with the completed neurologic injury, the unstable spine, and the desire to provide the patient with optimal early rehabilitation. As an ancillary, when anterior decompression has been performed, surgical posterior stabilization can permit full brace-free activity and rehabilitation when combined in a 360° approach.

The information provided in the 1980s by Edwards and Levine[24] remains effective in early stages to allow ligamentotaxis to decompress bony and disk elements via distraction. Although this procedure remains a viable option, the surgeon is cautioned to maintain awareness that 24- to 48-hour surgery with multisystem trauma is still beset with high incidences of complications, and a small number of spinal fractures with neurologic injury are in this category.

Summary

In treating thoracolumbar injuries, an accurate diagnosis of the structural injury to the spine is critical. I recommend the Allen classification,[2,3] but all classifications assist in obtaining an accurate understanding of the spine dynamics resulting from the injury. It is essential to remember that the majority of thoracolumbar injuries result from high-energy trauma. It is incumbent upon the spinal surgeon to ensure that multisystem trauma and life-threatening injuries, with the exception of a deteriorating neurologic injury, are cared for before embarking on spinal surgery. Even treatment of these injuries may have to be delayed if cardiovascular or abdominal hemorrhagic injuries take precedence.

A critically important piece of information is the neurologic diagnosis. I recommend the ASIA Motor Index[6] as the gold standard for diagnosing injuries and prognosticating outcome. Accurate neurologic diagnosis must be obtained prior to surgery. Finally, I recommend a firm

understanding and a good working relationship with the device system used for fixation. Other instructional course authors agree that whether the anterior or the posterior approach is used, familiarity with the device nuances, by not only the surgeon but also the operating team, is very helpful in achieving a successful uncomplicated implantation. If all of the above recommendations are followed, successful outcome and optimal patient recovery can be anticipated in most cases.

References

1. Denis F: The three column spine and its significance in the classification of acute thoracolumbar spinal injuries. *Spine* 1983;8:817–831.

2. Ferguson RL, Allen BL Jr: A mechanistic classification of thoracolumbar spine fractures. *Clin Orthop* 1984;189:77–88.

3. Allen BL Jr, Ferguson RL, Lehmann TR, O'Brien RP: A mechanistic classification of closed, indirect fractures and dislocations of the lower cervical spine. *Spine* 1982;7:1–27.

4. McAfee PC, Yuan HA, Fredrickson BE, Lubicky JP: The value of computed tomography in thoracolumbar fractures: An analysis of one hundred consecutive cases and a new classification. *J Bone Joint Surg* 1983;65A:461–473.

5. Frankel HL, Hancock DO, Hyslop G, et al: The value of postural reduction in the initial management of closed injuries of the spine with paraplegia and tetraplegia: I. *Paraplegia* 1969;7:179–192.

6. American Spinal Cord Injury Association: *Standards for Neurological and Functional Classification of Spinal Cord Injury*, Revised. Chicago, IL, American Spinal Cord Injury Association, 1992.

7. Waters RL, Yakura JS, Adkins RH, Sie I: Recovery following complete paraplegia. *Arch Phys Med Rehabil* 1992;73:784–789.

8. Waters RL, Adkins RH, Yakura JS, Sie I: Motor and sensory recovery following incomplete paraplegia. *Arch Phys Med Rehabil* 1994;75:67–72.

9. Waters RL, Adkins RH, Yakura JS, Sie I: Motor and sensory recovery following complete tetraplegia. *Arch Phys Med Rehabil* 1993;74:242–247.

10. Rimoldi RL, Zigler JE, Capen DA, Hu SS: The effect of surgical intervention on rehabilitation time in patients with thoracolumbar and lumbar spinal cord injuries. *Spine* 1992;17:1443–1449.

11. Waters RL, Adkins RH, Yakura JS, Sie I: Effect of surgery on motor recovery following traumatic spinal cord injury. *Spinal Cord* 1996;34:188–192.

12. Bohlman HH, Bahniuk E, Raskulinecz G, Field G: Mechanical factors affecting recovery from incomplete cervical spinal cord injury: A preliminary report. *Johns Hopkins Med J* 1979;145:115–125.

13. Delamarter RB, Sherman J, Carr JB: Pathophysiology of spinal cord injury: Recovery after immediate and delayed decompression. *J Bone Joint Surg* 1995;77A:1042–1049.

14. Marshall LF, Knowlton S, Garfin S, et al: Deterioration following spinal cord injury: A multicenter study. *J Neurosurg* 1987;66:400–404.

15. Keenen TL, Antony J, Benson DR: Noncontiguous spinal fractures. *J Trauma* 1990;30:489–491.

16. McLain RF, Sparling E, Benson DR: Early failure of short-segment pedicle instrumentation for thoracolumbar fractures: A preliminary report. *J Bone Joint Surg* 1993;75A:162–167.

17. Davis LA, Warren SA, Reid DC, Oberle K, Saboe LA, Grace MG: Incomplete neural deficits in thoracolumbar and lumbar spine fractures: Reliability of Frankel and Sunnybrook scales. *Spine* 1993;18:257–263.

18. Stambough JL: Cotrel-Dubousset instrumentation and thoracolumbar spine trauma: A review of 55 cases. *J Spinal Disord* 1994;7:461–469.

19. Akbarnia BA, Fogarty JP, Tayob AA: Contoured Harrington instrumentation in the treatment of unstable spinal fractures: The effect of supplementary sublaminar wires. *Clin Orthop* 1984;189:186–194.

20. Keene JS, Wackwitz DL, Drummond DS, Breed AL: Compression-distraction instrumentation of unstable thoracolumbar fractures: Anatomic results obtained with each type of injury and method of instrumentation. *Spine* 1986;11:895–902.

21. Cotler JM, Vernace JV, Michalski JA: The use of Harrington rods in thoracolumbar fractures. *Orthop Clin North Am* 1986;17:87–103.

22. Dickson JH, Harrington PR, Erwin WD: Results of reduction and stabilization of the severely fractured thoracic and lumbar spine. *J Bone Joint Surg* 1978;60A:799–805.

23. Jacobs RR, Asher MA, Snider RK: Thoracolumbar spinal injuries: A comparative study of recumbent and operative treatment in 100 patients. *Spine* 1980;5:463–477.

24. Edwards CC, Levine AM: Early rod-sleeve stabilization of the injured thoracic and lumbar spine. *Orthop Clin North Am* 1986;17:121–145.

Combined Anterior and Posterior Surgery for Fractures of the Thoracolumbar Spine

Alexander R. Vaccaro, MD

Introduction

The incidence of traumatic spinal injury has increased over the last several decades, with the majority of patients being males between the ages of 15 and 29 years.[1,2] In a multicenter review of more than 1,000 patients with thoracolumbar fractures, 16% of injuries occurred between the T1 and T10 levels, 52% between the T11 and L1 levels, and 32% between the L1 and L5 levels.[3] Nearly half of the injuries in this study were the result of motor vehicle accidents, with the remainder due to falls, sporting involvement, violence, and other miscellaneous causes.[2]

Significant 3-column injuries, including fracture-dislocations, make up approximately 50% of thoracolumbar fractures, with approximately 75% of these injuries resulting in a complete neurologic deficit.[4] Spinal injuries presenting with circumferential instability usually result from a combination of significant vector forces including, but not limited to, compression, extension, rotation, and shear. In most of these unstable injuries, surgical treatment is necessary to stabilize the spinal elements and allow early mobilization; moreover there is a frequent need to decompress the neural elements. The surgeon can gain access to the anterior and posterior spinal elements through a variety of approaches, depending on the anatomic level.

Occasionally, because of the degree of instability, the quality of the bony and ligamentous structures, and the location of neural impingement, a circumferential surgical approach may be necessary to accomplish the goals of surgical treatment. The sequence of surgical approaches, anterior then posterior, posterior then anterior, or simultaneous, is patient- and fracture-specific and should be determined on a patient-to-patient basis. Regardless of approach, the basic goals of surgical treatment remain the same: to maintain or improve the patient's neurologic status, to realign the spine, to relieve pain, and to allow early mobilization and rehabilitation.

Anterior Followed by Posterior Approach

An anterior followed by a posterior approach is often useful in an unstable 3-column injury of the upper thoracic or lower lumbar spine in the setting of canal occlusion and an incomplete neurologic deficit. An anterior decompression followed by bone grafting is then stabilized with a posterior compression or neutralization construct. In these locations, the use of anterior instrumentation is often contraindicated because of the close proximity of the great vessels (Figs. 1–3). An anterior followed by a posterior approach may be necessary in situations where anterior instrumentation may not sufficiently stabilize the involved levels, such as in the setting of an unstable burst or shear injury that reduces adequately in the sagittal plane with recumbency (Fig. 4). In this situation, an adjunctive posterior procedure is beneficial. Shiba and associates[5] presented a series of patients who were treated surgically with an anterior decompression and bone grafting followed by posterior transpedicular fixation for unstable thoracolumbar injuries, primarily of the burst type. The authors noted a 98% rate of fusion, with 65% of patients improving by at least one Frankel grade. No patients experienced worsening of their neurologic symptoms.

A combined anterior followed by a posterior procedure is also indicated when an anterior decompression and reconstruction is needed, but anterior instrumentation is contraindicated because of the presence of significant osteoporosis. This situation often occurs in elderly patients or in patients with metabolic bone disease and poor bone quality in whom

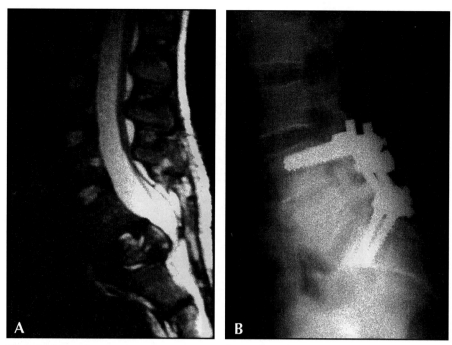

Fig. 1 A, A lateral magnetic resonance image of an L5 burst fracture in a patient with a unilateral L5 and S1 nerve root deficit. **B,** The patient underwent a posterolateral transpedicular decompression of the left L5 and S1 nerve roots and thecal sac followed by short segment posterior pedicular stabilization.

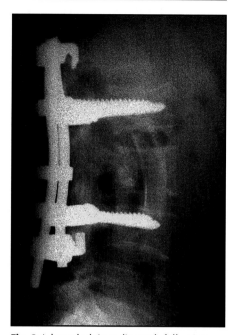

Fig. 2 A lateral plain radiograph following an anterior L3 corpectomy and strut grafting and posterior L1 to L4 hook and pedicular stabilization procedure. Anterior plate stabilization was not used because of the close proximity of the great vessels.

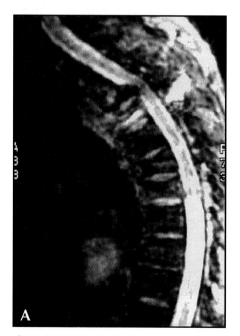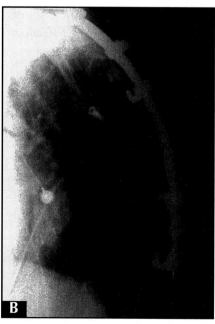

Fig. 3 A, A sagittal magnetic resonance image revealing a T3 burst fracture as well as T6 and T7 anterior compression fractures in a patient with an incomplete neurologic injury. **B,** A lateral plain radiograph following an anterior T3 carpectomy and fibula strut graft fusion with interference screw and a posterior rod hook compression and neutralization procedure. Anterior plate fixation could not be placed safely at the T2 to T4 level without risk of contact to the surrounding vasculature.

placement of anterior instrumentation carries the potential risk of screw, rod, or plate migration (Fig. 5).

Posterior Followed by Anterior Approach

A posterior followed by an anterior approach is often necessary in a significantly displaced fracture-dislocation of the thoracolumbar spine in a patient with an incomplete neurologic deficit. Adequate coronal and sagittal plane realignment is obtained through an initial posterior approach before decompressing the neural elements. Following this, the degree of canal occlusion may be assessed by intraoperative myelography, sonography, intracanal exploration, or postoperative imaging with computed tomography, myelogram, or magnetic resonance imaging. In a study by Edwards and Levine,[6] 4% of patients with an incomplete neurologic deficit who had been treated by a posterior indirect reduction had sufficient focal neurologic impingement remaining to warrant an immediate posterolateral or subsequent anterior decompression.

Occasionally, in a patient with a complete neurologic deficit, a posterior realignment procedure may result in significant loss of anterior column support and therefore not be adequately stabilized by a single-staged posterior procedure (Fig. 6). Sasso and Cotler[7] evaluated the efficacy of 3 different posterior internal fixation systems (Harrington rods and hooks, Luque rods with sublaminar wires, and AO dynamic compression plates with pedicle screws) used alone in the treatment of unstable fractures and fracture-dislocations of the thoracic and lumbar spine. At 12 months of follow-up, all 3 systems were found to be inadequate in maintaining sagittal balance, thereby illustrating the potential benefit of anterior column reconstruction and support.

Patients with ankylosing spondylitis or diffuse idiopathic skeletal hyperostosis who incur a traumatic distraction-extension injury may occasionally require a circumferential stabilization procedure (posterior, then anterior) to adequately stabilize the spine. Often, following posterior stabilization, a significant "fish mouth" anterior column defect is present, which may result in long-term instability if it is not reconstructed (Fig. 7). Also, in the setting of an open, unstable thoracolumbar injury, an initial posterior debridement followed by an anterior decompression and instrumentation fusion, if technically applicable, is recommended. Posterior instrumentation should not be used in this setting to avoid the risk of deep infection. Last, in a patient with an incomplete neurologic deficit an ante-

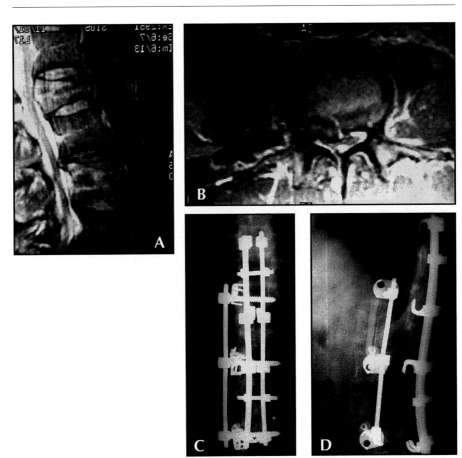

Fig. 4 A, A sagittal magnetic resonance image (MRI) of a 23-year-old man with an L1 and L3 burst fracture and an incomplete neurologic deficit. **B,** A transaxial MRI revealing the degree of canal encroachment at the L3 level. **C** and **D,** An anterior L1 and L3 corpectomy and strut graft fusion with instrumentation was followed by a neutralization and posterior stabilization because of the degree of instability. Note the single, not dual, rod application anteriorly because of the close proximity of the iliac vessels.

rior approach following an attempted posterior indirect reduction is occasionally necessary if sufficient canal clearance is not obtained during the posterior procedure. Several authors have advocated an additional anterior decompression procedure in this patient population if canal occlusion of 20% or greater is demonstrated by postoperative computed tomography scanning.[8]

Surgical Approach

In North America, a surgical team comprising of the spinal surgeon, anesthesiologist, electrophysiologist,

general or thoracic surgeon, and nursing staff work in a coordinated fashion to accomplish the aforementioned surgical goals with the least potential morbidity to the trauma patient. The possibility for intraoperative adverse events, such as loss of neurologic function with positioning or fracture reduction, great vessel injury, excessive blood loss due to the length of surgery, or instrumentation malpositioning, is increased with procedures that require circumferential stabilization because of the inherent instability of these procedures.

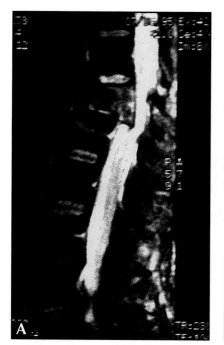
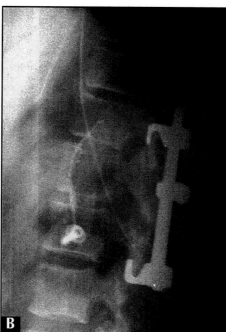

Fig. 5 A, A sagittal magnetic resonance image revealing an L1 flexion-compression burst fracture in a 68-year-old woman with significant osteoporosis. **B,** Because of the degree of osteoporosis and the potential for screw migration, an anterior plate was not applied following the corpectomy and bone grafting. A posterior compression hook and rod stabilization procedure followed the anterior procedure.

An experienced electrophysiologist using contemporary neurologic monitoring techniques greatly assists the surgeon in detecting the early onset of neurologic dysfunction. Additionally, an operating table that is equipped to rotate the patient's body axially without the need for repositioning further decreases the potential for any complications from patient movement. Most importantly, an experienced general or vascular surgeon is often of great use in anterior exposures that require exposure of the upper thoracic spine (transsternal or modified cervicothoracic approach) or lumbosacral region. Several useful posterior surgical approaches are available by which the spinal surgeon can gain access to the anterior spinal elements when a separate anterior approach is not desired. These include the posterior transpedicular approach and lateral extracavitary approach.

Lateral Extracavitary Approach

The lateral extracavitary approach[9] allows the spinal surgeon to access the anterior thecal sac and anterolateral vertebral elements throughout the thoracic and lumbar spine. However, this approach may be difficult above the level of T2 because of the presence of the scapula, and below the level of L4 because of the presence of the iliac crest (although this can be removed during the procedure and used for bone grafting). The approach consists of a "curved hockey stick" incision beginning in the midline approximately 3 vertebral levels above to 3 levels below the lesion. The incision is extended laterally with an abrupt curve toward the side of the approach for approxi-

mately 12 to 14 cm. The subcutaneous tissue and thoracodorsal fascia are then incised along the line of the skin incision and elevated from the midline laterally off the underlying musculature. If instrumentation is to be used, subperiosteal dissection is performed to expose the posterior vertebral elements.

Exposure of the thoracic and upper lumbar spine requires the removal of ribs for adequate visualization, and resection of a portion of the posterior iliac crest is necessary for visualization of the lumbar spine. During the exposure of the thoracic spine, a surgical plane is developed along the lateral aspect of the erectae spinae muscles in order to elevate them from the ribs and retract them medially. The laterally situated muscles—the latissimus dorsi, trapezius, and serratus groups—are retracted laterally. The intercostal muscles are then dissected away from the ribs, taking care not to injure the underlying neurovascular bundles that run along their inferior surface. The intercostal artery is routinely ligated, and the nerve may be divided or left intact at the discretion of the surgeon. The band of hypesthesia that results from sacrificing the intercostal nerve is rarely problematic and generally resolves over time. Following the proximal portion of the intercostal nerve allows identification of the neural foramen. The ribs that are to be removed (the rib at the level of the lesion and usually the adjacent caudal rib) are transected 7 to 10 cm lateral to the costovertebral junction, and they are then carefully disarticulated from their costovertebral and costochondral articulations. The transverse processes are also removed at these levels.

In lower lumbar lesions, the posterior, superior, and medial portion of the iliac crest is removed following dissection of surrounding mus-

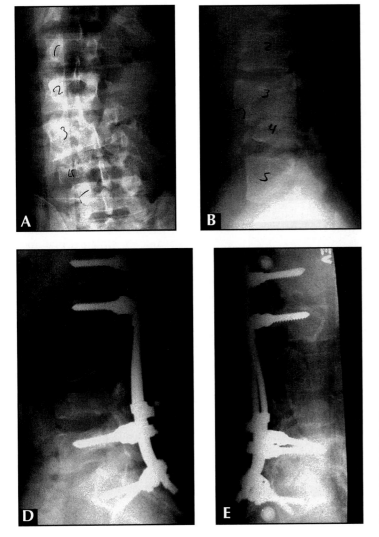

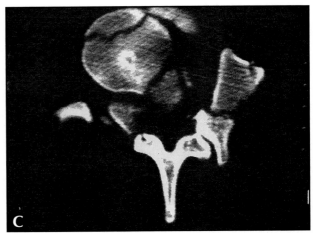

Fig. 6 A, anteroposterior and **B,** lateral plain radiographs of a severe rotational fracture-dislocation in a patient with a complete neurologic injury. **C,** A transaxial computed tomography scan revealed the presence of lateral vertebral subluxation as well as significant canal compromise. **D,** A lateral plain radiograph following an open posterior realignment and stabilization. **E,** Due to the degree of loss of anterior column support, an anterior L3 and L4 corpectomy and iliac crest graft reconstruction was performed.

culature and periosteum. The transverse process at the level of the lesion and the one caudal to it are dissected free of all contiguous soft-tissue structures and are removed to expose the exiting nerve roots. The nerve roots are subsequently mobilized and retracted laterally with nerve tapes and are again used to identify the neural foramen.

Subsequent to the soft-tissue exposure of the involved vertebrae, the vertebral periosteum is bluntly dissected off the ventrolateral aspect of the vertebral body and pedicle in preparation for spinal canal decompression.

Posterolateral Transpedicular Approach

The transpedicular approach may be selected in certain thoracolumbar injuries in which there is significantly lateralized or asymmetric anterior canal occlusion in a patient with symptomatic neural compression. This technique is most useful in lower lumbar injuries, in which anterior reconstructive procedures are often technically challenging and difficult to stabilize with instrumentation because of the close proximity of the great vessels. In the vast majority of cases with significant neural compression, the anterior approach provides optimal access to the anterior neural elements for decompression and reconstruction.

After posterior exposure of the involved vertebral level, the cephalad portion of the lamina, spinous process, supra-adjacent ligamentum flavum, and inferior lamina of the superior vertebrae are removed to expose clearly the medial and inferior boundaries of the pedicle to be decompressed. A burr is then used to remove the central portion of the pedicle into the fractured vertebral body. Using care to protect the transversing and exiting nerve roots, a rongeur or curette may be used to

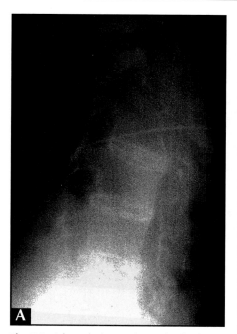 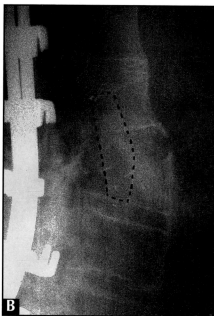

Fig. 7 A, A lateral plain radiograph of a distraction extension injury at the L1, L2 level in a patient with ankylosing spondylitis. **B,** Following a posterior stabilization procedure, an anterior column reconstruction was performed because of the presence of a large anterior "fish mouth" bony deficiency.

remove the medial cortex of the involved pedicle. A trough is then cut into the posterior portion of the vertebral body anterior to the medial pedicular wall decompression. Reverse-angled curettes are used to displace bony fragments out of the canal into the region of this trough. Large bony fragments may be removed posteriorly with gentle thecal sac retraction in the lower lumbar spine below the conus of the spinal cord.

Spinal Fixation

Spinal instrumentation allows the surgeon to manipulate the spinal elements efficiently in order to obtain proper alignment, to assist in indirectly decompressing the spinal elements, and to afford stability to allow for early mobilization. Commonly used spinal implants include hooks, screws, and wires attached to rods or plates posteriorly and screws attached to plates or rods as well as metallic

interbody spacers (cages) anteriorly. The choice of implant is determined by the nature, degree, or biomechanics of the existing instability, the quality of the spinal elements in terms of bone density or osteoporosis, and the medical condition of the patient. Hooks and rods are frequently used in posterior spinal applications for thoracolumbar injuries. Converging hook patterns allow the surgeon to apply compressing forces; diverging hook patterns allow distraction. A combination of hook patterns, such as the use of claw configurations with or without supplemental sublaminar wires, allows multisegmental rigid spinal fixation, especially when a long level arm is needed for spinal manipulation. Sublaminar wires are useful in the neurologically complete patient when multiple level segmental fixation is necessary. Pedicle screw fixation is useful in lower lumbar and sacral injuries where short segment

fixation is desirable as long as there is adequate anterior column support. The anatomic constraints of the pedicle in the mid and upper thoracic spine render pedicle screw applications less useful in these regions.

Techniques for anterior fixation usually involve plate and screw instrumentation. This form of fixation is generally chosen when a single approach (ie, anterior) is acceptable for neural decompression and stabilization. Circumferential procedures often use a single anterior rod and screw construct for added spinal and bone graft stability in addition to supplemental posterior instrumentation. Anterior spinal instrumentation, especially of the plating type, is generally not used in the lower lumbar and sacral region because of the close proximity of the great vessels.

Postoperative Care

Aggressive postoperative pulmonary and nutritional care is vital to the successful recovery of a patient undergoing a circumferential reconstructive procedure for an unstable thoracolumbar injury. The primary objective of such an involved procedure is to allow early patient mobilization so as to avoid the morbidity associated with recumbency. Nutritional supplementation assists in wound healing and provides the energy necessary for early patient rehabilitation.

If medically stable, patients who undergo a circumferential stabilization procedure may be mobilized in a chair on the first postoperative day. Increased mobility, either via a wheelchair or through ambulation, usually commences on approximately postoperative day 2 or at the time of chest tube removal. A standard thoracolumbosacral orthosis (TLSO) with a cervical extension is applied to fracture patterns cephalad to the T7 level. The cervical extension is used for approximately 6 weeks. Below T6, a standard TLSO is used. For fractures involving the L4, L5, or sacral levels, an additional thigh cuff attachment is used for approximately 6 weeks. The duration of brace wear ranges from 3 to 6 months, depending on the fracture type and degree of stability.

Routine upper and lower extremity range of motion and strengthening begin in the early postoperative period and are patient specific depending on the neurologic status. Following brace removal, truncal strengthening and range of motion are begun.

Outcomes

The literature is sparse on the outcomes of circumferential stabilization procedures for fracture-dislocations of the thoracolumbar spine. The obvious benefits of this procedure are the ability to decompress the anterior neural elements, provide anterior column support, and recreate or maintain sagittal balance with a variety of posterior instrumentation techniuqes. As anesthetic techniques improve and surgeons become more

experienced with circumferential stabilization techniques for thoracolumbar spinal injuries, the morbidity in terms of surgical time and blood loss will certainly be overshadowed by the satisfactory long-term outcomes of these procedures.

★At the time of this writing, bone screws placed posteriorly into vertebral elements have been cleared for use in this specific manner by the Food and Drug Administration (FDA) to provide immobilization and stabilization as an adjunct to fusion in the treatment of the following acute and chronic instability or deformities of the thoracic, lumbar and sacral spine; degenerative spondylolisthesis with objective evidence of neurological impairment; fracture; dislocation; scoliosis; kyphosis; spine tumor and failed previous fusion (pseudoarthrosis). In addition, anterior vertebral body screws (cervical, thoracic, and lumbar) are Class II devices and can be used as labeled in vertebral bodies.

References

1. Kraus JF, Franti CE, Riggins RS, Richards D, Borhani NO: Incidence of traumatic spinal cord lesions. *J Chronic Dis* 1975;28:471–492.

2. Price C, Makintubee S, Herndon W, Istre GR: Epidemiology of traumatic spinal cord injury and acute hospitalization and rehabilitation charges for spinal cord injuries in Oklahoma, 1988-1990. *Am J Epidemiol* 1994;139:37–47.

3. Gertzbein SD: Scoliosis Research Society: Multicenter spine fracture study. *Spine* 1992;17:528–540.

4. Bohlman HH: Treatment of fractures and dislocations of the thoracic and lumbar spine. *J Bone Joint Surg* 1985;67A:165–169.

5. Shiba K, Katsuki M, Ueta T, et al: Transpedicular fixation with Zielke instrumentation in the treatment of thoracolumbar and lumbar injuries. *Spine* 1994;19:1940–1949.

6. Edwards CC, Levine AM: Early rod-sleeve stabilization of the injured thoracic and lumbar spine. *Orthop Clin North Am* 1986;17:121–145.

7. Sasso RC, Cotler HB: Posterior instrumentation and fusion for unstable fractures and fracture-dislocations of the thoracic and lumbar spine: A comparative study of three fixation devices in 70 patients. *Spine* 1993;18:450–460.

8. Danisa OA, Shaffrey CI, Jane JA, et al: Surgical approaches for the correction of unstable thoracolumbar burst fractures: A retrospective analysis of treatment outcomes. *J Neurosurg* 1995;83:977–983.

9. Maiman DJ, Larson SJ: Lateral extracavitary approach to the thoracic and lumbar spine, in Rengachary SS, Wilkins RH (eds): *Neurosurgical Operative Atlas*. Park Ridge, IL, American Association of Neurological Surgeons (AANS), 1991, pp 153–161.

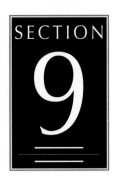

SECTION 9

Osteoporotic Spine

Osteoporotic Spine

With the progressive aging of the US population, the osteoporotic spine is becoming more prevalent, and necessarily, the prevention and management of osteoporotic compression fractures are becoming more common aspects of the practice of medicine. The challenges of caring for patients with an osteoporotic spine involve a wide array of issues, including the role of preventive medicine and the decisions regarding specific treatment approaches, namely minimally invasive procedures versus conventional open surgery. The articles in this section address the basic science of normal and osteoporotic bone, vertebral compression fractures, medical consequences of these fractures, and the current array of treatment options.

Dr. Thomas Einhorn covers the basic science of biomechanics and osteoporosis by eloquently defining key concepts and describing how the bony architecture of normal bone differs from that of osteoporotic bone. One definition of osteoporosis is the "absolute decrease in the amount of bone leading to an increase in the risk of fracture." The loss of bone is important to the structural properties of the vertebrae, but the importance of the microarchitecture of the trabecula should be noted as well. Trabecular "quality" involves both the percent of continuous trabecula as well as the thickness of the trabecular elements. The vertebral body trabeculae continuously remodel and are affected by both hormonal and cellular changes; these can result in differences in resistance to fracture even when bone density is relatively comparable. Dr. Einhorn's article highlights the importance of continued research in methods of improving bone quality as well as bone mineral density.

Dr. David Kim and associates provide a comprehensive review of osteoporotic vertebral compression fractures. This problem can be described as an epidemic: up to one quarter of all women over the age of 70 years in the United States has radiographic evidence of a vertebral compression fracture. Preventing osteoporosis is the best way to prevent these fractures, and preventing fractures is the best treatment. The World Health Organization defines osteoporosis as bone density that is 2.5 standard deviations below average as measured by dual-energy x-ray absorptiometry (DEXA). Osteoporosis has been classified as either type I or type II. Type I is a result of estrogen deficiency and is associated with a higher incidence of vertebral fractures. Type II osteoporosis is caused by inadequate lifetime calcium intake and is associated with proximal femur fractures. Dr. Kim and associates emphasize that the differences between the two types must be recognized to properly prevent and treat osteoporosis.

Dr. Eric Truumees updates what is known about the medical consequences of osteoporotic vertebral compression fractures. The conventional wisdom that most osteoporotic compression fractures are benign is changing. Most patients with acute compression fractures improve within 4 to 6 weeks; however, the severity and length of symptoms vary widely between patients. He points out that some patients have severe pain that requires hospitalization, while others have persistent pain for months. Nonsurgical treatment such as bracing is often ineffective. Limiting physical activity may be necessary for palliation, but this approach can aggravate the comorbidities common in the elderly. The progression of kyphosis, both segmental and global, may be related to chronic back pain and loss of self-esteem. Dr. Truumees also describes the adverse physiologic effects associated with fracture deformity. One thoracic compression fracture causes a 9% loss of forced vital capacity. Increased risk of pulmonary death from conditions such as pneumonia and chronic obstructive pulmonary disease also has been reported with increased thoracic kyphosis.

Dr. Frank Philips and associates describe vertebroplasty and kyphoplasty. The development of these minimally invasive methods for surgically treating vertebral compression fractures has been quite timely given the current increase in the mean age of the US population. Stabilization and correction of deformity are proven orthopaedic principles and have been associated with the benefits of early mobilization and restored function. Traditionally, vertebral compression fractures have been difficult to stabilize externally, and methods of open fixation have been too invasive and risky to offer to most patients. Percutaneous methods of stabilizing vertebral compression fractures are effective for a much larger group of patients.

Even though the relative merits of vertebroplasty and kyphoplasty have been debated, both are generally considered to be highly effective for the treatment of osteoporotic vertebral compression fractures. Contraindications for these procedures include infection, vertebral plana, neurologic compression, and inability to tolerate general anesthesia. Some authors believe that the injection of high-pressure, low-viscosity cement increases the risk of cement extravasation outside the vertebral body. Cement leakage into the epidural, disk, paravertebral, and intraforaminal spaces has been reported, but the rate of clinically significant complications is small in experienced hands. Kyphoplasty advocates believe that the use of a balloon tamp to create a space to fill with low-viscosity cement placed under low pressure may lead to fewer uncontrolled extravasations. The use of a balloon tamp also affords the opportunity to restore vertebral body height. On a technical note, simultaneous biplanar visualization with excellent fluoroscopic equipment is necessary for safe, efficient vertebroplasty or kyphoplasty. Despite the theoretical considerations, cement leakage is uncommon with both procedures, and both are considered safe and effective when performed correctly.

Drs. John Kostuik and Michael Shapiro discuss open surgical treatment of osteoporotic vertebral compression fractures. Open surgical treatment is rarely required, but indications include fractures associated with (1) neurologic compromise that requires decompression; (2) progressive deformity associated with intractable pain or progression of neurologic compromise; and (3) possibly some painful fractures that are not amenable to percutaneous cement techniques such as vertebral plana. Careful preoperative workup and maximum preoperative nutrition are necessary. Despite the most careful preparation, however, major reconstructive surgery in the elderly population has a high rate of complications, usually because of comorbidities and the difficulties associated with obtaining sufficient hold on the osteoporotic spine with instrumentation. The addition of cement to the vertebral body during insertion of pedicle screws can significantly improve pullout strengths of the screws. Special screws have been designed for the osteoporotic spine, including expandable screws and tapered screws.

Drs. Steven Glassman and Gary Alegre describe adult spinal deformity in the osteoporotic spine. De novo scoliosis develops in adults as a result of osteoporosis or degenerative changes. Often these patients are elderly, have poor bone quality, and present with symptoms attributable to stenosis. Underlying osteoporosis should be treated medically, and nonsurgical treatment of stenosis and back pain should be initiated. However, nonsurgical treatment fails in a significant percentage of patients, making surgical treatment a requirement. The surgical treatment of de novo scoliosis is one of the most challenging aspects of spine surgery. The general medical condition and life expectancy of the patient should be considered as the surgery is planned. Important factors to consider include global and regional balance, presence of lateral listhesis or anterolisthesis, severity of deformity, and location of stenosis.

In summary, these articles provide a useful review of the current state of the art in the diagnosis and management of spinal disorders of the osteoporotic spine. Clearly the newest developments have been vertebroplasty and kyphoplasty to treat vertebral compression fractures. The indications for these procedures are evolving, and proposed randomized control studies will be very helpful to better understand their benefits and limitations. Ongoing improvements in spinal fixation methods have been helpful in situations that require open spinal surgery.

S. Tim Yoon MD, PhD
Chief of Orthopaedics, Atlanta VAMC
Assistant Professor of Orthopaedic Surgery
Emory University School of Medicine
Decatur, Georgia

The Structural Properties of Normal and Osteoporotic Bone

Thomas A. Einhorn, MD

Abstract

Although numerous advances have been made in the diagnosis and treatment of osteoporosis, only a fraction of those patients with osteoporosis who receive orthopaedic care are actually treated or referred for treatment of their osteoporotic condition. A review of the basic anatomic and structural properties of normal and osteoporotic bones and how these properties influence the load-carrying capacity of the skeleton is important. Anatomic and mechanical risk factors for osteoporosis form the basis for an appreciation of the clinical risk of fracture among patients. Because vertebral fractures are the most common fractures seen in patients with osteoporosis, attention is focused on the biomechanics of the vertebrae. This information should assist orthopaedic surgeons in the evaluation of patients who have or who are at risk for developing osteoporosis and prepare them for a variety of interventions, both pharmacologic and surgical, that can improve patient care.

In 2001, Freedman and associates[1] reviewed a claims database of over 3 million patients enrolled in multiple health plans and found that of 1,162 women aged 55 years or older who had a distal radius fracture, only 33 (2.8%) underwent a bone density scan, and 266 (22.9%) were treated with a medication approved for the management of osteoporosis. Moreover, there was a significant decrease in the rate of treatment of osteoporosis that correlated with the increasing age of the patient at the time of fracture. These investigators concluded that current physician practice may be inadequate for the diagnosis and treatment of osteoporosis. Based on findings such as these, it is clear that orthopaedic surgeons could have a major impact on America's bone health by having a heightened awareness of the prevalence of osteoporosis and by either treating or referring patients for treatment or prophylaxis when it is apparent that they have or are at risk for developing this disease. To establish the fundamental principles that underlie the structural components of osteoporosis and to use these principles as a basis for determining how pharmaceutical agents and/or surgical treatments (for example, vertebroplasty and kyphoplasty) may influence this disease, this chapter will review the basic anatomic and mechanical properties that characterize osteoporotic bone.

Normal and Osteoporotic Bone Structure

Bone is a composite material composed of a protein matrix impregnated with a mineral phase. The bone matrix is composed largely of type I collagen and a variety of noncollagenous proteins, and the mineral component consists of a crystalline hydroxyapatite $(Ca_{10}(PO_4)_6OH_2)$. Although the composition of bone is consistent throughout the skeleton, it is distributed to two distinct envelopes, cortical and trabecular bone, each of which has a different structure and architecture. Cortical bone has four times the mass of trabecular bone, and the metabolic turnover rate of trabecular bone is much higher than that of cortical bone (bone turnover is a surface event, and trabecular bone has a greater surface area than cortical bone).[2] Trabecular bone is found principally at the ends of long bones and in cuboid bones, such as the vertebrae (Fig. 1). The internal beams or plates of trabeculae form a three-dimensional branching lattice that is oriented along lines of stress. Trabecular bone is subject to a complex set of stresses and strains, although it is best designed for resisting compressive loads. Cortical bone appears as an entirely different

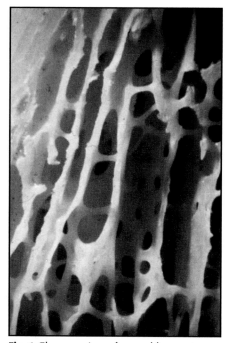

Fig. 1 Close-up view of normal human trabecular bone. Note that this structure is distributed as a three-dimensional branching lattice in which plates of bone are oriented at right angles to each other.

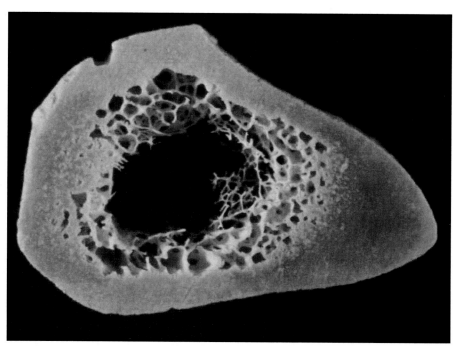

Fig. 2 Cross-section of cortical bone from the middiaphysis of the tibia. Note that cortical bone is a solid structure arranged not as interconnecting plates but as elliptoid cylinders. On the inner surface (endosteum), there is a structure that resembles that of trabecular bone. (Reproduced with permission from Lee CA, Einhorn TA: The bone organ system: Form and function, in Marcus R, Feldman D, Kelsey J (eds): *Osteoporosis*, ed 2. San Diego, CA, Academic Press, 2001, pp 3-20.)

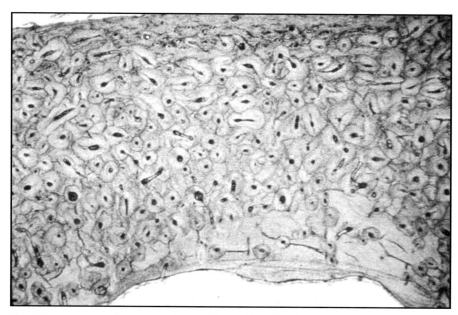

Fig. 3 Close-up view of a section of cortical bone. Note the distribution of vascular channels forming the osteons. (Reproduced with permission from Lee CA, Einhorn TA: The bone organ system: Form and function, in Marcus R, Feldman D, Kelsey J (eds): *Osteoporosis*, ed 2. San Diego, CA, Academic Press, 2001, pp 3-20.)

structure. It is solid and arranged not as interconnecting plates, but rather as cylinders that are elliptoid in cross-section (Fig. 2). Cortical bone is largely subjected to bending and torsional loads but experiences compressive loads as well. Although the regulation of bone mass is metabolically controlled by the effect of osteoblasts and osteoclasts that conduct their activities on the surface of trabecular bone, in cortical bone, the capillaries in the central canals, which are derived from the principal nutrient arteries of bone, are organized in haversian systems, and these structures form individual osteons that become the metabolic units of this compact structure[3] (Fig. 3).

Osteoporosis is defined as "an absolute decrease in the amount of bone leading to an increase in the risk of fracture."[3] For trabecular bone, the conversion of normal to osteoporotic bone consists of a change from a structure consisting of plates interconnected at right angles to one of spicules distributed in a delicate lattice framework (Fig. 4). This lattice is easily susceptible to failure under normal physiologic loads. Anatomically, the conversion of normal to osteoporotic trabecular bone occurs as a result of osteoclastic activity leading to thinning of the trabecular struts and a loss of horizontal interconnections between the vertical plates. Indeed, independent of the amount of bone mass present, the loss of horizontal interconnections can lead to a dramatic decline in the load-carrying capacity of the skeleton.[4]

Whereas cortical bone serves to encase trabecular bone in areas of the appendicular skeleton, its contribution to the mechanical properties will differ depending on the anatomic site. However, most long bones fail under a combination of axial compression, bending, and torsion, and the ability of cortical bone to support these loads will depend on its cross-sectional shape, length, and material properties. In cases of bending, the cross-sectional area is less important than the distribution of cortical bone in relation to its central axis of loading. Ideally, cortical bone should be distributed as far from this axis as possible; the geometric parameter used to describe this property is the areal moment of inertia. Similarly, in torsion, deformation is resisted more efficiently the farther bone is distributed from the torsional axis. The geometric parameter used to describe this property is polar moment of inertia.[5]

With aging, the outer cortical diameter of bone increases, and the cortical wall thickness declines. This set of changes results from the combined effects of increased endosteal resorption and periosteal bone apposition. Although the net effect may be cortical thinning, the increased diameter of the bone improves its resistance to bending and torsion and thus increases the areal and polar moment of inertia properties.[6] This may

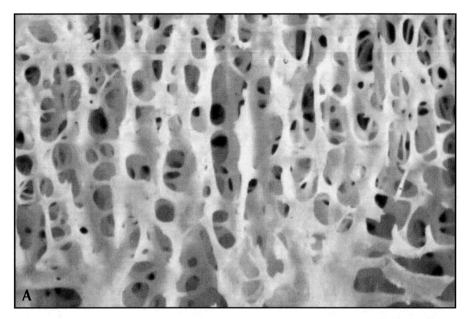

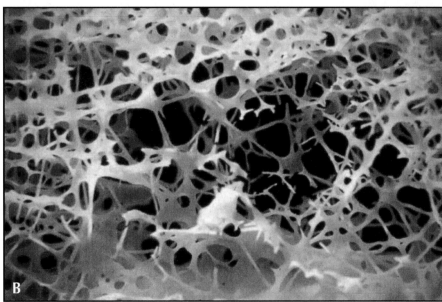

Fig. 4 A, Close-up view of normal human trabecular bone from the centrum of a vertebral body. **B,** Close-up view of osteoporotic human trabecular bone from the centrum of a vertebral body. Note the loss of trabecular mass and interconnections.

explain why cortical bone fractures in diaphyseal segments of the skeleton are surprisingly uncommon in elderly patients with osteoporosis.

Mechanisms of Bone Failure

As with other objects in nature, bone undergoes acceleration, deformation, or both when it experiences an externally applied load. In biomechanical terms, this load is known as a force.[7] If the force is sufficient to cause deformation in the bone, the bone will react by generating an internal resistance known as stress. Stress is equal in magnitude but opposite in direction to the applied force and is distributed over the cross-sectional area of the bone. It is generally expressed in units

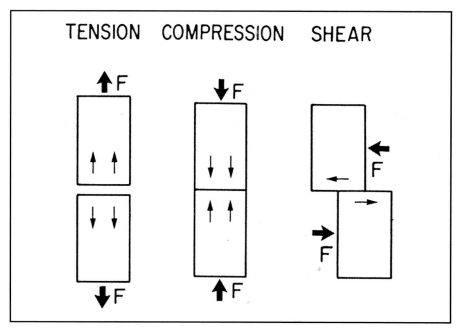

Fig. 5 The three basic types of stress into which all complex patterns can be resolved: tension, compression, and shear. F = force. (Reproduced with permission from Einhorn TA: Bone strength: The bottom line. *Calcif Tissue Int* 1992;51:333-339.)

of force per unit area (newtons per meters squared), and the standard international unit for stress is the pascal, (one newton of force distributed over one square centimeter).

Although an externally applied force can be directed at bone from any angle, producing complex stress patterns, all stresses can be resolved into the following three types: tension, compression, and shear[5] (Fig. 5). Tension is produced in bone when two forces are directed away from each other along the same line. Resistance to tensile forces comes from the intermolecular attractive forces that prevent the materials from being pulled apart; ultimate tensile strength is a measure of this cohesive force. Compression results from two forces, again acting along the same line, but directed toward each other. Compression is resisted by interatomic repulsive forces, which rise sharply at short interatomic distances. An excellent example of compression occurs when someone slips and falls backwards, landing on the buttocks, the

force of which transduces a compressive load along the axis of the spine via the vertebral bodies. Shear forces occur when two loads act in parallel but opposite directions of one another and can be oriented in either a linear or rotational fashion. Shear occurs in a vertebral body when the surface of the superior end plate is loaded anteroposteriorly that of the inferior end plate experiences a posteroanterior-directed load.

Most stress patterns are complex combinations of these three stress types.[8] Bending, for example, produces a combination of tensile forces on the convex side of a structure or material and compression on the concave side. This is the loading configuration that typically produces a femoral neck fracture in an elderly patient with osteoporosis. Torsion, or twisting, produces shear stresses along the entire length of a structure or material and can lead to a spiral fracture configuration. The measurement of deformation resulting from any of these stresses, when normalized by the original config-

uration of the specimen, is called strain.[7] Strain is dimensionless and therefore expressed as a percentage of change from the original dimensions of the bone.

Normal and shear strains experienced by bone will be influenced not only by the magnitude of the stresses generated by the applied loads, but also by the inherent material and structural properties of the anatomic part of the skeleton. Stresses applied to normal, well-mineralized bone will cause small strains, whereas the same stresses applied to osteoporotic bone will produce large strains.

Laboratory testing has been used to quantitate the biomechanical properties of the skeleton. By convention, stress is plotted on the ordinate (y axis) and strain on the abscissa (x axis). As three types of stress exist (tension, compression, and shear) and as these stresses are produced by different forces (tension, compression, bending, and torsion), the y axis could represent any of these loading conditions and the curve reflect any load-versus-deformation relationship. A standard stress-strain curve of bone loaded in bending can be used as an example to define and understand key terms used in characterizing the mechanical properties of bone (Fig. 6). The linear portion of the curve represents the elastic region, and the measured slope is used to derive the stiffness of the bone. Loading in this region will result in a nonpermanent deformation, and the energy returned by the bone when the load is removed is known as the resilience. The nonlinear portion of the curve represents the plastic region and indicates that the bone has been permanently deformed by the applied load. The point at which the linear region gives way to the nonlinear region (elastic region gives way to plastic region) is known as the yield point, and the stress at this point is known as the elastic limit. The maximum stress exhibited by the bone occurs at the point of failure, and a line extrapolated back to the ordinate provides a quantitative value known as the ultimate strength of the bone. The maximum strain at the point of failure gives a quantitative value that is the ductility of the bone. The area under the curve can be quantitated and represents the strain energy. The total energy stored at the point of fracture gives a value for the toughness of the bone.[5,7]

Osteoporotic Vertebral Compression Fractures

Vertebral fracture is the signature manifestation of osteoporosis. Although only half of the patients with osteoporosis have symptomatic fractures of their vertebrae, there is frequent disagreement among physicians as to whether a fracture is present.[9] This difficulty in deciding whether a vertebra is fractured results from variations in vertebral shape and also among individuals. Eastell and associates[9] classified vertebral fractures to one of the following three types: wedge, biconcavity, or compression. They further classified vertebral fractures by the degree of deformity (grade 1 or grade 2) (Fig. 7). By studying 195 postmenopausal women ranging in age from 47 to 94 years, these investigators showed that 40 (21%) had a vertebral fracture, wedge fractures were most common, and grade 2 fractures were more common than grade 1 fractures. Furthermore, bone mineral density of the lumbar spine was related to a mean fracture grade and fracture number.

The reduction in load-carrying capacity of the thoracic and lumbar vertebrae is a function of both bone mass and architecture. Because vertebrae are cuboid structures composed of trabecular bone encased in a cortical shell, the relative contribution of the cortex and trabeculae to the load-carrying capacity of the vertebrae has been a subject of investigation. Silva and associates[10] showed, using a finite-element model of vertebrae loaded in compression, that the cortical shell accounts for only approximately 10% of vertebral strength and that the trabecular

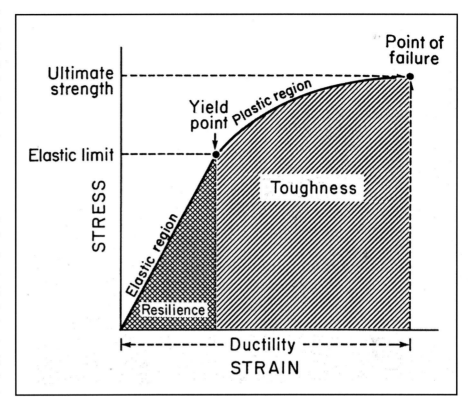

Fig. 6 A standard stress/strain curve of bone loaded in bending. (Reproduced with permission from Einhorn TA: Bone strength: The bottom line. *Calcif Tissue Int* 1992;51:333-339.)

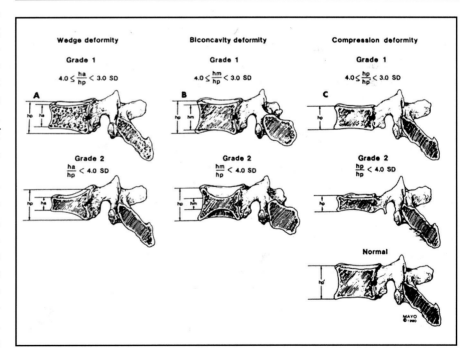

Fig. 7 Classification of vertebral fractures by type and grade. (Reproduced with permission from Eastell R, Cedel SL, Wahner HW, Riggs BL, Melton LJ: Classification of vertebral fractures. *J Bone Min Res* 1991;6:207-215.)

centrum is the dominant structural component of the vertebral body. In a subsequent report, these investigators used both direct tomography and CT to demonstrate that the cortical shells and end plates in vertebrae are porous and irregular and have an average thickness of approximately 0.35 mm.[11] They concluded that the cortical shell and end plate of the vertebral body behave more as thin membranes of fused trabeculae rather than as true cortices.

The distribution of trabecular and cortical bone in the vertebral bodies has also been a subject of investigation. Flynn and Cody[12] showed that the volume of bone in the vertebral cortex declines with age and at a slower rate than is observed for cancellous bone; however, the decline with age of cortical bone appears to vary substantially among subjects. Moreover, the amount of cortical bone in the anterior portion of the body is less than that in the lateral portion. Mizrahi and associates[13] used an isolated, human L3 vertebral body from an elderly subject to demonstrate how material properties and loading conditions influence end plate and cortical shell displacements and stresses. They demonstrated that a 50% reduction in trabecular bone modulus alone increases peak stresses in the end plate by 74% and that elimination of the cortical shell reduces these stresses by approximately 20%. When they adjusted the material properties to represent osteoporosis, with disproportionate reductions in trabecular (50% decrease) and cortical (25% decrease) bone moduli, compression of the anterior part of the vertebra increased peak stresses by up to 250% compared with uniform compression. They concluded that, for anterior compression, disproportionate modulus reductions in trabecular and cortical bone may substantially increase end-plate and cortical-shell stresses, suggesting a cause of age-related spinal fractures.

The dominant force on the human vertebral body is compression. Compressive forces, leading to compressive stresses, result in fractures that have an oblique configuration. Pure compression leads to an oblique fracture configuration and results in wedge fractures. Small variations in the directionality of the loading and the distribution of areas of trabecular deficiency can lead to biconcavity fractures. This anisotropic behavior of vertebrae is a function of both their cortical and trabecular bone compliment. Cortical bone is stronger in compression than in tension, and trabecular bone shows its greatest compressive strength along the vertical axis of the trabeculae.[14,15] Because of its greater porosity, trabecular bone has a lower modulus of elasticity than cortical bone; however, trabecular bone can typically withstand greater strains, fracturing at deformations of approximately 7%, and cortical bone can fail at strains as low as 2%.[16]

The Role of Bone Metabolism in the Development of Vertebral Compression Fractures

Cellular activity can play an important role in determining the mechanical properties of bone. This may partially explain the observation that not all patients with low bone mass experience osteoporosis. Although bone has a defined biochemical composition and structural form at a given point in time, these two properties are in a constant state of dynamic change, which will affect the ability of bone to respond to a load application. Under normal homeostatic conditions, bone undergoes breakdown and repair; thus, it may have reduced mechanical properties if homeostasis becomes uncoupled and bone resorption predominates. The resorptive activities produced by osteoclastic activity may act as stress risers for the initiation of crack propagation analogous to two brick walls of identical size and thickness, containing identical quantities of bricks and mortar in the same spatial array. When one wall undergoes continuous necessary repairs and bricks are occasionally lost or degraded, the mechanical integrity of the wall will be maintained. When the other wall undergoes the same degree of degradation but is not repaired until several bricks require attention, each site of degradation represents a stress riser and cracks may propagate throughout the structure, weakening the wall. Thus, bone in a state of high turnover, such as occurs with hyperparathyroidism, high-remodeling osteoporosis, or Paget's disease, may show a reduction in mechanical properties compared with bone that undergoes normal remodeling. Because this phenomenon is independent of bone mass, it is possible that two patients with equivalent vertebral bone density may have different risks for fracture based on differences in the control of their metabolic bone conditions.

Opportunities for Enhancing Vertebral Bone Properties in Osteoporosis

Several pharmaceutical agents are now available for the treatment of osteoporosis. Estrogens and estrogen-like compounds inhibit bone loss and, to varying degrees, increase bone formation. Bisphosphonates and calcitonins prevent bone loss and have minimal, short-range effects on enhancing bone mass. A new drug therapy, soon to be available for widespread use, is parathyroid hormone. This agent may have the ability to increase bone mass and provide substantial restoration to segments of the skeleton. Additionally, the surgical introduction of inert, nonbiologic materials, such as polymethylmethacrylate cement, has been shown to stabilize vertebral fractures and improve symptoms in a number of patients. Although this advance in treatment of osteoporosis requires further exploration, a basic understanding of the anatomic and mechanical properties of bone provides the necessary framework to assess therapeutic opportunities. Future technologies, such as the use of growth factors or gene therapy, hold the promise of providing actual cures for osteoporosis and related bone diseases.

Summary

Osteoporosis is a prevalent metabolic bone disease that leads to a decrease in bone mass and increased risk of fracture. Because the skeleton is distributed to two envelopes, trabecular and cortical bone, the anatomic and structural aspects of these two envelopes affect the mechanical properties of bone differently. Moreover, bone loss differs in trabecular and cortical bone and the effects of bone loss for both influence the type, frequency, and site of fracture. Although only three types of stresses (tension, compression, and shear) are generated in bone, combinations of these stresses are produced by different forces and lead to the ultimate failure of bone. Osteoporotic vertebral compression fractures are the most common fractures seen in patients with osteoporosis. Studies show that vertebrae are loaded in compression and approximately 90% of the structural integrity of the vertebral body is contributed by trabecular bone. Because trabecular bone has eight times the turnover rate of corti-cal bone, a small imbalance in bone homeostasis will affect trabecular bone dramatically. Knowledge of those events that control bone turnover will lead to a new understanding of how pharmaceutical interventions may prevent bone loss, strengthen the skeleton, and reduce the risk of fracture.

References

1. Freedman KB, Kaplan FS, Bilker WB, Strom BL, Lowe RA: Treatment of osteoporosis: Are physicians missing an opportunity? *J Bone Joint Surg Am* 2000;82:1063-1070.

2. Lee CA, Einhorn TA: The bone organ system: Form and function, in Marcus R, Feldman MD, Kelsey J (eds): *Osteoporosis*, ed 2. San Diego, CA, Academic Press, 2001, pp 3-20.

3. Riggs BL, Melton LJ III: The prevention and treatment of osteoporosis. *N Engl J Med* 1992;327:620-627.

4. Mosekilde L, Viidik A, Mosekilde L: Correlation between the compressive strength of iliac and vertebral trabecular bone in normal individuals. *Bone* 1985;6:291-295.

5. Einhorn TA: Bone strength: The bottom line. *Calcif Tissue Int* 1992;51:333-339.

6. Ruff CB, Hayes WC: Subperiosteal expansion and cortical remodeling of the human femur and tibia with aging. *Science* 1982;217:945-948.

7. Cullinane DM, Einhorn TA: Biomechanics of bone, in Bilezikian JP, Raisz LG, Rodan GA (eds): *Principles of Bone Biology*, ed 2. San Diego, CA, Academic Press, 2002, pp 17-32.

8. Carter DR, Spengler DM: Biomechanics of fractures, in Sumner-Smith G (ed): *Bone in Clinical Orthopedics: A Study in Comparative Osteology*. Philadelphia, PA, WB Saunders, 1982, pp 305-334.

9. Eastell R, Cedel SL, Wahner HW, Riggs BL, Melton LJ III: Classification of vertebral fractures. *J Bone Miner Res* 1991;6:207-215.

10. Silva MJ, Keaveny TM, Hayes WC: Load sharing between the shell and centrum in the lumbar vertebral body. *Spine* 1997;22:140-150.

11. Silva MJ, Wang C, Keaveny TM, Hayes WC: Direct and computed tomography thickness measurements of the human, lumbar vertebral shell and endplate. *Bone* 1994;15:409-414.

12. Flynn MJ, Cody DD: The assessment of vertebral bone macroarchitecture with X-ray computed tomography. *Calcif Tissue Int* 1993;53(suppl 1):S170-S175.

13. Mizrahi J, Silva MJ, Keaveny TM, Edwards WT, Hayes WC: Finite-element stress analysis of the normal and osteoporotic lumbar vertebral body. *Spine* 1993;18:2088-2096.

14. Burstein AH, Reilly DT, Martens MJ: Aging of bone tissue: Mechanical properties. *J Bone J Surg Am* 1976;58:82-86.

15. Galante J, Rostoker W, Ray RD: Physical properties of trabecular bone. *Calcif Tissue Res* 1970;5:236-246.

16. Nordin M, Frankel VH: Biomechanics of whole bones and bone tissue, in Frankel VH, Nordin M (eds): *Basic Biomechanics of the Skeletal System*. Philadelphia, PA, Lea and Febiger, 1980, pp 15-60.

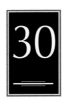

Osteoporotic Vertebral Compression Fractures

David H. Kim, MD
Jeffrey S. Silber, MD
Todd J. Albert, MD

Abstract

Osteoporotic vertebral compression fractures are a commonly encountered clinical problem. Although the majority of patients with this injury experience a benign and self-limited course of gradually resolving pain, a significant number continue to experience chronic pain and disability. In evaluating a patient with a vertebral compression fracture, the differential diagnosis must consider not only osteoporosis, but also various causes of osteomalacia, endocrinopathy, and malignancy. Accumulation of multiple compression fractures and increased thoracolumbar kyphosis are associated with a poor prognosis. Multiple medical treatments—including hormone replacement therapy, calcitonin, and bisphosphonates—are effective in maintaining or increasing bone mass and reducing the risk of compression fracture. Conventional treatment in the form of pain medication, activity limitation, and occasionally bracing is effective in returning most patients to their previous level of functioning. When therapies fail, patients may be considered for minimally invasive treatments such as vertebroplasty or kyphoplasty. Surgery, although enormously challenging because of poor underlying health status and structurally weak bone, may be the last resort for a small percentage of patients experiencing progressive deformity or neurologic deficit.

Vertebral compression fracture in the setting of osteoporosis is a frequently encountered clinical problem that is becoming even more common as the median age of the American population continues to increase. Although the majority of patients suffering with this injury remain minimally symptomatic, a large percentage experience significant pain and disability. Conventional treatment in the form of pain medication, activity limitation, and occasionally bracing is effective in returning most patients to their previous level of functioning. Patients who fail to respond to these therapies may be candidates for a variety of highly effective new techniques, including vertebroplasty and kyphoplasty. Surgery may be required in patients who experience progressive deformity or neurologic deficit; however, it is fraught with a high rate of complications.

Epidemiology

Osteoporosis is a highly prevalent disorder of bone characterized by decreased bone density, disruption of trabecular microarchitecture, and increased susceptibility to fractures. The World Health Organization has established standards for diagnosing low bone mass and osteoporosis using dual-energy x-ray absorptiometry (DEXA). Osteoporosis is defined as diminished bone density measuring 2.5 standard deviations below the average bone density of healthy 25-year-old same-sex members of the population.[1] Based on this definition, an estimated 25% of postmenopausal women and 35% of women over 65 years of age in the United States suffer from osteoporosis.[1]

The risk of proximal femur, distal radius, and proximal humerus fractures is significantly increased in postmenopausal women; however, vertebral compression fractures are the most common skeletal injury.[2,3] The incidence of osteoporotic fractures of the spine in the United States is greater than 500,000 per year, with women being affected twice as often as men.[4,5] One fourth of women reaching menopause can expect to suffer one or more vertebral compression fractures in their lifetime.[6] In the United States, 25% of women over the age of 70 years and 50% of women over the age of 80 years have radiographic evidence of vertebral compression fractures.[7]

Pathogenesis

Improvements in prevention and treatment of osteoporotic vertebral compression fractures will evolve from a more

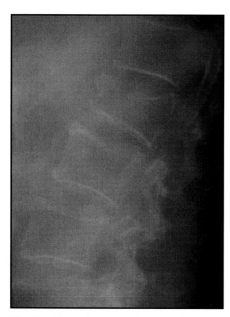

Fig. 1 Radiograph demonstrating wedge-shaped pattern characteristic of osteoporotic vertebral compression fracture. There is generalized osteopenia of bone. The involved vertebra shows loss of height anteriorly as a result of a fracture involving the anterosuperior portion. The posterior vertebral height is preserved, and the pedicle is not involved.

precise understanding of their etiology. Investigators have described two types of osteoporosis.[8] Type 2 osteoporosis is caused by inadequate lifetime calcium intake and is associated with an increased incidence of proximal femur fractures. Type 1 is attributed to estrogen deficiency and appears to be associated with a higher incidence of vertebral fractures.

Vertebral fractures in osteoporotic spines demonstrate a consistent (80%) wedge-shaped pattern in which there is gross collapse of the anterior portion of the vertebral body with relative preservation of height of the posterior body (Fig. 1). The morphology of osteoporotic compression fractures correlates with age-related patterns of trabecular bone loss. Oda and associates[9] examined pathologic specimens from 25 second lumbar vertebrae as well as radiographs of 99 patients with osteoporotic fractures of the second lumbar vertebra. The most fre-

quently observed deformity (42% of fractures) was a wedge-shaped vertebra with compression of the anterosuperior portion. This pattern correlated with selective trabecular atrophy and increased trabecular spacing in the anterosuperior portion of more aged specimens.[9]

Aging is also associated with predictable changes in the biomechanical environment of the functional spinal unit. Studies involving healthy disk have consistently revealed that the largest stress concentration occurs in the trabecular bone immediately underlying the central end plate.[10,11] With aging, however, end plate curvature increases and cortical thinning occurs.[12,13] Disk degeneration further alters the mechanics of end-plate loading and leads to primary load transfer via the anulus fibrosus with a selective increase of stress in the cortical shell.[10,11,14]

Mizrahi and associates[15] have attempted to resolve the complex biomechanical forces acting on the osteoporotic spine using a finite element method of stress analysis. Their model revealed that the superior end plate is loaded through axial compression and bending forces while the inferior end plate is loaded primarily through axial compression. Downward bending of the end plate, such as that which might occur during forward spinal flexion, leads to large compressive stress in the superior surface and tensile stress in the inferior surface. The asymmetric anatomy of the vertebral body creates maximum hoop stresses at the most anterior aspect of the superior cortical shell. Interestingly, this model was uniquely sensitive to disproportionate reductions in trabecular versus cortical bone moduli, a hallmark of osteoporotic bone loss.[15]

Osteoporosis is characterized by both cortical and trabecular bone loss; however, disruption of the microarchitecture of trabecular bone may be the critical factor predisposing osteoporotic vertebrae to fracture.[16] Loss of connectivity among tra-

becular plates is a shared feature in all examined specimens.[17] Unfortunately, analyzing the complex structure of trabecular bone has proved to be exceedingly difficult.[18-22] More recently, fractal geometry has been used to study the connectivity of trabecular bone in patients with and without osteoporotic vertebrae; this appears to provide more predictive value than measurements of bone area alone in identifying fracture risk.[23] It is possible that computer-assisted fractal analysis of bone biopsy specimens may offer an improvement over current histologic methods.

Prediction of Fracture Risk

Over 24 million Americans currently have osteoporosis and are at risk for spinal fracture.[8,24] Because medical costs and disability associated with osteoporotic vertebral fractures total billions of dollars per year, a large research effort is underway to develop more accurate and reliable predictors of fracture risk.

One of the strongest predictors of future vertebral fracture is a prior vertebral compression fracture. The risk of fracture in women who have already had an osteoporotic compression factor is five times that of women with no previous fracture.[3]

Iliac crest bone biopsy can provide a direct evaluation of bone status. Histologic examination of specimens from osteoporotic bone typically reveals clear alterations in trabecular architecture, including decreased trabecular number, width, and connectivity. The connectivity of the trabecular network in particular has been accorded principal importance in determining resistance to fracture. Trabecular bone mineral density can be measured indirectly using single-energy quantitative computed tomography (SE-QCT). Although only trabecular bone density is currently assessed by this method, a recent study of both cortical and trabecular bone using SE-QCT suggests that the measurement of both types of bone may provide stronger predictive value in assessing fracture risk.[25]

Diagnosis

Over 65% of patients with vertebral compression fractures are asymptomatic at the time of diagnosis.[26,27] However, a single compression fracture is associated with measurable height loss; accordingly, any patient reporting an apparent decrease in stature should be evaluated for vertebral fracture.[28] Patients who experience significant back pain as a result of an acute fracture often report pain onset during relatively atraumatic activities such as bending forward, standing from a seated position, or vigorous coughing or sneezing.[29] Most patients can recall the moment their back pain began but may have difficulty localizing the precise level of their back pain.[27] The pain is typically aggravated by the upright position and relieved by lying down. Coughing, sneezing, and the Valsalva maneuver may also worsen the pain.[27]

Physical examination often reveals the characteristic posture of increased thoracic kyphosis or flattening of the lumbar lordosis (Fig. 2). Accumulation of multiple vertebral compression fractures leads to a noticeable decrease in overall height. This height loss is caused by both height loss of individual vertebrae and increased spinal curvature. A normally proportioned individual stands with the fingertips at midthigh level. If the fingertips reach the lower thigh or knee, then spinal shortening should be suspected.[27] Localized spinal tenderness over the same-level spinous process is often present and does not necessarily signify involvement of the posterior elements. Percussion tenderness may be a particularly sensitive examination technique for identifying an acute compression fracture. There may be local tenderness and spasm of the paraspinal muscles. Forward flexion of the spine tends to cause more pain than does extension. Radicular pain or sensory changes are occasionally present and typ-

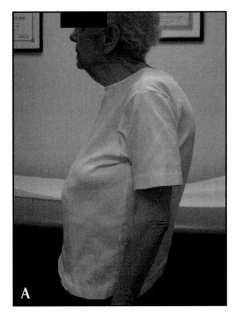
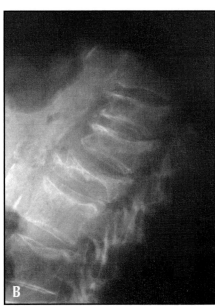

Fig. 2 A, 78-year old woman with thoracic hyperkyphosis creating a so-called "dowager's hump." **B,** Lateral radiograph of the same patient revealing multiple osteoporotic compression fractures.

ically radiate in a band-like distribution around the torso; however, significant neurologic deficit suggesting spinal cord or cauda equina injury is quite unusual and should prompt consideration of alternative diagnoses.[27] One retrospective review of 497 patients with osteoporotic vertebral compression fractures revealed only 10 patients (2%) with evidence of spinal cord compression.[30]

Clinical Evaluation

Diagnosis of a vertebral compression fracture in the setting of decreased bone density signifies the presence of severe osteoporosis according to World Health Organization guidelines. Evaluation and treatment of osteoporosis should be initiated and monitored by the patient's primary care physician. The initial work-up should include an accurate measurement of axial bone mass with technology such as DEXA. All major factors contributing to previous and ongoing bone loss should be identified and addressed. Common causes include menopause, glucocorticoid therapy, alcoholism, seizure medica-

tion, and excessive thyroid hormone levels.[5] Routine laboratory tests should include serum calcium, albumin, 25-hydroxyvitamin D, phosphorus, alkaline phosphatase, creatinine, blood urea nitrogen, and complete blood cell count with differential. Urine should be examined for levels of calcium excretion and markers for bone turnover such as collagen N-telopeptides.[31] Appropriate tests should be performed to rule out hyperthyroidism, hyperparathyroidism, hypogonadism, multiple myeloma, Cushing's syndrome, osteomalacia, and alcohol abuse as clinically indicated.[27] All men with osteoporosis should be considered for serum testosterone measurement because of the high incidence of asymptomatic hypogonadism.[27]

Because a rise in serum alkaline phosphatase occurs approximately 5 days after an acute fracture, a patient presenting earlier with a characteristic insufficiency fracture and an elevated alkaline phosphatase level should be suspected of osteomalacia.[32] A serum calcium and phosphate product below 25 is also sug-

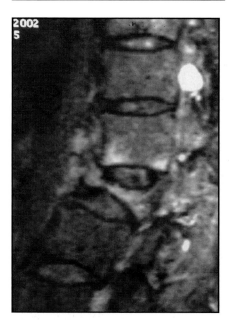

Fig. 3 T2-weighted MRI scan of a patient with an acute osteoporotic compression fracture.

gestive of osteomalacia, especially in the setting of elevated alkaline phosphatase.[27] The possibility of metastatic disease should also be considered.

Radiographic Evaluation

The occurrence of an osteoporotic vertebral compression fracture can usually be suspected based on the patient history and physical examination. However, assessment of the kyphosis angle and prediction of deformity progression require evaluation with plain radiography. CT with thin cuts through the level of injury can be useful in ruling out a more unstable burst fracture with involvement of the posterior vertebral body and the presence of bony fragments in the spinal canal. If the diagnosis remains in doubt following plain radiography, MRI is more useful than bone scan for identifying minimally displaced fractures, distinguishing acute from chronic fractures, and recognizing infection or tumor (Fig. 3).

Osteoporotic vertebral compression fractures typically involve the thoracolumbar junction. The most frequently involved vertebra is L1 (33%), followed by T12 (20%), L2 (19%), and T11 and L3 (each 6% to 7%). Increased incidence also occurs in the midthoracic region at either T7 or T8 (10%).[30] Pain severity and duration correlate poorly with the degree of collapse visualized on radiography.[30] In addition to vertebral height loss and kyphotic deformity, radiographs should be examined carefully for interpedicular widening, involvement of the posterior cortex, or laminar fracture; these features suggest the diagnosis of a potentially unstable vertebral burst fracture rather than a simple compression fracture.

Although the most common etiology of atraumatic thoracic compression fracture is osteoporosis, as many as 35% of these fractures in patients older than 50 years may be associated with metastatic disease or multiple myeloma.[33] MRI is frequently used to help discriminate between benign and malignant compression fractures. Decreased signal intensity on T1-weighted images and increased signal intensity on T2-weighted images is sensitive for tumor involvement but is not very specific. Normal marrow intensity on T1 images nearly excludes the possibility of tumor. Signal changes extending into the pedicle or a soft-tissue mass strongly suggest tumor involvement.[34] Within 1 to 3 months, a healed benign compression fracture on T1-weighted spin echo images should have equal or increased signal compared with adjacent normal vertebrae because of the return of fat cells.[35]

Diffusion-weighted MRI is a new technique that provides excellent discrimination between osteoporotic and tumor-associated compression fractures. This technique is based on the mobility of water molecules in interstitial tissue and was originally used in brain imaging to study infarction and tumors. Pathologically, benign osteoporotic compression fractures are associated with increased free interstitial water as a result of acute marrow edema. Compression fractures through tumor-infiltrated bone lead to compaction of tumor cells and less free interstitial water. As a result, with diffusion-weighted MRI, benign compression fractures have equal or decreased signal compared with adjacent normal vertebrae, while tumor-involved fractures demonstrate increased signal.[36]

Natural History

Conventional teaching maintains that the majority of isolated osteoporotic vertebral compression fractures demonstrate a benign natural history with relatively rapid resolution of acute pain over 6 to 8 weeks and perhaps occasional episodes of recurrent minor aching pain.[5,37] Follow-up studies, however, suggest that many patients experience persistent functional and psychological impairment as a result of these injuries. Retrospective interviews of women with healed osteoporotic compression fractures reveal a surprisingly high rate of persistent pain, disability, and diminished self-esteem.[38-40] A recent case study of patients with an average of four compression fractures each revealed a significant decrease in maximal trunk extension torque, thoracic and lumbar spine sagittal plane motion, functional reach, mobility skills, and 6-minute walk distance.[41] Moreover, population studies suggest that survival may be decreased nearly 20% in women with vertebral compression fractures; increased mortality rates appear to correlate with increasing numbers of fractured vertebrae.[42,43]

Patient prognosis is definitely worse with the accumulation of multiple compression fractures (Fig. 4). Several studies have identified a correlation between severity of kyphosis and the occurrence of more frequent and severe back pain.[39,44-47] Even in the absence of severe pain, patients may experience difficulty standing still for any period of time, bending forward, descending stairs, reaching for objects, and lifting.[5] With progressive spinal collapse, the costal margin falls toward the iliac crests, the abdomen becomes protuberant with the appearance of characteristic horizontal skin folds, and intra-abdominal volume decreases. Patients may experience significant gastrointestinal disturbance characterized by bloating and early satiety, which in turn may further aggravate already present nutritional deficits. Potentially more worrisome, smaller abdominal volume may lead to limitation of diaphragmatic excursion with compromise of pulmonary function, decrease in exercise tolerance, and potential destabilization of coexisting cardiopulmonary disease. Pulmonary function testing in patients with severe osteoporotic spinal deformity has demonstrated significant decreases in functional lung capacity.[48,49]

Although individual compression fractures tend to occur as temporally discrete events, one text notes that compression fractures occasionally "cluster in groups of two or three within a few months, with many years of freedom between clusters."[50] Patients taking corticosteroid medication long-term may be particularly susceptible to the rapid accumulation of five or more vertebral fractures over a period of a few months. This clustering phenomenon was observed in eight patients who had recently undergone an increase in steroid dose for exacerbation of associated illness.[51] Although these patients experienced persistent back pain for up to 8 months, all were able to discontinue narcotic medication within 3 months of the last fracture. Use of a lightweight hyperextension orthosis was found to be helpful.[51]

We have observed that clinical outcomes tend to be less favorable in patients who had more pronounced thoracic kyphosis prior to the occurrence of a vertebral compression fracture and suspect that a patient's native sagittal alignment is an important prognostic factor. If this association is confirmed by further investigation, it may allow more accurate identification of patients at risk for poor outcome and may suggest more aggressive intervention in those cases.

Treatment

Postmenopausal women with a diagnosis of osteoporosis should be advised to take 1,500 mg of elemental calcium and 400 IU of vitamin D daily. Calcium citrate is preferable to calcium carbonate in elderly patients because of its improved absorption and decreased risk of nephrolithiasis. Maintaining a healthy lifestyle is essential. Cigarette smoking should be prohibited, and alcohol consumption must remain moderate. A daily exercise program should be designed by a trained physical therapist or health care professional educated in the treatment of osteoporosis.[5] Patients should also be counseled in fall prevention strategies.

Although calcium and vitamin D supplementation can help maintain appendicular skeletal mass, axial bone mass will continue to decline in postmenopausal women without the addition of hormone replacement therapy. Estrogen supplementation leads to an increase in bone mass of 2% per year and may decrease vertebral fracture risk between 50% and 70%.[5,52] Risks of estrogen replacement include thrombophlebitis and uterine and breast cancer. To monitor the skeletal effects of hormone replacement therapy, N-telopeptide elimination should be measured. This typically declines by 30% within 3 to 6 months of initiating appropriate doses of estrogen replacement. A cutoff N-telopeptide level of 39 nm bone collagen equivalents/mM creatinine or above has been proposed as indicating the need for antiresorptive therapy.[53] Very thin patients and patients who smoke often require higher estrogen doses.

Calcitonin therapy is another treatment alternative. Recent studies of inhaled calcitonin at a dose of 200 units daily reveal increases in spinal bone mass and a 37% decrease in the incidence of vertebral compression fractures.[54] An added benefit of calcitonin is moderate analgesia

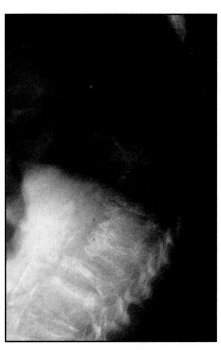

Fig. 4 Severe osteoporosis and multiple compression fractures throughout the thoracolumbar spine, resulting in significant kyphotic deformity.

when taken in the setting of painful acute osteoporotic compression fractures.[55]

Patients with significant osteoporosis should also be considered candidates for treatment with a bisphosphonate. Alendronate, the first bisphosphonate approved by the Food and Drug Administration for treatment of osteoporosis, increases spinal bone mass and decreases the risk of vertebral compression fractures.[56-58] In a prospective randomized trial involving patients with preexisting vertebral compression fractures and decreased bone density, alendronate reduced the risk of additional fractures by 50%.[59] Studies reveal that even larger gains in bone density can be attained through a combination of estrogen and alendronate therapy.[60] At this time, the National Osteoporosis Foundation recommends that all female patients with vertebral compression fractures be treated with hormone replacement therapy, alendronate, or calcitonin.[61]

Pain Medication

The acute pain associated with a new vertebral compression fracture typically resolves over a period of 6 to 8 weeks.[5,37] During this time, analgesic medication should be administered to reduce pain and improve activity tolerance. First-line medication consists of acetaminophen or salicylates.[5] If this is inadequate for pain relief, the next choice is a nonsteroidal anti-inflammatory drug (NSAID). Elderly patients should be warned of the risk of gastrointestinal bleeding and renal insufficiency as well as the theoretical risk of inhibiting fracture healing with NSAIDs and salicylates. Mental status changes may occur in a patient with a history of dementia or confusion. Narcotic medication may be necessary for severe pain. Although concerns regarding respiratory depression and addiction have tempered enthusiasm for prescribing narcotic medication, often leading to undertreatment of pain, studies have demonstrated that patients nearly always discontinue narcotic medication once the acute pain has resolved.[51] In those patients who have difficulty taking narcotics, calcitonin can lead to significant pain reduction.[55]

Painful paravertebral muscle spasms can be treated with cyclobenzaprine or diazepam.[51] The addictive potential of these medications has been recognized, and treatment should not be prolonged. Adynamic ileus and constipation are among the most frequent complaints in the acute period, and all patients should be advised to drink plenty of fluids as well as maintain a diet high in fiber.[51]

Bracing

After an acute vertebral compression fracture, a short period of bed rest is appropriate, but prolonged bed rest beyond a few days should be avoided.[43] Early mobilization can often be achieved with the assistance of a spinal orthosis. Fracture of thoracic vertebrae may be treated in a molded thoracolumbar spinal orthosis (TLSO), but involvement above the T6 level requires a cervical extension.[62] Bracing is typically necessary only during the initial 6 to 8 weeks, until the acute pain resolves. Thereafter, intermittent use of the brace may provide symptomatic relief during long rides or periods requiring prolonged standing.[5]

We treat all symptomatic patients with some form of bracing. A well-fitting brace provides substantial and predictable pain relief during the acute postinjury period. For fractures of L1 or above, fitting a Jewett or Cash-type extension brace should be considered. TLSOs tend to be poorly tolerated by elderly patients and are extremely difficult to put on alone. We reserve TLSO use for the patient with refractory pain despite the use of other braces. For the rare patient with fracture of the L2 vertebra or below, we use a lumbosacral orthosis.

Exercise

Once the acute pain period ends, patients should begin a carefully designed exercise program to enhance their axial muscle strength. As the body ages, a disproportionate loss of muscle strength occurs axially, compared with peripherally. One prospective study further suggested that back-strengthening exercises can improve kyphotic deformity.[63]

Back-extension exercises are preferable to abdominal-flexion exercises. In a study comparing radiographs of patients before and after enrollment in two different exercise programs, patients engaged in flexion exercise demonstrated an 89% incidence of new compression fractures compared with only a 16% incidence in patients performing extension exercises.[64]

Patients should be warned that certain activities might also be associated with increased risk in patients with osteoporosis. The popularity of golf among the elderly may be of particular concern. Several cases of acute vertebral compression fracture in osteoporotic women have been reported as occurring during midswing while playing golf.[65]

Vertebroplasty and Kyphoplasty

Although most patients recover from the acute pain associated with a new vertebral compression fracture, a minority continues to experience persistent or recurrent episodes of chronic pain. These patients may be candidates for treatment with vertebroplasty or kyphoplasty. Vertebroplasty is a minimally invasive treatment designed to relieve chronic pain and stabilize the spine following vertebral compression fractures. Originally developed in France in the late 1980s to treat compression fractures associated with aggressive hemangiomas and osteolytic tumors, the technique was soon applied successfully to the treatment of vertebral fractures associated with osteoporosis.[66]

Kyphoplasty is a newer alternative facilitated by the US Food and Drug Administration's approval of use of the inflatable balloon tamp in 1998. Purported advantages of kyphoplasty over vertebroplasty include correction of deformity and decreased potential for cement leakage. Vertebroplasty and kyphoplasty are discussed in detail in chapter 48.

Pain Clinic Treatment

If vertebroplasty or kyphoplasty fail to provide relief from chronic pain, patients may be candidates for referral to specialized pain clinics. A variety of strategies have been developed for the local or regional administration of analgesia. In general, epidural injections and somatic nerve root blocks have not provided sustained pain relief for this problem.[67] Long-term intrathecal infusion of bupivacaine with or without buprenorphine has been successfully relieved intractable pain associated with vertebral compression fractures.[68] Long-term epidural infusion has also been successful, and offers the advantages of decreased infection risk and the ability to treat patients on an ambulatory basis.[69] Most recently, a technique for performing gray ramus communicans nerve block has been described.[67] A retrospective review of 52 cases reported a 75% high or medium patient satisfaction rate.[67]

Surgery

The surgical treatment of osteoporotic vertebral compression fractures is complicated by the deficient mechanical properties of osteoporotic bone, which may not withstand the local application of forces through structural grafts and instrumentation.[70] Absolute indications for surgical intervention have not been strictly defined, but general indications are thought to include progressive neurologic loss and significant deformity.[71]

A retrospective study of 497 patients with osteoporotic vertebral compression fractures included 10 patients (2%) with evidence of spinal cord compression and canal compromise.[30] Indications for surgery included progression of neurologic deficit or absence of neurologic recovery within 1 week. Nine of 10 patients met these requirements and underwent anterior decompression through either a thoracotomy or retroperitoneal approach. The decompressed level was reconstructed using structural iliac crest for one level or fibular graft for more than one level. Postoperatively, patients were maintained on bed rest for 1 to 2 weeks and then mobilized in a spinal extension brace for 8 weeks. The authors reported that all patients returned to independent ambulatory status with a cane or walker but none regained full lower extremity strength. Bowel and bladder functional recovery was reportedly satisfactory.

The appearance of paraplegia may be delayed, and in these cases, weakness tends to steadily progress to the point of severe paraplegia.[72] Historically, surgical approaches to this problem have included laminectomy, laminectomy with posterior fusion, anterior decompression with posterior fusion, and anterior decompression with anterior fusion.[72-77] It is now known that laminectomy without fusion contributes to local instability and should be avoided. Most investigators currently appear to favor some form of anterior decompression and reconstruction.[77]

Difficulty may be encountered maintaining correction following anterior spinal reconstruction due to settling of graft into weak osteoporotic bone. Although improved results may be obtained with the addition of anterior instrumentation,[77] fixation points for anterior instrumentation are limited by intrinsic bone weakness and perhaps should be avoided. An excellent alternative to anterior surgery for an acute kyphus is a pedicle subtraction or "eggshell" osteotomy, performed from an entirely posterior approach. In this procedure, bone is removed from the vertebral body through a transpedicular approach followed by a measured resection of bone from the posterior elements. Subsequently, a posterior instrumental fusion stabilizes the correction and alignment. Recently, a variation on the posterior spinal shortening procedure has been developed and applied with apparent success.[78]

In our experience, fusion and instrumentation of the osteoporotic spine is among the most challenging tasks in adult spine surgery. The key to maximizing favorable outcomes is judicious patient selection. A thorough assessment of the patient's preoperative health status must be made. A complete discussion with the patient should delineate a realistic description of treatment goals as well as risks and benefits. In terms of surgical approaches, anterior surgery is appropriate for performing decompression or obtaining additional anatomic release to improve correction of kyphosis. However, we believe that anterior-only surgery carries a high risk of failure, even with the addition of anterior instrumentation, and recommend that consideration be given to the addition of posterior fusion and instrumentation as well. Both anterior and posterior instrumentation may fail because of the structural weakness of osteoporotic bone, but the risk can be minimized by more generous use of multiple fixation sites and occasionally cement augmentation.

Recently approved by the US Food and Drug Administration for use in the thoracic spine, pedicle screws may provide safe and secure fixation in the osteoporotic spine when applied properly. Theoretically, sublaminar hooks may provide superior resistance to pullout, the primary mode of failure following correction of the kyphotic spine. In the setting of osteoporotic bone, however, migration of hooks through soft laminar bone frequently occurs, and the versatility of pedicle screws is clearly advantageous. The use of thoracic pedicle screws should be restricted to surgeons with a thorough knowledge of thoracic spinal anatomy as well as experience with modern insertion techniques. For local kyphosis correction, we prefer posterior segmental instrumentation using double rods with or without the addition of anterior decompression and fusion. We favor the use of pedicle screws where allowed by local anatomy and reinforcement with sublaminar hooks or wires at the cranial and caudal ends (Fig. 5).

The potential for new compression fractures adjacent to the fusion mass has been suggested and may be addressed through prophylactic vertebroplasty of adjacent levels. Mismatch in elastic modulus between metal and bone or between an anterior structural graft and adjacent native bone is poorly tolerated in the osteoporotic patient. Autologous fibular strut grafts in this sense may be a less favorable graft choice, and we prefer autologous iliac crest graft when possible. Of course, osteoporosis may similarly weaken the mechanical properties of the iliac crest bone, yeilding no perfect solution for graft material.

Education

Perhaps the most effective treatment strategy is patient education. Patients should be well informed about their dis-

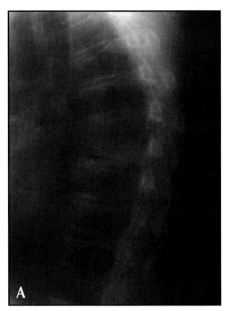 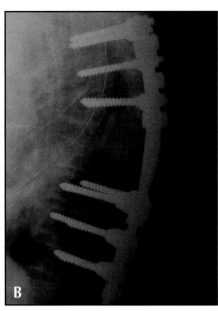

Fig. 5 Two-level osteoporotic compression fractures in a 65-year-old patient with severe unrelenting back pain. **A,** Preoperative radiograph shows increased thoracolumbar kyphosis. **B,** Postoperative radiograph after instrumented reduction and fusion using pedicle screw fixation. The patient experienced excellent symptomatic relief. (Courtesy of Alexander R. Vaccaro, MD.)

ease and understand that significant improvements in their quality of life can be achieved through a thoughtful combination of medication, exercise, and minimal lifestyle changes. Daily activities should be modified to incorporate strategies for fall prevention. In order to reduce episodes of severe coughing, patients should be encouraged to receive a pneumococcal vaccine and undergo yearly influenza vaccination.[5] The National Osteoporosis Foundation provides extensive instructional literature and videotapes for the general public and organizes many local support groups.

Summary

Vertebral compression fractures are the most common clinical manifestation of osteoporosis and represent a significant public health problem. Decreased bone density and disruption of trabecular bone architecture predispose osteoporotic vertebrae to fracture. The vast majority of clinically significant fractures can be diagnosed with a thorough history and physical examination. Nevertheless, additional laboratory testing and radiographic evaluation is often indicated to rule out other processes such as malignancy. Although the majority of compression fractures are initially clinically silent, recent follow-up studies suggest that the natural history for many patients is not as favorable as once thought. Despite conventional treatment with pain medication, activity modification, and bracing, many patients experience persistent pain and deformity that results in significant functional and psychological impairment. For these patients, a variety of new and effective therapeutic techniques have become available, including vertebroplasty and kyphoplasty. In a few patients suffering progressive deformity or neurologic deficit, surgery may be the only option; however, fusion and instrumentation of the osteoporotic spine is a technical challenge that carries a high risk for complications. The most cost-effective treatment of this problem remains prevention through patient education and accurate identification of the at-risk population.

References

1. Assessment of fracture risk and its application to screening for postmenopausal osteoporosis. World Health Organization, 1994, pp 1-129.

2. Melton LJ, Kan SW, Frye MA, Wahner HW, O'Fallon WM, Riggs BL: Epidemiology of vertebral fractures in women. *Am J Epidemiol* 1989;129:1000-1011.

3. Ross PD, Davis JW, Epstein RS, Wasnigh RD: Pre-existing fracture and bone mass may predict vertebral fracture incidence in women. *Ann Internal Med* 1991;114:919-923.

4. Cooper C, Atkinson EJ, O'Fallon WM, Melton LJ: Incidence of clinically diagnosed vertebral fractures: A population-based study in Rochester, Minnesota. *J Bone Miner Res* 1992;7:221-227.

5. Lyles KW: Management of patients with vertebral compression fractures. *Pharmacotherapy* 1999;19(suppl):S21-S24.

6. Melton LJI: Epidemiology of spinal osteoporosis. *Spine* 1997;22:S2-S11.

7. Kanis JA, McCloskey EV: The epidemiology of vertebral osteoporosis. *Bone* 1992;13(suppl 2): S1-S10.

8. Riggs BL, Melton LJ: Involutional osteoporosis. *N Engl J Med* 1992;326:357-362.

9. Oda K, Shibayama Y, Abe M, Onomura T: Morphogenesis of vertebral deformities in involutional osteoporosis. *Spine* 1998;23:1050-1056.

10. Kurowski P, Kubo A: The relationship of degeneration of the intervertebral disc to mechanical loading conditions on lumbar vertebrae. *Spine* 1986;11:726-731.

11. Shirazi-Adl SA, Shrivastava SC, Ahmed AM: Stress analysis of lumbar disc-body unit in compression. *Spine* 1984;9:120-134.

12. Barnett E, Nordin BEC: The radiological diagnosis of osteoporosis: A new approach. *Clin Radiol* 1960;11:166-174.

13. Doyle FH, Gutteridge DH, Joplin GF, Fraser R: An assessment of radiologic criteria used in the study of spinal osteoporosis. *Br J Radiol* 1967;40:241.

14. Horst M, Brinckmann P: Measurement of the distribution of axial stress on the end-plate of the vertebral body. *Spine* 1981;6:217-232.

15. Mizrahi J, Silva MJ, Eng M, Keaveny TM, Edwards WT, Hayes WC: Finite-element stress analysis of the normal and osteoporotic lumbar vertebral body. *Spine* 1993;18:2088-2096.

16. Parfitt AM: Implications of architecture for the pathogenesis and prevention of vertebral fracture. *Bone* 1992;13:S41-S47.

17. Mellish RWE, Garrahan NJ, Compston JE: Age-related changes in trabecular width and spacing in human iliac crest biopsies. *Bone Miner* 1989;6:331-338.

18. Vesterby A: Star volume of marrow space and trabeculae in iliac crest: Sampling procedure and correlation to star volume of first lumbar vertebra. *Bone* 1990;11:149-155.

19. Kimmel DB, Recker RR, Gallagher JC, Vaswani AS, Aloia JF: A comparison of iliac bone histomorphometric data in postmenopausal osteoporotic and normal subjects. *Bone Miner* 1990;11:217-235.

20. Mellish RWE, Ferguson-Pell MW, Cochran GVB, Lindsay R, Dempster DW: A new manual method for assessing two-dimensional cancellous bone structure: Comparison between iliac crest and lumbar vertebra. *J Bone Miner Res* 1991;6:689-696.

21. Hahn M, Vogel M, Pompesius-Kempa M, Delling G: Trabecular bone pattern factor: A new parameter for simple quantification of bone microarchitecture. *Bone* 1992;13:327-330.

22. Feldkamp LA, Goldstein SA, Parfitt AM, Jesion G, Kleerekoper M: The direct examination of three dimensional bone architecture in vitro by computed tomography. *J Bone Miner Res* 1989;4:3-11.

23. Weinstein RS, Majumdar S: Fractal geometry and vertebral compression fractures. *J Bone Miner Res* 1994;9:1797-1802.

24. Resnick NM, Greenspan SL: Senile osteoporosis reconsidered. *JAMA* 1989;261:1025-1029.

25. Andresen R, Werner HJ, Schober H-C: Contribution of the cortical shell of vertebrae to mechanical behaviour of the lumbar vertebrae with implications for predicting fracture risk. *Br J Radiol* 1998;71:759-765.

26. Lane JM, Riley EH, Wirganowicz PZ: Osteoporosis: diagnosis and treatment. *J Bone Joint Surg Am* 1996;78:618-632.

27. Glaser DL, Kaplan FS: Osteoporosis: Definition and clinical presentation. *Spine* 1997;22:17S-24S.

28. Ross PD: Clinical consequences of vertebral fractures. *Am J Med* 1997;103:305-325.

29. Gallagher JC, Aaron J, Horsman A, et al: The crush fracture syndrome in postmenopausal women. *Clin Endocrinol Metab* 1973;2:293-297.

30. Lee YL, Yip KMH: The osteoporotic spine. *Clin Orthop* 1996;323:91-97.

31. Eyre D: Biochemical markers. *Spine* 1997;22(suppl):S17-S24.

32. Lane JM, Russell L, Khan SN: Osteoporosis. *Clin Orthop* 2000;372:139-150.

33. Biyani A, Ebraheim NA, Lu J: Thoracic spine fracture in patients older than 50 years. *Clin Orthop* 1993;328:190-193.

34. Rupp RE, Ebraheim NA, Coombs RJ: Magnetic resonance imaging differentiation of compression spine fractures or vertebral lesions caused by osteoporosis or tumor. *Spine* 1995;20:2499-2504.

35. Baker LL, Goodman SB, Perkash I, Lane B, Enzmann DR: Benign versus pathologic compression fractures of vertebral bodies: Assessment with conventional spin-echo, chemical shift, and STIR MR imaging. *Radiology* 1990;174:495-502.

36. Baur A, Stabler A, Bruning R, et al: Diffusion-weighted MR imaging of bone marrow: Differentiation of benign versus pathologic compression fractures. *Radiology* 1998;207:349-356.

37. Silverman SL: The clinical consequences of vertebral compression fracture. *Bone* 1992;13:S27-S31.

38. Leidig G, Minne HW, Sauer P, et al: A study of complaints and their relation to vertebral destruction in patients with osteoporosis. *Bone Miner* 1990;8:217-229.

39. Ettinger B, Block JE, Smith R, Cummings SR, Harris ST, Genant WK: An examination of the association between vertebral deformities, physical disbilities and psychosocial problems. *Maturitas* 1988;10:283-296.

40. Cook DJ, Guyatt GH, Adachi JD, et al: Quality of life issues in women with vertebral fractures due to osteoporosis. *Arthritis Rhem* 1993;36:750-756.

41. Lyles KW, Gold DT, Shipp KM, Pieper CF, Martinez S, Mulhausen PL: Association of osteoporotic vertebral compression fractures with impaired functional status. *Am J Med* 1993;94:595-601.

42. Cooper C, Atkinson EJ, Jacobsen SJ, O'Fallon WM, Melton LJI: Population-based study of survival following osteoporotic fractures. *Am J Epidemiol* 1993;137:1001-1005.

43. Kado DM, Browner WS, Palermo L, et al: Vertebral fractures and mortality in older women. *Arch Intern Med* 1999;159:1215-1220.

44. Ross PD, Ettinger B, Davis JW, et al: Evaluation of adverse health outcomes associated with vertebral fractures. *Osteoporosis Int* 1991;1:134-140.

45. Ettinger B, Black DM, Nevitt MC, et al: Contribution of vertebral deformities to chronic back pain and disability. *J Bone Miner Res* 1992;7:449-456.

46. Nicholson PH, Haddaway MJ, Davie MW, et al: Vertebral deformity, bone mineral density, back pain and height loss in unscreened women over 50 years. *Osteoporosis Int* 1993;3:300-307.

47. Ensrud KW, Black DM, Harris F, et al: Correlates of kyphosis in older women. *J Am Geriatr Soc* 1997;45:688-694.

48. Leech JA, Dulberg C, Kellie S, Pattee L, Gay J: Relationship of lung function to severity of osteoporosis in women. *Am Rev Respir Dis* 1990;141:68-71.

49. Schlaich C, Minne HW, Bruckner T, et al: Reduced pulmonary function in patients with spinal osteoporotic fractures. *Osteoporosis Int* 1998;8:261-267.

50. Rothman RH, Simeone FA: *The Spine.* Philadelphia, PA, WB Saunders, 1975.

51. Kaplan FS, Scherl JD, Wisneski R, Cheatle M, Haddad JG: The cluster phenomenon in patients who have multiple vertebral compression fractures. *Clin Orthop* 1993;297:161-167.

52. Lindsey R, Bush TL, Graly D, Speroff L, Lobo RA: Therapeutic controversy: Estrogen replacement therapy in the treatment of osteoporosis. *J Clin Endocrinol Metab* ;81:3829-3838.

53. Chestnut CH, Bell NH, Clark GS, et al: Hormone replacement therapy in postmenopausal women: Urinary N-telopeptide of type I collagen monitors therapeutic effect and predicts response of bone mineral density. *Am J Med* 1997;102:29-37.

54. Cardona JM, Pastor E: Calcitonin versus etidronate for the treatment of postmenopausal osteoporosis: A meta-analysis of published clinical trials. *Osteoporosis Int* 1997;7:165-174.

55. Siminoski J, Josse RG: Prevention and management of osteoporosis: Consensus statements from the Scientific Advisory Board of the Osteoporosis Society of Canada. *Can Med Assoc J* 1996;155:962-965.

56. Bernstein DS, Sadowsky N, Hegsted DM, Guri CD, Stare FJ: Randomized trial of effect of alendronate on risk of fracture in women with existing vertebral fractures. *Lancet* 1996;348:1535-1541.

57. Cummings SR, Eckert S, Kreuger KA, et al: Effect of alendronate on risk of fracture in women with low bone density but without vertebral fractures. *JAMA* 1998;280:2077-2082.

58. Leiberman UA, Weiss SR, Broll J, et al: Effect of oral alendronate on bone mineral density and the incidence of fracture in postmenopausal osteoporotic women. *N Engl J Med* 1995;333:1437-1443.

59. Black DM, Cummings SR, Karpf DB, et al: Randomized trial of effect of alendronate on the risk of fracture in women with existing vertebral fractures. *Lancet* 1996;348:1535-1541.

60. Lindsey R, Cosman F, Lobo RA, et al: Addition of alendronate to ongoing hormone replacement therapy in the treatment of osteoporosis. *J Clin Endocrinol Metab* 1999;84:3078-3081.

61. National Osteoporosis Foundation: *Osteoporosis: Physician's Guide to Prevention and Treatment of Osteoporosis.* Belle Mead, NJ, Excerpta Medica, 1998.

62. Paneda SJ, Bauerle W, McAfee PC: Thoracic spine fractures, in Cotler JM, Simpson JM, An HS, Silveri CP (eds): *Surgery of Spinal Trauma.* Philadelphia, PA, Lippincott-Williams & Wilkins, 2000, pp 257-268.

63. Itoi E, Sinaki M: Effect of back-strengthening exercise on posture in healthy women 49 to 65 years of age. *Mayo Clin Proc* 1994;69:1054-1059.

64. Sinaki M, Mikkelson BA: Postmenopausal spinal osteoporosis: Flexion versus extension exercises. *Arch Phys Med Rehabil* 1984;65:593-596.

65. Ekin JA, Sinaki M: Vertebral compression fractures sustained during golfing: Report of three cases. *Mayo Clin Proc* 1993;68:566-570.

66. Deramond H, Darrason R, Galibert P: Percutaneous vertebroplasty with acrylic cement in the treatment of aggressive spinal angiomas. *Rachis* 1989;1:143-153.

67. Chandler G, Dalley G, Hemmer J, Seely T: Gray ramus communicans nerve block: Novel treatment approach for painful osteoporotic vertebral compression fracture. *South Med J* 2001;94:387-393.

68. Dahm PO, Nitescu PV, Appelgren LK, Curelaru ID: Intrathecal infusion of bupivacaine with or without buprenorphine relieved intractable pain in three patients with vertebral compression fractures caused by osteoporosis. *Reg Anesth Pain Med* 1999;24:352-357.

69. Aldrete JA, Ghaly R, Zapata JC, Aldrete VT: Ambulatory, pain-free treatment of compressed vertebral fractures from osteoporosis: A preliminary report. *Pain* 1998;8:26-31.

70. Hu SS: Internal fixation in the osteoporotic spine. *Spine* 1997;22:S43-S48.

71. Bostrom MPG, Lane JM: Augmentation of osteoporotic vertebral bodies. *Spine* 1997;22:S38-S42.

72. Kempinsky WH, Morgan PP, Boniface WR: Osteoporotic kyphosis with paraplegia. *Neurology* 1958;8:181-186.

73. Maruo S, Tatekawa F, Nakano K: Paraplegia caused by vertebral compression fractures in senile osteoporosis. *Z Orthop Ihre Grenzgeb* 1987;125:320-323.

74. Salomon C, Chopin D, Benoist M: Spinal cord compression: An exceptional complication of spinal osteoporosis. *Spine* 1988;13:222-224.

75. Shikata J, Yamamuro T, Iida H, et al: Surgical treatment for paraplegia resulting from vertebral fracture in senile osteoporosis. *Spine* 1990;15:485-489.

76. Arciero RA, Leung KYK, Pierce JH: Spontaneous unstable burst fracture of the thoracolumbar spine in osteoporosis. *Spine* 1989;14:114-117.

77. Kaneda K, Ascano S, Hashimoto T, et al: The treatment of osteoporotic-posttraumatic vertebral collapse using the Kaneda device and a bioactive ceramic vertebral prosthesis. *Spine* 1992;17(suppl):S295-S303.

78. Saita K, Hoshino Y, Kikkawa I, Nakamura H: Posterior spinal shortening for paraplegia after vertebral collapse caused by osteoporosis. *Spine* 2000;25:2832-2835.

Medical Consequences of Osteoporotic Vertebral Compression Fractures

Eeric Truumees, MD

Abstract

Osteoporotic vertebral compression fractures are an increasingly common source of morbidity and mortality in the aging population. Previously, these fractures were assumed to be benign, self-limited entities with few, if any, significant sequelae. More recently, however, individual cohorts and population-wide analyses demonstrate high rates of chronic pain, functional decline, physiologic disorder, psychosocial dysfunction, and early mortality among patients with osteoporotic vertebral body compression fractures.

Osteoporotic vertebral compression fractures (VCFs) result from a collapse or implosion of weakened and discontinuous trabecular bone. Previously, VCFs were thought to be benign, self-limited injuries with few, if any, significant, long-term sequelae. This conception arose from the large percentage of reported subclinical fractures. However, current estimates indicate that as many as two thirds of VCFs are never reported by patients to their physicians.[1-5] Furthermore, in many of those cases brought to medical attention, symptoms respond rapidly to simple nonsurgical treatment.[6]

Yet, as the osteoporotic patient population grows, it is becoming clear that VCFs have many far-ranging consequences. Today, spinal compression fractures serve as sentinel markers in the epidemiologic study of osteoporosis.[2,7,8]

Moreover, fracture incidence is a benchmark by which new therapies are measured.[7,9] Thus, during the development of new medical therapies for osteoporosis, large study populations have allowed close evaluation of VCF sequelae.

Earlier literature suggested that mild deformities were not associated with losses in physical function or emotional status. In these studies, back pain and functional decline increased only with larger deformities.[10] Based on recent population-wide studies, however, it is becoming increasingly evident that any VCFs can have significant functional and physiologic impact, including acute and chronic pain, recurrent fracture, kyphotic deformity, gastrointestinal dysfunction, pulmonary dysfunction, functional decline, increased hospitalization, and increased mortality.[4]

Economics

Cost data provide one measure of the enormous social impact of osteoporosis. In 1995, direct expenditures for osteoporotic fractures in the United States exceeded $13.8 billion, or $38 million per day.[11] With the aging population, these costs are expected to rise. By 2030, annual direct costs are projected to exceed $60 billion, or $164 million per day. Previously, the majority of these costs were assumed to stem from hip fracture care. Earlier estimates attributed only 36.9% of the costs of osteoporosis care to fractures at skeletal sites other than the hip. More recent reports suggest that the contribution of spine fractures to both the substantial morbidity and costs associated with osteoporosis have been underestimated.[12,13]

Data characterizing the indirect costs of VCFs have not been readily available. Lost productivity of patients and family members and earlier transitions into assisted-living and nursing home settings likely multiply the true financial impact of these injuries.

Pain Cycle

Most acute VCFs are painful. However, the severity of this acute pain is highly

Table 1
Association of VCFs With Increased Back Pain and Back-Related Disability[4]

	Increased Back Pain		Increased Back-Related Disability	
	Women (%)	Odds Ratio (95% CI)	Women (%)	Odds Ratio (95% CI)
No baseline fracture				
No incident fracture (n = 5,629)	23	1.0	15	1.0
≥ 1 incident fracture (n = 178)	43	2.4 (1.7-3.3)	34	2.6 (1.9-3.7)
1 incident fracture (n = 145)	41	2.2 (1.6-3.2)	28	1.8 (1.2-2.7)
≥ 2 incident fractures (n = 33)	52	3.1 (1.5-6.3)	63	10.8 (5.1-23.1)
≥ 1 baseline fracture				
No incident fracture (n= 1,223)	22	1.0	21	1.0
≥ 1 incident fracture (n = 193)	34	2.0 (1.4-2.8)	39	2.2 (1.5-3.1)
1 incident fracture (n = 139)	34	1.9 (1.3-2.8)	35	1.8 (1.2-2.7)
≥ 2 incident fracture (n = 54)	35	2.1 (1.1-3.9)	51	3.6 (2.0-6.6)

n = number of women
(Reproduced with permission from Nevitt MC, Ettinger B, Black DM, et al: The association of radiologically detected vertebral fractures with back pain and function: A prospective study. *Ann Intern Med* 1998;128:793-800.)

variable. Some patients require hospitalization for intractable pain. Others report only mild and transient symptoms. Furthermore, the period of acute pain can persist in some patients for months. On the other hand, most patients report significant symptomatic improvement with treatment in the first 4 weeks.

During the initial painful interval, those patients presenting to their physicians are typically offered pain medications and braces. Limited activity and sometimes bed rest are recommended or self-imposed. Unfortunately, at least 150,000 compression fractures per year are refractory to these measures and require hospitalization, with protracted periods of bed rest and the administration of intravenous narcotics.[14]

As these fractures heal, the acute pain subsides (Table 1). However, many patients report ongoing, chronic pain. Sources of this pain are diverse and occasionally unknown. In some patients with thoracic hyperkyphosis, the rib cage rubs on the ilium, causing pain.[6] In others,

spinal imbalance leads to muscular pain and palpable spasm. Additional spinal pain may arise from microfractures. With kyphosis, the weight-bearing axis moves anteriorly over the already compromised anterior vertebral body. This unfavorable mechanical environment may account for the increased risk of additional fractures as well as increased rates of painful microfractures.[15] The risk of developing chronic pain increases with the number of VCFs.[16-19] This pain may be intensified with many typical daily activities, such as maintaining a given position in 95%, bending in 88%, and standing in 72% of patients.[20]

In many of these patients, standing tolerance decreases to only a few minutes. Pain is relieved upon lying down, but the increase in bed rest, as in patients with acute fractures, only serves to accelerate bone loss.

Prevalence of Fractures

In patients with VCFs, hospitalization rates for nonskeletal diagnoses also increase with the number of prevalent fractures.[16] In one study, an age-matched control group of women with no prior fractures had an average of seven hospitalizations per 100 patient-years; in women with three or more fractures, 12

Table 2
Association of VCFs With Bed Rest and Limited-Activity Days During Follow-Up of The Study of Osteoporotic Fractures Cohort[4]

Fracture Status	Back Pain		Back Disability		≥ 1 Day of Bed Rest Per Year		≥ 7 Limited-Activity Days Per Year	
	Women (%)	Odds Ratio (95% CI)	Women (%)	Odds Ratio (95% CI)	Women (%)	Odds Ratio (95% CI)	Women (%)	Odds Ratio (95% CI)
No incident fracture (n = 6849)	23	1.0	16	1.0	4	1.0	13	1.0
≥ 1 incident fracture and no clinical spinal fracture (n = 270)	37	2.0 (1.5-2.6)	31	1.8 (1.4-2.4)	16	4.9 (3.3-7.1)	32	2.7 (2.0-3.7)
≥ 1 incident fracture and ≥ 1 clinical spinal fracture (n = 101)	43	2.7 (1.8-4.1)	52	4.1 (2.7-6.3)	38	7.5 (4.2-13.5)	65	7.4 (4.8-11.5)

n = number of women
(Reproduced with permission from Nevitt MC, Ettinger B, Black DM, et al: The association of radiologically detected vertebral fractures with back pain and function: A prospective study. *Ann Intern Med* 1998;128:793-800.)

hospitalizations per 100 patient-years were reported.[21] Outside of the hospital, a greater number of incident spinal deformities correlates with greater back-related disability, annual number of bed-days, and annual number of limited-activity days.[4] Thus, in most patients, a period of relative or complete bed rest follows a VCF whether self-imposed or physician mandated (Table 2). In the osteoporotic population, such bed rest is associated with an additional 4% loss of bone mineral density (BMD).[22]

With age, axial strength declines more rapidly than appendicular strength. Increased kyphosis and VCF are also associated with decreased truncal strength[23,24] (Figs. 1 and 2). In a study that reviewed outcomes in cohorts of women totaling 100,000 patient-years, results showed that osteoporotic vertebral fractures lead to periods of inactivity that increase weakness, accelerate bone loss, and thereby compound the risk of additional fractures.[1] The increased weakness and bone loss that occur after spinal fractures underscore their role in a vicious cycle of pain, recurrent fracture, and ultimately increased mortality.

In fact, several studies demonstrate this increased risk of subsequent fractures with the number of prevalent fractures.[25,26] Lindsay and associates[24] collated fracture risk data from several drug trials involving patients with osteoporosis[9] (Fig. 3). In a group of patients taking vitamin D and calcium supplements, the overall risk of fracture was 6.6%. The presence of one or more fractures at baseline led to a fivefold increase in the likelihood of sustaining a new fracture in the following year. In another series, women with low bone mass had a sevenfold increase in the risk of a VCF when compared with women with normal BMD. The risk of fracture increased 25-fold in women with low BMD and a single previous fracture.[27]

Prevalent VCFs also increase the risk of sustaining nonspinal fractures.[26]

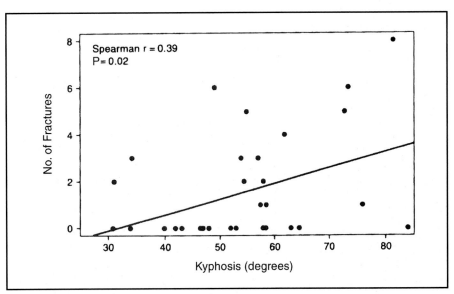

Fig. 1 Correlation of the number of VCFs with the degree of kyphosis in women with osteoporosis. (Reproduced with permission from Sinaki M, Wollan PC, Scott RW, Gelczer RK: Can strong back extensors prevent vertebral fractures in women with osteoporosis? *Mayo Clin Proc* 1996;71:951-956.)

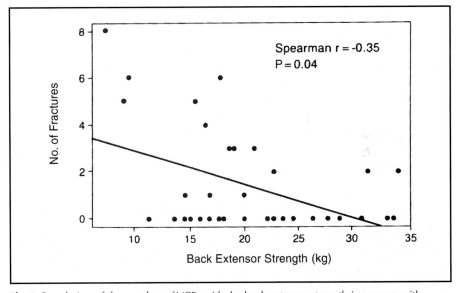

Fig. 2 Correlation of the number of VCFs with the back extensor strength in women with osteoporosis. (Reproduced with permission from Sinaki M, Wollan PC, Scott RW, Gelczer RK: Can strong back extensors prevent vertebral fractures in women with osteoporosis? *Mayo Clin Proc* 1996;71:951-956.)

Lauritzen and Lund[28] found that the relative risk (RR) of hip fracture after lumbar VCF was increased by 4.8. This association was stronger than for osteoporotic fractures of the olecranon (RR, 4.1), knee (RR, 3.5), and ankle (RR, 1.5). Kinoshita and associates[29] characterized prior lumbar vertebral fractures in 120 patients with femoral neck fracture. They compared a group of 19 men and 101 women with age- and sex-matched controls with no evidence of femoral neck frac-

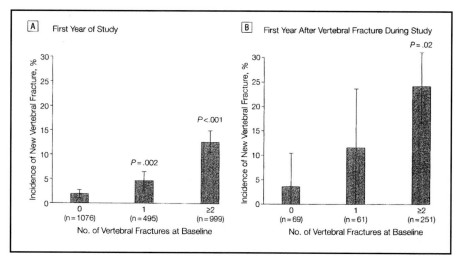

Fig. 3 Incidence of VCFs as a function of previous fractures. The increased number of baseline fractures increases risk of additional fractures. (Reproduced with permission from Lindsay R, Silverman SL, Cooper C, et al: Risk of new vertebral fracture in the year following a fracture. *JAMA* 2001;258:320-323.)

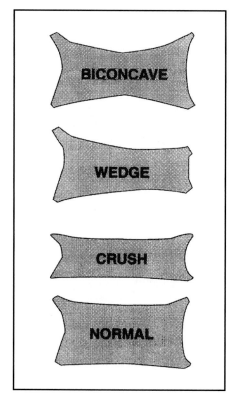

Fig. 4 Morphology of various common types of osteoporotic VCFs. (Reproduced with permission from Tamayo-Orozco J, Arzac-Palumbo P, Peon-Vidales H, Mota-Bolfeta R, Fuentes F: Vetebral fractures associated with osteoporosis: Patient management. *Am J Med* 1997;103:44S-48S.)

ture. The incidence of VCF was significantly higher in the femoral neck fracture group than in the control group (65.0% versus 41.0%). Furthermore, after calculating the extent of height loss in the fractured vertebrae, the authors concluded that multiple and more severely deformed vertebral fractures present an even higher risk for femoral neck fracture, particularly in patients younger than 79 years.

Physiologic Consequences of Fracture Deformity

VCFs have been categorized morphologically (Fig. 4). Biconcave or codfish vertebra, seen mainly in the lumbar spine, result in loss of lordosis and decreased spinal column height. Wedge vertebrae, common in the anterior or posterior aspect of thoracic spine, cause increased kyphosis and decreased spinal column height. Crush vertebrae involve anterior, posterior, and central elements and are associated with spinal column height loss of greater than 50% and may be seen in either the thoracic or lumbar spine. Crush fractures often have posterior retropulsion of bone into the spinal canal.

The deformity associated with each of these fracture types may have multiple physiologic implications. Taken together, the osteoporotic body habitus is characterized by loss of height and thoracic hyperkyphosis (dowager's hump). Abdominal protuberance and loss of lumbar lordosis may also be noted. Many otherwise active, elderly patients complain about the cosmetic effects of these changes.

Beyond the cosmetic changes, compression on the abdominal viscera by the rib cage or by loss of height through the lumbar spine leads to decreased appetite, early satiety, and weight loss.[1,5] Similarly, thoracic hyperkyphosis leads to compression of the lungs and, subsequently, decreased pulmonary function and an increased risk of pulmonary death. Lung function, as measured by forced vital capacity and forced expiratory volume, is significantly reduced in patients with thoracic or lumbar fractures.[30] One thoracic VCF causes a 9% loss of forced vital capacity.[31] Kado and associates[32] found that the degree of kyphosis is significantly related to the risk of pulmonary death from pneumonia and obstructive disease. These authors reported an age-adjusted RR of 2.0 (95% confidence interval [CI], 1.4 to 2.9). Their findings were independent of tobacco and steroid use.

In the absence of population-wide studies, the precise risk of neurologic deficit after VCF is not known. Lee and Yip[33] reviewed 497 patients admitted for osteoporotic spinal fracture and found that 10 had neurologic involvement requiring surgical decompression. Other case series describe from 3 to 27 patients with significant neurologic impairment.[34-36] Interestingly, late neurologic decline may occur up to 18 months after the initial injury. These late neurologic changes are thought to represent dysfunction of the spinal cord as it drapes over the apex of kyphosis. Neurologic involvement is certainly uncommon with osteoporotic VCFs, but is probably not as rare as was first thought.

Increasing deformity and sagittal-plane spinal imbalance have other effects, including an increased risk of falls. The incidence of both hip fracture and subdural hematoma also rise among patients with these problems. In rare cases, chin-on-chest deformities may occur.

Finally, patients with VCFs have an unexplained, increased risk of death from other diseases.[32,37] For example, a 35% to 40% increase in cancer deaths occurs independently of smoking history among those with VCFs. Stroke and myocardial infarction risk, however, is not increased. Whether this increased risk of death represents an epiphenomenon or a common etiology between cancer and osteoporosis remains unknown.

Psychologic Effects

Women sustaining osteoporotic VCFs report a number of debilitating psychologic effects.[38] These women have a poor body image and decrease in self-esteem.[39] The number of prevalent vertebral deformities is also associated with significant increases in the number of depressive symptoms and the percentage of women with clinical depression, as defined by a global depression score greater than six.[40] In one study, 40% of the patients with VCFs were clinically depressed.[20]

Patients who sustain one or more compression fractures experience increased anxiety.[8,41] In particular, patients report a fear of falling, additional fracture, and loss of independence. These psychologic effects alone, especially in older patients, may have major functional implications.[38,41] Patients with VCFs become more reclusive and fearful of activity. These behavioral changes can lead to earlier moves into assisted-living facilities and nursing homes.

Function and Quality of Life

The global impact of VCFs on pain, physical and psychologic functioning, and social independence can be measured with a variety of new quality of life instruments that are sensitive to outcomes that assess pain, physical functioning, and emotional status (including self-image and fear of falling). The validated instruments that are available include the Osteoporosis Assessment Questionnaire (OPAQ), the Quality of Life Instrument of the European Foundation for Osteoporosis (QUALEFFO), and the Osteoporosis Targeted Quality of Life Instrument.[8,42-44]

Using QUALEFFO scores, Oleksik and associates[17] found that an increasing number of VCFs lead to progressively worse pain, physical and social functioning, and mental health scores. They also found that lumbar fractures were more debilitating than thoracic fracture. Matthis and associates[45] found that limitations caused by back pain decreased the ability to perform activities of daily living and that poorer health increased among patients with prevalent fracture deformities.

In a study by Leidig-Bruckner and associates,[20] patients with VCFs reported lower functional status when compared with an age-matched control group with low back pain but without fractures. Physical function tests that assessed walking, bending, dressing, carrying bags, climbing stairs, rising from a supine position, and rising from a seated position were also performed, and it was reported that 13% of patients with VCFs were able to accomplish these activities without difficulty, 40% had difficulty, and 47% required assistance to accomplish these tasks. In 69% of patients, doing housework or rising from a supine position required assistance.

In the MacArthur Study, the results of eight physical performance tests were measured at baseline and at follow-up, including turning a circle and walking fast and performing chair stands, timed taps, tandem stands, and single-leg stands. Grip strength and balance were also assessed.[46] In the group that sustained a VCF during the follow-up period, a statistically significant ($P < 0.05$)

decline in the scores for seven of the eight performance tests was reported. Individuals with a hip and shoulder fracture showed similar global declines in physical performance, whereas those with wrist fractures demonstrated no physical performance decrements.

In the Multiple Outcomes of Raloxifene Evaluation study, the physical consequences of VCFs were studied in 1,395 women.[39] Walking/bending, standing/sitting, dressing/reaching, household/self-care, and transfers were tested. Symptom dimension, including back pain and fatigue, was also recorded using the OPAQ. Women with even one prevalent VCF were found to have significantly lower OPAQ scores than women without fractures ($P < 0.01$). Additional fractures led to further declines, with a particularly steep change occurring after the third fracture.

The number and severity of prevalent VCFs correlates with frailty and poor functional status by multiple validated quality of life instruments[47,48] (Fig. 5). Moreover, an increased number of prevalent fractures predict for greater impairments in activities of daily living and increased physician visits.[15] These combined physical and emotional effects lead to loss of independence.[49] This effect is more pronounced in older patients and in those with thoracolumbar burst fractures.[50]

Increased Mortality

The 5-year survival rate is significantly worse for those with VCFs than for age-matched controls without VCFs (61% versus 76%) and is comparable to survival rates after hip fracture[51] (Fig. 6). In patients with hip fractures, the death rate returns to baseline after 2 years. The survival rate after VCFs declines steadily after the fracture.[37] Population-based studies reveal that even women who are unaware of their fractures are subject to increased mortality (RR, 1.13; 95% CI, 1.03 to 1.32).[32]

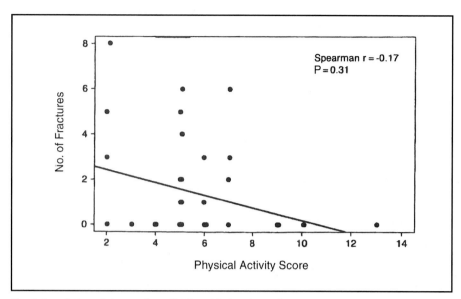

Fig. 5 Correlation of the number of VCFs with the physical activity score in women with osteoporosis. (Reproduced with permission from Sinaki M, Wollan PC, Scott RW, Gelczer RK: Can strong back extensors prevent vertebral fractures in women with osteoporosis? *Mayo Clin Proc* 1996;71:951-956.)

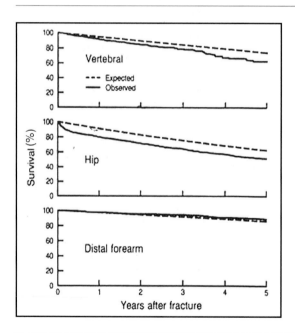

Fig. 6 Increased mortality rates after VCFs. Both hip and vertebral fractures lead to increase in mortality when compared with age-matched control patients. Distal radius fractures have no significant effect on mortality. (Reproduced with permission from Cooper C, Atkinson EJ, Jacobsen SJ, O'Fallon WM, Melton LJ III: Population-based study of survival after osteoporotic fractures. *Am J Epidemiol* 1993;137:1001-1005.)

patients with VCFs was pulmonary disease, including chronic obstructive pulmonary disease and pneumonia.

In the Fracture-Intervention Trial, patients with VCFs had an age-adjusted mortality risk of 2.15 (95% CI, 1.36 to 3.42).[52] Center and associates[53] reported that after VCFs a decline in life expectancy of 6.1 years was observed in men age 60 to 69 years. The effect was smaller in older men, with a 1.4-year decline in those older than 80 years. The authors also reported that the decline in life expectancy was smaller among women, and that women age 60 to 69 years lost only 1.9 years and women older than 80 years lost only 0.4 years. Another multi-center, population-based survey of vertebral osteoporosis in Europe found little significant difference in the mortality risk among patients with osteoporosis.[54]

Summary

With the aging of the population, osteoporotic VCFs are increasingly common. While these fractures were previously thought to be benign, self-limited entities, the explosion in interest in osteoporosis and its effects has led to a dramatically revised concept of these injuries over the last 5 years. According to the literature, 35 of 47 relevant studies into VCF outcomes were published since 1996. These studies almost uniformly portray significant and wide-ranging physical, functional, and psychologic consequences of osteoporotic VCFs. Because the quality of life has shown to decrease and mortality rates to increase after the first VCF and because the spiral of decline accelerates among those with three or more VCFs, primary and secondary prevention of osteoporosis and early, aggressive management of these injuries is essential.

References

1. Silverman SL: The clinical consequences of vertebral compression fracture. *Bone* 1992;13(suppl 2):S27-S31.

In the population-based, prospective study of 9,575 women followed for more than 8 years conducted by Kado and associates,[32] one VCF increased mortality rates by a range of 23% to 34%. Mortality was reported to have increased with the number of fractures. A death rate of 20 to 25 per 1,000 patient-years was reported in the group with two or fewer VCFs. In the group with five or more VCFs, a death rate of 40 to 50 per 1,000 patient-years was observed. This increased mortality was independent of tobacco use, BMD, self-reported health status, and other fractures, such as rib and hip fractures. The most common cause of death in

2. O'Neill TW, Felsenberg D, Varlow J, Cooper C, Kanis JA, Silman AJ: The prevalence of vertebral deformity in European men and women: The European Vertebral Osteoporosis Study. *J Bone Miner Res* 1998;11:1010-1018.

3. Tamayo-Orozco J, Arzac-Palumbo P, Peon-Vidales H, Mota-Bolfeta R, Fuentes F: Vertebral fractures associated with osteoporosis: Patient management. *Am J Med* 1997;103:44S-50S.

4. Nevitt MC, Ettinger B, Black DM, et al: The association of radiographically detected vertebral fractures with back pain and function: A prospective study. *Ann Intern Med* 1998;128: 793-800.

5. Cooper C, Atkinson EJ, O'Fallon WM, Melton LJ III: Incidence of clinically diagnosed vertebral fractures: A population-based study in Rochester, Minnesota 1985-1989. *J Bone Miner Res* 1992;7:221-227.

6. Rapado A: General management of vertebral fractures. *Bone* 1996;18(suppl 3):191S-196S.

7. Faciszewski T, McKiernan F: Calling all vertebral fractures: Classification of vertebral compression fractures: A consensus for comparison of treatment and outcome. *J Bone Miner Res* 2002;17:185-191.

8. Silverman SL: The Osteoporosis Assessment Questionnaire (OPAQ): A reliable and valid disease-targeted measure of health-related quality of life (HRQOL) in osteoporosis. *Qual Life Res* 2000;9:767-774.

9. Black DM, Reiss TF, Nevitt MC, Cauley J, Karpf D, Cummings SR: Design of the fracture intervention trial. *Osteoporos Int* 1993;(suppl 3):S29-S39.

10. Ettinger B, Block JE, Smith R, Cummings SR, Harris ST, Genant HK: An examination of the association between vertebral deformities, physical disabilities and psychosocial problems. *Maturitas* 1988;10:283-296.

11. *Michigan Osteoporosis Strategic Plan.* Lansing, MI, Michigan Department of Community Health, 1999.

12. Ray NF, Chan JK, Thamer M, Melton LJ III: Medical expenditures for the treatment of osteoporotic fractures in the United States in 1995: Report from the National Osteoporosis Foundation. *J Bone Miner Res* 1997;12:24-35.

13. Tosteson AN: Quality of life in the economic evaluation of osteoporosis prevention and treatment. *Spine* 1997;22(suppl 24):58S-62S.

14. Riggs BL, Melton LJ III: The worldwide problem of osteoporosis: Insights afforded by epidemiology. *Bone* 1995;17(suppl 5):505S-511S.

15. Myers ER, Wilson SE: Biomechanics of osteoporosis and vertebral fracture. *Spine* 1997;22(suppl 24):25S-31S.

16. Huang C, Ross PD, Wasnich RD: Vertebral fracture and other predictors of physical impairment and health care utilization. *Arch Intern Med* 1996;156:2469-2475.

17. Oleksik A, Ott SM, Vedi S, Bravenboer N, Compston J, Lips P: Health-related quality of life in postmenopausal women with low BMD with or without prevalent vertebral fractures. *J Bone Miner Res* 2000;15:1368-1375.

18. Ettinger B, Black DM, Nevitt MC, et al: Contribution of vertebral deformities to chronic back pain and disability: The Study of Osteoporotic Fractures Research Group. *J Bone Miner Res* 1992;7:449-456.

19. Huang C, Ross PD, Wasnich RD: Vertebral fracture and other predictors of back pain among older women. *J Bone Miner Res* 1996;11:1026-1032.

20. Leidig-Bruckner G, Minne HW, Schlaich C, et al: Clinical grading of spinal osteoporosis: Quality of life components and spinal deformity in women with chronic low back pain and women with vertebral osteoporosis. *J Bone Miner Res* 1997;12:663-675.

21. Ensrud KE, Thompson DE, Cauley JA, et al: Prevalent vertebral deformities predict mortality and hospitalization in older women with loss bone mass: Fracture Intervention Trial Research Group. *J Am Geriatr Soc* 2000;48:241-249.

22. Heaney RP: The natural history of vertebral osteoporosis: Is low bone mass an epiphenomenon? *Bone* 1992;13(suppl 2):S23-S26.

23. Sinaki M, Wollan PC, Scott RW, Gelczer RK: Can strong back extensors prevent vertebral fractures in women with osteoporosis? *Mayo Clin Proc* 1996;71:951-956.

24. Lindsay R, Silverman SL, Cooper C, et al: Risk of new vertebral fracture in the year following a fracture. *JAMA* 2001;285:320-323.

25. Wasnich RD: Vertebral fracture epidemiology. *Bone* 1996;18(suppl 3):179S-183S.

26. Black DM, Arden NK, Palermo L, Pearson J, Cummings SR: Prevalent vertebral deformities predict hip fractures and new vertebral deformities but not wrist fractures: Study of Osteoporotic Fractures Research Group. *J Bone Miner Res* 1999;14:821-828.

27. Ross PD, Davis JW, Epstein RS, Wasnich RD: Pre-existing fractures and bone mass predict vertebral fracture incidence in women. *Ann Intern Med* 1991;114:919-923.

28. Lauritzen JB, Lund B: Risk of hip fracture after osteoporosis fractures: 451 women with fracture of lumbar spine, olecranon, knee or ankle. *Acta Orthop Scand* 1993;64:297-300.

29. Kinoshita T, Ebara S, Kamimura M, et al: Nontraumatic lumbar vertebral compression fracture as a risk factor for femoral neck fractures in involutional osteoporotic patients. *J Bone Miner Metab* 1999;17:201-205.

30. Schlaich C, Minne HW, Bruckner T, et al: Reduced pulmonary function in patients with spinal osteoporotic fractures. *Osteoporo Int* 1998;8:261-267.

31. Leech JA, Dulberg C, Kellie S, Pattee L, Gay J: Relationship of lung function to severity of osteoporosis in women. *Am Rev Respir Dis* 1990;141:68-71.

32. Kado DM, Browner WS, Palermo L, Nevitt MC, Genant HK, Cummings SR: Vertebral fractures and mortality in older women: A prospective study: Study of Osteoporotic Fractures Research Group. *Arch Intern Med* 1999;159:1215-1220.

33. Lee YL, Yip KM: The osteoporotic spine. *Clin Orthop* 1996;323:91-97.

34. Kaplan PA, Orton DF, Asleson RJ: Osteoporosis with vertebral compression fractures, retropulsed fragments, and neurologic compromise. *Radiology* 1987;165:533-535.

35. Heggeness MH: Spine fracture with neurological deficit in osteoporosis. *Osteoporos Int* 1993;3:215-221.

36. Baba H, Maezawa Y, Kamitani K, Furusawa N, Imura S, Tomita K: Osteoporotic vertebral collapse with late neurological complications. *Paraplegia* 1995;33:281-289.

37. Cooper C, Atkinson EJ, Jacobsen SJ, O'Fallon WM, Melton LJ III: Population-based study of survival after osteoporotic fractures. *Am J Epidemiol* 1993;137:1001-1005.

38. Gold DT: The clinical impact of vertebral fractures: Quality of life in women with osteoporosis. *Bone* 1996;18(suppl 3):185S-189S.

39. Silverman SL, Minshall ME, Shen W, Harper KD, Xie S: Abstract: The relationship of health-related quality of life to prevalent and incident vertebral fractures in postmenopausal women with osteoporosis: Results from the Multiple Outcomes of Raloxifene Evaluation Study. *Arthritis Rheum* 2001;44:2611-2619.

40. Silverman SL, Minshall ME, Shen W, Harper KD, Xie S: Abstract: The association between vertebral fracture and depression as measured by the Affective Rating Scale (ARS): Results from the Multiple Outcomes of Raloxifene Evaluation Study. *J Bone Miner Res* 1999;14(suppl 1);S261.

41. Gold DT: The nonskeletal consequences of osteoporotic fractures: Psychologic and social outcomes. *Rheum Dis Clin North Am* 2001;27:255-262.

42. Randell AG, Bhalerao N, Nguyen TV, Sambrook PN, Eisman JA, Silverman SL: Quality-of-life in osteoporosis: Reliability, consistency and validity of the Osteoporosis Assessment Questionnaire. *J Rheumatol* 1998;25:1171-1179.

43. Lips P, Cooper C, Agnusdei D, et al: Quality of life in patients with vertebral fractures: Validation of the Quality of Life Questionnaire of the European Foundation for Osteoporosis (QUALEFFO): Working Party for Quality of Life of the European Foundation for Osteoporosis. *Osteoporos Int* 1999;10:150-160.

44. Silverman SL, Cranney A: Quality of Life measurement in osteoporosis. *J Rheumatol* 1997;24:1218-1221.

45. Matthis C, Weber U, O'Neill TW, Raspe H: Health impact associated with vertebral deformities: Results from the European Vertebral Osteoporosis study (EVOS). *Osteoporos Int* 1998;8:364-372.

46. Greendale GA, DeAmicis TA, Bucur A, et al: A prospective study of the effect of fracture on measured physical performance: Results from the MacArthur Study (MAC). *J Am Geriatr Soc* 2000;48:546-549.

47. Pluijm SM, Tromp AM, Smit JH, Deeg DJ, Lips P: Consequences of vertebral deformities in older men and women. *J Bone Miner Res* 2000;15:1564-1572.

48. Burger H, Van Daele PL, Grashuis K, et al: Vertebral deformities and functional impairment in men and women. *J Bone Miner Res* 1997;12:152-157.

49. Lyles KW, Gold DT, Shipp KM, Pieper CF, Martinez S, Mulhausen PL: Association of osteoporotic vertebral compression fractures with impaired functional status. *Am J Med* 1993;94:595-601.

50. Ryan PJ, Blake G, Herd R, Fogelman I: A clinical profile of back pain and disability in patients with spinal osteoporosis. *Bone* 1994;15:27-30.

51. Cooper C: The crippling consequences of fractures and their impact on quality of life. *Am J Med* 1997;103:12S-19S.

52. Cauley JA, Thompson DE, Ensrud KC, Scott JC, Black D: Risk of mortality following clinical fractures. *Osteoporos Int* 2000;11:556-561.

53. Center JR, Nguyen TV, Schneider D, Sambrook PN, Eisman JA: Mortality after all types of osteoporotic fracture in men and women: An observational study. *Lancet* 1999;353:878-882.

54. Ismail AA, O'Neill TW, Cooper C, et al: Mortality associated with vertebral deformity in men and women: Results from the European Prospective Osteoporosis Study (EPOS). *Osteoporos Int* 1998;8:291-297.

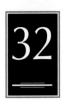

Minimally Invasive Treatments of Osteoporotic Vertebral Compression Fractures: Vertebroplasty and Kyphoplasty

Frank M. Phillips, MD
Bernard A. Pfeifer, MD
Isador H. Lieberman, BSc, MD, FRCSC
Eubulus J. Kerr III, MD
In Sup Choi, MD
Artemis G. Pazianos, MD

Abstract

Although nonsurgical treatment of osteoporotic vertebral compression fractures, including medication, exercise, bracing, and bed rest, have been reasonably effective, vertebroplasty and kyphoplasty have evolved as valuable adjunctive treatment options. Over the past decade, vertebroplasty, which involves the percutaneous injection of bone cement directly into the fractured vertebral body, has been used as a treatment for painful osteoporotic vertebral body compression fractures, a leading cause of morbidity in the elderly.

Kyphoplasty, another minimally invasive procedure that allows for correction of spinal deformity and for controlled cement filling of the fractured vertebral body, involves the percutaneous cannulation of the vertebral body followed by the placement of an inflatable bone tamp. Reported results for both vertebroplasty and kyphoplasty suggest rapid improvement in pain and physical functioning in patients with osteoporotic vertebral compression fractures. Kyphoplasty allows for low-pressure cement injection and affords the opportunity to correct spinal deformity. Further study is required to define the precise indications, timing, and relative merits of these techniques.

Traditionally, acute osteoporotic vertebral compression fractures (VCFs) are treated nonsurgically, except in rare cases in which the fracture is associated with neurologic compromise or advanced spinal instability. Spinal surgery in the osteoporotic patient is fraught with risk related to the patient's advanced age and comorbidities and the difficulties in securing fixation in osteoporotic bone. Thus, the treatment of most patients with painful VCFs includes bed rest, analgesic medications, bracing, antiosteoporotic drugs, or some combination thereof.[1-4] Although these treatments appear to be reasonably effective, anti-inflammatory and narcotic medications are often poorly tolerated by the elderly and may lead to confusion, increased fall risk, and adverse effects on the gastrointestinal tract. Bed rest can lead to an overall physiologic deconditioning and acceleration of bone loss. Bracing often is not well tolerated by older patients, is expensive, and may further restrict diaphragmatic excursion. Furthermore, none of these treatments directly addresses the fracture causing the pain or the spinal deformity.

Orthopaedic fracture care should emphasize restoring anatomy, correcting deformity, and preserving function. The treatment of osteoporotic VCFs ideally should address both the fracture-related pain and the kyphotic deformity. This should be accomplished in a minimally invasive fashion without subjecting the patient to inordinate risks or excessive surgical trauma. Over the past decade, vertebroplasty, the percutaneous injection of polymethylmethacrylate (PMMA) directly into a fractured vertebral body, has been used for the treatment of osteoporotic VCFs. Substantial pain relief is reported in a majority of patients treated with vertebroplasty.[1,5-13] Kyphoplasty is a minimally invasive orthopaedic procedure designed to address kyphotic deformity and fracture pain. This operation involves the percutaneous insertion of an inflatable bone tamp into a fractured vertebral body under fluoroscopic guidance. Inflation of the bone tamp elevates the end plates and reduces the vertebral body back toward its original height, and creates a cavity to be filled with bone-void filler. Early results of kyphoplasty suggest significant pain relief as well as the ability to increase the height of the collapsed vertebral body and reduce spinal kyphosis.[3,13-16]

Vertebroplasty

Percutaneous vertebroplasty involving augmentation of the vertebral body with bone cement was first described by Galibert and associates[17] in 1987. The procedure was first reported in the United States by Deprister-Debussche and associates[18] in 1993. Since then, this technique has been used widely.

Biomechanics

The pain relief brought about by vertebroplasty is probably secondary to fracture stabilization. The injected cement prevents painful micromotion at the fracture site. In studies by Belkoff and associates,[19] a relatively small amount of injected PMMA was needed to restore the prefracture strength in the cadaveric vertebra; 4.4 mL in the lumbar spine, 3.1 mL in the thoracolumbar spine, and 2.5 mL in the thoracic levels were sufficient to restore the prevertebroplasty strength to the vertebra. A study by Wilson and associates[20] showed that augmentation by vertebroplasty reduced flexion-extension compliance by 23% and lateral bending compliance by 26%. Augmentation restored more than half of the stiffness lost to the fracture, and there was a 40% increase overall in the stiffness of the vertebral segments. In this study, no difference was shown between the mechanical restoration of compliance from vertebroplasty or kyphoplasty. Eriksson and associates[21] believed that the exothermic reaction that occurs with the polymerization

of the cement causes heat trauma to the surrounding tissues, thereby providing relief of pain. They report that during the polymerization, temperatures may reach 122°C for large quantities of cement.

Indications

The indications for vertebroplasty are evolving. It was first believed that the ideal patient had a semiacute fracture with nonimproving pain that was less than 60% compressed and required tenderness over the spinous process of the affected vertebra and a radiographic study to prove that the fracture is still active. Vertebroplasty is not indicated for patients whose pain is improving. When there is more than 60% compression, the procedure is technically arduous; however, with experience, vertebrae with severe compression can be treated. Suggested indications for vertebroplasty include stabilization of painful osteoporotic vertebral fractures, painful vertebra as a result of osteolytic metastases or multiple myeloma, Kummell's disease, painful vertebral hemangioma, and debilitating pain and loss of mobility that was unresponsive to medical treatment with the pain thought to be coming from the uninvolved vertebra.

In addition to plain radiographs, a study to indicate the activity of the fracture is needed before performing vertebroplasty. When a patient has a pacemaker in place, then technetium Tc 99m scintigraphy is sufficient. MRI sagittal short tau inversion recovery (STIR) sequencing is reliable and shows very clearly the edema that is seen in a healing or acute compression fracture. Baker and associates[22] showed that a benign compression fracture appears hypointense with T1-weighted imaging and hyperintense with STIR imaging.

Contraindications

Contraindications to vertebroplasty include infection, vertebral plana, neural compression, and uncorrectable coagu-

lopathy. Additional contraindications may include the inability to tolerate general anesthesia and a prone position for an extended period. A burst fracture is a relative contraindication to vertebroplasty.

The limitations of vertebroplasty are related to the inability of the procedure to correct spinal deformity and also the risk of extravertebral cement extravasation during injection. During vertebroplasty, the high-pressure injection of low-viscosity cement directly into cancellous bone makes it difficult to control cement flow in the vertebral body, which creates an unpredictable risk of cement extravasation outside of the vertebral body.[15] In fact, extravertebral cement extravasation commonly occurs during vertebroplasty, and leak rates of up to 65% have been reported.[10] However, the proponents of vertebroplasty have reported infrequent clinical sequelae of the leakage. Cotten and associates[23] noted 15 epidural cement leaks, 8 intradiscal leaks, 2 venous leaks, and 21 paravertebral leaks in 20 of 37 patients (40 fractures) treated with vertebroplasty. Two of the foraminal leaks required decompressive surgery, and one soft-tissue femoral neuropathy was treated with steroids. Cortet and associates[10] reported extravertebral cement extravasation in 13 of 20 vertebrae treated with vertebroplasty for osteoporotic fractures. Cement leaked into the paravertebral soft tissues in six patients, into the peridural space in three, into the disk space in three, and into the lumbar venous plexus in one. Cyteval and associates[11] noted extravertebral cement extravasation in 8 of 20 patients who underwent vertebroplasty, with leakage into the intervertebral disk in 5 patients, into the neural foramen in 2, and into the lumbar venous plexus in 1. Chiras and associates[7] reported radiculopathy in 4% of patients undergoing vertebroplasty, which was likely related to intraforaminal cement leakage and frequent leaks of PMMA into the perivertebral veins. A recent study reported that 3 of 35 patients treated with vertebroplasty had extravasation of cement into the epidural space, necessitating open surgical decompression in 2 patients.[24] In this series, an additional two patients had cement pulmonary emboli. Cases of symptomatic and lethal PMMA pulmonary embolism with vertebroplasty have also been reported.[25-28]

In an effort to reduce the risk of extravertebral cement leak, intravertebral contrast injection studies may be performed before cement injection in an attempt to predict potential egress of cement from the vertebral body. McGraw and associates[29] reported that intraosseous venography predicted the flow of PMMA during vertebroplasty in 83% of cases. Using similar intravertebral contrast injection studies, Phillips and associates[30] have shown significantly higher rates of transcortical and intravenous contrast leak for vertebroplasty when compared with kyphoplasty. Others have argued that intravertebral contrast injections are not useful and that discontinuing cement injection once cement leaks out of the vertebral body or fills the perivertebral veins remains the best technique for reducing the risk of complications. This may, however, lead to less than adequate vertebral fill or the need for multiple injections.

In spite of the limitations, vertebroplasty has been shown to be an effective and relatively inexpensive technique for improving pain associated with osteoporotic VCFs. As vertebroplasty is frequently performed by interventional radiologists in a radiology suite, it is essential that adequate support is available to deal with any complications, such as pulmonary embolism or neural compromise.

Technique

During vertebroplasty, bone cement is injected directly into the fractured vertebral body using a transpedicular or extrapedicular approach with a large-bore needle under multidirectional fluoroscopy.

PMMA has been the bone cement most widely used for vertebroplasty, although it is not approved by the US Food and Drug Administration for use in the spine. Clinically, vertebroplasty has been shown to provide lasting partial or complete pain relief within 72 hours of the procedure in the majority of patients. Reported follow-up periods after vertebroplasty have ranged from a few months to more than 10 years.[1,5-13] The reported vertebroplasty complication rate is low, with most complications resulting from extravertebral cement leakage that causes spinal cord or nerve root compression or pulmonary embolism.[1,5-13]

A percutaneous transpedicular approach can be done through either one or both pedicles, depending on whether the cement will flow across midline and completely fill the vertebral body. An alternative approach in the lumbar spine is the lateral approach such as one would use for a diskogram, and in the thoracic spine, an approach between the rib head and the pedicle.[31] Reports on pedicle screw fixation provide the best anatomic nuance for performing vertebroplasty via a transpedicular approach, particularly the technique described by Krag.[32]

Although the procedure has been and can be performed with the patient under general anesthetia, vertebroplasty is more typically performed with the patient under monitored anesthesia care to allow for the patient to report any symptoms of neural encroachment. The patient can be placed in either the prone or direct lateral position.

All patients undergo a standard preoperative assessment and are cleared for general anesthesia. An intravenous line is placed, and the patient is placed prone on bolsters.

Adequate imaging is paramount to the safe accomplishment of vertebroplasty. The patient must be in a true AP position with the spinous processes aligned midway between the pedicles on the radiographic view. For the lateral view,

the C-arm should be aligned along the end plate so that a true profile is obtained. Oblique images can be obtained as needed. Local anesthesia is infiltrated over the portal that is selected and a small incision is made. A thin-gauge spinal needle is used to plan a trajectory. An 11-gauge trocar and cannular system bone biopsy needle is then advanced via the pedicular approach to the junction of the anterior middle third of the vertebra. At this time, a transosseous phlebograph can be obtained by injecting contrast through the cannula, and assessment of the path of filling and epidural or other venous drainage can be carried out. However, the path taken by the cement (because it has different rheologic properties) may be more contracted than that taken by the less viscid contrast. With increased experience of the operator, the phlebograph may be optional.

The PMMA cement mixture can consist of Cranioplastic (Codman and Surtleff, Raynham, MA, off-label use) contained in the commercial kit, sterile barium, and injectable tobramycin. This is mixed until a dull sheen consistency is achieved. This mixture sets within 20 minutes and achieves 90% of its ultimate strength within in 1 hour of injection, as shown by the studies of Mathis.[33] By storing the mixture in an ice saline bath prior to injection, polymerization of the cement is delayed and up to 2 hours of working time obtained. The injection is done in very small boluses and is nonpressurized. Small, 1-mL syringes are used to reduce the complication of cement emboli. Additionally, small amounts of cement to "plug off" paraspinal or intraspinous veins can be used. The flow path of the cement can be random and variable. Angling the cannula tip in the direction of the intended cement path allows for a more targeted placement. Vertebral body filling should be maximized. The end point of injection as reported by Centenera and associates[34] is either filling to the posterior quarter of

Table 1
Vertebroplasty Results

Authors	Year	No. of Patients (No. of vertebra)	Good to Excellent Results (%)
Weill et al[35]	1996	37 (50)	73
Cotten et al[23]	1996	37 (40)	97
Martin et al[36]	1997	40 (68)	70
Jensen et al[37]	1997	29 (126)	90
Gangi et al[38]	2000	187 (289)	78
Barr et al[39]	2000	38 (70)	95

the vertebra, or incipient filling of the epidural or paraspinal veins, or filling of the intervertebral disk space through an end-plate fracture.

Digital subtraction angiography can be very helpful, especially when injecting the second side of a vertebral body. If digital subtraction angiography is not available, then cannulas should be placed in both sides and controlled injection performed in each side until the vertebral body is filled from anterior to posterior. Gangi and associates[6] have described CT-guided vertebroplasty. In addition, Hirsch described a vertebroplasty technique using a combination of portable CT and biplane fluoroscopy (Boston, MA, unpublished data, 2001). However, these techniques can be time consuming and cumbersome.

Results
A review of the results of vertebroplasty shows that between 73% and 97% of patients have good to excellent pain relief[24,35-39] (Table 1). These results have been demonstrated to be long lasting by Grados and associates[40] in a 4-year follow-up study of 25 patients (35 vertebrae) treated with vertebroplasty. Mean preoperative visual analog pain scale (VAS) scores of 80 decreased to 37 at 3 months and to 34 at 48 months, which was statistically significant ($P < 0.05$). Moreover, no progression of fractures, of the injected vertebrae was shown to have

occurred. Cortet and associates,[10] using the VAS and the Nottingham pain profile in a study published in 1999, showed statistically significant improvement in VAS scores and the pain, physical mobility, emotion, energy, and social isolation scales of the Nottingham pain profile. No change in the sleep scale was noted. Levine and associates[26] concluded in the meta-analysis that although no prospective randomized studies have been done, one could expect 80% of patients treated with vertebroplasty to have significant pain relief.

Complications
Serious complications have been reported as the result of vertebroplasty, including spinal cord damage and complications caused by injection of cement either around the neural elements or intravenously. Increased pain, minor leakages, rib fractures, venous thromboembolism, infection, bleeding, and adverse reaction to PMMA have also been reported. The risk of complication increases with the vascularity of the lesion and when injecting more liquid cement in the presence of cortical destruction. Therefore, power injection of cement is not advised. To minimize complications, vertebroplasty must be carried out in an appropriate environment with excellent visualization, and surgical backup should be readily available if a complication occurs.

One complication of particular con-

cern is a contiguous or new fracture. Grados and associates[38] showed that 52% of patients undergoing vertebroplasty experienced a new fracture over the 4-year study period. The odds ratio for the fracture to occur adjacent to the treated vertebra was 2.3 versus 1.4 for a nonadjacent vertebra. Watts and associates[41] reported that one in five patients who underwent vertebroplasty would have a second fracture. Another study showed that 12% of 177 patients treated with vertebroplasty had a subsequent compression fracture, two thirds of which occurred within 30 days. Sixty-six percent of these fractures occurred in an adjacent vertebra and 33% in a nonadjacent vertebra.[42] Because the reported 1-year risk of a second vertebral fracture after a first documented fracture is almost 20%,[43] the 12% rate reported may relate to the fact that all patients treated were seen by an endocrinologist to assure maximal medical treatment. It would seem to negate the effect of residual wedging and lack of sagittal contour change. Although some authors have advocated performing vertebroplasty for multiple levels to avoid causing contiguous or new fractures, overtreating a large number of vertebrae can be inappropriate. Although PMMA is the vertebral augmentation material that is currently used to perform vertebroplasty, better materials are needed that more closely match the mechanical characteristics of bone, have better flow characteristics, and are osteoinductive.

Kyphoplasty
Kyphoplasty is a newer minimally invasive technique, having evolved from the marriage of vertebroplasty and balloon angioplasty (Figs. 1 and 2). Kyphoplasty has a number of potential advantages, including lower risk of cement extravasation and better restoration of vertebral body height.[44] A cannula is introduced into the vertebral body, via a transpedicular or extrapedicular route. Next, an inflatable bone tamp is inserted, which

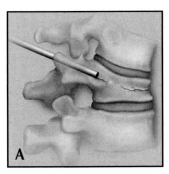 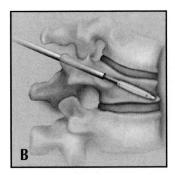 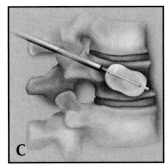 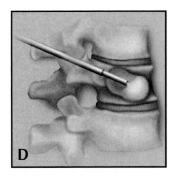

Fig. 1 Steps in kyphoplasty procedure. **A,** Vertebral body cannulation. **B,** Balloon placement. **C,** Balloon deployment. **D,** Cement fill.

when deployed, reduces the compression fracture and restores the vertebral body toward its original height. This scenario then creates a cavity to be filled with bone cement. The cement augmentation can now be completed with more control into the low-pressure environment of the preformed cavity with viscous, partially cured cement. The procedure can be performed under general anesthesia or local anesthesia with intravenous sedation; some patients are able to return home the same day of the procedure.

Indications

Kyphoplasty is indicated for any progressive and/or painful osteoporotic or osteolytic vertebral compression fracture. In the typical elderly patient with a VCF, a clear distinction must be made between the pain and fracture progression associated with the VCF versus the pain or progressive deformity that may result from degenerative disease or a degenerative scoliosis.

Fracture progression after a VCF may be an indication for kyphoplasty and implies any loss of sagittal alignment or increased focal angulation at the index vertebral body. Progression may be monitored using parameters such as loss of measured true standing height, and/or changes noted on sequential diagnostic imaging (such as radiograph, CT, or MRI). Progression may be anticipated in those patients with DEXA "T" scores of –2.5 or greater, metabolic bone disease

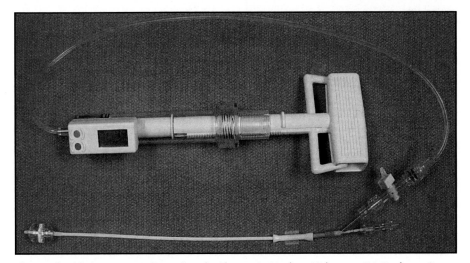

Fig. 2 Inflatable bone tamp. (Reproduced with permission from Lieberman IH, Dudeney S, Reinhardt M-K, Bell G: Initial outcome and efficacy of "kyphoplasty" in the treatment of painful osteoporotic vertebral compression fractures. *Spine* 2001;26:1631-1638.)

(such as osteomalacia or amyloid) or osteolysis secondary to tumors (for example, multiple myeloma and lytic breast cancer metastases). Progression of the fracture may be considered an indication for kyphoplasty.

Pain after VCF may be associated with direct tenderness over the vertebral level, increased symptoms with range of motion testing, and/or loss of patient mobility. Pain may be attributable to one or all of the following factors: microarchitectural fracture progression, altered load-bearing capacity of the anterior column (ie, vertebral body), altered tensile or compressive loads on the posterior column (ie, facets), progression of degenerative spondylolisthesis above or below

the fracture level in response to kyphotic posturing, or movement between fractured end plates of an established vertebral body pseudarthrosis. In addition, nonhealing of the fracture may be implied by increased activity on technetium bone scan and/or altered signal intensity (marrow edema) on MRI (T1, T2, and STIR T2 images).

Like hip fracture surgery, kyphoplasty may also be considered as prophylaxis against any extraskeletal physiologic consequences associated with immobility or prolonged bed rest, such as the development of deep vein thrombosis, the deterioration of pulmonary function, the increased incidence of urinary tract infections, and decubitus ulcers.

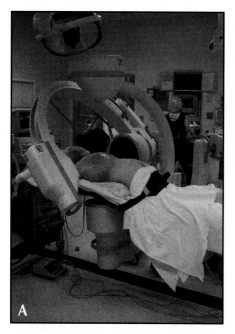

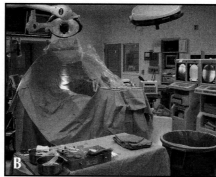

Fig. 3 Operating room setup. **A,** C-arms positioned for AP and lateral views. **B,** The surgical field draped.

Kyphoplasty is contraindicated in patients with burst fracture configurations (retropulsed bone and/or neurologic deficit) in nonosteoporotic bone. This scenario is typical of the young trauma patient, in whom the ability of the inflatable bone tamp to actually create a cavity is cause for concern, along with the use of cement to stabilize physiologically normal bone. Burst fracture configurations do occasionally occur with osteoporotic bone but tend to be the exception. Under most circumstances, when intervention is indicated, treatment of burst fracture configurations in osteoporotic bone should be governed by traditional treatment principles. Wedge compression fractures might also occur in the younger population (younger than age 40 years), but are the exception rather than the rule. These fractures of the superior end plate tend not to be progressive, typically go on to heal in a slightly kyphotic posture, and are more likely to be symptomatic from disk disruption as opposed to collapsing bone.

Kyphoplasty is not indicated in the treatment of osteoblastic, matrix, or tissue-producing solid tumors, where once again the ability of the inflatable bone tamp to create a cavity has not been proven. Vertebral collapse secondary to osteomyelitis is another contraindication to kyphoplasty.

Technique (DVD-48.1)

With the patient under general or local anesthesia in the prone position on a radiolucent spinal frame, two fluoroscopic C-arms are positioned for AP and lateral fluoroscopic images (Fig. 3). Once in position the C-arms and patient are not moved to ensure repeatable images throughout the procedure. Two 3-mm incisions are made at the vertebral level, parallel to the pedicles in both planes. Next, a guide wire or biopsy needle is advanced into the vertebral body via a transpedicular or extrapedicular approach, depending on fracture configuration and the patient's anatomy. The guide wire is then exchanged for the working cannula using a series of obturators. Once the working cannula is positioned, a corridor is reamed out to accommodate the inflatable bone tamp, which is positioned under the collapsed end plate. The inflatable bone tamp is deployed slowly under

fluoroscopic guidance until maximum fracture reduction is achieved or the balloon reaches a cortical wall (Fig. 4). At this point the bone tamp is deflated and removed, the cement mixed, and the cement cannulae prefilled, allowing the cement to partially cure in the cement cannulae. Next, the cement cannulae are positioned through the working cannulae into the center of the cavity created by the bone tamp. The PMMA is then slowly extruded into the vertebral body under continuous lateral fluoroscopic guidance (Fig. 5). This technique permits a low-pressure fill. In most instances, the volume of cement can slightly exceed that of the bone cavity to interdigitate PMMA from the central bolus with the surrounding bone. Once filling is complete and the cement has hardened, the cannula is removed and the 3-mm incisions are closed.

During the perioperative period, the patient is observed for 2 to 6 hours before being discharged. If significant comorbid issues are present, overnight monitoring at the hospital may be warranted. All patients are encouraged to resume their normal activities as soon as possible. Oral analgesics are issued as necessary. Patients who were bedridden prior to surgery may require a short course of rehabilitation and physical therapy to reestablish mobility.

Results

Kyphoplasty has been slowly advanced through a number of surgical centers participating in a multicenter study begun in 1999. A Phase I efficacy study of 70 consecutive kyphoplasty procedures in 30 patients with painful, progressive osteoporotic/osteolytic VCFs was recently completed.[41] Mean duration of symptoms was 5.9 months. Symptomatic levels were identified by correlating the clinical data with MRI findings. Preoperative and postoperative radiographs were compared to calculate the percentage of height restored. Outcome was further assessed by comparing the preoperative and latest

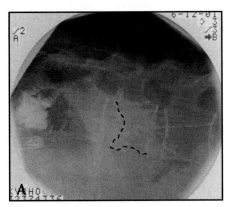
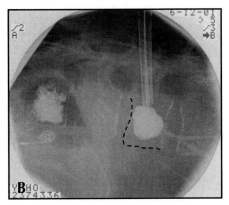
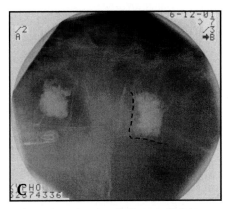

Fig. 4 Typical osteoporotic compression fracture. **A,** Collapsed vertebrae. **B,** Reduction of fracture and creation of cavity. **C,** Cement PMMA augmentation.

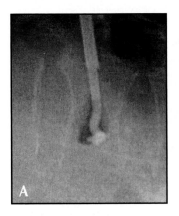
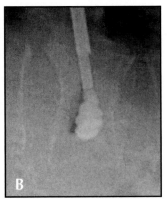
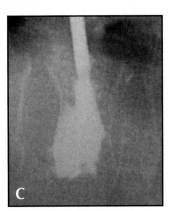

Fig. 5 Stepwise PMMA cement fill of the cavity. (Reproduced with permission from Lieberman IH, Dudeney S, Reinhardt M-K, Bell G: Initial outcome and efficacy of "kyphoplasty" in the treatment of painful osteoporotic vertebral compression fractures. *Spine* 2001;26:1631-1638.)

postoperative survey of patient's self-reported health status using the 36-item Short Form Health Survey (SF-36).[45] In 70% of the vertebral bodies, kyphoplasty restored, on average, 47% of the lost vertebral height (P = .001). SF-36 scores for bodily pain (P = .0001), physical function (P = .002), and vitality (P = .001) were among the subscales that showed substantial and significant improvement (Fig. 6). Complications were infrequent. One patient experienced perioperative pulmonary edema and a myocardial infarction secondary to intraoperative fluid overload; two patients suffered rib fractures as a result of incorrect positioning during the procedure. Cement leakage occurred at 6 of 70 treated levels (8.6%); however, no complications were directly related to selection of this technique or to the use of the inflatable bone tamp. In an

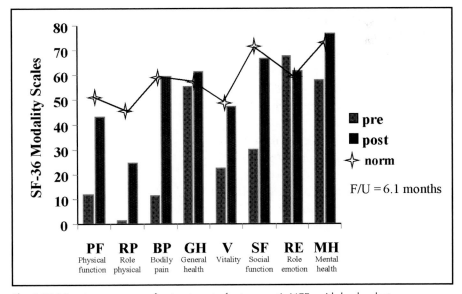

Fig. 6 SF-36 outcome scores after treatment of osteoporotic VCFs with kyphoplasty. (Reproduced with permission from Lieberman IH, Dudeney S, Reinhardt M-K, Bell G: Initial outcome and efficacy of "kyphoplasty" in the treatment of painful osteoporotic vertebral compression fractures. *Spine* 2001;26:1631-1638.)

ongoing evaluation, the results of this initial series have been maintained in the most recent follow-up of over 100 consecutive patients after 14 months. Phillips and associates[46] confirmed the ability of kyphoplasty to improve spinal alignment and reported a mean improvement of local kyphosis of 14° in VCFs that were considered reducible.

Summary

Over the past decade, physicians have become aware of the devastating consequences of osteoporotic VCFs. Vertebroplasty has been popularized as a reliable minimally invasive technique for relieving pain associated with VCFs and represents a significant step forward in the management of these patients. Kyphoplasty appears to be the next step in the evolution of the management of VCFs, allowing for low-pressure insertion of cement into the fractured vertebra thereby reducing the risk of cement leak and allowing for correction of spinal deformity. Further study is required to define the role for each of these procedures in the spinal physician's armamentarium and to determine the optimal indications for intervention in patients with osteoporotic VCFs.

Prevention of osteoporotic VCFs with a combination of pharmacologic agents and timely reinforcement of at-risk osteoporotic vertebrae is the ultimate goal aside from prevention of osteoporosis itself. New osteoconductive synthetic agents will figure more prominently as an emerging alternative to cement. Advances in minimally invasive surgical techniques, imaging, and synthetic engineering are rapidly changing the treatment protocols available for osteoporotic VCF.

References

1. Rapado A: General management of vertebral fractures. *Bone* 1996;18(suppl 13):191S-196S.

2. Lukert BP: Vertebral compression fractures: How to manage pain, avoid disability. *Geriatrics* 1994;49:22-26.

3. Eck JC, Hodges SD, Humphreys SC: Vertebroplasty: A new treatment strategy for osteoporotic compression fractures. *Am J Orthop* 2002;31:123-128.

4. Meunier PJ, Delmas PD, Eastell R, et al: Diagnosis and management of osteoporosis in postmenopausal women: Clinical guidelines: International Committee for Osteoporosis Clinical Guidelines. *Clin Ther* 1999;21:1025-1044.

5. Lapras C, Mottolese C, Deruty R, Lapras C Jr, Remond J, Duquesnel J: Percutaneous injection of methyl-metacrylate in osteoporosis and severe vertebral osteolysis: Galibert's technic. *Ann Chir* 1989;43:371-376.

6. Gangi A, Kastler BA, Dietemann JL: Percutaneous vertebroplasty guided by a combination of CT and fluoroscopy. *Am J Neuroradiol* 1994;15:83-86.

7. Chiras J, Depriester C, Weill A, Sola-Martinez MT, Deramond H: Percutaneous vertebral surgery: Technics and indications. *J Neuroradiol* 1997;24:45-59.

8. Jensen ME, Evans AJ, Mathis JM, Kallmes DF, Cloft HJ, Dion JE: Percutaneous polymethylmethacrylate vertebroplasty in the treatment of osteoporotic vertebral body compression fractures: Technical aspects. *Am J Neuroradiol* 1997;18:1897-1904.

9. Mathis JM, Petri M, Naff N: Percutaneous vertebroplasty treatment of steroid-induced osteoporotic compression fractures. *Arthritis Rheum* 1998;41:171-175.

10. Cortet B, Cotten A, Boutry N, et al: Percutaneous vertebroplasty in the treatment of osteoporotic vertebral compression fractures: An open prospective study. *J Rheumatol* 1999;26:2222-2228.

11. Cyteval C, Sarrabere MP, Roux JO, et al: Acute osteoporotic vertebral collapse: Open study on percutaneous injection of acrylic surgical cement in 20 patients. *Am J Roentgenol* 1999;173:1685-1690.

12. Hardouin P, Grados F, Cotten A, Cortet B: Should percutaneous vertebroplasty be used to treat osteoporotic fractures? An update. *Joint Bone Spine* 2001;68:216-221.

13. Watts NB, Harris ST, Genant HK: Treatment of painful osteoporotic vertebral fractures with percutaneous vertebroplasty or kyphoplasty. *Osteoporos Int* 2001;12:429-437.

14. Garfin SR, Yuan HA, Reiley MA: New technologies in spine: Kyphoplasty and vertebroplasty for the treatment of painful osteoporotic compression fractures. *Spine* 2001;26:1511-1515.

15. Wong W, Reiley MA, Garfin S: Vertebroplasty/kyphoplasty. *JWI* 2000;2:117-124.

16. Theodorou DJ, Theodorou SJ, Duncan TD, Garfin SR, Wong WH: Percutaneous balloon kyphoplasty for the correction of spinal deformity in painful vertebral body compression fractures. *Clin Imaging* 2002;26:1-5.

17. Galibert P, Deramond H, Rosat P, Le Gars D: Preliminary note on the treatment of vertebral angioma by percutaneous acrylic vertebroplasty. *Neurochirurgie* 1987;33:166-168.

18. Deprister-Debussche C, Deramond H, Fardellone P, et al: Percutaneous vertebroplasty with acrylic cement in the treatment of osteoporotic vertebral crush fractures syndrome. *Neuroradiology* 1991;33(suppl):149-152.

19. Belkoff SM, Mathis JM, Fenton DC, Scribner RM, Reiley ME, Talmadge K: An ex vivo biomechanical evaluation of an inflatable bone tamp used in the treatment of compression fracture. *Spine* 2001;26:151-156.

20. Wilson DR, Myers ER, Mathis JM, et al: Effect of augmentation on the mechanics of vertebral wedge fractures. *Spine* 2000;25:158-165.

21. Eriksson RA, Albrektsson T, Magnusson B: Assessment of bone viability after heat trauma: A histological, histochemical and vital microscopic study in the rabbit. *Scand J Plast Reconstr Surg* 1984;18:261-268.

22. Baker LL, Goodman SB, Perkash I, Lane B, Enzmann DR: Benign versus pathologic compression fractures of vertebral bodies: Assessment with conventional spin-echo, chemical-shift, and STIR MR imaging. *Radiology* 1990;174:495-502.

23. Cotten A, Dewatre F, Cortet B, et al: Percutaneous vertebroplasty for osteolytic metastases and myeloma: Effects of the percentage of lesion filling and the leakage of methyl methacrylate at clinical follow-up. *Radiology* 1996;200:525-530.

24. Moreland DB, Landi MK, Grand W: Vertebroplasty: Techniques to avoid complications. *Spine J* 2001;1:66-71.

25. Amar AP, Larsen DW, Esnaashari N, Albuquerque FC, Lavine SD, Teitelbaum GP: Percutaneous transpedicular polymethylmethacrylate vertebroplasty for the treatment of spinal compression fractures. *Neurosurgery* 2001;49:1105-1115.

26. Levine SA, Perin LA, Hayes D, Hayes WS: An evidence-based evaluation of percutaneous vertebroplasty. *Manag Care* 2000;9:56-63.

27. Padovani B, Kasriel O, Brunner P, Peretti-Viton P: Pulmonary embolism caused by acrylic cement: A rare complication of percutaneous vertebroplasty. *Am J Neuroradiol* 1999;20:375-377.

28. Perrin C, Jullien V, Padovani B, Blaive B: Percutaneous vertebroplasty complicated by pulmonary embolus of acrylic cement. *Rev Mal Respir* 1999;16:215-217.

29. McGraw JK, Heatwole EV, Strnad BT, Silber JS, Patzilk SB, Boorstein JM: Predictive value of intraosseous venography before percutaneous vertebroplasty. *J Vasc Interv Radiol* 2002;13:149-153.

30. Phillips FM, Wetzel FT, Lieberman I, Cambell-Hupp M: An in vivo comparison of the potential for extra-vertebral cement leak after vertebroplasty and kyphoplasty. *Spine* 2002;27:2173-2177.

31. Wood GW II: Lower back pain and disorders of the intervertebral disk, in Canale ST (ed): *Campbell's Operative Orthopaedics*, ed 9. St. Louis, Mosby, 1998, pp 3030-3036.

32. Krag MH: Biomechanics of thoracolumbar spinal fixation: A review. *Spine* 1991;16(suppl 3):S84-S99.

33. Mathis JM, Barr JD, Belkoff SM, et al: Percutaneous vertebroplasty: A developing standard of care for vertebral compression fractures, *Am J Neuroradiology* 2001;22:373-381.

34. Centenera LV, Choi S, Hirsch JA: Percutaneous vertebroplasty treats compression fractures: *Diagn Imaging* 2000;22:147-153.

35. Weill A, Chiras J, Simon JM, Rose M, Sola-Martinez T, Enkaoua E: Spinal metastases: Indications for and results of percutaneous injection of acrylic surgical cement. *Radiology* 1996;199:241-247.

36. Martin JB, Jean B, Sugiu K, et al: Vertebroplasty: Clinical experience and follow-up results. *Bone* 1999;25(suppl 2):11S-15S.

37. Jensen ME, Evans AJ, Mathis JM, Kallmes DF, Cloft HJ, Dion JE: Percutaneous polymethyl-methacrylate vertebroplasty in the treatment of osteoporotic vertebral body compression fractures: Technical aspects. *Am J Neuroradiol* 1997;18:1897-1904.

38. Gangi A, Dietemann JL, Guth S, Stelb JP, Roy C: Computed tomography and fluoroscopic guided vertebroplasty: Results and complications in 187 patients. *Semin Intervent Radiol* 1999;16:137-142.

39. Barr JD, Barr MS, Lemley TJ, McCann RM: Percutaneous vertebroplasty for pain relief and spinal stabilization. *Spine* 2000;25:923-928.

40. Grados F, Depriester C, Cayrolle G, Hardy N, Deramond H, Fardellone P: Long-term observations of vertebral osteoporotic fractures treated by percutaneous vertebroplasty. *Rheumatology (Oxford)* 2000;39:1410-1414.

41. Watts NB, Harris ST, Genant HK: Treatment of painful osteoporotic vertebral fractures with percutaneous vertebroplasty or kyphoplasty. *Osteoporos Int* 2001;12:429-437.

42. Uppin AA, Hirsch JA, Centinara LV, Pfeifer BA, Pazianos A, Choi II: New vertebral body compression fracture occurrence after percutaneous vertebroplasty in osteoporotic patients. *Radiology*, in press.

43. Lindsay R, Silverman SL, Cooper C, et al: Risk of new vertebral fracture in the year following a fracture. *JAMA* 2001;285:320-323.

44. Lieberman IH, Dudeney S, Reinhardt M-K, Bell G: Initial outcome and efficacy of "kyphoplasty" in the treatment of painful osteoporotic vertebral compression fractures. *Spine* 2001;26:1631-1638.

45. Ware JE Jr, Gandek B: Overview of the SF-36 Health Survey and the International Quality of Life Assessment (IQOLA) Project. *J Clin Epidemiol* 1998;51:903-912.

46. Phillips FM, Ho E, Campbell-Hupp M, et al: Balloon kyphoplasty for the treatment of painful spinal deformity resulting from osteoporotic vertebral compression fractures. *Spine J* 2002;2:121.

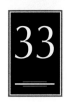

Open Surgical Treatment of Osteoporotic Fractures and Deformity of the Spine

John P. Kostuik, MD
Michael B. Shapiro, MD

Abstract

Osteoporotic fractures of the spine are an increasing major international health concern. The number of osteoporotic spinal fractures both in the United States and worldwide continue to increase. Early recognition is important in successful treatment.

The National Osteoporosis Foundation (NOF) reports that of 44 million Americans affected by osteoporosis, 80% are women. It is estimated that 10 million Americans already have osteoporosis and another 34 million are osteopenic.[1] By the year 2020, it is estimated that roughly 33% of the United States population will be age 65 years or older. As the population ages, the number of patients afflicted with osteoporosis and osteoporosis-related fractures will certainly increase. The NOF reports that one in two women and one in eight men will sustain an osteoporosis-related fracture in their lifetime and that the total number of fractures incurred secondary to osteoporosis will top 1.5 million, with vertebral fractures accounting for 700,000 fractures. Osteoporosis has not only led to significant patient morbidity and mortality, but has an overwhelming economic impact on the United States. It is estimated that total expenditures secondary to osteo-

porosis and related fractures topped $17 billion in 2001.[1] The projected cost of treatment of osteoporotic-related fractures is $200 billion in the year 2050.

There are several misconceptions regarding osteoporotic vertebral fractures. One of the myths regarding osteoporotic vertebral fractures is that they are not painful. In fact, in the United States, 260,000 of 700,000 patients per year will have severe pain requiring narcotic medication and 150,000 will require hospitalization. Patients later become disabled and morbidity and mortality increase. Women with one or more fractures have a 23% increase in mortality when compared with age-matched patients without fractures.[2] In patients with five or more severe fractures, the mortality rate increases 34%.[2] With one fracture there is a 12° increase in kyphosis at that level and a 9% decrease in forced vital capacity.[3] The risk of death secondary to pulmonary complications is increased 300%, espe-

cially in patients with kyphosis.[2] The risk of future fracture at other levels in the spine increases 500%.

Treatment

The recognition of osteoporosis as a world health and economic concern has led to interventions to prevent osteoporosis and osteoporotic fractures. Educational programs that inform patients on how to build and maintain skeletal mass starting at a young age are a key component of prevention. Weight-bearing exercise, diet (rich in calcium and vitamin D), smoking cessation, minimal alcohol intake, and bone density testing with appropriate interventions make up a well-balanced defense against osteoporosis.[4] To date, there is no cure for osteoporosis but many medicines have been approved for its prevention and treatment, including hormone replacement therapies (estrogen preparations), alendronate, calcitonin, raloxifene, and risedronate.[5]

Patients with osteoporotic fractures of the spine now have more treatment options. Nonsurgical treatment includes bed rest and cast/brace use. Patients will experience less pain with bed rest; however, they will lose up to 10% of their bone mass within 2 weeks. Elderly patients have difficulty complying with casting or bracing. Skin irritation and breakdown may result from prolonged brace use. Newer, less invasive techniques include vertebroplasty and kyphoplasty. Barr and associates[6] have reported excellent pain relief in almost two thirds of patients treated (24 of 38) and moderate pain relief in another 32% of patients (12 of 38) with minimal complications.[4] In a study by Amar and associates,[7] 74% of patients undergoing vertebroplasty had improved quality of life. Kyphoplasty has been used to not only treat pain but to reduce the deformity at the level of fracture. In recent reports on the use of kyphoplasty, 95% of patients had a good to excellent result at 1 week to 2 years and kyphosis was improved 50% if the fracture was treated within 3 months of the injury.[8,9] These techniques will only be discussed herein in combination with open techniques.

Maximally invasive treatment consists of open approaches to the spine. An anterior, posterior, or combined approach can be used.

Indications for Open Surgical Treatment

Indications for open treatment include osteoporotic vertebral compression fractures (VCFs) with neurologic injury that would require decompression and reconstruction. VCFs with neurologic compromise are uncommon. In a study of 497 VCF patients admitted to a hospital, 10 had significant neurologic deficit requiring surgery.[10] Patients may also present with late neurologic deficit secondary to progressive collapse, instability, and spinal stenosis. Patients with painful fractures not amenable to vertebroplasty or kyphoplasty (vertebra plana fractures) may benefit from open treatment. Patients in whom vertebroplasty or kyphoplasty has failed and continue to have pain and/or deformity, along with osteoporotic patients who have progressive scoliotic and/or kyphotic deformity with intractable pain are candidates for open procedures.

A complete workup that includes evaluation of the patient's medical conditions, including nutritional status, must be done prior to the start of any open surgical procedure. Determination of preoperative and postoperative nutritional status is important because nutritionally depleted patients have higher mortality rates and diminished healing potential.[11,12]

Studies evaluating complications associated with major reconstructive spinal surgery show a high rate of major complications that are age-related (JY Chang, JP Kostuik, MD, A Sieber, MD, DB Cohen, MD, unpublished data, Switzerland, 2002). Many patients who have osteoporosis often have significant comorbidities such as heart disease, respiratory disease, and high blood pressure. Although age is not a contraindication to spinal fusion, morbidity increases significantly if two or more comorbid conditions are present.[13] The surgeon must be aware of and prepared for several critical surgical concepts in order to avoid intraoperative problems. The bone in this group of patients has greatly decreased mechanical strength, and the pedicle is the strongest point of fixation. Anterior cortex fixation is important in the sacrum and far cortex purchase is important for anterior screw fixation in the vertebral bodies. The surgeon must be prepared to augment fixation with methylmethacrylate and to use alternate points of fixation, including the sacral promontory or alar or pelvic fixation.

When the decision to proceed with surgery is made, the surgical plan must be individualized to each patient, taking into account patient age, comorbidities, and type and age of the fracture.

Anterior Approach

The anterior approach is useful when a fracture has an associated neurologic deficit that would benefit from anterior decompression. The anterior approach allows for direct decompression of the neural elements, and anterior column

reconstruction. Many fractures occur at the thoracolumbar junction and hence have increased surgical morbidity if the diaphragm needs to be taken down during the approach. In these cases, an eggshell (pedicle subtraction) procedure may be beneficial. The disadvantages include poor fixation and graft/host modulus mismatch. Graft options for reconstruction of the anterior column include autograft, allograft, vertebral body replacement, and cement (polymethylmethacrylate, PMMA). The modulus of elasticity of bone changes with age. It is important to best match the modulus while gaining strength. Failure to recognize modulus mismatch will lead to fractures at adjacent levels. Patients will develop topping off and/or bottoming off syndrome (compression fractures above or below the construct leading to kyphosis) with recurrent deformity and pain. Autogenous iliac crest bone graft will provide the best modulus match. Femoral ring allografts will provide a stable environment, and augmenting the adjacent levels with PMMA can be done to decrease fractures at those levels in conjunction with anterior fixation (Fig. 1). Vertebral body PMMA supplementation can enhance screw fixation. The alternate is a combined anterior-posterior approach.

Posterior Approach

The posterior approach is advantageous because it provides the best points of fixation in the pedicles (Fig. 2). The disadvantages are that it allows for limited or indirect decompression of the neural elements and the potential for tension band failure. A recent study[14] describes a posterior decompression via a pedicle subtraction osteotomy, which allowed for adequate decompression of the spinal cord while improving the biomechanical environment for the posterior instrumentation. Longer constructs must be used for the posterior approach because shorter constructs fail in osteoporotic bone. Failure can be avoided by using multiple points of fixation and not ending constructs in kyphotic areas of the spine.[15]

Combined Approaches

A combined anterior-posterior approach to the spine is advantageous because it allows for direct decompression of the neural elements and three-column reconstruction. On the other hand, patient morbidity and potentially mortality are increased. Therefore, whether the risks of surgery are greater than the disease itself is a topic of debate. Neurologic compromise and the potential for increased deformity correction, increased stability, decreased hardware failure, and increased fusion rate are reasons to use a combined approach. Three-column reconstruction can be carried out through separate anterior and posterior approaches to the spine or a combined approach. The level of injury and patient comorbidities aid in the decision on whether to use a combined approach. Combined approaches place a significant metabolic demand on the patient that some elderly patients cannot tolerate. Fractures at the thoracolumbar junction that would require the diaphragm to be taken down using an anterior approach may better be treated with an eggshell (pedicle subtraction) procedure because taking down the diaphragm can increase the potential for significant morbidity, especially if significant preexisting pulmonary disease is present (Fig. 3). Posterior-anterior-posterior surgery gives the surgeon several options for reconstruction of the three columns of spine. A pedicle subtraction osteotomy restores alignment and reduces biomechanical forces on the posterior instrumentation, diminishing the risk of posterior instrumentation failure. Posterior procedures can be combined with intraoperative kyphoplasty to restore alignment and reconstruct the anterior column, therefore diminishing biomechanical forces on posterior instrumentation without the added morbidity of a separate anterior exposure (Fig. 4).

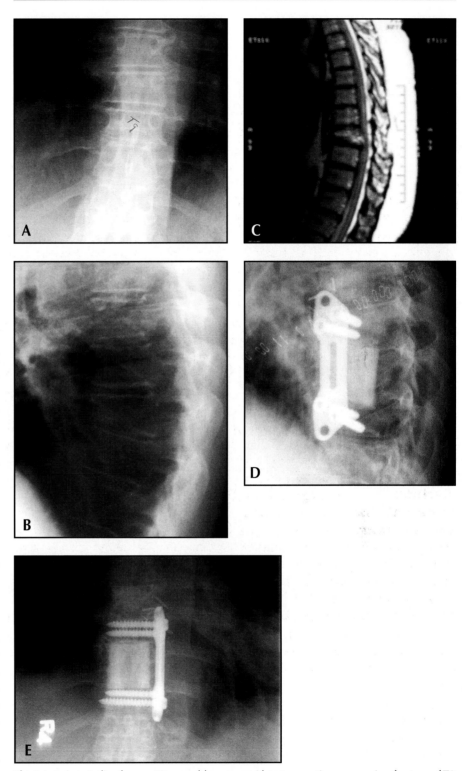

Fig. 1 Imaging studies from a 60-year-old woman with osteoporotic compression fracture of T9 treated conservatively. Progressive deformity and stenosis developed later. **A**, Preoperative AP radiograph shows loss of height. **B**, Preoperative lateral radiograph. **C**, Preoperative MRI scan. Postoperative lateral (**D**) and AP (**E**) radiographs show postoperative anterior corpectomy and reconstruction using an allograft and anterior fixation.

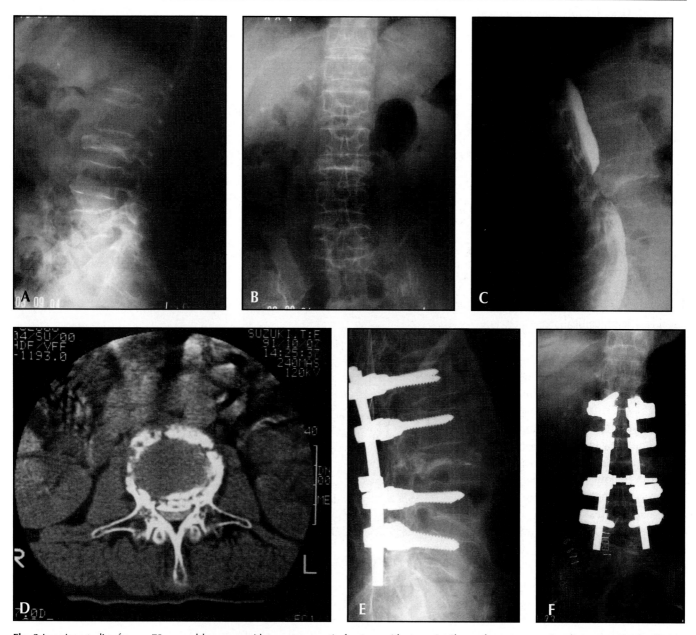

Fig. 2 Imaging studies from a 73-year-old woman with an osteoporotic fracture with stenosis. She underwent posterior decompression and fusion. A, Preoperative lateral radiograph indicating compression burst type fracture. B, Preoperative AP radiograph indicates a burst fracture with vertebral body widening. C, Preoperative myelogram of the fracture with block. D, Preoperative CT myelogram with block. Postoperative lateral (E) and AP (F) radiographs showing reconstruction with decompression posterolaterally and fusion with cement-augmented pedicle screws.

Open Techniques With Vertebroplasty/Kyphoplasty

Open maximally invasive techniques are more commonly being combined with newer, less invasive methods including both vertebroplasty and kyphoplasty. Patients who are severely osteoporotic may derive some benefit. When performed in patients with severe osteoporosis, vertebroplasty done at adjacent levels may lessen the stress riser effect and diminish the chance of topping off and/or bottoming off syndrome. Vertebral fractures proximal or distal to a fusion may occur in up to 20% of cases. Preoperative vertebroplasty at levels adjacent to a spinal fracture to allow for augmentation of instrumentation is an attractive use of this technique (Fig. 5). The indications for adjunctive kyphoplasty are less clear. When the weight-bearing nature of the anterior column needs to be restored and an anterior approach avoided, a kyphoplasty combined with a posterior fusion is an attractive option (Fig. 4). The role of kyphoplasty and vertebroplasty as an adjunct to open procedures continues to evolve. More studies to evaluate long-term outcome need to be performed. Further investigations into the effects of cement on regional spinal biology, end-plate perfusion, and disk nutrition are needed, along with studies into a percutaneous biologic solution to enhance fixation, promote healing, and restore anatomy.

Fixation Augmentation

Because of the known complications associated with instrumentation fixation in the osteoporotic spine, developments in both pedicle screw design and biologic enhancement are advancing rapidly. Expandable screws, conical screws, alternative thread designs, and biologically enhanced screws are all currently under investigation. There are expandable screws on the market, which have shown increased pullout strength in many studies. Biomechanical testing of a new two-fin expandable screw (alligator screw, DePuy Acromed, Raynham, MA) shows a 22% increase in pullout strength when tested in osteoporotic bone (D Cohen, MD, J Elias, MD, JP Kostuik, MD, A Sieber, MD, New York, NY, unpublished data, 2002). With the alligator screw, PMMA cement can be added through the open central canal of the screw to the tip (Fig. 6). Biomechanical testing of four-fin expansion screws shows an increase in pullout strength of 30%. In osteoporotic bone the pullout strength was increased 50%. The tip of the expansion screw expands 2 mm at its tip.[16] Clinical follow-up of patients treated with the expansion screw reveals a 91% fusion rate, with five implant-related postoperative complications—two misplaced screws, local pain above the implant, and two broken screws. The patient with the broken screws has a solid arthrodesis and has returned to work.[17] An 89% fusion rate and one instance of screw breakage has been reported when osteoporosis cases

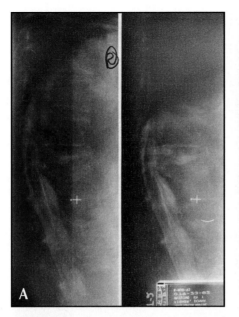
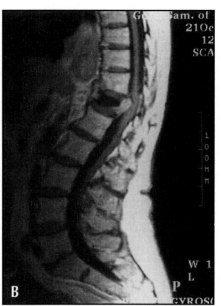
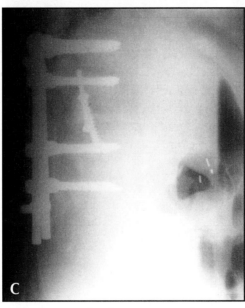
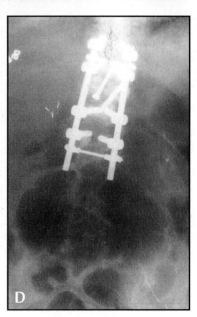

Fig. 3 Imaging studies from a patient with osteoporotic fracture of the spine for whom conservative treatment failed. Posterior pedicle subtraction osteotomy kyphectomy and fusion were performed. Preoperative lateral radiograph and myelogram **(A)** and preoperative MRI scan **(B)** show cord compression from an osteoporotic burst fracture. Postoperative lateral radiograph **(C)** and postoperative AP radiograph **(D)** showing decompression with kyphectomy. Anterior column reconstruction using screws and PMMA cement together with pedicle screw cement augmentation and bone fusion was done at posterior L4.

are singled out.[18] Conical screws have a theoretical advantage over cylindrical screws in that they compact bone as they are inserted. Conical screws have been shown to have better mechanical fixation to the vertebral body, increased insertion-

al torque, and improved pullout strength than conventional cylindrical screws when inserted in a triangulated fashion.[19] Kwok and associates[20] have shown that insertional torque is increased with conical screws, but pullout strength is not

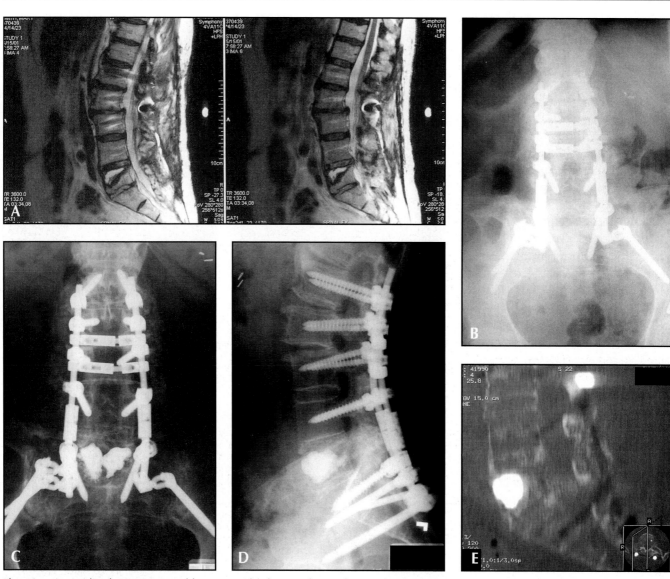

Fig. 4 Imaging studies from a 70-year-old woman with a history of L2-L4 fusion. She developed pain after a fall and a compression fracture of L5. Posterior extension of fusion to the pelvis and kyphoplasty were performed to restore anterior column support. **A,** Preoperative MRI scan showing fracture at L5. **B,** Postoperative AP radiograph with posterior instrumentation and prekyphoplasty. **C,** Postoperative AP radiograph showing instrumentation to pelvis and kyphoplasty. **D,** Postoperative/kyphoplasty lateral radiograph. **E,** Postoperative CT showing kyphoplasty.

increased when compared with conventional cylindrical screws. The authors point out that fixation stability in osteoporotic patients depends more on bone quality than screw design. Screw hole preparation and the maintenance of the dorsal cortex are important factors in improving pedicle screw fixation.[21,22] Hydroxyapatite-coated screws have shown improved pullout strength in animal studies.[23] Hydroxyapatite augmentation

of both the vertebral body and of pedicle screws has been shown to improve fixation in the osteoporotic spine. Hydroxyapatite-coated screws have been shown to have significantly more bone surrounding the screw threads than noncoated screws in the sheep model.[24] The role of hydroxyapatite-coated pedicle screws has not been elucidated in the clinical setting but has shown promise in laboratory studies; however, its potential clinical use

remains controversial. PMMA cement augmentation of pedicle fixation, both intraoperative and preoperative, has been shown to improve pullout strength. Bone mineral density has been shown to be the best bone mineral density predictor of screw fixation.[25] For each 0.100 g/cm² increase in bone mineral density, pullout has been shown to increase 120 Nm. In the osteoporotic spine, the addition of 2 cc of PMMA via direct injection into the

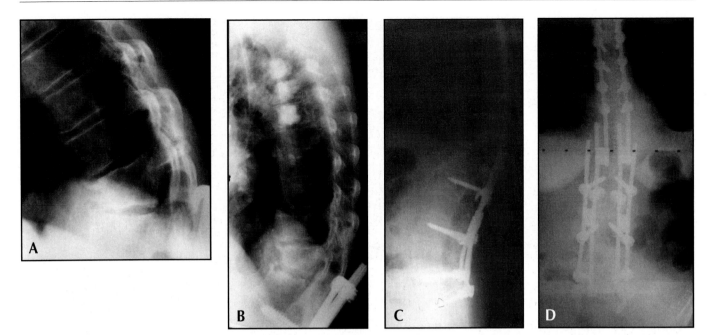

Fig. 5 A patient who developed topping off syndrome at cranial aspect of fusion. The radiographs in **A** and **B** show preoperative vertebroplasty (6-7-8 levels proximal) done prior to extension of fusion. **A,** Compression fracture above fusion. **B,** Compression and preoperative vertebroplasty at proximal aspect of fusion extension. **C,** Postoperative lateral radiograph with extension and vertebroplasty. **D,** Postoperative radiograph showing extension and vertebroplasty.

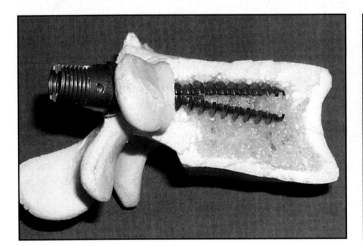

Fig. 6 Alligator screw expanded in sawbone model.

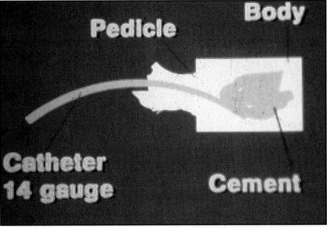

Fig. 7 Schematic representation of cement introduction into the pedicle. Liquid cement placed in 20 cm³ syringe that is drilled out with a 3.2-mm drill. A 14-gauge catheter is used to introduce the cement.

pedicle (Fig. 7) increased pullout strength 500% over that of controls; 3 cc increased pullout strength 600% over that of controls. This degree of pullout strength was greater than a 7-mm screw in normal density bone for both the 2 cc and 3 cc group (DB Cohen, MD, D Cullinane, MD, M Iizuka, MD, N Walk, MD, A Sieber, MD, JP Kostuik, MD, Edinburgh, Scotland, unpublished data, 2001). The use of PMMA is clearly beneficial when used to augment fixation (Fig. 8). However, it may have a detrimental effect on the local biologic environment. Newer materials, including calcium phosphate bone cements, offer advantages over PMMA. Calcium phosphate cements are replaceable by local bone and curing is not an exothermic reaction. Calcium phosphate augmentation has shown an average 68% improve-

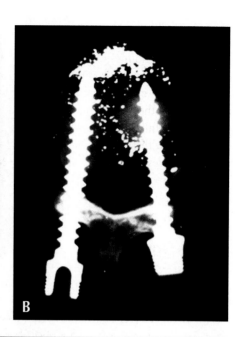

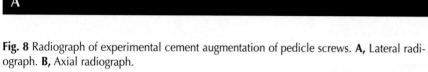

Fig. 8 Radiograph of experimental cement augmentation of pedicle screws. **A,** Lateral radiograph. **B,** Axial radiograph.

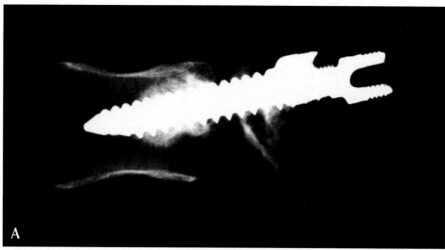

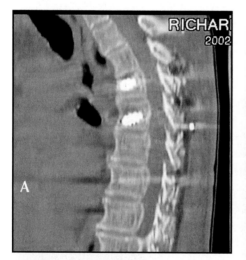

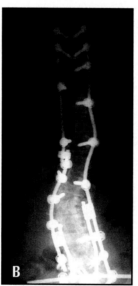

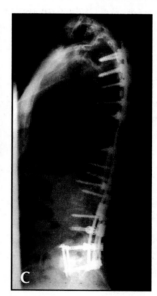

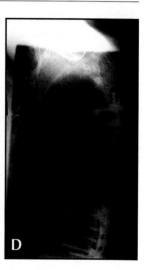

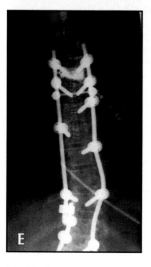

Fig. 9 Imaging studies from a 61-year-old woman who underwent AP spinal fusion for deformity with osteoporotic compression fracture at the uppermost instrumented level 4 weeks after surgery. The patient complained of pain and deformity; kyphoplasty was performed at the affected level with 50% correction of deformity and resolution of pain postoperatively. **A,** Postoperative CT scan showing collapse at the uppermost level. **B,** Prekyphoplasty AP radiograph. **C,** Prekyphoplasty lateral radiograph. **D,** Postkyphoplasty lateral radiograph. **E,** Postkyphoplasty AP radiograph.

ment in pullout strength when used to augment osteoporotic pedicles in the laboratory.[26] The bending rigidity in the anterior spine was initially increased 58% and 125% after cyclic loading.[27] In the clinical setting, the use of calcium apatite cement augmentation has proved safe and effective, with 1 of 16 anterior screws being loose despite augmentation and 4 of 48 posterior augmentations having cement leakage with no postoperative sequela.[28]

Spinal Deformity and Osteoporosis

Osteoporosis and its relationship to spinal deformity has been an area of much interest. Thevenon and associates[29] correlated the degree of kyphosis with low bone mineral density of the spine and scoliosis with low bone mineral content of the femoral neck. Healey and Lane[30] studied 50 women with osteoporosis; 48% had structural scoliosis greater than 10° and average kyphosis of 70°. There were 140 fractures in 47 women. The authors concluded that scoliosis in the elderly is a marker of osteoporosis and compression fractures. More recent studies have correlated the degree of spinal deformity and number of osteoporotic fractures with the extent of osteoporosis.[31] Patients with adolescent idiopathic scoliosis have been shown to have lower bone mineral density than patients without scoliosis. This lower bone mineral density has been shown to be permanent in duration.[32] Patients with adolescent idiopathic scoliosis should be followed closely and their osteoporosis treated aggressively. Adults with spinal deformity have increased risk of topping and bottoming off syndromes as well as sustaining fractures of their fusion masses (Fig. 5). Prevention of an osteoporotic fracture proximal to the fusion mass necessitates extension of fusion to a stable area proximal to the thoracic apex and stiffening of vertebral bodies proximal and distal to the fusion. Assessment of the fu-

sion mass in patients with osteoporosis is difficult; patients with fractures may experience instrumentation loosening and bony resorption. Tomographic imaging may identify a fracture. Persistent pain may be the only symptom exhibited by a patient with a fracture. Fractures of the most proximal or distal instrumented body may occur and lead to progressive deformity (Fig. 9). Fractures of this type are elusive and may be difficult to identify. A high index of suspicion and the comparison of postoperative radiographs at each office visit is important. Imaging of the spine with CT scan with sagittal reconstruction is often necessary to identify this problem. Patients who develop osteoporotic problems above, below, or within their fusions need to be thoroughly evaluated and treated along the same principles described.

Summary

The increasing age of the population along with the increasing incidence of osteoporosis has made the surgical reconstruction of osteoporotic vertebral compression fractures a subject of paramount interest. The developments in the procedures of vertebroplasty and kyphoplasty have resulted in significant advances in the surgical treatment of osteoporotic vertebral body fractures. However, some fractures require open surgical reconstruction. The techniques available for open surgical reconstruction continue to evolve along with indications for their use.

References

1. Fast Facts on Osteoporosis. Available at: http://www.nof.org/osteoprosis/stats.htm. Accessed March 11, 2002.

2. Kado DM, Browner WS, Palermo L, Nevitt MC, Genant HK, Cummings SR: Vertebral fractures and mortality in older women: A prospective study: Study of Osteoporotic Fractures Research Group. *Arch Intern Med* 1999;159:1215-1220.

3. Leech JA, Dulberg C, Kellie S, Pattee L, Gay J: Relationship of lung function to severity of osteoporosis in women. *Am Rev Respir Dis* 1990;141:68-71.

4. Miller PD: Management of osteoporosis. *Dis Mon* 1999;45:21-54.

5. Ettinger B, Black DM, Mitlak BH, et al: Reduction of vertebral fracture risk in postmenopausal women with osteoporosis treated with raloxifene: Results from a 3-year randomized clinical trial: Multiple Outcomes of Raloxifene Evaluation (MORE) Investigators. *JAMA* 1999;282:637-645.

6. Barr JD, Barr MS, Lemley TJ, McCann RM: Percutaneous vertebroplasty for pain relief and spinal stabilization. *Spine* 2000;25:923-928.

7. Amar AP, Larsen DW, Esnaashari N, Albuquerque FC, Lavine SD, Teitelbaum GP: Percutaneous transpedicular polymethylmethacrylate vertebroplasty for the treatment of spinal compression fractures. *Neurosurgery* 2001;49:1105-1115.

8. Garfin SR, Yuan HA, Reiley MA: New technologies in spine: Kyphoplasty and vertebroplasty for the treatment of painful osteoporotic compression fractures. *Spine* 2001;26:1511-1515.

9. Lieberman IH, Dudeney S, Reinhardt MK, Bell G: Initial outcome and efficacy of "kyphoplasty" in the treatment of painful osteoporotic vertebral compression fractures. *Spine* 2001;26:1631-1638.

10. Lee YL, Yip KM: The osteoporotic spine. *Clin Orthop* 1996;323:91-97.

11. Hu SS, Fontaine F, Kelly B, Bradford DS: Nutritional depletion in staged spinal reconstructive surgery: The effect of total parenteral nutrition. *Spine* 1998;23:1401-1415.

12. Lapp MA, Bridwell KH, Lenke LG, Baldus C, Blanke K, Iffrig TM: Prospective randomization of parenteral hyperalimentation for long fusions with spinal deformity: Its effect on complications and recovery from postoperative malnutrition. *Spine* 2001;26:809-817.

13. Fujita T, Kostuik JP, Huckell CB, Sieber AN: Complications of spinal fusion in adult patients more than 60 years of age. *Orthop Clin North Am* 1998;29:669-678.

14. Saita K, Hoshino Y, Kikkawa I, Nakamura H: Posterior spinal shortening for paraplegia after vertebral collapse caused by osteoporosis. *Spine* 2000;25:2832-2835.

15. Hu SS: Internal fixation in the osteoporotic spine. *Spine* 1997;22(suppl 24):43S-48S.

16. Cook SD, Salkeld SL, Whitecloud TS III, Barbera J: Biomechanical evaluation and preliminary clinical experience with an expansive pedicle screw design. *J Spinal Disord* 2000;13:230-236.

17. Cook SD, Salkeld SL, Whitecloud TS III, Barbera J: Biomechanical testing and clinical experience with the OMEGA-21 spinal fixation system. *Am J Orthop* 2001;30:387-394.

18. Cook SD, Barbera J, Rubi M, Salkeld SL, Whitecloud TS III: Lumbosacral fixation using expandable pedicle screws: An alternative in reoperation and osteoporosis. *Spine* 2001;1:109-114.

19. Ono A, Brown MD, Latta LL, Milne EL, Holmes DC: Triangulated pedicle screw construct technique and pull-out strength of conical and cylindrical screws. *J Spinal Disord* 2001;14:323-329.

20. Kwok AW, Finkelstein JA, Woodside T, Hearn TC, Hu RW: Insertional torque and pull-out strengths of conical and cylindrical pedicle screws in cadaveric bone. *Spine* 1996;21: 2429-2434.

21. Daftari TK, Horton WC, Hutton WC: Correlations between screw hole preparation, torque of insertion, and pullout strength for spinal screws. *J Spinal Disord* 1994;7:139-145.

22. Oktenoglu BT, Ferrara LA, Andalkar N, Ozer AF, Sarioglu AC, Benzel EC: Effects of hole preparation on screw pullout resistance and insertional torque: A biomechanical study. *J Neurosurg* 2001;94(suppl 1):91-96.

23. Sanden B, Olerud C, Larsson S: Hydroxyapatite coating enhances fixation of loaded pedicle screws: A mechanical in vivo study in sheep. *Eur Spine J* 2001;10:334-339.

24. Sanden B, Olerud C, Johansson C, Larsson S: Improved bone-screw interface with hydroxyapatite coating: An in vivo study of loaded pedicle screws in sheep. *Spine* 2001;26:2673-2678.

25. Soshi S, Shiba R, Kondo H, Murota K: An experimental study on transpedicular screw fixation in relation to osteoporosis of the lumbar spine. *Spine* 1991;16:1335-1341.

26. Lotz JC, Hu SS, Chiu DF, Yu M, Colliou O, Poser RD: Carbonated apatite cement augmentation of pedicle screw fixation in the lumbar spine. *Spine* 1997;22:2716-2723.

27. Bai B, Kummer FJ, Spivak J: Augmentation of anterior vertebral body screw fixation by an injectable, biodegradable calcium phosphate bone substitute. *Spine* 2001;26:2679-2683.

28. Wuisman PI, Van Dijk M, Staal H, Van Royen BJ: Augmentation of (pedicle) screws with calcium apatite cement in patients with severe progressive osteoporotic spinal deformities: An innovative technique. *Eur Spine J* 2000;9: 528-533.

29. Thevenon A, Pollez B, Cantegrit F, Tison-Muchery F, Marchandise X, Duquesnoy B: Relationship between kyphosis, scoliosis, and osteoporosis in the elderly population. *Spine* 1987;12:744-745.

30. Healey JH, Lane JM: Structural scoliosis in osteoporotic women. *Clin Orthop* 1985;195: 216-223.

31. Antoniou J, Nguyen C, Lander P, Hadjipavlou A: Osteoporosis of the spine: Correlation between vertebral deformity and bone mineral density in postmenopausal women. *Am J Orthop* 2000;29:956-959.

32. Cheng JC, Guo X, Sher AH: Persistent osteopenia in adolescent idiopathic scoliosis: A longitudinal follow up study. *Spine* 1999;24:1218-1222.

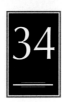

Adult Spinal Deformity in the Osteoporotic Spine: Options and Pitfalls

Steven D. Glassman, MD

Gary M. Alegre, MD

Abstract

Osteoporosis has received heightened attention over the past 2 decades because of its overwhelming cost to society. It is one of the most common diseases affecting both men and women. The key to treatment is early prevention accompanied by modification of risk factors and impact-oriented exercise, optimal medical management with antiresorptive medications, and addressing the complications of this disease such as compression fractures and spinal deformities. Most osteoporotic vertebral compression fractures can be treated nonsurgically, but new techniques such as vertebroplasty and kyphoplasty are producing good early clinical results with low complication profiles. The surgical treatment of deformities such as kyphosis and scoliosis can be very challenging given the poor bone quality and propensity for instrumentation cutout. The surgical treatment of spinal stenosis in the face of deformity in these patients requires keen surgical planning and a clear identification of the source of the patient's complaints—be it the deformity, the stenosis, or both. Several advances in instrumentation, such as the use of laminar fixation (if available), multisegment fixation, limited correction of the deformity, and augmentation of pedicle screw purchase through biologic and nonbiologic fillers have been developed.

Osteoporosis plays a major role in the development of adult spinal deformity and has become a growing concern among the medical community as epidemiology, natural history, treatment options, and economic and social cost associated with the condition are better understood. Along with hypertension and diabetes mellitus, osteoporosis is one of the most common chronic diseases. It is estimated that 30% of postmenopausal white women in the United States have osteoporosis, according to the World Health Organization definition (bone mineral density of more than 2.5 standard deviations below the mean in young, healthy people).[1] The lifetime risk of sustaining a clinically diagnosed vertebral fracture is about 15% in women, with a loss of 1 standard deviation in bone mineral density giving rise to a twofold risk of spine fractures.[2,3] This number has varied depending on the definition used for vertebral fractures and the method of data collection. There is a widespread misconception that osteoporosis is a disease of women. Recent data have shown that the rates of vertebral fractures in men are as high as those in women, with adjustments being made for the longer life span of women.[4]

Medical Management of Osteoporosis
Prevention

The first step in the treatment of osteoporosis is prevention. Major risk factors for osteoporosis are a personal history of a fracture as an adult or a history of a fracture in a first-degree relative.[3] Minor risk factors include Caucasian race, advanced age, female gender, dementia, and poor health or fragility. The major risk factors that can be modified are current cigarette smoking and low body weight (less than 127 lb). The minor risk factors that can be modified include estrogen deficiency, low calcium intake, alcoholism, impaired eyesight, recurrent falls, inadequate physical activity, and poor health and fragility depending on the cause.

Peak bone mass is known to be achieved at approximately 20 to 25 years of age. An initial approach at prevention is achieving a high peak bone mass at this early age. Adequate intake of calories coupled with sufficient calcium levels approaching 1,200 to 1,500 mg from age

11 to 24 years is required, along with daily intake of vitamin D (800 IU). In women, achieving regular menstrual cycles and maintaining acceptable body weight, along with avoiding excessive exercise, are paramount. Once peak bone mass has been achieved the next goal is to maintain this peak bone mass into menopause. Lower doses of calcium (less than 1,000 mg/day) and limited vitamin D intake are then required for menopausal women and for men up to age 65 years. Optimal calcium intake for postmenopausal women taking estrogen and men older than 65 years is then 1,000 mg/day.[5] A regular exercise program and adequate caloric intake are also essential to maintain bone mass. In premenopausal and perimenopausal women, antiresorptive agents such as estrogen, bisphosphonates, and possibly calcitonin should be considered to achieve an appreciable decrease in bone density.[6] These preventive measures, along with addressing modifiable risk factors, maintaining adequate caloric intake, and a regular impact-oriented exercise program, should be the first step in addressing this disease.

Treatment

The diagnosis of primary osteoporosis is made using bone density studies and by ruling out secondary causes such as endocrinopathies, excessive alcohol intake, osteomalacia, and multiple myeloma. Once osteoporosis is diagnosed, collagen breakdown products such as N-telopeptide or the pyridinoline peptides can be measured in urinary assays to guide treatment decisions.[6-9] The most appropriate treatment for patients with high levels of these breakdown products is with antiresorptive agents such as estrogen, selective estrogen receptor modulators, bisphosphonates, and calcitonin. Estrogen supplementation at doses of 0.625 mg per day will convert bone loss in the spine to a bone gain of approximately 1% to 2% per

year.[6] The benefits of estrogen therapy must be weighed against the increased risk of uterine and breast cancer. For women younger than 65 years of age receiving estrogen for more than 5 years, the risk of breast cancer is expected to increase to up to 30%. There is an increased risk of uterine cancer with unopposed estrogen administration, but the coadministration of progesterone can lower this risk. In addition, newer selective estrogen receptor modulators have been developed to address these concerns; however, the value of these medications currently is controversial.

Bisphosphonates are the second line antiresorptive agents that act by preventing osteoclastic bone resorption. A second-generation bisphosphonate, alendronate, is highly effective and has been shown to reduce the risk of spine fractures by 50%. Calcitonin, a third-line antiresorptive agent available in a nasal formulation, is effective in ameliorating pain from an acute osteoporotic vertebral fracture. Its role in preventing fractures is not well established.

Bone-stimulating agents include fluoride and parathyroid hormone. There are no approved agents for the direct stimulation of osteoblasts in the treatment of osteoporosis. Caution is urged when using these agents because of an increased risk of hip fractures seen with high doses of fluoride[10] and the high rate of osteosarcoma in laboratory animals exposed to parathyroid hormone.[11] Slow-release forms of fluoride and parathyroid hormone are currently under investigation by the Food and Drug Administration (FDA).

Osteoporotic Vertebral Compression Fractures
Presentation

Osteoporotic vertebral compression fractures are characterized by the acute onset of back pain that is often the result of minor trauma such as lifting a heavy object, sneezing, bending, coughing, or a

minor fall. The patient may have incapacitating back pain with spinous process tenderness on examination, difficulty sitting or standing, and plain radiographs showing one or multiple wedge-shaped vertebral fractures. Another common scenario is the patient who presents with the insidious onset of back pain and progressive deformity such as kyphosis or scoliosis presumably resulting from a series of microfractures. These patients often have no history of acute onset of back pain or trauma. In both cases the patient should be evaluated for the possibility of other pathologic conditions such as an infectious process, tumor, or other metabolic disease. Laboratory data such as complete blood count, erythrocyte sedimentation rate, blood urea nitrogen and creatinine, urinalysis, calcium, phosphate, or alkaline phosphatase levels, thyroid function studies, liver function studies, and protein electrophoresis can be helpful in ruling out other metabolic processes and multiple myeloma.[12] A bone scan can be helpful in differentiating between acute and old fractures and is also useful to screen for metastatic tumor. Several MRI characteristics have been described to help differentiate osteoporotic fractures from tumor-related compression fractures.[13]

Occasionally a patient with an osteoporotic vertebral compression fracture can present with a neurologic deficit[14-16] (Fig. 1). Lee and Yip,[14] in their study of 497 patients admitted with acute osteoporotic vertebral compression fractures, reported a 2% incidence of cord compression presenting as back pain, lower extremity weakness, and numbness together with sphincter disturbances. Neurologic recovery, although incomplete, is generally satisfactory.

Natural History

Two natural histories have been presented for acute vertebral osteoporotic fractures.[17] The most common presentation is characterized by acute pain with radiographic evidence of vertebral collapse or wedging. In this scenario, the pain usually resolves over 4 to 8 weeks. In the presence of multiple microfractures the pain is less intense with a shorter duration and the radiographic evidence of fracture is less evident, but repeated bouts of pain episodes are more common.

Long-term effects of osteoporotic vertebral compression fractures have been well studied.[18-20] In women with osteoporotic compression fractures, functional limitations, increased episodes of back pain, and impaired quality of life are more common than in patients without a history of compression fractures. In addition, there is a 23% increase in mortality in women older than 65 years with osteoporotic vertebral compression fractures compared to age-matched controls, and this mortality rate increases with the number of vertebrae fractured.[21] Men with osteoporotic vertebral compression fractures are more likely to complain of back pain and greater loss of height, and have poorer scores for energy, pain, emotion, sleep, and physical mobility compared to controls.[22]

Nonsurgical Treatment

Nonsurgical treatment, such as the use of analgesics, calcitonin nasal spray, and orthotic devices, for acute osteoporotic vertebral fractures without neurologic deficit is the conventional approach and is the safest and most effective method of treatment for most patients.

Initially, the treatment of an acute fracture begins with analgesics. Narcotics should be used with caution in elderly patients because of the risk of disorientation, which can be associated with an increased risk of falls. Tylenol with codeine, or low doses of oxycodone, or pentazocine can be effective if used sparingly. Calcitonin as a nasal spray, 200 IU intranasally daily for 1 to 2 weeks, has analgesic properties and does not interfere with fracture healing. It is generally well tolerated but on rare occasions can

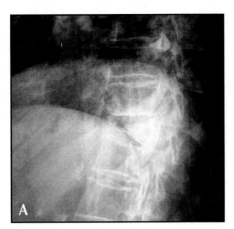 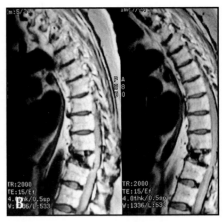

Fig. 1 A, Lateral radiograph showing a 3-week-old osteoporotic vertebral compression fracture in a 71-year-old woman who is unable to walk. **B,** Sagittal MRI showing canal compromise.

produce dry nares and an allergic reaction. An intradermal test dose is recommended prior to commencing therapy.

Brace treatment for identified acute fractures allows for relief of pain through mechanical means and permits early mobilization by unloading the fractured anterior column. The most desirable orthotic devices are the least cumbersome, lightweight, and easy to use. Fractures up to the level of T6 can be generally managed with a thoracolumbosacral orthosis. Fractures more cephalad to T6 require a cervical extension to a thoracolumbosacral orthosis in order to effectively immobilize this area. Noncompliance can be an issue in the fragile patient with little social support; therefore, a rehabilitation facility with ancillary services should be considered.

Semisurgical Treatment

Semisurgical treatment options such as vertebroplasty and kyphoplasty recently have been introduced for the treatment of painful osteoporotic compression fractures. These modalities offer the potential to reduce the deformity and add immediate stability to a compressed osteoporotic vertebrae. Vertebroplasty, which provides stabilization and pain relief without improving the deformity of vertebral fractures, requires the injec-

tion of polymethylmethacrylate (PMMA) into the compressed vertebral body at moderate pressure through one or two biopsy needles (Fig. 2). Kyphoplasty offers the advantage of correcting the deformity and at lower pressures of PMMA by inserting a bone tamp/balloon into the vertebral body under image guidance. The balloon is then inflated with radiocontrast material to reexpand the vertebral body, and the expanded cavity is then filled with PMMA under low pressure.

Although no randomized controlled studies on the use of vertebroplasty or kyphoplasty exist, the early results of prospective studies are promising. The literature on percutaneous vertebroplasty reports success rates in pain relief of approximately 70% to 90%, but most of these studies have only small numbers of patients and limited follow-up.[23-26] Kyphoplasty has only been used actively since 1998, when the FDA approved the use of inflatable bone tamps. Prospective studies have shown a 90% rate of symptomatic and functional improvement, with kyphosis correcting by over 50% if kyphoplasty is performed within 3 months from the onset of fracture or pain.[27,28] There is equal clinical improvement, although not as much improvement in vertebral body height, if the pro-

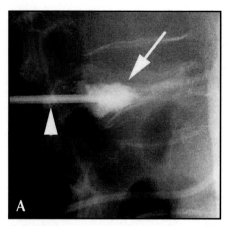

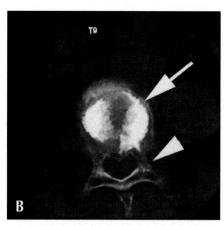

Fig. 2 A, Lateral radiograph showing the injection of PMMA into an osteoporotic vertebral fracture during a vertebroplasty (*arrow*). **B,** Axial CT scan obtained after vertebroplasty (*arrow*).

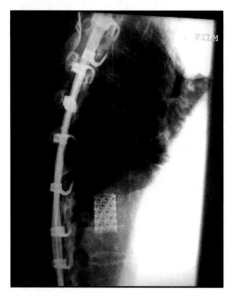

Fig. 3 Radiograph showing paraparesis following an osteoporotic vertebral compression fracture that was treated with an anterior corpectomy and cage strut along with a posterior spinal instrumentation and fusion.

cedure is performed after 3 months.

Vertebroplasty and kyphoplasty are not without complications. The reported incidence of significant complications associated with vertebroplasty is less than 10% and includes increased pain, radiculopathies, spinal cord compression, pulmonary embolism, infection, and rib fractures.[24,26,29-31] Cement leakage is reported to occur in 30% to 67% of patients but does not generally lead to clinical complications. It is seen more commonly in the treatment of pathologic fractures resulting from malignancy. In the largest reported series, the rate of radiculopathy was 4%, the rate of cord compression was less than 0.5%, and the majority of the reported symptoms were transient.[23] Concern over the potential for thermal injury from heat proliferation from PMMA has prompted the study of biodegradable calcium phosphate bone substitute as an alternative to PMMA.[32] Although the biomechanical results are promising, there are no clinical trials to date on its use as an alternative to PMMA during vertebroplasty.

Compared to vertebroplasty, kyphoplasty is associated with a lower complication rate and a lower incidence of cement leakage. In a recent study, there were no major complications related directly to the use of this technique in 70 kyphoplasty procedures.[27] Cement leakage occurred at a rate of 8.6%. To date there have been four important complications in four patients treated with this technique.[28] Two patients had neurologic deficits related to improper positioning of the device or a vertebral fracture during inflation of the device. In another patient, hypoxia and hypotension developed after placement of the liquid PMMA, and an epidural hematoma developed in the fourth patient when heparin bolus was administered postoperatively.

Surgical Treatment

Indications for the surgical treatment of osteoporotic compression fractures are limited, particularly when bracing and injection techniques are both safe and effective. A clear indication for surgical intervention is an osteoporotic fracture causing neurologic compromise (Fig. 3). When neurologic deficits are present, the neurologic elements should be decompressed anteriorly.[14] Once the spinal cord or thecal sac is decompressed and the anterior column is supported with a strut, the patient can use a brace or a posterior stabilization can be performed. Kaneda and associates[33] reported good neurologic recovery and restored spinal stability using anterior instrumentation and a bioresorbable ceramic vertebral prosthesis in a one-stage procedure to address instability and cord compression. Posterior decompressive laminectomy without fusion is not recommended because it further destabilizes the spine. Laminectomy and instrumented fusion can be considered but it is difficult because it requires a long posterior fusion in pathologic bone.

A painful kyphotic deformity that is not responsive to conservative measures is another indication for surgical treatment. When caused by multiple compression fractures, these kyphotic deformities can be stabilized with posterior spinal fusion and instrumentation. If caused by a single compression fracture, kyphoplasty or vertebroplasty may be a better alternative. Limited correction of the deformity from a posterior approach can be expected because these curves are often rigid (Fig. 4). The goals of surgery are prevention of further deformity, limited correction of the curve, and pain relief. In the absence of a neurologic deficit, there is little indication for an anterior release given the added morbidi-

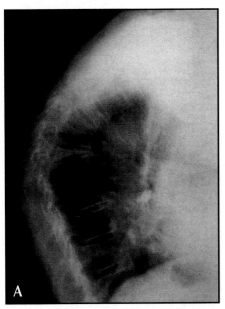
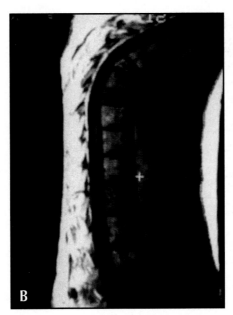
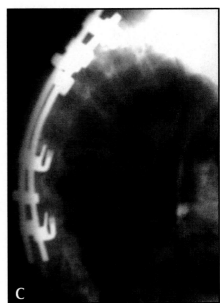

Fig. 4 A, Radiograph showing painful kyphotic deformity that was not responsive to conservative treatment. **B,** Preoperative MRI. **C,** Radiograph showing limited correction with posterior spinal fusion and instrumentation.

ty in this population. Fixation into osteoporotic bone can be a challenge, and hardware failure or instrumentation cutout is a significant risk.

Scoliosis
Presentation
There is an association between osteoporosis and scoliosis. In two separate studies, the incidence of scoliosis was found to be 36% and 48% in osteoporotic women.[34,35] Most of these scoliotic curves were found to be associated with vertebral compression fractures. Adult idiopathic scoliosis involves progression of a preexisting curve based on osteoporotic compression in the involved vertebral bodies. De novo scoliosis involves the development of a new scoliosis in an adult, arising from either osteoporosis or degenerative changes.[34-37] The age at which de novo scoliotic curves develop is difficult to determine. The patient's history may be unreliable because small lumbar curves are difficult to recognize. These curves may occur after age 40 years.[34] There are conflicting reports as to whether or not vertebral rotation is a sig-

nificant factor in the development of these curves.[34,35]

The presenting complaint in patients with significant osteoporotic curves is often that of spinal stenosis rather than scoliosis itself (Fig. 5). Patients may present with mechanical back pain, radiculopathy, neurogenic claudication, or problems with balance and alignment. At times an osteoporotic compression fracture either within or outside the curve itself may alter the dynamics of an otherwise compensated lumbar stenosis. A clear understanding of the time course of the patient's symptoms as well as the extent of disability will be critical to appropriate treatment decisions.

Natural History
The natural history of osteoporotic scoliotic curves is not well characterized. Particularly, the rate of curve progression has not been widely reported as with adolescent idiopathic scoliosis. It is certainly clear that many patients have a well compensated spinal deformity with significant but adequately controlled symptoms. In general, patients who undergo a

symmetric collapse will experience a stabilization of their symptoms, which bodes well for the success of nonsurgical treatment. Patients who undergo an asymmetric collapse of their deformity often develop progressive symptoms and may be less responsive to conservative care. Progressive lateral listhesis is often associated with neurogenic complaints of claudication or radiculopathy. These patients may also experience rapid deterioration in standing balance with symptoms of mechanical back pain and functional disability. A significant component of kyphoscoliosis is also associated with poorer outcomes. Deterioration in pulmonary function, although typically associated with thoracic deformity, can also be seen in association with significant lumbar curves.[38,39]

Nonsurgical Treatment
As compared with the nonsurgical treatment of osteoporotic kyphosis, which is almost always successful, the nonsurgical treatment of osteoporotic scoliosis is more difficult and less reliable. Initially, it is important to ensure that the underly-

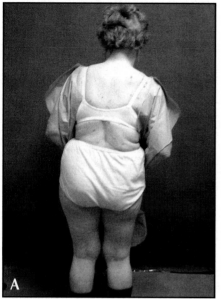
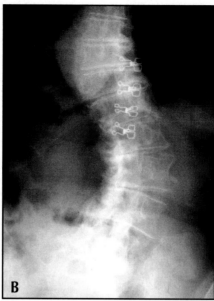
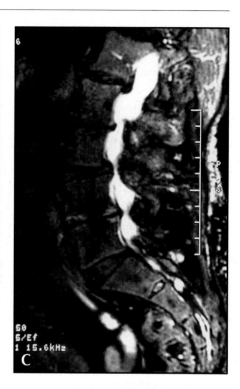

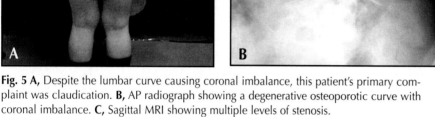

Fig. 5 A, Despite the lumbar curve causing coronal imbalance, this patient's primary complaint was claudication. **B,** AP radiograph showing a degenerative osteoporotic curve with coronal imbalance. **C,** Sagittal MRI showing multiple levels of stenosis.

ing osteoporosis is being treated to as great a degree as possible. It is worthwhile to review the patient's antiosteoporotic regimen to be sure that this avenue of treatment is not overlooked.

Because surgical management of patients with significant osteoporosis is difficult at best, nonsurgical treatment should be used aggressively. If the primary symptoms are neurogenic, initial treatment should include anti-inflammatory medications with cyclo-oxygenase II inhibitors being most appropriate for older patients at risk for gastrointestinal toxicity. Epidural steroids are also an appropriate option for patients with symptoms unresponsive to oral medication. External control of the deformity either by physical therapy and strengthening or bracing may be helpful for radicular symptoms that are exacerbated on weight bearing. Although standard physical therapy is poorly tolerated in older patients, alternative therapies such as water aerobics may elicit a better response. In most instances the magnitude of the spine deformity preexisted the

onset of neurogenic claudication or radicular symptoms, and the deformity should not be considered as a prohibitive factor for successful nonsurgical treatment.

Patients who present with significant deterioration in standing balance associated with severe mechanical back pain or neurogenic symptoms are often more resistant to nonsurgical treatment. Initial treatment may require more extensive bracing for support and aggressive strengthening exercises in an effort to control the deformity. Adjunctive pain management is helpful in that residual symptoms often persist despite moderately successful conservative care. Given the risks associated with surgical intervention, acceptance of chronic medical management including low-dose narcotics may be necessary.

Surgical Treatment

Failure of nonsurgical care and a disabling level of symptoms requiring surgical treatment are unfortunately not uncommon in patients with significant osteoporosis and scoliosis. These patients

tend to be older, with multiple medical comorbidities, and are at high risk for perioperative complications. Proper planning is therefore critical, along with a clear indication for surgical treatment. It is important to determine whether the scoliosis itself is an etiologic factor in the patient's symptoms or whether the curve is at issue based on the need for a decompressive procedure, which will then render the deformity unstable.

If the patient is well balanced when in a standing position and the curve is not the primary problem, then every effort should be made to minimize the surgical procedure. For the occasional patient with single nerve root involvement and no major back pain, unilateral root decompression may be indicated. Decompression alone within a significant scoliosis is often unsuccessful either because the decompression is inadequate or the extent of bone resection leads to progressive spinal collapse and exacerbation of neural symptoms.[40] A limited fusion within the deformity can be successful particularly if the rotation is not severe or if the segment of high-grade stenosis lies outside of the apical region of the curve.

If the patient has significant mechanical symptoms or the stenosis is more extensive, then fusion may be required over the extent of the scoliotic deformity. In this situation, the modest deformity correction obtained with prone positioning and decompression is usually sufficient (Fig. 6). A posterior decompression and fusion with instrumentation can be undertaken without a preceding anterior release. If anterior interbody fusion is required because of the number of levels involved or for extension of the fusion to the sacrum, the interbody fusion can be undertaken after the posterior procedure.

If symptoms such as severe mechanical back pain, deterioration in standing balance, or impingement of the ribs on the pelvis suggest that the deformity itself is a major etiologic component of the patient's complaints, then correction of the deformity is a primary goal of the surgical procedure. In this instance, anterior release should precede a posterior stabilization procedure. The quality of the bone may limit the magnitude of reduction obtained even with anterior diskectomy. Staged procedures may be necessary based on the extent of blood loss and the patient's anesthetic risks. Interbody grafting is important to restore lordosis and maintain alignment, although some degree of settling is common based on the osteoporotic bone and difficulty in maintaining integrity of the end plate. The posterior procedure is often used to correct additional deformity because the facets are generally osteophytic and therefore limit the initial correction. Often a relatively limited correction of the deformity is sufficient to restore balance and yields adequate symptomatic relief.

Regardless of the specific procedure, these patients typically have a long and difficult recovery. Perioperative complications are not infrequent and inpatient rehabilitation is often required. The rate of

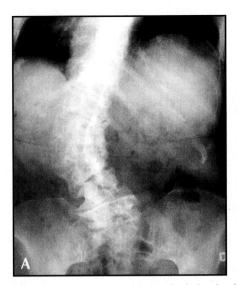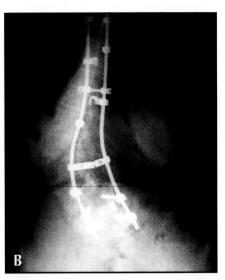

Fig. 6 A, Radiograph showing multiple levels of stenosis within an osteoporotic curve. The patient's symptoms were neurogenic claudication and severe back pain that did not respond to epidural injections, nonsteroidal anti-inflammatory drugs, or physical therapy. **B,** Postoperative AP radiograph showing modest correction of the curve, but the decompression and stabilization provided adequate relief of her symptoms.

complications is significantly greater in patients older than 60 age years.[41] Patients should be prepared preoperatively for postoperative recovery of 6 months to 1 year, based on Short Form-36 evaluation.[42]

Overall, surgical management of scoliosis associated with osteoporosis is difficult, but the patients often have severely incapacitating symptoms preoperatively and therefore are willing to accept a significant intervention to relieve symptoms. Limited procedures, particularly in patients whose primary symptoms are neurogenic, are a reasonable consideration. It is important to recognize, however, that procedures that yield an inadequate decompression or destabilize the deformity are counterproductive.

Technical Issues in Osteoporosis
Fixation
Spinal instrumentation is generally necessary to obtain satisfactory results when treating deformity and instability in osteoporotic patients. Although the added benefits of instrumentation are well demonstrated, the weak link in the reconstruction is the bone-hardware interface. Certain principles, including the use of multiple sites of fixation, acceptance of lesser degrees of deformity correction, and avoidance of ending the instrumentation within kyphotic segments, should be observed when considering instrumentation in osteoporotic patients.[43]

The most pressing concern with spinal instrumentation in osteoporotic bone is hardware pullout (Fig. 7). In an in vitro study comparing the load to failure of transpedicular screws, laminar hooks, and spinous process wires, Coe and associates[44] found that laminar hooks were the strongest means of fixation against pullout. In addition, they concluded that there was no significant correlation between load to failure and bone mineral density with laminar hooks in contrast to pedicle screws. With pedicle screws there is a strong correlation between bone density and screw pullout because osteoporosis primarily affects trabecular bone and pedicle fixation relies primarily on cancellous bone for purchase.[44-48]

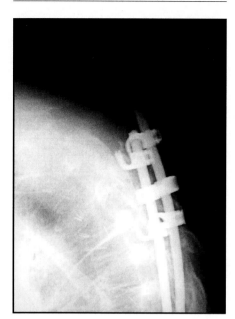

Fig. 7 Radiograph showing superior hook cutout in a patient with osteoporosis.

It is not always possible to use laminar fixation because of laminectomies. Several solutions to the problem of pedicle fixation in osteoporotic bone have been devised, including the use of larger diameter screws, penetration into the anterior vertebral cortex, use of PMMA or bioresorbable cement, and the use of offset laminar hooks at the caudal end of instrumentation.[49-59]

Larger diameter screws have been proposed as a salvage screw in the case of poor cancellous purchase.[49,50,60] The problem with larger diameter screws is the accompanying risk of pedicle fracture. Hirano and associates,[61] in a study using osteoporotic cadaveric vertebrae, found that 24% of the pedicles fractured with the placement of pedicle screws. When the pedicle screw was greater than 70% of the outer pedicle diameter, the fracture rate was 41%. They recommended the pedicle screw diameter not exceed 70% of the outer diameter of the pedicle in osteoporotic bone to lower the fracture risk.

Depth of pedicle penetration and pedicle preparation are two additional areas that have been studied in osteoporotic bone. Zindrick and associates[51] demonstrated in an in vitro model that pullout strength could be increased by 30% by placing pedicle screws to penetrate the anterior cortex. The benefit of tapping the pedicle hole was also studied. They found no benefit in tapping in osteoporotic bone. Halvorson and associates[48] found that either an untapped or undertapped hole was stronger in pullout than a hole tapped to the size of the pedicle screw.

PMMA augmentation of pedicle screw fixation has been studied as a solution to pedicle screw failure in osteoporotic bone. Kleeman and associates[52] found PMMA-augmented pedicle screws had more than twice the pullout strength as nonaugmented screws. Zindrick and associates[51] found that pedicle screw pullout strength was increased only if the cement was pressurized. The problem with PMMA is the reported neurologic deterioration with the inadvertent injection of cement into the canal and the heat necrosis damage caused by the exothermic reaction that is needed to solidify the cement.[62-64] Alternatives to PMMA are calcium apatite cement and milled or matchstick allograft bone. Calcium apatite cement has shown promise in both biomechanical and human studies and offers the advantage of being both nonexothermic and the potential to be biologic.[54,55] Milled or matchstick allograft bone used as a pedicle filler has been shown to restore more than half of the initial screw pullout strength.[53]

The use of offset laminar hooks in conjunction with pedicle fixation, also known as pediculolaminar fixation, has been studied at length as a solution to pedicle screw pullout.[48,56-59] Halvorson and associates[48] found an increased pullout strength using a two-hook compression construct with an infralaminar hook at the level of the pedicle screw and a supralaminar hook one to two levels cephalad. They found no benefit with the use of a single laminar hook to supplement a pedicle screw. In a vertebrectomy model, Margulies and associates[56] found no benefit to inferior laminar hooks at the caudal end of the construct when the level was supported by two pedicle hooks. Studying the bending moment on the pedicle screw, Chiba and associates[57] did find a decreased bending moment on the pedicle screw using offset laminar hooks. They concluded that using offset laminar hooks would protect osteoporotic bone from failure. Similarly, Hasegawa and associates[59] found increased stiffness using a combination of a pedicle screw and an offset laminar hook. Hilibrand and associates[58] used a specially modified pedicle screw/supralaminar hook combination and found it to restore nearly all the intact pedicle screw pullout strength. Despite the biomechanical studies supporting use of pediculolaminar fixation, clinical use of this fixation technique is not widespread.

Reduction of Deformity
Correction of the deformity is limited because of weak bone anchors, and suboptimal radiographic outcome should be expected. Multiple points of fixation are needed to maximize bone purchase. Because of extensive collapse and degeneration of the motion segments, reduction techniques used in adolescent idiopathic scoliosis and juvenile kyphosis generally do not work. Sublaminar wires using multiple points of fixation that can be repeatedly tightened do have a role in deformity correction in the osteoporotic spine.[43] Drawbacks of sublaminar wires are limited axial control, potential for neurologic injury, and problems with junctional kyphosis.

Fusion
There is no clear indication that osteoporosis interferes with the ability to heal bone. There are no studies to suggest that the rate of fusion is any less in osteoporotic bone than in normal bone. What

is generally seen is poor quality bone graft from autogenous harvest. Osteoporotic patients have bone with less trabeculae and more fatty marrow, so that osteoinductive and osteoconductive factors will be available in less quantity. Allograft and other bone graft expanders may be used as supplements in these patients, and growth factors may have a useful role in the future.

Summary

The medical management of osteoporosis begins with early prevention and modification of risk factors. Osteoporotic vertebral compression fractures and scoliosis are osteoporosis-related conditions that can be treated with surgery, but surgical management takes careful planning and is difficult at best. It is hoped that advances in the use of antiresorptive agents and surgical techniques will lead to more options for treatment.

References

1. Melton LJ III: How many women have osteoporosis now? *J Bone Miner Res* 1995;10:175-177.

2. Dennison E, Cooper C: Epidemiology of osteoporotic fractures. *Horm Res* 2000;54(suppl 1): 58-63.

3. Lane JM, Russell L, Khan SN: Osteoporosis. *Clin Orthop* 2000;372:139-150.

4. Melton LJ III: Epidemiology of spinal osteoporosis. *Spine* 1997;22(suppl 24):2S-11S.

5. Eriksen EF, Kassem M, Langdahl B: European and North American experience with HRT for the prevention of osteoporosis. *Bone* 1996;19(suppl 5):197S-183S.

6. Lane JM: Osteoporosis: Medical prevention and treatment. *Spine* 1997;22(suppl 24):32S-37S.

7. Lane JM, Riley EH, Wirganowicz PZ: Osteoporosis: Diagnosis and treatment. *J Bone Joint Surg Am* 1996;78:618-632.

8. Price CP, Thompson PW: The role of biochemical tests in the screening and monitoring of osteoporosis. *Ann Clin Biochem* 1995;32:244-260.

9. Eyre DR: Bone biomarkers as tools in osteoporosis management. *Spine* 1997;22(suppl 24):17S-24S.

10. Riggs BL, Hodgson SF, O'Fallon WM, et al: Effect of fluoride treatment on the fracture rate in postmenopausal women with osteoporosis. *N Engl J Med* 1990;322:802-809.

11. FDA advisory panel recommends hormone treatment for osteoporosis. *Nagelberg News*, Monday, July 30, 2001.

12. Mankin HJ: Metabolic bone disease. *68th Annual Meeting Proceedings.* Rosemont, IL, American Academy of Orthopaedic Surgeons, 2001, p 229.

13. Rupp RE, Ebraheim NA, Coombs RJ: Magnetic resonance imaging differentiation of compression spine fractures or vertebral lesions caused by osteoporosis or tumor. *Spine* 1995;20:2499-2504.

14. Lee YL, Yip KM: The osteoporotic spine. *Clin Orthop* 1996;323:91-97.

15. Arciero RA, Leung KY, Pierce JH: Spontaneous unstable burst fracture of the thoracolumbar spine in osteoporosis: A report of two cases. *Spine* 1989;14:114-117.

16. Heggeness MH: Spine fracture with neurological deficit in osteoporosis. *Osteoporos Int* 1993;3:215-221.

17. Lyritis GP, Mayasis B, Tsakalakos N, et al: The natural history of the osteoporotic vertebral fracture. *Clin Rheumatol* 1989;8(suppl 2):66-69.

18. Hall SE, Criddle RA, Comito TL, Prince RL: A case-control study of quality of life and functional impairment in women with long-standing vertebral osteoporotic fracture. *Osteoporos Int* 1999;9:508-515.

19. Nevitt MC, Ettinger B, Black DM, et al: The association of radiographically detected vertebral fractures with back pain and function: A prospective study. *Ann Intern Med* 1998;128:793-800.

20. Cortet B, Houvenagel E, Puisieux F, Roches E, Garnier P, Delcambre B: Spinal curvatures and quality of life in women with vertebral fractures secondary to osteoporosis. *Spine* 1999;24:1921-1925.

21. Kado DM, Browner WS, Palermo L, Nevitt MC, Genant HK, Cummings SR: Vertebral fractures and mortality in older women: A prospective study: Study of Osteoporotic Fractures Research Group. *Arch Intern Med* 1999;159:1215-1220.

22. Scane AC, Francis RM, Sutcliffe AM, Francis MJ, Rawlings DJ, Chapple CL: Case-control study of the pathogenesis and sequelae of symptomatic vertebral fractures in men. *Osteoporos Int* 1999;9:91-97.

23. Chiras J, Depriester C, Weill A, Sola-Martinez MT, Deramond H: Percutaneous vertebral surgery: Technics and indications. *J Neuroradiol* 1997;24:45-59.

24. Cortet B, Cotten A, Boutry N, et al: Percutaneous vertebroplasty in the treatment of osteoporotic vertebral compression fractures: An open prospective study. *J Rheumatol* 1999;26:2222-2228.

25. Deramond H, Depriester C, Galibert P, Le Gars D: Percutaneous vertebroplasty with polymethylmethacrylate: Technique, indications and results. *Radiol Clin North Am* 1998;36:533-546.

26. Jensen ME, Evans AJ, Mathis JM, Kallmes DF, Cloft HJ, Dion JE: Percutaneous polymethylmethacrylate vertebroplasty in the treatment of osteoporotic vertebral body compression fractures: Technical aspects. *AJNR Am J Neuroradiol* 1997;18:1897-1904.

27. Lieberman IH, Dudeney S, Reinhardt MK, Bell G: Initial outcome and efficacy of "kyphoplasty" in the treatment of painful osteoporotic vertebral compression fractures. *Spine* 2001;26:1631-1638.

28. Garfin SR, Yuan HA, Reiley MA: New technologies in spine: Kyphoplasty and vertebroplasty for the treatment of painful osteoporotic compression fractures. *Spine* 2001;26:1511-1515.

29. Cotten A, Dewatre F, Cortet B, et al: Percutaneous vertebroplasty for osteolytic metastases and myeloma: Effects of the percentage of lesion filling and the leakage of methyl methacrylate at clinical follow-up. *Radiology* 1996;200:525-530.

30. Padovani B, Kasriel O, Brunner P, Peretti-Viton P: Pulmonary embolism caused by acrylic cement: A rare complication of percutaneous vertebroplasty. *AJNR Am J Neuroradiol* 1999;20:375-377.

31. Tohmeh AG, Mathis JM, Fenton DC, Levine AM, Belkoff SM: Biomechanical efficacy of unipedicular versus bipedicular vertebroplasty for the management of osteoporotic compression fractures. *Spine* 1999;24:1772-1776.

32. Bai B, Jazrawi LM, Kummer FJ, Spivak JM: The use of an injectable, biodegradable calcium phosphate bone substitute for the prophylactic augmentation of osteoporotic vertebrae and the management of vertebral compression fractures. *Spine* 1999;24:1521-1526.

33. Kaneda K, Asano S, Hashimoto T, Satoh S, Fujiya M: The treatment of osteoporotic-posttraumatic vertebral collapse using the Kaneda device and a bioactive ceramic vertebral prosthesis. *Spine* 1992;17(suppl 8):S295-S303.

34. Vanderpool DW, James JI, Wynne-Davies R: Scoliosis in the elderly. *J Bone Joint Surg Am* 1969;51:446-455.

35. Healey JH, Lane JM: Structural scoliosis in osteoporotic women. *Clin Orthop* 1985;195:216-223.

36. Grubb SA, Lipscomb HJ, Coonrad RW: Degenerative adult onset scoliosis. *Spine* 1988;13:241-245.

37. Epstein JA, Epstein BS, Jones MD: Symptomatic lumbar scoliosis with degenerative changes in the elderly. *Spine* 1979;4:542-547.

38. Leech JA, Dulberg C, Kellie S, Pattee L, Gay L: Relationship of lung function to severity of osteoporosis in women. *Am Rev Respir Dis* 1990;141:68-71.

39. Schlaich C, Minne HW, Bruckner T, et al: Reduced pulmonary function in patients with spinal osteoporotic fractures. *Osteoporos Int* 1998;8:261-267.

40. Benner B, Ehni G: Degenerative lumbar scoliosis. *Spine* 1979;4:548-552.

41. McDonnell MF, Glassman SD, Dimar JR II, Puno RM, Johnson JR: Perioperative complications of anterior procedures on the spine. *J Bone Joint Surg Am* 1996;78:839-847.

42. Albert TJ, Purtill J, Mesa J, McIntosh T, Balderston RA: Health outcome assessment before and after adult deformity surgery: A prospective study. *Spine* 1995;20:2002-2005.

43. Hu SS: Internal fixation in the osteoporotic spine. *Spine* 1997;22(suppl 24):43S-48S.

44. Coe JD, Warden KE, Herzig MA, McAfee PC: Influence of bone mineral density on the fixation of thoracolumbar implants: A comparative study of transpedicular screws, laminar hooks, and spinous process wires. *Spine* 1990;15:902-907.

45. Okuyama K, Sato K, Abe E, Inaba H, Shimada Y, Murai H: Stability of transpedicle screwing for the osteoporotic spine: An in vitro study of the mechanical stability. *Spine* 1993;18:2240-2245.

46. Soshi S, Shiba R, Kondo H, Murota K: An experimental study on transpedicular screw fixation in relation to osteoporosis of the lumbar spine. *Spine* 1991;16:1335-1341.

47. Yuan HA, Garfin SR, Dickman CA, Mardjetko SM: A historical cohort study of pedicle screw fixation in thoracic, lumbar, and sacral spinal fusions. *Spine* 1994;19(suppl 20):2279S-2296S.

48. Halvorson TL, Kelley LA, Thomas KA, Whitecloud TS III, Cook SD: Effects of bone mineral density on pedicle screw fixation. *Spine* 1994;19:2415-2420.

49. Krag MH, Beynnon BD, Pope MH, DeCoster TA: Depth of insertion of transpedicular vertebral screws into human vertebrae: Effect upon screw-vertebra interface strength. *J Spinal Disord* 1988;1:287-294.

50. Zdeblick TA, Kunz DN, Cooke ME, McCabe R: Pedicle screw pullout strength: Correlation with insertional torque. *Spine* 1993;18:1673-1676.

51. Zindrick MR, Wiltse LL, Widell EH, et al: A biomechanical study of intrapeduncular screw fixation in the lumbosacral spine. *Clin Orthop* 1986;203:99-112.

52. Kleeman B, Gerhart T, Hayes W: Augmenting screw fixation in osteoporotic trabecular bone, in *Transactions of the Society of Biomaterials Annual Meeting*. Birmingham, AL, Society for Biomaterials, 1987.

53. Pfeifer BA, Krag MH, Johnson C: Repair of failed transpedicle screw fixation: A biomechanical study comparing polymethylmethacrylate, milled bone, and matchstick bone reconstruction. *Spine* 1994;19:350-353.

54. Yerby SA, Toh E, McLain RF: Revision of failed pedicle screws using hydroxyapatite cement: A biomechanical analysis. *Spine* 1998;23:1657-1661.

55. Wuisman PI, Van Dijk M, Staal H, Van Royen BJ: Augmentation of (pedicle) screws with calcium apatite cement in patients with severe progressive osteoporotic spinal deformities: An innovative technique. *Eur Spine J* 2000;9:528-533.

56. Margulies JY, Casar RS, Caruso SA, Neuwirth MG, Haher TR: The mechanical role of laminar hook protection of pedicle screws at the caudal end vertebra. *Eur Spine J* 1997;6:245-248.

57. Chiba M, McLain RF, Yerby SA, Moseley TA, Smith TS, Benson DR: Short-segment pedicle instrumentation: Biomechanical analysis of supplemental hook fixation. *Spine* 1996;21:288-294.

58. Hilibrand AS, Moore DC, Graziano GP: The role of pediculolaminar fixation in compromised pedicle bone. *Spine* 1996;21:445-451.

59. Hasegawa K, Takahashi HE, Uchiyama S, et al: An experimental study of a combination method using a pedicle screw and laminar hook for the osteoporotic spine. *Spine* 1997;22:958-963.

60. McLain RF, Fry MF, Moseley TA, Sharkey NA: Lumbar pedicle screw salvage: Pullout testing of three different screw designs. *J Spinal Disord* 1995;8:62-68.

61. Hirano T, Hasegawa K, Washio T, Hara T, Takahashi H: Fracture risk during pedicle screw insertion in osteoporotic spine. *J Spinal Disord* 1998;11:493-497.

62. Wilkes RA, Mackinnon JG, Thomas WG: Neurological deterioration after cement injection into a vertebral body. *J Bone Joint Surg Br* 1994;76:155.

63. McAfee PC, Bohlman HH, Ducker T, Eismont FJ: Failure of stabilization of the spine with methylmethacrylate: A retrospective analysis of twenty-four cases. *J Bone Joint Surg Am* 1986;68:1145-1157.

64. Sturup J, Nimb L, Kramhoft M, Jensen JS: Effects of polymerization heat and monomers from acrylic cement on canine bone. *Acta Orthop Scand* 1994;65:20-23.

Index

S